Tiana T

Handbook of Evidence-Based
Treatment Manuals for Children and Adolescents

Handbook of Evidence-Based Treatment Manuals for Children and Adolescents

Second Edition

Edited by Craig Winston LeCroy

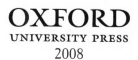

UNIVERSITY PRESS
2008

OXFORD
UNIVERSITY PRESS

Oxford University Press, Inc., publishes works that further
Oxford University's objective of excellence
in research, scholarship, and education.

Oxford   New York
Auckland   Cape Town   Dar es Salaam   Hong Kong   Karachi
Kuala Lumpur   Madrid   Melbourne   Mexico City   Nairobi
New Delhi   Shanghai   Taipei   Toronto

With offices in
Argentina   Austria   Brazil   Chile   Czech Republic   France   Greece
Guatemala   Hungary   Italy   Japan   Poland   Portugal   Singapore
South Korea   Switzerland   Thailand   Turkey   Ukraine   Vietnam

Published by Oxford University Press, Inc.
198 Madison Avenue, New York, New York 10016
www.oup.com

Oxford is a registered trademark of Oxford University Press

Library of Congress Cataloging-in-Publication Data
Handbook of evidence-based treatment
manuals for children and adolescents / edited by Craig Winston LeCroy.
        p.   cm.
    Rev. ed. of : Handbook of child and adolescent treatment manuals.
c1994.
    Includes bibliographical references and index.
    ISBN 978–0–19–517741–1
    1. Child psychotherapy—Handbooks, manuals, etc.   2. Adolescent psychotherapy—
Handbooks, manuals, etc.   3. Evidence-based psychiatry—Handbooks, manuals, etc.
    I. LeCroy, Craig W.   II. Handbook of child and adolescent treatment manuals.
    RJ504.H356   2008
    618.92'8914—dc22   2007034431

9 8 7 6 5 4 3 2 1

Printed in the United States of America
on acid-free paper

Contents

Contributors

Craig Winston LeCroy, PhD, MSW, is professor of social work at the Arizona State University School of Social Work. Dr. LeCroy received his PhD from the University of Wisconsin–Madison. He has been the Zellerbach Visiting Professor at the University California–Berkeley, visiting professor at the University of Wisconsin–Madison, and visiting professor at the University of Christchurch, New Zealand. He has published nine books including: *Social Skills Training for Children and Youth; Case Studies in Child, Adolescent, and Family Treatment; The Call to Social Work; Empowering Adolescent Girls; The Go Grrrls Workbook;* and *Handbook of Prevention and Intervention Programs for Adolescent Girls* and is the author of more than 100 chapters and journal articles. Dr. LeCroy has directed several child and adolescent projects including a National Institute of Mental Health Training grant for children and adolescents; Youth Plus, a substance abuse prevention program for youth; Go Grrrls, a primary prevention program for adolescent girls; Healthy Families Arizona, a home visitation program; and a research program for investigating substance abuse among American Indian adolescents.

ELIZABETH M. BANISTER, RN, PhD
School of Nursing, University of Victoria

DEBORAH L. BEGORAY, PhD
Faculty of Education, University of Victoria

RINAD S. BEIDAS, MA
Temple University

MICHELE S. BERK, PhD
Harbor-UCLA Medical Center
  UCLA School of Medicine

CAROLINE L. BOXMEYER, PhD
Center for the Prevention of Youth Behavior Problems,
  University of Alabama

GREGORY K. BROWN, PhD
University of Pennsylvania

EDWARD R. CHRISTOPHERSEN, PhD
Children's Mercy Hospitals and Clinics
  University of Missouri at Kansas City
  School of Medicine

KARA MARIE DEAN-ASSAEL, MSW
Mount Sinai School of Medicine, New York

RALPH J. DICLEMENTE, PhD
Emory University, Rollins School of Public Health Center for AIDS Research

CARLA ELIA, PhD
Center for Community Health, University of California, Los Angeles

AMY ELKAVICH, MA
Center for Community Health, University of California, Los Angeles

ROBERT D. ENRIGHT, PhD
University of Wisconsin–Madison

JEANETTE KNUTSON ENRIGHT, PhD
International Forgiveness Institute, Inc. Madison, WI

EVA L. FEINDLER, PhD
Long Island University, C.W. Post Campus

LYDIA MARIA FRANCO, LMSW
Mount Sinai School of Medicine, New York

MEGHANN GERBER, MA
Long Island University, C.W. Post Campus

COURTNEY HAIGHT, MA
University of Nevada, Las Vegas

JAMES A. HALL, PhD
University of Iowa

GREGG R. HENRIQUES, PhD
James Madison University

CHRISTOPHER A. KEARNEY, PhD
University of Nevada, Las Vegas

PHILIP C. KENDALL, PhD, ABPP
Temple University

CRAIG WINSTON LECROY, PhD, MSW
Arizona State University

DANIEL LE GRANGE, PhD
Department of Psychiatry and Behavioral Sciences, University of Chicago

PATRICIA LESTER, MD
Center for Community Health, University of California, Los Angeles

JOHN E. LOCHMAN, PhD
Center for the Prevention of Youth Behavior Problems, University of Alabama

JAMES LOCK, MD, PhD
Department of Psychiatry and Behavioral Sciences, Stanford University School of Medicine

MARY MCKERNAN MCKAY, PhD, LCSW
Mount Sinai School of Medicine, New York

JOANNE PEDRO-CARROLL, PhD
Children's Institute, University of Rochester

JENNIFER L. PODELL, MA
Temple University

NICOLE POWELL, PhD, MPH
Center for the Prevention of Youth Behavior Problems, University of Alabama

ERIC RICE, PhD
Center for Community Health, University of California, Los Angeles

MARY JANE ROTHERAM-BORUS, PhD
Center for Community Health, University of California, Los Angeles

DOUGLAS C. SMITH, PhD
University of Iowa

STEPHANIE STOWMAN, MA
University of Nevada, Las Vegas

SUSAN MORTWEET VANSCOYOC, PhD
Children's Mercy Hospitals and Clinics University of Missouri at Kansas City School of Medicine

ADRIANNA WECHSLER, MA
University of Nevada, Las Vegas

AMY WENZEL, PhD
University of Pennsylvania

JULIE K. WILLIAMS, PhD
University of Iowa

GINA M. WINGOOD, ScD, MPH
Emory University Rollins School of Public Health Center for AIDS Research

Preface

The primary purpose of the *Handbook of Evidence-Based Treatment Manuals for Children and Adolescents* is to provide practitioners, researchers, and students with up-to-date descriptions and detailed procedures used in clinical practice with children and adolescents. Although treatment is a complex process, a good place to start when unpacking treatment procedures is the treatment manual. Indeed, the *treatment manual* has become part and parcel of today's evidence-based practice procedures.

I am happy to bring to readers a wide assortment of treatment manuals and make them available to practitioners and students interested in furthering their knowledge and skills in working with children and adolescents. Although there are many state-of-the-art books on child and adolescent treatment, this book approaches treatment from a different vantage point—that of the treatment manual itself. Rather than address conceptual, theoretical, or practical matters in child and adolescent treatment, I wanted to compile detailed procedural descriptions that can be used in the prevention and intervention of childhood behavior problems.

The *Handbook* attempts to survey some broad and emerging areas of treatment with children and adolescents. It is intended to be comprehensive and consistent with some new developments in the field. The contents are divided into three major areas—treatment manuals used in the prevention of child and adolescent behavior problems, treatment manuals used to address many of the significant social problems facing youth, and treatment manuals used in the clinical intervention of children and adolescents with behavior problems.

Although the treatment manuals were selected to reflect many of the major areas of treatment when working with children and adolescents, there are some clear omissions. First, on a practical level, treatment manuals have become quite popular and many individuals are publishing them as separate monographs. Unlike the previous edition of this book, current efforts to obtain agreements to reproduce treatment manuals were more difficult. Therefore, a special thanks is extended to all authors who agreed to have their material included in the *Handbook*. Their effort to share their work in a combined handbook benefits students and practitioners who are committed to learning the difficult skills of doing effective work to help children and adolescents.

While many new areas are included in the manual, I was not able to secure treatment manuals in some areas that would have added significant value to the effort such as depression,[1] grief, and attention deficit disorder. In addition to these clinical problems, the *Handbook* does not include material on prevention such as preventing teen pregnancy or substance abuse or any material on victims of child abuse. Perhaps a future edition can be more comprehensive and provide a rich assortment of treatment manuals that addresses these areas and more.

However, this edition does include some very important new work being done across the country. And as the child and adolescent field has grown so has the procedural details describing how we implement treatments. The wide range of treatment manuals presented here will give individuals a complete perspective on what many of the major preventive and therapeutic activities look like.

In a general sense, the *Handbook* can provide practitioners with excellent models of how to design a complete and comprehensive treatment manual. Many practitioners must develop new treatments for purposes of remediation or prevention. Unfortunately, there is little information on how to design interventions, much less, treatment manuals. Examining the treatment manuals in this *Handbook* can provide a framework for others who are interested in developing procedural guidelines for interventions.

All of the chapters in this book have a degree of evidence supporting their effectiveness. For the most part, I left it up to the authors to understand that this publication was to focus on *evidence-based treatments* and to make the case for the evidence involving their treatment manual. The research supporting treatments in this book was not reviewed prior to acceptance of the treatment manual. An important role for readers is to make their own assessment of that evidence. If I had applied a conservative standard of evidence for treatment manuals to be included in this book there very likely would be no book.

It is important to acknowledge that the criteria for defining what constitutes evidence-based practice are far from clear. Many groups, such as the American Psychological Association (APA) task force, the What Works Clearinghouse, and RAND, list effective programs that all approach evidence-based practice from different perspectives. For example, for some, randomized trials are critical and for others, clinical practice and expert clinical judgment need to be included. The debate between *research-based* treatment and *community-based* treatment emerges but increasingly there is recognition that both standards are needed for endorsement of treatments likely to produce reliable outcomes. As the field becomes more focused, researchers and practitioners will have to struggle with unclear definitions and different conclusions about evidence. One suggestion has been to create a national clearinghouse from the various databases listing the different criteria from various organizations. Whatever solutions emerge from this it is clear that managing the evidence will be a major challenge.

The introductory chapter discusses the issues in using treatment manuals and reviews current perspectives about treatment manuals. It provides an important orientation about treatment manuals and what can and can not be expected with their use. This book does not intend to imply that treatment manuals can be easily picked up and used for clinical purposes. It is fully recognized that professional help is complex and that treatment manuals do not address many of the important nuances in effective treatment. In many cases the authors of the treatment manuals may provide training and supervision in their approach and I would encourage readers to contact them if further training is desired. Also, in some cases the treatment manuals reflect just one aspect of a treatment model and a more complete book can be purchased that describes in more detail the treatment approach and methods. The chapters that follow are each of the treatment manuals organized into three sections: prevention, social problems, and clinical problems. As readers will see, the treatment manuals vary in terms of how they are written and the procedural detail they contain. Depending on how they were developed and how they have been used, each manual is organized in a different fashion. For example, a manual being used in an early research project might describe the bare essentials of how treatment is to be conducted. It may have been heavily supplemented with supervision and included extensive training prior to use. Other manuals may have been refined and work more effectively for practitioners who have less exposure to the treatment procedures. As such, there is no consistency across the different manuals. Because each of the author or authors designed the manual to their specifications and for their use it would not make sense to impose an organization to the manuals that wasn't intended. Please review the manuals with this in mind.

In summary, the contents of the *Handbook* represent a comprehensive effort to address critical child and adolescent behavior problems. My hope is that the *Handbook* contains enough knowledge about how to treat many of the major behavior problems seen by professionals that it can serve as a useful reference volume.

I would like to acknowledge, first and foremost, those who contributed to this book. The individuals who made a contribution to this book are people who wanted to push practice forward and who were unselfish in providing all of us access to their treatment manual. It is only with their kindness and effort that this book is possible. This book became a successful project under the direction of Maura Roessner at Oxford University Press and I appreciate her support of the book. Throughout the effort of putting this book together, my spouse, Kerry Milligan, and son, Skyler, have supported this endeavor and I owe them gratitude.

Note

1. An excellent treatment manual for adolescent depression (adolescents coping with depression manual) can be accessed on the Internet at http://www.kpchr.org/public/acwd/acwd.html.

Craig Winston LeCroy
River Toad Ranch
In the Sonoran Desert outside Tucson, Arizona

Handbook of Evidence-Based
Treatment Manuals for Children and Adolescents

Chapter 1

Evidence-Based Treatment Manuals: Some Practical Considerations

Craig Winston LeCroy, MSW, PhD

Practitioners, researchers, mental health directors, and policy makers have recently joined together in a growing commitment to integrate evidence and practice. Researchers are making great progress in developing and testing interventions for effectiveness, practitioners are searching for guidance on using evidence-based treatments, mental health directors are responding to federal and local pressure to use resources for what works, and policy makers are influencing legislatures to bring science to bear on social problems. Much of the discussion at conferences, staff meetings, and special interest group meetings centers on integrating practice and evidence. What evidence supports the different treatments being used or proposed? If we are to fulfill the ideal of providing the best available treatment to remedy different psychosocial problems for children and adolescents these conversations are critical. However, such discussion is not without debate and disagreement and most would agree that progress toward this ideal is modest at best. Chorpita argues that "the frontier of evidence-based

practice is yet to be mapped, and much still stands in the way of forging sustainable connections between research and clinical service" (2003, p. 42).

If effective practice is going to be realized an essential ingredient is describing, in a detailed manner, what constitutes practice. In today's child and adolescent clinical practice that translates to a treatment manual. Because researchers needed to standardize treatment and make sure it was consistently applied, treatment manuals became the mechanism to accomplish this goal. The treatment manual is, for all practical purposes, the definition of the treatment.

TREATMENT FIDELITY

One of the major advantages of treatment manuals is that they move us closer to treatment fidelity. Treatment fidelity has to do with the extent to which the treatment as described was actually provided. Treatment fidelity is also referred to as treatment delivered with *integrity.* To discover if the treatment was responsible for the outcomes observed in an experimental trial the research needs to document that there was treatment fidelity. If practitioners administering treatment are acting exclusively on their clinical judgment rather than a proscribed set of treatment procedures we could not conclude that it was the treatment procedures that produced the outcome. Researchers recognized the need to be clear about the procedures that represented the *treatment* and needed to ensure that all practitioners implementing the treatment did so in a relatively consistent manner. Hence, the birth of treatment manuals.

Kazdin (2000) describes a model for developing effective treatments and "specification of treatment" is one of eight key steps in that model. He describes specification as:

> Operationalize the procedures, preferably in manual form, that identify how one changes the key processes. Provide material to codify the procedures so that treatment integrity can be evaluated and that treatment can be replicated in research and practice. (Kazdin, 2000, p. 133)

The treatment manual also clarifies in an open source manner what the developer means when they say the treatment is *cognitive behavioral* or based on *acceptance and commitment.* This distinction is crucial otherwise we may be assuming a type of treatment represents something that it is not. As Ollendick, King, and Chorpita note "there are many interventions and there are many variations of those interventions that fall under any one type of psychotherapy" (2006, p. 503). Chambless makes this point clear: "the brand names are not the critical identifiers the manuals are" (1996, p. 6).

ISSUES IN THE USE OF MANUALIZED TREATMENT

While I am arguing for the advantages of manualized treatment, it is not without critics. The mere idea of manualizing treatment has not been accepted by many practitioners (Kendall, 1998). Fundamental to this argument is that treatment needs to be individualized and that treatment procedures are not amenable to a set of written instructions. Criticism such as "promoting a cookbook mentality" (Smith, 1995), "paint by numbers" (Silverman, 1996), "more of a straightjacket than a set of guidelines" (Goldfried & Wolfe, 1996), and "analogous to cookie cutters" (Strupp & Anderson, 1997) are aptly summarized by Ollendick and King (2004) and Ollendick, King, and Chorpita (2006) who say that "use of treatment manuals might lead to mechanical, inflexible interventions and that such 'manually driven' treatments might stifle creative and innovation in the therapy process."

In support of treatment manuals many argue that these critiques represent a misunderstanding of how manuals can be used in practice. Wilson believes that "the use of standardized, manual-based treatments in clinical practice represents a new and evolving development with far reaching implications for the field of psychotherapy" (1998, p. 363). Kazdin is more direct in his response to the criticism: "At this time there is no alternative to the manualization of treatment. It is a convenient straw man to argue that manuals are too rigid for clinical use or that they ignore individual differences of the patient (or therapist), but this claim is spurious" (2000, p. 136). Kendall (2006) proposes research on the process of using manuals to address empirically the concerns about manualized treatment. He argues that manuals can be used with flexibility, quality manuals, he says, "provide the structure, organization, sequence, and duration of the program, and note the goals of each session" (p. 19). And more emphatically he asserts, "when actually applied, a treatment manual permits therapist creativity and is not rule-bound, but the treatment is provided within the proscribed strategic approach" (p. 20).

Practitioners find treatment manuals helpful because they offer a proscriptive approach to treatment. If you want to learn how to implement a treatment, the manual is your first step. Still, there is a lot of wiggle room in treatment implementation. How long do I focus on one aspect of the treatment manual? What do I do if the child is responding more to one aspect of the treatment—keep that focus or move on? Can I skip certain parts of the treatment protocol and still expect to obtain treatment outcomes? If the treatment prescribes 18 sessions and I can only provide 12 sessions should I just pick the sessions I think are most relevant? The questions can be endless and suggest the need to carefully study real world implementation of evidence-based treatment manuals.

The focus on treatment manuals raises a number of questions about how we implement evidence-based practice. Many of the manuals were developed in universities and under a more restricted setting than routine service delivery. As noted by Kratochwill and Hoagwood, "the ironic consequence is that there is almost no evidence base to guide implementation of evidence-based practices into routine care and services" (2006, p. 12).

TRANSPORTABILITY

Future research is needed to examine not just what treatments lead to evidence-based outcomes but how evidence-based practice is implemented in applied settings. Transportability is becoming the issue that needs to be addressed in order to realize the goals of empirically supported or evidence-based practice.

A critical question aptly raised by Kendall (2006) is described as follows: "even if practitioners in service clinics are willing to accept that an EBT/EST can be applied flexibly and that there are client-driven individualizations that are proper and preferred, will the transportation of an EST from a research clinic to a service clinic be without speed bumps?" His answer: probably not.

Kendall recommends more research and critique of the implementation of manualized treatments. He notes that future efforts should focus on two aspects, studying the process of implementing an empirically supported treatment, and the writing of manuals that reflect flexible application.

A key in understanding the effective implementation of manualized treatment is likely to be more studies on therapeutic process. As Kendall (2006) asserts, we need to understand the moment-to-moment features of interaction between child and practitioners that are important for positive change. He provides an example. The factor, "child involvement," defined as a child's participation in treatment activities, has been found to predict both improvement and treatment gains (Chu & Kendall, 2004). Such relationship-building strategies are likely an important part of how manualized treatments can be more effectively implemented.

In a similar manner, Ollendick et al. (2006) discuss moving away from the use of highly specific treatment manuals and instead identifying and selecting common elements of evidence-based protocols. For example, certain practice elements such as time out can be reliably coded and empirically factored into groupings that represent particular approaches. This

model could address many of the current criticisms leveled against treatment manuals but has not been tested and raises additional issues.

Lastly, it is noteworthy that Chorpita, Taylor, Francis, Moffitt, and Austin (2004) have experimented with the application of a modular intervention for childhood anxiety. This approach is manualized but allows for the systematic adaptation of the protocol to client characteristics (Chorpita, Daleiden, & Weisz, 2005). Each practice technique is an independent module that is integrated with the other modules. A flowchart is used to help guide the selection of appropriate modules. Depending on the client's circumstances, a different combination of treatment modules are applied to the case.

CONDUCTING MANUAL-BASED TREATMENT

Can someone take a book such as this one and apply the manual in the treatment of a child or adolescent? Critics and supporters of manual-based treatments would both agree that treatment is more complex than the simple application of a treatment manual to a case situation. But, think about how far we have come from 10–20 years ago. In the past there were no treatment guidelines, no detailed treatment manuals, and rarely did student practitioners even get to witness an expert providing a type of treatment. Researchers and practitioners struggled with the black box of treatment. It didn't take long for many professionals to realize that we could not advance the field without a greater understanding of what really happens in treatment. So, yes, manual-based treatment is limited but it represents significant progress in the field. Many manual authors agree that what they have described cannot be used in a cookbook style. Often noted is the need for extensive preimplementation training for the manual to be used appropriately (Chorpita, 2002; Henggeler & Schoenwald, 2002). Further, there are additional clinical considerations in every case that need to be considered.

We are beginning to learn more about treatment implementation based on manuals. Singer (2004) points to many relevant issues in his article, "Bambi Meets Godzilla, or a Practicing Community Clinician Attempts to Apply a Manualized Treatment in the Field." He identifies several issues such as: Under what conditions is it clear that the treatment manual fits the client problem? Does the order of treatment procedures need to be followed when, depending on the client, that order may not make sense? Singer also notes that many manuals call for certain materials (checklists or assessments) to be used but may not include these materials in the manual. Policy and procedural difficulties can interfere with implementation (e.g., requiring the practitioner to meet individually with the child and individually with the parent when the agency policy is that children can't be left alone in the waiting room). Godley, White, Diamond, Passetti, and Titus (2001) conducted a study of practitioners who had used a manualized treatment of marijuana abuse for a randomized trial. The overall feedback was that the manuals were helpful and useful additions to their implementation of the treatment. More specifically they noted that the manuals were easy to use, provided needed structure to the treatment process, helped the practitioner focus their treatment, and allowed for some creativity and flexibility. The practitioner commented on the following difficulties in implementing the manualized treatment: managing behavioral problems not addressed in the manuals, adapting material that was perceived as too complex for the clients, need for additional guidance not offered in the manual, and maintaining the child's focus when conducting social skills training procedures. Singer (2004, p. 17) concludes his experience in using manualized treatment with four basic recommendations for practitioners.

1. Review the treatment manual for missing components (e.g., assigned homework), or handouts that are not in copy-ready format.
2. Discuss the manual with supervisors or a peer supervision group.
3. Identify the theoretical base and determine if it is congruent with your practice framework. Although many clinicians claim to be eclectic, there is a danger in mixing and matching theoretically different approaches.
4. Determine if the treatment manual is compatible with agency requirements.

Despite some clear limitations, treatment manuals are a great beginning to learning the process of implementing a certain treatment and with supervision and practice can become an important part of advancing the field.

References

Chambless, D. L. (1996). In defense of dissemination of empirically supported psychological interventions. *Clinical Psychology: Science and Practice, 3,* 230–235.

Chorpita, B. (2002). Treatment manuals for the real world: Where do we build them? *Clinical Psychology: Science and Practice, 66,* 431–433.

Chorpita, B. (2003). The frontier of evidence-based practice. In A. E. Kazdin & J. R. Weisz (Eds.), *Evidence-based psychotherapies for children and adolescents.* New York: Guilford Publications.

Chorpita, B., Daleiden, E., & Weisz, J. R. (2005). Modularity in the design and application of therapeutic interventions. *Applied and Preventive Psychology, 11,* 141–156.

Chorpita, B., Taylor, A. A., Francis, S. E., Moffitt, C. E., & Austin, A. A. (2004). Efficacy of modular cognitive behavior therapy for childhood anxiety disorders. *Behavior Therapy, 35,* 263–287.

Chu, B., & Kendall, P. C. (2004). Positive association of child involvement and treatment outcome within a manual-based cognitive-behavioral treatment for children with anxiety. *Journal of Consulting and Clinical Psychology, 72,* 1–11.

Godley, S. H., White, W. II, Diamond, G., Passetti, L., & Titus, J. C. (2001). Therapist reactions to manual-guided therapies for the treatment of adolescent marijuana users. *Clinical Psychology: Science and Practice, 8,* 405–417.

Goldfried, M. R., & Wolfe, B. E. (1996). Psychotherapy practice and research: Repairing a strained alliance. *American Psychologist, 51,* 1007–1016.

Henggeler, S. W., & Schoenwald, S. K. (2002). Treatment manuals: Necessary, but far from sufficient. *Clinical Psychology: Science and Practice, 9,* 419–420.

Kazdin, A. E. (2000). *Psychotherapy for children and adolescents: Directions for research and practice.* New York: Oxford University Press.

Kendall, P. C. (1998). Directing misperceptions: Researching the issues facing manual-based treatments. *Clinical Psychology: Science and Practice, 58,* 729–740.

Kendall, P. C. (2006). Flexibility within fidelity: Advocating for and implementing empirically-based practices with children and adolescents. *Children and Family Policy Review, 2,* 17–21.

Kratochwill, T. R., & Hoagwood, K. E. (2006). Evidence-based interventions and system change: Concepts, methods, and challenges in implementing evidence-based practices in children's mental health. *Child and Family Policy Review, 2,* 12–16.

Ollendick, T. H., & King, N. J. (2004). Empirically supported treatments for children and adolescents: Advances toward evidence-based practice. In P. M. Barrett & T. L. Ollendick (Eds.), *Handbook of interventions that work with children and adolescents: Prevention and treatment.* Hobokin, NJ: Wiley.

Ollendick, T. H., King, N. J., & Chorpita, B. (2006). Empirically supported treatments for children and adolescents. In P. C. Kendall (Ed.), *Child and adolescent therapy: Cognitive-Behavioral procedures.* New York: Guilford Publications.

Silverman, W. H. (1996). Cookbooks, manuals, and paint-by-numbers: Psychotherapy in the 90's. *Psychotherapy, 33,* 207–215.

Singer, J. B. (2004, December 20). Bambi meets Godzilla, or a practicing community clinician attempts to apply a manualized treatment in the field. Unpublished manuscript.

Smith, E. W. L. (1995). A passionate, rational response to the "manualization" of psychotherapy. *Psychological Bulletin, 33,* 36–40.

Strupp, H. H., & Anderson, T. (1997). On the limitations of therapy manuals. *Clinical Psychology: Science and Practice, 4,* 76–82.

Wilson, G. T. (1998). Empirically validated treatments: The clinical application of research findings. *Behavior Research and Therapy, 34,* 295–314.

Part I

Treatment Manuals for Prevention

Chapter 2

Social Problem-Solving Skills Training: Sample Module from the Coping Power Program

Nicole Powell, PhD, MPH,
Caroline L. Boxmeyer, PhD,
and John E. Lochman, PhD

The Coping Power Program (Lochman, Wells, & Lenhart, in press; Wells, Lochman, & Lenhart, in press) is an indicated preventive intervention designed to address malleable risk factors for aggression, delinquency, and substance abuse in at-risk children prior to the middle school transition. Manualized child and parent group components feature intervention activities that target distal and proximal risk factors for children's aggressive behavior. This chapter will describe the contextual social-cognitive model of risk for aggression on which the Coping Power Program is based, provide an overview of the program and its empirical support, and present manualized session-by-session content on social problem solving from the child component module.

The material in this chapter is adapted with permission from *Coping Power: Child Group Program, Facilitator Guide*, published by Oxford University Press (2008). For the complete program, please visit the TreatmentsThatWork companion Web site at http://www.oup.com/us/ttw.

Contextual Social-Cognitive Model. Developmental psychopathology research indicates that two sets of factors mediate the onset and maintenance of externalizing behavior problems in children: child level social cognitive factors and contextual parenting characteristics. Lochman's (2006) contextual social-cognitive model summarizes these factors. Aggressive children have difficulty at a number of levels of social information processing. They tend to pay more attention to negative social cues and to misattribute others' intent as hostile. When they reach the problem solution stage, aggressive children generate fewer and less adaptive solutions to perceived problems and expect that aggressive solutions will work for them. The family context in which children develop plays a critical role in shaping these social-cognitive processes. Several parental risk factors have been directly linked to childhood aggression, including low involvement in the child's life and an overly harsh and inconsistent disciplinary style (Hawkins, Catalano, & Miller, 1992). The Coping Power Program seeks to address these child and parenting risk factors directly, as well as to impact more distal contextual risk factors, including parental stress, the level of social support that parents receive, and interparent conflict.

Overview of Child Component. The Coping Power Child Component (Lochman et al., in press) includes 34 manualized sessions centered on building social cognitive competencies to address the deficits described previously. The sessions are designed to be delivered in a group format, typically including four to six students and two coleaders. A range of topics are covered during the child group sessions, including: (1) behavioral and personal goal-setting; (2) organization and study skills; (3) emotion recognition; (4) anger management training; (5) perspective taking and attribution retraining; (6) social problem-solving; and (7) positive peer affiliation and resistance to peer pressure. Sessions run 45–60 minutes and include a variety of interactive games, role-plays, and activities to facilitate active practice of new social-emotional and coping skills.

To promote generalization of skills outside the group setting, students set weekly personal behavior goals. Classroom teachers are asked to provide input on appropriate behavioral goals at the beginning of the program. Students are responsible for obtaining daily feedback on goal completion from their teachers while the program is underway. The students earn tangible reinforcers during group sessions for goal and homework completion, positive participation, and following group rules. To promote retention of information across sessions, students are asked to recall the main topics discussed during the previous meeting at the start of each session. At the close of each session, students are offered an opportunity to purchase prizes with points they have earned. To end on a positive note and to further reinforce gains made, each student is also asked to identify a specific behavioral improvement that he or she has made and that one other group member has made at the close of each session.

Overview of Parent Component. The Coping Power Parent Component (Wells et al., in press) consists of 16 manualized parent group sessions offered over the same 15- to 18-month period as the child group. Parent meetings last approximately 90 minutes each and are typically run with groups of up to 10 parents or parent dyads and two coleaders. The parent program is derived from social learning theory-based behavioral parent training programs. It focuses on teaching parents to: (1) identify and reinforce positive child behaviors; (2) give effective instructions and establish age-appropriate rules and expectations; (3) ignore minor disruptive behaviors; (4) apply effective consequences following disruptive child behaviors; (5) foster family cohesion; and (6) establish ongoing structures for family communication and parental monitoring of child behavior.

In addition to these behavioral parenting skills, parents learn additional skills that support the social-cognitive and problem solving skills that children learn in the Coping Power Child Component. The parents learn to apply the same problem-solving model that the children are taught to resolve family problems more effectively at home. Parents also learn to support their child's academic work by establishing a structure for ongoing communication with their child's teacher, establishing a contract for homework completion, and supporting the organizational skills that their child is learning. Finally, the parents practice mood and stress management skills to better allow them to cope with the stress of parenting and to create more positive relationships with their children. The parent sessions are also designed to be highly interactive and to include group discussions, role plays, and homework assignments. The parents are frequently updated about what the children are learning in their group and are encouraged to facilitate their children's use of newly emerging skills at home.

Empirical Support for Coping Power. The efficacy and effectiveness of the Coping Power Program have been examined in a number of randomized controlled trials.

Children participating in Coping Power have been shown to have statistically significant reductions in aggressive behavior and improvements in social cognitive processes by the end of the intervention (Lochman & Wells, 2002b). In two different studies, positive program effects on reduced delinquency, substance use, and school behavior problems were still present one year following the end of the intervention (Lochman & Wells, 2003, 2004). The combined child and parent intervention had more significant effects on adolescents' delinquency and substance use than the child-only intervention at one-year follow-up (Lochman & Wells, 2004). It is important to note that program-induced changes in key target behaviors, including children's hostile attributions, outcome expectations, and locus of control, and parents' consistent use of positive parenting strategies, have been shown to mediate long-term child behavioral improvements (Lochman & Wells, 2002a).

The Coping Power Program has also been effectively implemented with clinically disordered youths in psychiatric outpatient clinics (Van de Wiel, Matthys, Cohen-Kettenis, Maassen, Lochman, et al., 2007; Zonnevylle-Bender, Matthys, Van de Wiel, & Lochman, 2007) and in residential facilities for specialized populations such as deaf children (Lochman, FitzGerald, Gage, Kannaly, Whidby, et al., 2001). Van de Wiel, Matthys, and Cohen-Kettenis (2003) found Coping Power to be a more cost-effective intervention method than other care-as-usual procedures. Coping Power has been successfully disseminated to a range of real world clinic and school providers. We are currently examining how level and type of training and individual and organizational factors affect intervention fidelity and outcomes. Further information regarding the Coping Power Program and the steps to obtaining training is available at www.copingpower. com, or by contacting the authors directly.

INTRODUCTION TO THE MANUAL

To illustrate the structure and content of the Coping Power Program, six sessions from the Child Component manual (Lochman et al., in press) are presented in the following section. These sessions were selected as representative of one of the core foci of the Coping Power Program: addressing aggressive children's characteristic deficits in social-problem solving skills. Toward this end, the Coping Power Program instructs students to use the PICC model, a structured sequence of steps to apply to problem situations (Problem Identification, Choices, and Consequences). Students learn to accurately identify problem situations, to generate a variety of possible solutions, to identify and evaluate possible consequences associated with each solution, and to choose the solution with the most favorable consequences. Leaders play an active role in helping students to come up with adaptive solutions (e.g., verbal assertions, compromise) and to recognize the negative consequences associated with unfavorable solutions (e.g., aggression, overly dependent on adult intervention).

The first session presented here is also the first session in the full Child Component manual and is designed to introduce students to the purpose and structure of the intervention. The remaining five sessions are drawn from Coping Power's 14 social problem-solving sessions (the numbering of the sessions reflects their placement in the full manual). Social problem-solving sessions that are not included here provide additional opportunities for practice (e.g., through creation of a group video) and application of the model in a variety of contexts (e.g., to conflicts with teachers, siblings, and peers).

The following sessions have been slightly modified so that they may be used as a stand-alone module. Using these sessions, clinicians might conduct a brief intervention to enhance the problem-solving skills of an at-risk group of students; clinicians conducting longer-term group work may wish to incorporate some of the ideas and activities from these sessions while retaining their group's preexisting structure. An important caveat to the use of these sessions is that dismantling research has not been conducted on the Coping Power Program, and it cannot be assumed that the program's documented empirical support translates down to individual portions of the curriculum. For maximum benefit to students and families, our recommendation is that both the child and parent components be implemented in their entirety.

References

Hawkins, J. D., Catalano, R. F., & Miller, J. Y. (1992). Risk and protective factors for alcohol and other drug problems in adolescence and early adulthood: Implications for substance abuse prevention. *Psychological Bulletin, 112,* 64–105.

Lochman, J. E. (2006). Translation of research into interventions. *International Journal of Behavioral Development, 31,* 31–38.

Lochman, J. E., & Wells, K. C. (2002a). Contextual social-cognitive mediators and child outcome: A test of the theoretical model in the Coping Power Program. *Development and Psychopathology, 14*(4), 945–967.

Lochman, J. E., & Wells, K. C. (2002b). The Coping Power Program at the middle school transition: Universal and indicated prevention effects. *Psychology of Addictive Behaviors, 16*(4S), S40–S54.

Lochman, J. E., & Wells, K. C. (2003). Effectiveness study of Coping Power and classroom intervention with aggressive children: Outcomes at a one-year follow-up. *Behavior Therapy, 34,* 493–515.

Lochman, J. E., & Wells, K. C. (2004). The Coping Power Program for preadolescent boys and their parents: Outcome effects at the 1-year follow-up. *Journal of Consulting and Clinical Psychology, 72*(4), 571–578.

Lochman, J. E., Wells, K.C., & Lenhart, L. A. (in press). *COPING POWER: Child group Facilitator's Guide.* New York: Oxford University Press.

Lochman, J. E., FitzGerald, D. P., Gage, S. M., Kannaly, M. K., Whidby, J. M., Barry, T. D., et al. (2001). Effects of social-cognitive intervention for aggressive deaf children: The Coping Power Program. *Journal of the American Deafness and Rehabilitation Association, 35*, 39–61.

Van de Wiel, N. M. H., Matthys, W., & Cohen-Kettenis, P. (2003). Application of the Utrecht Coping Power Program and care as usual to children with disruptive behavior disorders in outpatient clinics: A comparative study of cost and course of treatment. Special issue: Behaviorally oriented interventions for children with aggressive behavior and/or conduct problems. *Behavior Therapy, 34*(4), 421–436.

Van de Wiel, N. M. H., Matthys, W., Cohen-Kettenis, P. T., Maassen, G. H., Lochman, J. E., & van Engeland, H. (2007). The effectiveness of an experimental treatment when compared to care as usual depends on the type of care as usual. *Behavior Modification, 31*(3), 298–312.

Wells, K. C., Lochman, J. E., & Lenhart, L. A. (in press). *COPING POWER: Parent Group Facilitator's Guide.* New York: Oxford University Press.

Zonnevylle-Bender, M. J. S., Matthys, W., Van de Wiel, N. M. H., & Lochman, J. (2007). Preventive effects of treatment of Disruptive Behavior Disorder in middle childhood on substance use and delinquent behavior. *Journal of the American Academy of Child and Adolescent Psychiatry, 46*(1), 33–39.

Session 1: Establish Structure of the Group and Behavioral Goal Setting Procedure

Materials Needed

- Handouts 1.1–1.4
- Folder for each group member
- Posters for rules, point system, and recording points
- Ball (optional)
- Prize box with a variety of items ranging in value

Session Outline

- Discuss group purpose and structure
- Outline group rules
- Discuss the Point System and the Three Strike System
- Engage children in an activity to build group cohesion
- Begin discussion of behavioral goal setting

General Purpose and Structure of the Program

Introduce yourself and your coleader to group members and provide a brief overview of what the children can expect to experience over the course of the intervention (e.g., talk about the general purpose of the group, provide details about length and frequency of meetings, and the expectations that will be placed on them).

For example, you may say something like the following:

> Group meetings will last for approximately one hour, and will occur once each week this year for approximately 22 weeks. You will also meet with a group in sixth grade once per week for approximately 12 weeks. We will not meet on holidays or days on which you will attend meetings, assemblies, or field trips. One of us will meet with each of you individually once a month to discuss how things are going. These individual meetings let us spend time with each of you helping you to brainstorm about ways that you can make positive changes in your life. When you are in the group, we hope that you will feel comfortable talking amongst yourselves and with us. During each group you will be provided the opportunity to earn points, all of which are based on your level of participation. We will talk more about this later.

The following paragraph is an example of how you or your coleader may introduce the purpose of the group:

> We will be working with you in this group to improve your ability to cope with strong feelings and with difficult situations (such as peer pressure, tough schoolwork, and hard-to-get-along-with teachers). One of the goals of the group is to provide you with enough information so that you are better equipped to make a smooth and successful transition to middle school next year. As part of the group you will learn new ways to handle your anger and how to solve problems that come up at school, in your neighborhood, and at home. Have any of you heard the term "coping" before?

If the answer is yes ask, "What does coping mean to you?" Elicit or shape a response from group members for the definition of the term *coping*. For example, assist children in stating that coping may mean being able to manage or handle stressful situations when they arise without becoming too angry or upset. Ask children, "Why do you think this is called the Coping Power Program?" Elicit or shape a response that would indicate that they could increase or strengthen their coping skills in this group.

Explain that over the course of the next few weeks, the group will work on helping members recognize when they are angry and develop skills to handle their angry feelings in a positive way.

We are not going to teach you to stop being angry, but we will teach you new ways to respond so that you can make smarter choices.

Identify situations that make you (leaders) feel angry and convey the idea that feeling angry is a natural experience that everybody has. Emphasize that choosing effective responses to anger provoking situations is what is important, not the emotion itself.

Have group members discuss situations that are difficult for them or ones that trigger an angry response. Try to have each member talk about what makes them angry and how they respond. If the child has difficulty generating answers, ask them to tell you what his or her parent or teacher might suggest. Be sure to record children's responses for use in the goal setting section of today's session.

Group Rules

Next, talk to children about the need for group rules. Ask them for their ideas of what some of the rules should be. Have one child go to the poster paper that is taped to the wall and ask him or her to record the rules that the group generates (you will retain this poster for display at subsequent meetings). If possible, select a child who does not have writing difficulties. You may choose to select a particularly quiet child or one whom you are concerned may not become involved in the group process. This may facilitate positive group interaction. Leaders can also have the group members take turns recording the rules that are generated. Try to make sure that all group members participate in generating rules. If a child offers a strange, unclear, or silly rule, try to reframe this into a useful rule. General rules for the group should include:

- No physical contact
- No name calling
- No swearing
- Arriving on time
- Having a positive attitude
- Not interrupting each other
- Keeping everything private (confidential)
- Following directions

If these general group rules have not been generated, you and your coleader should suggest them. Define the confidentiality rule for group members as: "What we say in here, stays in here." Let children know that this rule applies to both the group leaders and other group members. Note that the children can talk to their parents about group discussions but should not talk to other children.

Provide Handout 1.1 (Group Rules) and ask the children to record the rules on this form so that they have their own copy. Ask them to place the forms in their folders.

Point System

Prior to this meeting, leaders should create a poster describing the Point and Strike Systems and a poster for recording students' points (a sample Point Tracking System follows the handouts for this session). These should also be displayed during this and every subsequent group meeting. Direct the students' attention to the Point and Strike System poster and provide them with Handout 1.2 (Point System), then describe the procedures as follows.

Group members can earn *one point* for:

- Following rules
- Positive participation

Group members can earn *two points* for:

- Completing homework assignments

Group members can earn up to *five points* for:

- Meeting their weekly goal.

Following Rules and the Three Strike System

This system should be used for dealing with problem behavior displayed during the meetings or, if appropriate, outside of the meetings (e.g., breaking the confidentiality rule). Members are given three chances or warnings before losing a point for not following rules. If a child breaks a rule once, that is *strike one*. If a child breaks a rule twice, that is *strike two*, and if a child breaks a rule a third time, that is *strike three*. On strike three the child loses a point.

Leader Note

If a child receives three strikes during one group session, he or she may need to leave group for that day if he or she is not able to regain control of his or her behavior.

Positive Participation

Discuss with the children the concept of positive participation and how they can use it to earn points. Ask group members, "What do you think positive participation means?" Elicit or shape a definition that indicates that behaviors, such as responding meaningfully to questions from leaders or other children, raising important points related to the discussion, and engaging in activities, are examples of positive participation. Inform the children that you and your group leader will let them know if they have earned the positive participation point at the end of each session.

Prize Box

Group leaders should then explain how the points can be used.

> You will be able to use the points you earn to purchase items in this box (show the prize box). We will talk with you at the end of each group and tell you how many points you have earned for that group. We will keep track of the total number of points you have earned and spent on this poster (draw the students' attention to the Point Tracking poster). You can spend your points immediately or save your points to buy specific prizes. There are small prizes and big prizes; if you would like to purchase a bigger prize, you will have to save your points.

Provide group members with Handout 1.3 (Prize Box Menu) and ask them to place it in their folder.

Getting Acquainted/Achieving Group Cohesion

The following activities can help the children get to know one another and build group cohesion.

Pass the ball: Have group members throw a ball to each other. Ask them to identify the person (by name) to whom they threw the ball, identify one thing that is the same about the two of them, and identify one thing that is different about the two of them.

Group naming task: Have group members decide on a name for their group (e.g., using a combination of their first initials to form a word). Have group members generate several alternative names and vote on the name they would like to use.

Goal Setting

Discuss with children the idea of setting goals. Ask them for their ideas about what goals are and the purpose of setting goals. Elicit a response indicating that a goal is something you work toward meeting. Explain to children that people set goals in order to improve something in themselves or so that they have a better idea about what they would like to achieve in the future. A goal provides a person with structure for the future and allows him or her to plan ahead.

Inform members that each of them will be choosing weekly goals based on input obtained from their teacher, counselor, or parent. Be sure to tell them that, at times, more than one person may be working on the same goal (e.g., being quiet during class), but that meeting this goal may be easy for one person but difficult for another. Introduce the idea that the group will be using goal sheets to keep track of their success with meeting their goals. Provide the students with Handout 1.4 (Goal Sheet) and discuss how points are earned on the goal sheet.

You can earn one point a day for each day that you meet your goal. If you meet your goal for the entire week you will earn five points.

In the full Coping Power Program, Goal Sheets are not distributed until after the second session, during which the concept of goal setting is explored in detail. Leaders conducting an abbreviated form of the program may wish to initiate the goal sheet procedure after the first session. With input from the leaders, students should come up with a goal for the week and write it on their goal sheet (Handout 1.4). Leaders should help the group members describe their goals in terms of observable behavior in order to help minimize their use of subjective statements as goals. For example, "being good in class" is very subjective. This goal can be behaviorally defined in terms of "not talking back to the teacher," "no physical contact with other kids," and so on. It is important to select a goal that is relevant and is not too difficult so that the child's initial experiences with the goal-setting procedures will be positive. Based on the student's performance, it may be necessary to increase or decrease the level of difficulty of the chosen goals at subsequent sessions.

Rules for the goal-setting procedure include the following.

- Each child is responsible for his or her goal sheet.
- Each child is responsible for getting his or her goal sheet signed by the teacher.
- Each child is responsible for returning the goal sheet to group each week.

Remind students that they must have their teachers sign the goal sheet to earn points and that the goal sheet must be presented at the beginning of each group meeting. Problem solve with group members about how they can remember to have their goal sheet signed and to bring it back to the group the following week. Some ideas may include the following.

- Putting a sticker on their desk that will serve as a reminder.
- Asking students to remind one another.
- Making sure that they leave it at school in a place that is visible.

Positive Feedback

Toward the end of each session, group leaders should ask each group member to identify one positive thing about himself or herself and/or one positive thing about another group member. Try to have the children avoid complimenting one another on their clothing or other non-behavioral or status oriented things. Work toward having group members provide positive feedback to peers on group-related behaviors or positive examples outside of group that they observed at school during the week. To assist in this process, group leaders can model appropriate compliments or positive feedback. If time permits, ask each child to identify one thing that he or she learned during the group. Praise the group for any positive achievements they may have made during the session.

Prize Box

At the end of each group meeting, complete the point tracking form while discussing with students whether they earned their positive participation and following rules points. Provide feedback to students who do not earn one or both points. Tally the points earned for each child in the group and allow them to select prizes from the prize box (if applicable).

Free Time

This is an *optional* (time permitting) free play period (5–10 minutes). Each student who has earned at least one point during group is eligible for free time. Group leaders should be aware of any potential problems that arise between group members during this free play time and use it as an opportunity to practice problem solving in action. Attempt to have each person involved in the situation discuss the problem and try to come to a resolution. Try to develop a plan to prevent this type of problem from occurring again. It is helpful to follow up with these issues individually and/or at the beginning of the next group session. The leaders should view this problem-solving opportunity as a process to be worked on over the course of the entire program. When possible, the first step would be to have each child discuss the problem individually with the group leader and then to work toward having the children discuss the problem situation with each other. During the discussion, the leaders should have the children accurately identify the problem, talk about possible misinterpretations, generate several solutions for the problem, discuss the consequences of these solutions, and determine which solution would best achieve the goal of getting along with the peer.

GROUP RULES

1. _____

2. _____

3. _____

4. _____

5. _____

6. _____

7. _____

8. _____

9. _____

10. _____

_____

As a member of this group I agree to follow the rules outlined above.

Signature:

_____

HANDOUT 1.2
POINT SYSTEM

GOAL SHEETS

0 days = 0 points
1 day = 1 point
2 days = 2 points
3 days = 3 points
4 days = 4 points
5 days = 5 points

POSITIVE PARTICIPATION

1 point per session

* Active Listening
* Engaging in Activities

FOLLOWING THE RULES

1 point per session
"3 Strikes and you lose 1 point"

* If you follow the rules that you and your leader agreed upon, you will earn 1 point.
* During each session you will get 2 warnings about breaking the rules. The third time that the leader has to warn you, the point is lost.

SAMPLE PRIZE BOX MENU

Item	Cost
Pencils (for 3)/Pen (for 1)	4 points
Eraser (2 SMALL OR 1 LARGE)	4 points
Folders	6 points
Hair Clips	8 points
Nail Polish	10 points
Lip Gloss	10 points
Yo-Yo	10 points
Gloves	10 points
Playing Cards	10 points
Jewelry	15 points
Small Nerf Balls	15 points
Harry Potter Cards	18 points
Softball	20 points
Magnetic Game	20 points
Frisbee	20 points
Wallet	25 points
Football/Soccer ball/Basketball	35 points
CD Wallet	40 points
Disposable Camera	50 points
Clock Radio	75 points

HANDOUT 1.4

GOAL SHEET

For: _____

Week of: ___/___/___

Goal: _____

_____

Monday	Y N	_____
Tuesday	Y N	_____
Wednesday	Y N	_____
Thursday	Y N	_____
Friday	Y N	_____

(Students earn 1 point for each day they meet their goal.)

<u>Teacher:</u> Please sign your name on the line provided and indicate whether or not the goal was met by circling Y (Yes) or N (No). If the child did not meet the goal, please provide a brief explanation as to why.

I, _____, have chosen the above goal and am responsible for doing my best to meet this goal and having my teacher sign this sheet daily.

Table 1.1
Coping Power Point Tracking System

NAME	SESSION #	SESSION #	SESSION #	SESSION #	SESSION #	SESSION #	SESSION #	SESSION #	SESSION #	SESSION #
	Remaining from Last week:	Remaining from Last week:	Remaining from Last week:	Remaining from Last week:	Remaining from Last week:	Remaining from Last week:	Remaining from Last week:	Remaining from Last week:	Remaining from Last week:	Remaining from Last week:
	THIS WEEK Earned: Spent: Remaining:	THIS WEEK Earned: Spent: Remaining:	THIS WEEK Earned: Spent: Remaining:	THIS WEEK Earned: Spent: Remaining:	THIS WEEK Earned: Spent: Remaining:	THIS WEEK Earned: Spent: Remaining:	THIS WEEK Earned: Spent: Remaining:	THIS WEEK Earned: Spent: Remaining:	THIS WEEK Earned: Spent: Remaining:	THIS WEEK Earned: Spent: Remaining:
	Remaining from Last week:	Remaining from Last week:	Remaining from Last week:	Remaining from Last week:	Remaining from Last week:	Remaining from Last week:	Remaining from Last week:	Remaining from Last week:	Remaining from Last week:	Remaining from Last week:
	THIS WEEK Earned: Spent: Remaining:	THIS WEEK Earned: Spent: Remaining:	THIS WEEK Earned: Spent: Remaining:	THIS WEEK Earned: Spent: Remaining:	THIS WEEK Earned: Spent: Remaining:	THIS WEEK Earned: Spent: Remaining:	THIS WEEK Earned: Spent: Remaining:	THIS WEEK Earned: Spent: Remaining:	THIS WEEK Earned: Spent: Remaining:	THIS WEEK Earned: Spent: Remaining:
	Remaining from Last week:	Remaining from Last week:	Remaining from Last week:	Remaining from Last week:	Remaining from Last week:	Remaining from Last week:	Remaining from Last week:	Remaining from Last week:	Remaining from Last week:	Remaining from Last week:
	THIS WEEK Earned: Spent: Remaining:	THIS WEEK Earned: Spent: Remaining:	THIS WEEK Earned: Spent: Remaining:	THIS WEEK Earned: Spent: Remaining:	THIS WEEK Earned: Spent: Remaining:	THIS WEEK Earned: Spent: Remaining:	THIS WEEK Earned: Spent: Remaining:	THIS WEEK Earned: Spent: Remaining:	THIS WEEK Earned: Spent: Remaining:	THIS WEEK Earned: Spent: Remaining:
	Remaining from Last week:	Remaining from Last week:	Remaining from Last week:	Remaining from Last week:	Remaining from Last week:	Remaining from Last week:	Remaining from Last week:	Remaining from Last week:	Remaining from Last week:	Remaining from Last week:
	THIS WEEK Earned: Spent: Remaining:	THIS WEEK Earned: Spent: Remaining:	THIS WEEK Earned: Spent: Remaining:	THIS WEEK Earned: Spent: Remaining:	THIS WEEK Earned: Spent: Remaining:	THIS WEEK Earned: Spent: Remaining:	THIS WEEK Earned: Spent: Remaining:	THIS WEEK Earned: Spent: Remaining:	THIS WEEK Earned: Spent: Remaining:	THIS WEEK Earned: Spent: Remaining:
	Remaining from Last week:	Remaining from Last week:	Remaining from Last week:	Remaining from Last week:	Remaining from Last week:	Remaining from Last week:	Remaining from Last week:	Remaining from Last week:	Remaining from Last week:	Remaining from Last week:
	THIS WEEK Earned: Spent: Remaining:	THIS WEEK Earned: Spent: Remaining:	THIS WEEK Earned: Spent: Remaining:	THIS WEEK Earned: Spent: Remaining:	THIS WEEK Earned: Spent: Remaining:	THIS WEEK Earned: Spent: Remaining:	THIS WEEK Earned: Spent: Remaining:	THIS WEEK Earned: Spent: Remaining:	THIS WEEK Earned: Spent: Remaining:	THIS WEEK Earned: Spent: Remaining:
	Remaining from Last week:	Remaining from Last week:	Remaining from Last week:	Remaining from Last week:	Remaining from Last week:	Remaining from Last week:	Remaining from Last week:	Remaining from Last week:	Remaining from Last week:	Remaining from Last week:
	THIS WEEK Earned: Spent: Remaining:	THIS WEEK Earned: Spent: Remaining:	THIS WEEK Earned: Spent: Remaining:	THIS WEEK Earned: Spent: Remaining:	THIS WEEK Earned: Spent: Remaining:	THIS WEEK Earned: Spent: Remaining:	THIS WEEK Earned: Spent: Remaining:	THIS WEEK Earned: Spent: Remaining:	THIS WEEK Earned: Spent: Remaining:	THIS WEEK Earned: Spent: Remaining:
	Remaining from Last week:	Remaining from Last week:	Remaining from Last week:	Remaining from Last week:	Remaining from Last week:	Remaining from Last week:	Remaining from Last week:	Remaining from Last week:	Remaining from Last week:	Remaining from Last week:
	THIS WEEK Earned: Spent: Remaining:	THIS WEEK Earned: Spent: Remaining:	THIS WEEK Earned: Spent: Remaining:	THIS WEEK Earned: Spent: Remaining:	THIS WEEK Earned: Spent: Remaining:	THIS WEEK Earned: Spent: Remaining:	THIS WEEK Earned: Spent: Remaining:	THIS WEEK Earned: Spent: Remaining:	THIS WEEK Earned: Spent: Remaining:	THIS WEEK Earned: Spent: Remaining:

Session 2: Introduction to Problem Solving

Materials Needed

- Handout 1.4 (Goal Sheet)
- List of possible problem situations and solutions
- Prize box

Session Outline

- Review goal sheets and main points from previous session
- Introduce problem solving
- Introduce the PICC model
- Teach children how to break problems down into solvable steps using the Pick it Apart method

Review Goal Sheets and Main Points from Previous Session

Begin the group by asking students to produce the goal sheet distributed during the last meeting. Review each student's sheet and award one point for each day that the student's teacher indicated that the goal was met. Engage each student in a discussion of the goal-setting process: "What goal did you set for yourself? How did you do with meeting this goal? What made it easy/difficult to reach the goal you set for yourself?"

If the goal set last week was too difficult, break it down into smaller more manageable steps; if goal was easily achieved, assess the need for setting a goal that will be a little more challenging; share with students the idea of goal-setting as a process.

Also, begin this and each subsequent session by asking each child to recall one point from the previous group meeting, using reminders as needed. As each session in the curriculum builds on the previous one, the review process enhances the opportunity for students to retain the material being covered from one week to the next. Recapping the primary message from each group meeting is one way of meeting this objective.

Problem Identification

Introduction to Problem Solving

Problem identification will be discussed as a component of the problem solving process. Explain to children that over the next several weeks, the group will talk about problem solving and how to make good choices when they have problems with their friends, or other people in their lives. Before you start, ask the group to define what a problem is. Encourage students to provide a definition but do not force the issue. If they are unable to describe it, you may use the following sample dialogue to define problems.

A problem exists when there is something that gets in the way of a goal that we want to reach or something that keeps us from getting where we want to be. There are many examples of problems, some of which are individual problems (e.g., your bike gets a flat tire and you are miles away from home) or some are group problems (e.g., your boy scout troop is having trouble raising money for a field trip). A problem can also exist if two people want different goals and both goals cannot be met with the same solution.

For example, you have homework to do but you really want to watch your favorite TV show first. Your mother wants you to get your homework done before you can watch TV. People can sometimes tell when there is a problem, because they will feel angry or sad. Can you think of any examples of problems?

Wait for the students to respond. If they do not spontaneously offer examples, ask them to think of a problem that they have experienced in school during the last week. You may want to use one of these examples to demonstrate how to think through the steps of problem solving.

Introduction to PICC Model

Start the discussion by asking group members what they think the first step to solving a problem is. Guide them toward creating the words associated with the PICC model. P = Problem, I = Identification, C = Choices, and C = Consequences. The PICC outline represents the main problem-solving steps schematically and will be used throughout the problem-solving sessions. Write the PICC schematic on the dry erase board or flipchart. PICC follows the form of:

Problem Identification _____
Choices   Consequences

Defining a Problem in Solvable Steps

After the discussion about problem solving in general, introduce the notion of *picking it apart*. You may use the following sample dialogue.

Great! You have some really good ideas about getting started with problem solving. Let's use the PICC chart (this should have already been drawn on the dry erase board or flipchart) to "pick apart" a problem and to "pick" good choices that really work for you. Let's look at an example of breaking down a problem into smaller parts.

Choose one of the following exercises to demonstrate the process of picking apart a problem.

Exercise 1: My Car Is Not Working!

I had my car towed into the automotive shop and all of you were mechanics who worked at the shop. One of you asked me to describe the reason that I had my car towed to the shop. I replied, "Because it won't run." Would my answer be helpful to you? Would it help you to figure out what is wrong?

Wait for the children to respond and then continue. Refer to the PICC chart on display and write "Pick it Apart = Ask Questions" underneath the words "Problem Identification." Leave enough room below to write the children's responses.

Problem Identification _____
Pick it Apart = "Ask Questions"

Continue by asking the group, "What kinds of things would you need to know to figure out what was wrong with the car?" As the children generate questions, try to reframe these questions into more general categories, such as

- How often has it happened?
- In what situations does it happen?
- What happened just before the problem occurred?
- What is not affected by the problem?

Make sure that responses included things like

- It will not run after leaving my parking lights on all night (a battery or electric problem).
- I have not been to the gas station in a long time (car ran out of gas).

- There was a loud crash under the car and since then there has been a loud noise (muffler problem).

After sufficient additional information has been obtained, ask children to think about what caused the problem with your car. Instruct the group to solicit suggestions for what caused the problem and how understanding what the problem is helps us to understand the cause of the problem.

Then, talk to children about your goal.

There is one other thing you probably want to ask me before you start to work on my car. You will want to know what my goal is. For example, you might ask me if I want the car fixed no matter what the cost or if I am only willing to pay a certain amount of money.

Instruct the group to solicit information that would help to identify what your goal is and then, in response to the group's questions, you can state that you want it fixed only if the repairs cost less than $500.00, since the car is pretty old. If the repairs cost more than $500.00, your goal would be to get rid of the car and try to sell it as-is. Be sure to discuss how considering the goal changes how you think about the problem. Frame these under the terms Choices and Consequences (e.g., you choose to only fix the muffler but the transmission needs to be overhauled— the consequence would be that you may not get much money when you try to sell it).

Exercise 2: My Video Game Is Not Working!

Let's say that your brother wants to play a video game, but it isn't working. He comes to you and tells you that the game does not work. Does this help you to figure out what is wrong? What kinds of things would you ask to figure out what the problem is?

Again, as children are generating questions, try to reframe these questions into more general categories such as

- When does the problem occur?
- What are some of the specific difficulties encountered?

Now, I want you to pretend that you are a videogame repairman while I play the role of your brother. Try to get a better idea of why the game is not working by asking me some questions.

Encourage one group member to take on the role of the videogame repairman. Following are some of the questions that you would like this person to ask so that they get a better idea as to what is happening.

Problem Identification_____
Pick it Apart = "Ask Questions"

- Is the power light on? (not plugged in, no electricity to operate the machine)
- Does the picture come on the screen but you cannot move the figures? (the joy stick is not plugged in correctly)
- Is the TV screen on but the game does not show up on the screen? (cartridge is not all the way in)
- Does the TV work fine when the game is not plugged in? (the video game machine is probably broken)
- Is the TV on the wrong channel? (needs to be on the right channel)

Ask the child playing the role of the repairman if now that he or she has more information about the problem, he or she also has a better idea about what might have caused the problem. Solicit suggestions for what caused the problem and how understanding what the problem is helps us to understand the cause of the problem. Then, explain that once the problem and the cause of the problem have been identified, it is time to think about what you (the brother) want. What is your goal? For example, do you want to have the machine fixed no matter how much it costs, or would you rather buy a new machine if the expense will be too great? Instruct the group to solicit information that would help to identify what your goal is. Note how consideration of the goal changes how you think about the problem. Once again, frame these under the terms Choices and Consequences (e.g., you choose to get the game working no matter what the cost and the problem is that the cartridge is jammed—the consequence might be that you need to take the game to a repairman and this would cost a lot of money. An option would be to see if a new game would cost less money than getting the old one repaired).

Set Weekly Goals

Remind each student to set a new weekly goal (or continue with their current goal if it has yet to be achieved) and complete the Goal Sheet in the workbook (Handout 1.4). Remind children to bring their signed Goal Sheets to next week's session.

Positive Feedback

See Session 1.

Prize Box

See Session 1.

Free Time

See Session 1.

Session 3: Social Problem Solving: Part I

Materials Needed

- Handout 1.4 (Goal Sheet)
- Prize box

Session Outline

- Review goal sheets and main points from previous session (Session 2)
- Complete introduction to problem solving from the previous session (Session 2)
- Engage group in a problem-solving exercise

Review Goal Sheets and Main Points from Previous Session

See Session 2.

Problem Identification

Continue last week's discussion about problem solving and the PICC model.

> Last time we met we talked about the PICC model. Can anyone tell me what that refers to? (Wait for responses and prompt students as needed.) Remember how we talked about the importance of really knowing what a problem is before we try to solve it? (Wait for responses and prompt as needed.)

Put the PICC model on the dry erase board or flipchart so that all group members can see it.

Problem Identification _____
Pick it Apart = "Ask Questions"
Choices   Consequences

Choose one of the following two exercises to illustrate how to pick apart a problem.

Exercise 1: My Friends Won't Let Me Play!

Engage in the Pick it Apart procedure with a vague social problem. Introduce to the students the problem of a child not wanting to play with them. Using the PICC chart, try to determine more explicitly what the problem is.

> Here is the problem. My name is Tim and I have a friend named Bob. I see Bob walking in front of my house and I run outside to ask him if he wants to play with me. When I asked him he responded by saying "No" and kept on walking. Can you help me to figure out what the problem is? What questions should I ask myself?

Make it appear as though you think that Bob doesn't like you so you have decided that you are never going to ask him to play again. Obviously, this is not a good solution. Ask group members to help you come up with a different interpretation to the problem; ask them to provide you with a list of possible questions that you could ask so that you could be sure of what the problem is. For example:

- When are the times he will not play with you (e.g., dinner time)?
- Is this all the time or only sometimes?

- What is he doing when he will not play with you?
- Are there other people around when you ask him to play?
- How do you ask him to play with you?
- Did he use to play with you?

Offer responses to these questions and create a scenario in which the only times that Bob will not play are when he has to get home for dinner or when you ask him to play tennis, which is a game that Bob does not like. Point out that one way to solve the problem would be to ask him to do something else besides play tennis—find out what games he likes to play or to approach him after dinner is over.

Exercise 2: Parent–Child Conflict

Role play a situation that involves a parent–child conflict. Either you or your coleader can play the part of the parent while one of you takes on the role of the child. The basic scenario to portray is one in which the child asks the parent if he can go to the mall or stay up an hour later to watch a TV show, and the parent says, "No! I asked you to clean your room today, and your room is still a mess." Ask group members to define the problem in the situation. If the child suggests the problem is that "Mom is not fair" or that "I never get to do what I want," discuss how this problem definition may actually hinder problem solving, because there is little that the child can do to resolve the problem. Here are some suggested questions to ask the group members.

- What is the problem according to the mom?
- What is the problem according to the child?
- When would this be a problem?
- How did this problem emerge?
- What is the child's goal?
- What is the parent's goal?

Problem Identification and Solution Formation

Introduce the relationship between problem identification and solution generation by having the children play a game. The goal of the game is for students to come up with 10 solutions to a problem in five minutes. If they can come up with 10 solutions, each group member earns one extra point for the session; if they can't, the group does not earn any extra points. You may use the following sample dialogue to introduce the game:

Now we are going to have you play a game. What we want you to do is to try to think of 10 different solutions to this problem: "You are out on the playground and you see a boy in your class named Dan sitting on the ground holding his head. Another boy from your class, Tom, is standing over him, threatening to hit him. We want you to think of as many solutions to this problem as you can. We want you to do this as fast as you can—the solutions can be good solutions or bad solutions, it doesn't matter. We will write down your solutions as you come up with them. Ready? Go!"

Either you or your coleader should record the solutions as they are generated and keep them in list format on the far side of the dry erase board or flipchart. You will use the rest of the board for the second part of the exercise. Possible solutions include:

1. Try to get the two boys to talk to each other.
2. Help his friend Dan by hitting Tom.
3. Go tell a teacher that there is a fight on the playground.
4. Convince Dan that it is not worth getting in trouble and they should just leave.
5. Go get a basketball and see if they will play a game and become friends again.
6. Refer the boys to peer mediation.

7. Tell Tom he will get his brother to beat him up if he hits Dan again.
8. Say to Tom that they do not like to be hit by other kids.
9. Ask Dan if he wants to come over to his house and get away from this place.
10. Begin to talk about the fun things that they did at school that day.

Following this exercise, categorize the solutions students generated into more general solution types. For example, you can use the following categories to help the children understand that there are some general ways to classify solutions.

- Help seeking
- Verbal assertion
- Direct action
- Physical aggression
- Verbal aggression
- Compromise or bargaining
- Avoidance or nonconfrontation

This type of categorization will help students to develop more complete ideas of how problems can be solved, and they will learn that there are several different types of solutions within each category. Write down the general categories on the dry erase board or flipchart.

Positive Feedback

See Session 1.

Prize Box

See Session 1.

Free Time

See Session 1.

Session 4: Social Problem Solving: Part II

Materials Needed

- Handout 1.4 (Goal Sheet)
- Handouts 4.1 and 4.2
- Prize box

Session Outline

- Review goal sheets and main points from previous session (Session 2)
- Identify and evaluate consequences for solutions
- Demonstrate the difference between automatic thinking and deliberate thinking
- Assign homework

Review Goal Sheets and Main Points from Previous Session

See Session 2.

Review Weekly Goal Sheets

Check that children completed their weekly goal sheets.

Identifying Consequences for Solutions

To begin today's session, ask the group for a definition of a consequence.

So far, we have talked a lot about how we should define a problem. We have said that we need to look at problems from many different angles or viewpoints so that we can get a complete understanding of what is going on. We have also talked about the importance of generating many solutions for a problem so that we can evaluate the solutions and choose the best one. What we haven't talked about is how we actually evaluate our choices. How do we know which choice is the best one?

Wait for the group to respond. Praise anyone who comes up with the notion of looking at consequences or outcome. If nobody comes up with an answer ask the group the following question: "Has anyone heard of the word consequence?" If yes, "Tell the group what that word means." If not, explain that a consequence is what happens as a result of something you do, or it is what happens after you do something. Provide a simple example of a consequence such as, "what happens if you leave a chocolate bar in the car on a hot day?" (Answer: It melts.) Melting is the consequence that is associated with your behavior of leaving your chocolate bar in the car on a hot day.

Leaders should provide a hypothetical problem that lends itself well to this activity or elicit a real-life problem situation from students. Have students brainstorm solutions (good and bad) using the PICC format.

Problem *I*dentification_____
Pick it Apart = "Ask Questions"
Choices   Consequences

Once all of the solutions have been generated, ask group members to identify what the consequences are for each solution. It is also useful to ask group members to state what the goal is for each of the solutions and to encourage their recognition of the relationship between problem definition, the goal being pursued, and the solutions that are generated. Following are examples of questions to be asked during the discussion.

- What would be the consequence for this solution?
- What would happen after this solution was used?
- What else might happen?
- What else might the other person do?
- What else might the other person feel?

Several consequences for each solution should be generated.

The point of the preceding exercise is to introduce the idea that there are often several consequences for one solution and, if you want to make a good decision, you must think of all of the possible consequences.

Evaluating Consequences

Using the consequences that have been generated to the problem situation just described, ask group members, "How can you tell if a consequence is 'good' or 'bad?' What makes a consequence good versus bad?" Introduce the idea that a consequence is good if it helps the person to reach an important goal. It may be useful to discuss the difference between long-term and short-term goals (e.g., fighting may help to reach the short-term goal of feeling strong or important or tough but may get in the way of reaching the long-term goals of doing well in school, having a good job, and staying out of trouble).

Using the PICC chart with consequences listed, ask group members to rate each of the consequences as good (++), okay (+), or bad (–). Then ask group members to indicate which of the possible solutions generated would be the best solution based on the consequences. This further illustrates the idea that there may be several options or choices in every situation, and there may be several consequences for each solution. "When making a decision, it is useful to think about all the consequences and think about what you want to have happen and make your choice based on which solution will help you achieve that goal."

The point of this exercise is to convey to the group members that, in order to make good choices, we must evaluate the consequences of our choices.

Provide Handout 4.1 (Problem Solving: PICC Model) and review with the group.

Automatic Responding versus Thinking Ahead: Part I

The following exercises are designed to teach children to recognize the difference between solutions that are generated in an automatic mode of responding and those that are generated when people think before responding. It is important to convey to the students the idea that if they are able to stop and think before responding, they will often be able to think of better solutions.

Engage the children in a game where they think of as many possible solutions to a problem as they can. Instruct group members to respond to you as quickly as possible, giving you every possible solution they can think of. Children should say the first thing that pops into their heads, regardless of whether the solution is right or wrong or good or bad. Use a real-life or hypothetical problem situation. Either you or your coleader should record all of the responses on the dry erase board or flipchart. Do not evaluate any of the solutions offered, but instead ask for clarification if a solution is not clearly delineated (e.g., "Why do you think that would solve the problem?" or "How would that solve this problem?"). If a child offers a solution that is a variation of a solution previously mentioned, point out that this is a variation and then list it with the solutions generated.

After generating a long list of solutions, ask group members to identify the consequences for these solutions and evaluate the consequences in terms of being good (++), okay (+), or bad (–).

Leader Note

You will need a copy of the solutions and the consequence ratings so that you can compare them to the new ones that will be generated in a similar exercise to be conducted next week. Be sure to write them down and have them available for next week.

Assign Homework

Provide group members with Handout 4.2 (Problem Solving Worksheet). Ask that they complete this form for the next session. Remind group members that they will receive *two points* for completing the assignment. The target problem can be one experienced at home, in school, or in the community. The solution should be carried out and the consequences noted in the space provided. Encourage group members to think before responding and to evaluate all available options.

Positive Feedback

See Session 1.

Prize Box

See Session 1.

Free Time

See Session 1.

HANDOUT 4.1

Problem Solving—PICC Model

PROBLEM IDENTIFICATION (P.I.)

(a) Perspective Taking
* Identify what the problem is based on **each** person's perspective of the situation.
* No blaming, name-calling or put-downs in stating the problem.

(b) Individual Goals
* Identify your goal in the situation.
* Identify the other person's goal in the situation.
* Look toward cooperation and compromise.

IDENTIFY CHOICES (C)

* Brainstorm all possible solutions to the problem. What are your choices?
* Do not evaluate the solutions in terms of outcome, just list all possible choices.

IDENTIFYING CONSEQUENCES (C)

* Identify what the consequences would be for each solution.
* Provide ALL possible consequences, both positive and negative.

CHOOSE THE BEST SOLUTION

* Choose the best solution based on a review of all the consequences.
* Weigh out the positives and negatives → choose the one that has the fewest negatives.
* Choose a backup solution in case the first solution does not work.
* Try out your solution.

HANDOUT 4.2
PROBLEM SOLVING WORKSHEET

My problem is:

_____
_____
_____

Possible choices/solutions: **Consequences of the choices/solutions:**

_____   _____
_____   _____
_____   _____
_____   _____
_____   _____
_____   _____

The solution I chose is:

_____
_____
_____

The consequences of my solution were:

_____
_____
_____

Session 5: Social Problem Solving: Part III

Materials Needed

- Handout 1.4 (Goal Sheet)
- List of solutions generated by the group during Session 4 (recorded by a group leader)
- Pictures or object representations for use with boat activity (optional)
- Prize box

Session Outline

- Review goal sheets and main points from previous session (Session 2)
- Complete discussion of the value of thinking ahead
- Illustrate how decisions are made based on consequences

Review Goal Sheets and Main Points from Previous Session

See Session 2.

Review the Homework Assignment

Review the homework assignment (Handout 4.2, Problem Solving Worksheet). Group members who completed their homework should receive *two points*. Discuss the target problems, choices, and consequences.

Automatic Responding versus Thinking Ahead: Part II

Remind children of last week's discussion regarding generating solutions to problems and the game they played in which the group generated multiple solutions to a particular problem. Explain to children that today the group is going to play a similar game, but instead of generating all of the answers that they can possibly think of, they are going to think about the consequences of each solution and identify only those that they think will have good outcomes. Stress the importance of thinking through the consequences of the solutions before choosing one. Choose the same problem that was used during the previous session's activity.

After solutions have been generated, ask group members to look at the two lists of solutions (one from today and one from the previous session) and decide which list has better ideas on it. Ask group members to generate the consequences for each of the solutions offered in today's exercise and then rate the consequences as good (++), okay (+), or bad (−). Point out that, in general, people can come up with better solutions if they stop to think about the following things.

- What is the problem?
- What do I want to see happen?
- What are my choices for solving this problem?

This sequence usually produces better results than if the person simply responded without thinking about the choices first.

Remind group members to use breathing techniques or other methods to help them calm down before they make a decision. Inform them that, right now, the focus is on their ability to stop and think, rather than their ability to think quickly. This is because they are at the early stages of learning how to make good decisions and, because of this, they need to proceed slowly. As children get better at making good decisions they will be able to do so faster and the whole process will not seem as tedious and difficult. One way to explain this to the group is to use the metaphor of learning to play a new video game.

Learning how to make good decisions is like learning to play a new videogame. The first few times you play a new game you need to really think about what you are doing and how to win the game. You make mistakes and you learn from those mistakes. After playing the game for a while, you can play without thinking very much, and your playing becomes much more automatic. It is the same for solving problems. First you will have to really stop and think about what options are available and what the consequences are for each solution. But, after a while, your responding will become much more automatic and you will not have to think as much as you do now.

Trouble at Sea Exercise

This exercise is designed to introduce and extend the concept of consequence identification and to assist students in better understanding the problem solving process. Explain that the group as a whole will be discussing a situation and that they must come to some agreement regarding items to keep and items to discard. (An optional way to complete this activity is to give the list of items to all the students and ask them to decide which items they would keep and which items they would throw overboard.) Having pictures of, or the actual objects themselves to help demonstrate this exercise, generally heightens the level of interest and participation amongst the group members. Explain the story as follows.

You are all members of a fishing party on a boat which has run into bad weather and some engine trouble several miles from shore. The captain of the ship has told you that because of the rough weather, the boat needs to be lighter in order to make it through the storm and to avoid sinking. You as members of the crew need to decide which items to keep and which items to throw overboard. You need to decide as a group the order in which you throw the following items overboard.

1. Box of matches
2. Radio (ship to shore)
3. Compass
4. Navigational map
5. 10 gallons of water
6. Signal flares
7. Life rafts
8. 100 feet of rope
9. Flashlight
10. Life jackets

Allow group members five minutes to discuss the problem and decide which items would be thrown overboard first. Encourage students to identify the consequences for throwing each item overboard, and to use the identified consequences in their decisions about which items to keep and which items to discard. Ask group members:

- What was the problem in this situation?
- Did different people have different ideas about which items to throw overboard?
- How did you decide which items to keep and which ones to throw overboard?
- Did thinking about the consequences help you decide which items to keep?

Positive Feedback

See Session 1.

Prize Box

See Session 1.

Free Time

See Session 1.

Session 6: Application of Social Problem Solving to Teacher Conflict

Materials Needed

- Handout 1.4 (Goal Sheet)
- Handout 6.1
- Materials for Top 10 game
- Prize box

Session Outline

- Review goal sheets and main points from previous session (Session 2)
- Enhance perspective-taking ability
- Discuss teacher's perspective
- Practice problem solving with teacher conflicts

Review Goal Sheets and Main Points from Previous Session

See Session 2.

Understanding the Teacher's Perspective

Inform the students that you and your coleader have interviewed their teachers and questioned them about their expectations. Divide the group in half and ask each group to come up with the top 10 responses they think teachers gave to the question. What do you (teachers) expect from students in the classroom? Write the responses generated by the group on the dry erase board or flipchart. After they have provided their answers, discuss with students why teachers may have selected these specific responses and how these items may impact a teacher in the classroom. Discuss the importance of understanding the needs and desires of others (teachers), in order to develop and improve relationships. (If you want, you can conduct this exercise in a *Family Feud* game show format and have the answers already prepared on slips of cardboard. When a student lists one of the top ten answers, you turn over that slip and display the answer.)

The top 10 answers in our survey were:

1. To be involved, working and learning something.
2. To be happy or excited about learning something.
3. To participate.
4. To be prepared and ready to work.
5. To be respectful.
6. To work to their best ability.
7. To follow the rules.
8. To be creative and have fun.
9. To pay attention and understand the material.
10. To seek out answers to questions they have.

If audiotapes are available from the teacher interviews conducted, you may replay portions of these interviews for the students to hear.

Use the Problem-Solving Model
to Discuss Teacher Issues

Problem Identification

Have group members brainstorm about differences of opinion that have occurred or could occur between a teacher and a student, as well as possible differences in the perspectives of teachers and students. Try to focus this discussion on the teacher's expectations for students in the classroom. You may use the following sample dialogue.

What do teachers expect students to do in the classroom? If they expect you to do your work independently, how can you ask teachers for help when you need it? What do teachers expect from students in terms of homework? You may think that homework is boring or takes away from your free time, but your teachers probably think that home-work is a great way to help you retain what you have learned in class.

Provide each child with Handout 25.1 (Problem Solving Worksheet) and ask them to write down a problem that they have with a teacher and use the worksheet to help generate solu-tions to that problem. Make sure that the form is filled out completely. You can go over this as a group activity, or have each person complete the form independently and review each one and assist as needed.

Consequence Evaluation

Have group members rate each consequence in terms of whether it is a good (++), okay (+), or bad (−) consequence. Record the rating next to each consequence.

Develop a Plan

Have group members decide what the best solution would be and then discuss possible ob-stacles for that solution. Repeat until you have discussed three or more possible solutions and their associated obstacles.

Role Play

Have group members role play the problem situation and several alternatives. Ask each of them to choose a solution that has been rated (++) or (+), and ask them to enact the solution with another group member acting as the teacher in the role play.

Positive Feedback

See Session 1.

Prize Box

See Session 1.

Free Time

See Session 1.

HANDOUT 6.1
PROBLEM SOLVING WORKSHEET

My problem is:

_____

_____

_____

Possible choices/solutions: **Consequences of the choices/solutions:**

_____   _____

_____   _____

_____   _____

_____   _____

_____   _____

_____   _____

_____

The solution I chose is:

_____

_____

_____

The consequences of my solution were:

_____

_____

_____

Chapter 3

Mentoring Adolescent Girls: A Group Intervention for Preventing Dating Violence

Elizabeth M. Banister, RN, PhD, and Deborah L. Begoray, PhD

RATIONALE AND DEVELOPMENT

Research has shown that the health status of adolescent girls has not improved in recent years (King, Boyce, & King, 1999). Adolescent girls face a number of serious health issues related to sexuality and relationships. Unplanned pregnancies, HIV/AIDS, and sexually transmitted infections (STIs) are major public health concerns (Health Canada, 2002). In the United States, the Centers for Disease Control and Prevention (CDC) identified risky sexual behavior as one of six health behaviors most associated with mortality, morbidity, and social problems among youth (CDC, 2004). In 2003, nearly 46.7% of high school students in the United States had engaged in sexual intercourse, while 37% who were sexually active had not used a condom at last sexual intercourse (CDC, 2004). Conflicting social pressures continue to affect adolescents' abilities to make decisions about contraceptive use and safe sex and contribute to risk-taking behaviors in heterosexual intimate relationships. For example, Hutchinson (1998) found that for 59% of young women sexual risk history was not discussed with their partners prior to having sexual relations for the first time. Furthermore, relationship violence is a leading cause of injuries in both adult and adolescent women. Reported rates of dating violence in high school students range from 9% to 45% (Downey, Bonica, & Rincon, 1999) with significant numbers of students continuing in such relationships despite the abuse. A national U.S. survey reveals that almost one in four (23%) women aged 18–24 were assaulted by a date, boyfriend, acquaintance, or stranger (U.S. Department of Justice, 1997). Problematic romantic relationships can have multiple negative effects such as those on adolescents' self-esteem (Ackard, Neumark-Sztainer, & Hannan, 2003) and emotional health (Compian, Gowen, & Hayward, 2004).

The study was made possible by the generous funding of the Social Sciences and Humanities Council of Canada (SSHRC) and Canadian Institutes of Health Research (CIHR).

Despite considerable funding, few intervention programs have resulted in a substantial increase in postponing sexual initiation or curtailing pregnancy among adolescents. For example, programs that advocate saying no to having sex assume that young women have an assertive sexual identity and confidence in negotiating safe sex. Asking young women to talk about sex in advance and to produce condoms can carry a heavy cost for this population. Youth are reticent to initiate conversations about issues such as sex and need health-related educators who are willing to broach sensitive topics in a gender sensitive, direct, nonjudgmental, and open manner.

Evidence for Using Mentoring Intervention

Mentoring programs are becoming an integral component of youth services programs (Rhodes & Roffman, 2002). The increased use of mentoring programs reflects in part the reduced availability of informal adult support in our society. The importance of relationships between adult women and girls for girls' healthy development has been emphasized by many researchers (Pastor, McCormick, & Fine, 1996). Evaluations suggest that volunteer mentoring relationships promote positive development through role modeling and emotional support, facilitate improvements in adolescents' attitudes, self-perceptions, and behaviors (Walker & Freedman, 1996), and reduce risky sexual behavior among adolescent women (Taylor-Seehafer & Rew, 2000). Connection with a caring adult in a mentoring program setting can contribute to a mutual sense of trust and of being understood and respected. Meaningful relationships with nonparent adults can facilitate changes in youths' perceptions of self and of close relationships (Rhodes & Roffman, 2002).

Introduction to the Mentoring Program

Our program emerged from a community-based mentorship study that focused on understanding adolescent women's dating health concerns and best practices for addressing them (Banister & Leadbeater, 2007). Forty participants were accessed through three public, urban high schools, an urban youth health clinic, and a rural Aboriginal secondary school. Initially, participants were 14 to 16 years of age and White ($N = 30$) or Aboriginal ($N = 10$). The majority were from families with low socioeconomic status and were at risk for dropping out of school. The staff and ado-

lescents at each site took adolescent women's dating-related health concerns seriously and were motivated to learn more about such concerns.

The study was conducted in two phases. In phase one, two to three consecutive focus groups were conducted with five groups of girls (one at each site) to obtain ethnographic data on their dating health concerns. Findings from the focus groups provided the foundation for the development of the mentoring program used in phase two. We designed the initial focus groups to create space so that participants could be an audience for each other while at the same time co-construct meaning of their dating experiences. Examples of issues identified by participants included substance abuse, having unprotected sex, and physical and emotional intimate partner abuse.

Results of the analyses of the focus group phase one data are reported in more detail elsewhere (Banister, Jakubec, & Stein, 2003); however, themes detected the complex interaction of power dynamics and socialization processes in the girls' relationships with men. Girls frequently blamed themselves for their boyfriends' abuse and lack of commitment and this, in turn, impeded their ability to speak in their own interests.

During the second phase of the study, with the same girls who participated in the focus groups, we conducted a weekly mentoring program for 16 weeks in 1.5-hour sessions. Each intervention group was composed of approximately eight girls, an adult woman mentor, and a research assistant. Building on data generated in phase one helped to ensure program relevance for the participants. The four school sites incorporated the program into their regular school hours, facilitating a low attrition rate (only two girls dropped out because of scheduling conflicts). Following policies at three of the sites (the rural Aboriginal school, an urban high school, and the local youth clinic), a staff member was included as the mentor. Researchers have reported on the central role of youth–staff relationships in a variety of youth development programs (Rhodes & Roffman, 2002). It has been suggested that, to effectively change behaviors of high-risk youth, program designs should include messages delivered by those who have similar life experiences (Villarruel, Sweet-Jemmott, Howard, Taylor, & Bush, 1998). In particular, having a safe place to discuss dating health concerns in the presence of a caring adult was an important part of the program. One participant reported:

Like, adults don't want to listen to you about telling them about drugs; they don't want to listen if you tell them you have an STI or you're pregnant or something. A lot of kids are scared to say something, right? And I think that it's really good to incorporate all of that [into the program] because kids are looking for someone to talk to and adults are the wisest and if a kid is telling you something and an adult is listening and not judging, that can be the best thing for them.

Many of the participants reported positive changes in their self-worth as a result of program participation. Furthermore, some reported leaving dating relationships that were emotionally and/or physically abusive. This chapter outlines strategies that were used in our mentorship program for enhancing adolescent relationships.

Issues to Consider When Conducting the Intervention

Although in early sessions of the program, youth may not be comfortable sharing personal information, in later sessions they may over-disclose. Youth may have limited experience in making decisions about what is safe to talk about within the intervention context (Banister & Daly, 2006). We found that the adolescent participants were less likely to self-censor when in a group with their peers. Participants need to be reminded at the beginning of the intervention to share only that which is comfortable.

"Watertight confidentiality" (Christians, 2000, p. 139) cannot be guaranteed in the group setting. Even though group rules are created to build safety in the group, participants need to be reminded that they do not have control over information that may be disclosed by others outside of the group setting.

Using staff members as mentors for the group raises the issue of dual role relationships. Dual roles can emerge when the mentoring role is confused with the mentor's service roles (e.g., as nurses and teachers). Group participants need assurance that the mentor or service provider will maintain confidentiality within the legal limits.

Training of facilitators is important for creating a safe group environment and reducing the potential for harm. Facilitators require well-developed group facilitation skills and experience working with adolescents. For example, facilitators need to be aware when girls are over-disclosing and model respect-

ful ways to help girls set limits on this. Keeping the focus on thoughts rather than on feelings will help girls contain some of the emotional content that may emerge. Groups of new facilitators can get together and do role playing, asking appropriate questions, and so forth, to prepare them for managing situations that may emerge.

MENTORING PROGRAM

Program Elements: People

Adolescent Girls

The peer group number should be small enough to inspire participation, yet large enough to promote social competencies and incorporate a variety of perspectives. We recommend a maximum of 10 girls.

Facilitators and Mentors

It is recommended that a group format for the girls' mentoring program be comprised of a small peer group of adolescent girls along with a female group facilitator and a female mentor. *Note:* When circumstances do not allow for two adult leaders to take on the roles of facilitator and mentor, it is suggested that these roles be combined into one facilitator/mentor role.

Group Mentor. A primary role of the group mentor is to help create an environment of encouragement and support within the group and to provide the girls with a positive and understanding role model.

Group Facilitator. The facilitator is responsible for leading and facilitating each session. The facilitator can also have a list of community resources available. Examples of resources are families, counselors, physicians, nurses, educators, artists, elders, crisis lines, and other community agencies available for consultation as needed.

Establishing the Environment

Establishing a safe, trusting, and respectful atmosphere is of critical importance for building dynamic interrelationships with and among the group as a whole. Participation in the girls' mentoring program is voluntary. Group members are invited to take part in all of the activities; however, it is ultimately the decision of each individual when and in what way they wish to participate.

Time

The recommended time frame for the adequate facilitation of this program is weekly, two-hour sessions carried out over a period of 13 weeks for a total of 26 hours. The timing for this project could be altered to accommodate diverse scheduling needs.

Space

To provide a safe and trusting atmosphere, it is recommended that the space allocated to facilitate discussions and activities be warm, welcoming, and free of outside noise or interruption. A circle format is suggested for discussion, and adequate floor and table space is required for hands-on activities.

Snack

It is recommended that a healthy snack (e.g., fruit) be provided to group members during each two-hour session. Individuals can also be encouraged to bring water bottles to each session.

Common Elements of Each Session

Each session follows the same basic format, which is outlined here.

Opening

Free Expression Journals. Each session opens individually. Free expression is an independent stream-of-consciousness activity that allows individuals to explore and articulate personal thoughts, feelings, and experiences prior to sharing them in or out of the group. Through journaling, sketching, poetry, or any other form of literary expression, this activity creates a safe space to free the mind and spirit so that girls can then engage in the group session more fully. Free expression can be very effective in helping raise girls' self-awareness, emotional literacy, trust in themselves and others, confidence, and communication skills. Because it is an independent activity, it takes away the peer influence of a discussion and gives them time to think freely and independently (Banister & Begoray, 2004). We recommend that the free expression activity be initiated at the beginning of each group meet-

ing as much as possible for approximately 10 minutes. Routines need to be established for the use of journals. The following choices can be discussed with girls and one alternative chosen.

- Collect and store journals after each session to ensure availability each week.
- Journals are taken home and used throughout the week, with a reminder to bring them to the following week's session.
- Two journals are provided: one for in-session use and one for out-of-session use.

Because journaling is a personal and reflective activity, the mentor/facilitator reminds girls that

- There are no preconceived notions of what individuals should be feeling or experiencing;
- Writing should be done freely without concern for spelling, grammar, content, or neatness; and
- Journals are personal and will be kept confidential—girls keep their journals private as a strategy for learning to set personal boundaries.

Closing

Each session closes with the group in a circle. While closing activities vary, we recommend choosing one or more from the following list.

- *Group reflection.* Use questions such as: What worked well today? What could we improve?
- *Appreciations or acknowledgments.* Take time to thank guest speakers, group members who lead discussions, or others who did special work to aid the group.
- *Review of goals and strategies.* Use questions such as: What did you learn today? What will you remember from today's session?
- *Reminders for upcoming sessions.* Make announcements and ask for group member input as well.

Question Box

Finally, a question box and slips of paper are provided to group members at the end of each session. This box provides girls the opportunity to ask questions anonymously. Girls are invited to write out a question that they have about the group, about relationships, or other issues on a small piece of paper and anonymously place it in the box. Responses from the mentor and facilitator will be provided as time allows during future sessions.

Materials and Resources Required

Each session also requires the following materials.

- Talking stick or sharing symbol (special rock, stone, feather, etc.)
- Journal (one or two per group member)
- Pencils, pens, other colored pencils or markers
- Flip chart with markers
- Healthy snack

Assessment

Facilitators need to evaluate the success of each session by systematic observation of their participation and behavior within the discussion, free writing, activities, and question box. Observations should be recorded as soon as possible after each session. Discussion can be assessed by quantity and quality of participation of each member in speaking, active listening, initiating ideas, responding to others, disagreeing respectfully. Free writing is evaluated by the quantity written and monitoring girls' comments on writing (for those who volunteer their comments). The question box is assessed by the number and kinds of questions.

Session 1: Building Community

A safe and collaborative forum is fostered in this first session as participants, including girls and mentor/facilitator, introduce themselves and work together to create group guidelines that will be revisited and used throughout all of the sessions.

The mentor and facilitator will

- foster dialogue among group members,
- co-construct group guidelines with participants, and
- offer the context and directions for the program and coming weeks.

The participants will

- understand group process,
- co-construct group guidelines and free write in their journal, and
- cooperate in group activities.

Procedures, Processes, and Activities

Introduction

In this first session only, the session opens with a group activity in a circle to provide building of community through an ice breaker activity. In a circle, the facilitator introduces herself and shares something interesting about her name. She then invites each member in turn to share around the circle as the talking stick is passed from hand to hand.

Free Expression

To begin the first session, each group member is given a journal, pencils, pens, or colored pencils. They are then invited to personalize the first page and reflect on their thoughts and feelings through writing, printing, calligraphy, poetry, sketching, or any other form of personal expression. The mentor or facilitator leads the discussion on use of journals, that is, in-session and/or out-of-session as described previously.

Discussion

To promote further discussion and dialogue, the mentor or facilitator poses the following question(s): What kinds of concerns might girls at your age have about relationships? To encourage expansion of ideas, also ask Why? after responses emerge. Wait time is especially important in these opening sessions. Counting silently to 10 will give girls time to formulate an answer. If none is forthcoming, try What problems do girls in this community face? Avoid personal questions, such as What is your concern/problem?

Snack Break

Group Guidelines

To begin, all participants are asked to define the things (principles) that are important to them in order to feel comfortable in their group. Facilitators should have a list of questions to help generate discussion.

The mentor and facilitator play a key role in promoting clear communication, clarification, and consensus between the girls. While words or phrases such as *honesty, confidentiality,* or *treating each other respectfully* may come up often in discussion, it should not be assumed that everyone has the same understanding of what these terms mean. Asking questions such as What would respect look like? or How would you know if someone was treating you respectfully? will help to generate greater understanding and clarity among group members.

All guidelines are recorded on chart paper in the front of the room. The group is then asked to decide upon a title for their guidelines such as "Our Group Rules."

The following suggestions may help to ensure that the constructed guidelines are held accountably by group members throughout each session.

- Group members write these guidelines into their journals. They become a reminder for positive group conduct.
- Before the next session, the facilitator can make a large, clear record of the agreed on principles and have it posted in the room in a prominent location. These can be revisited and revised as needed throughout the upcoming sessions.
- The mentor or facilitator can copy the principles in a document format and distribute to each group member in the following session.

Closing

Closing exercises can include a short closing (in the circle format) that is facilitated in which girls are invited to share one thing they found useful about the session. These comments can be made orally or recorded in their journals. Girls are reminded to bring a personal artifact to the next session—something that is meaningful for her and something she is comfortable introducing to the group.

Question Box

The mentor or facilitator introduces the question box. For this first session, everyone is provided with a slip of paper to submit to the box even if the submission is blank or a general comment rather than a question.

Assessment

The mentor or facilitator will evaluate the success of this session by recording observations. Some groups or members are reticent to participate in early sessions.

Session 2: How Do I See Myself?

Session 2 enhances self-identity and self-awareness. Group members are encouraged to explore and connect with inward perceptions of self and begin to differentiate between what is perceived from the inside and what is projected to others on the outside.

The mentor or facilitator will

- address some of the questions from the question box,
- revisit group guidelines, and
- lead activities to enhance girls' awareness of self and others.

The participants will

- engage in personal and collective reflection and discussion.

Procedures, Processes, and Activities

Free Expression

As group members arrive, they are encouraged to take a few minutes to reflect in their journals (refer to the Session 1 guidelines on Free Expression).

Sharing

Group members are invited to share their personal artifacts and why they represent something of meaning and significance.

Question Box

Time should be allocated to address any questions that girls have put in the question box at the end of Session 1. Depending on the number and content of questions, they can be grouped together in terms of similarity or interest. The mentor or facilitator needs to lead the discussion and provide information as appropriate such as One question that was submitted concerned . . .

Revisit Group Guidelines

The group reads over the group guidelines that were constructed the previous session (from chart paper). This provides a reminder for group conduct as well as an opportunity for girls to add or alter the agreed on principles.

"I See Myself As . . ."

This discussion provides a warm-up for developing self-awareness, which is the prominent theme for the next session (Session 3). The girls are invited to respond in writing one or all of the following questions using concentric circles.

- I see myself as . . . (inner circle)
- My friends and family think of me as . . . (middle circle surrounding first one)
- Society expects me to be . . . (outer circle surrounding the middle and first circle)

Depending on the time, facilitators may want to have the girls write their thoughts down first, then share, or just ask each question directly to the group. The mentor or facilitator provides a list of personality traits for girls to consider as descriptions of themselves. Discuss each word with an example from girls, for example, 'Independent' means to rely on yourself. How would you recognize an independent girl?

Once all of the "I see myself as ..." statements have been read aloud to the group, questions such as the following are posed for individuals to reflect on discrepancies between what was written down in the middle and outer circles and what the girl sees as her authentic or true self.

- What are some of the differences among the circles in how you see yourself?
- What accounts for the differences?

Snack Break

Closing

The mentor or facilitator leads a short closing (in the circle format) as previously described. Group members can be reminded about their journals; however, the routine is to be established (i.e., hand in, use over the week, remember to bring next week, see previous description).

Question Box

The mentor or facilitator will address questions from Session 1 that were placed in the question box.

Assessment

The mentor or facilitator evaluates the session as described in Session 1.

Session 3: Gender Stereotypes

Through discussion and awareness activities, girls examine gender stereotypes and confront the challenges they are faced with as adolescent girls who try to fit in. They also have the opportunity to participate in action planning to confront these issues and to make a difference in their lives and the lives of others.

The mentor or facilitator will

- respond to the question box questions,
- support members in examining and challenging gender stereotypes, and
- support the girls' action projects that confront stereotypes.

The participants will

- participate in activities,
- list and describe gender stereotypes, and
- plan and practice ways to subvert stereotypes.

Materials and Resources Required

In addition to the usual materials, two large poster boards, magazines, and glue sticks are required.

Procedure, Process, and Activities

Free Expression

See Session 1.

Check-In

At the beginning of the session, the mentor or facilitator invites the girls to state briefly how *present* they are for the group at that time. This encourages collective mutuality and empathy. It is important to limit the time to approximately one minute per girl to promote mutual respect for each other's opportunity to be heard.

Question Box

The mentor or facilitator will address questions from Session 2.

Activity 1: Drawing the "Perfect" Male and Female

The mentor or facilitator posts the definition on flip chart paper and invites discussion: A stereotype is a popularly held belief about a type of person or a group of people that does not take into account individual traits or differences. Stereotypes are often hurtful and damaging. One or two volunteers are asked to come up to the front of the room and draw a picture of the physically perfect man on one piece of flip chart paper (or on the board) and the perfect woman on the other. The rest of the group assists by calling out physical characteristics they think should be included (characteristics that are based on gender stereotypes). Alternatively or additionally, a number of magazine pictures can be used. After the drawings are complete, other volunteers are asked to draw a box around each drawing. Inside the box, words and phrases are written that represent gender stereotypes, that is, how males and females are portrayed in society.

Discussion

The mentor or facilitator asks: What happens if a boy or girl doesn't "fit in the box"? Outside each box, words and phrases are written by the mentor or facilitator that represent the names that people are called and the challenges they face if they are different from the gender stereotype.

The mentor or facilitator leads further discussion.

- How many of us really fit this stereotype?
- What do girls do if they don't fit with these pictures?
- Why do we accept stereotypes?
- What are other ways people are stereotyped?

Facilitators share the following with the group:

Stereotypes suggest that women and men have specific roles they must perform well and portray certain images they should aspire to. Boys aren't born to have violent or unhealthy attitudes towards girls. Girls aren't born to be passive or to wait for boys to make all the decisions (including when, where, and how to have sex). When we adopt a stereotype, we lose our authentic power. Stereotypes take away our personal choices in determining our own image, interests, and skills, and discourage us from pursuing roles and careers that we are interested in and capable of doing. (Adapted from http://www.media-awareness.ca/).

The final question the mentor or facilitator asks is How can we challenge stereotypes?

Snack Break

Additional Debriefing Questions

The mentor or facilitator leads a discussion asking the following questions as appropriate.

- What is sexy? What is the stereotype of sexy for males? females?
- What's the story about being sexy? Who is? Who isn't? Why? Who says?
- What's the story about being male or female?
- How does the media influence our decisions?
- Who gains? Who loses from allowing these stereotypes to control our reactions to other people?
- How do you or your friends fit into the stereotype? What happens if you or they don't?
- How does the media affect the way we think about relationships?

Closing

The mentor or facilitator encourages reflection by asking:

- What did you learn about yourself?
- What stood out for you today? What will you take with you today?
- How does today's discussions relate to how you are in relationships?

The mentor or facilitator completes closing by expressing an appreciation for individuals or the group and reminds members about journal entries.

Question Box

See Session 1.

Assessment

See Session 1.

Additional Resources

The Girls' Speak Out Web site is http://www.girlsspeakout.org/. To access a column by Andrea Johnston (author of Girls' Speak Out) go to http://www.feminist.com/resources/artspeech/girls/girlsspeak.html.

Session 4: Sex and Sexuality

Session 4 focuses on girls' understanding of sexual health and ways of communicating about their sexual health needs.

The facilitators will

- help girls identify a range of sexual activities,
- open discussion about choice and consent regarding sexual activity,
- explore notions of abstinence and safe, protected sex, and
- help girls develop a *no condom, no sex* mantra.

The participants will

- identify a range of sexual activities and through role playing will practice communicating and asserting themselves in challenging, sexual health situations.

Procedure, Process, and Activities

Free Expression

See Session 1.

Sharing

See Session 2.

Question Box

The mentor or facilitator will address questions from Session 3.

Activity 1: What Is Sex?

This session sets the stage for discussion about sexual health. Girls are invited to respond to a few general questions about sexual activities. A line is drawn across a blackboard or a flip chart paper with the left end of the line labeled *least intimate* and the right end of the line labeled *most intimate*.

Pose the questions:

- What are sexual kinds of activities?
- What do people do when they are being sexual?
- What are sexy activities that don't involve touching or genitals?

Girls are invited to call out different types of sexual activity and say where each one fits along the continuum of relationships from least to most intimate.

Discussion

The mentor or facilitator asks:

- At what point might any of these activities become assault?

If someone says or implies no to anything, anywhere along the continuum, from holding hands to oral sex to intercourse and they are forced to against their will, it is assault? Consent means saying yes to an activity, every time.

The mentor or facilitator leads further discussion.

- If you agree to any activity on the continuum, are you allowed to say no in the future?
- No one can assume that, just because you agreed to do something yesterday, you will want to do it again today. Every one has the right to say no.
- How would it feel to claim this right for you?

Snack Break

Activity 2: Saying No

Abstinence, negotiating condom use, and communication skills are integral to this program; a no condom, no sex message is reinforced through activities that promote choice and commitment.

Role Play

Brainstorm situations in which girls feel uncomfortable asserting their needs or saying no. These do not need to be conflicts about sex; it is useful to use a broad spectrum of examples including but not limited to sexual issues.

The facilitator or mentor role plays a scenario agreed on by the girls: "as it happened" and then "as she would have liked it to happen" (with another facilitator or a volunteer). Group members are invited to role play different scenarios and ways of safely saying no to sexual activity.

Ideas for role play can include:

- Asking for a date: Is it okay for a girl to ask a guy out?
- Practicing saying yes and no.
- Giving clear messages.

The Mantra

Group members cocreate a no condom, no sex mantra. Examples of a mantra may include messages such as:

- Take care of ourselves and each other.
- Don't have sex if we are not ready.
- When in doubt, run!
- Use condoms every time.
- Abstinence is still the safest choice.

Demonstration: Condom Use

Girls need to learn how to use condoms effectively. Condoms are important for birth control and sexually transmitted infection (STI) and HIV protection regardless of other birth control methods. If leaders are uncomfortable with condom demonstration, a trained professional (such as a nurse) from the community would be an excellent resource.

Closing

The mentor or facilitator leads a short closing (in the circle format) as previously described. Group members can be reminded of their journals.

Question Box

See Session 1.

Assessment

See Session 1.

Session 5: Values, Goals, and Relationships

Girls examine the relationships between core values and goal setting and how these provide the foundation for pursuing positive actions and relationships.

The mentor or facilitator will

- assist girls to develop personal values and goals, and
- assist girls to make connections between values, goals, and relationships.

The participants will

- develop personal values and goals,
- differentiate between values and strategies, and
- make connections between values, goals, and relationships.

Procedure, Process, and Activities

Free Expression

See Session 1.

Question Box

The mentor or facilitator will address questions from Session 4.

Activity 1: Identifying Values

The mentor or facilitator provides a definition of *value* and *strategy* on flip chart paper. Values are the beliefs and standards that we live by; strategies are what we do to achieve the things we value. Provide an example of a value from the following list: connection, safety, loyalty, security, and acceptance. Then ask How can a person achieve connection? (a possible response: spend more time with friends).

The mentor or facilitator leads a brief brainstorming activity. Provide basic brainstorming rules: quantity is important, the more ideas the better, no judgments, all ideas are accepted. Girls then brainstorm values that are important to them with the mentor or facilitator serving as recorder (it is important to use the girls' exact words as much as possible).

Once brainstorming is over, each girl individually chooses and writes down the five most important values in her journal. Alert girls that their chosen values will be shared with others. In pairs, girls discuss their values. The mentor or facilitator directs pairs to return to the circle and lead discussion of values commonly held.

Activity 2: Identifying Goals

The mentor or facilitator leads a brief brainstorming session of long-term goals (following brainstorming rules outlined above) by asking the following questions.

- What are your most important goals?
- Which of your goals will help you fulfill your potential/realize your dreams?

Girls write down these goals in their journals.

Setting Short-Term Goals

The mentor or facilitator displays and discusses a goal setting box.

1. Set a goal you really want, not just something that sounds good.
2. Write your goal in the positive instead of the negative.
3. Write your goal out in complete detail.
4. Make your goal short-term, achievable, and measurable.
5. Close your eyes and visualize the goal you have identified.
6. Write down your goal in your journal.
7. Review and visualize your goal each morning and night.

Girls are then asked to identify one personal, health-related goal they can track between group sessions and report on regularly to the group. For some girls, the idea of creating and having responsibility for the direction of their lives may be inconceivable. Begin with What could you set as a goal for the week? The goal can be revised or changed as needed as the group sessions unfold. Possible examples of short-term goals are: to come to school every day, to ride a bike to school every day for a week, to smoke half a pack of cigarettes instead of a whole pack in a week.

The mentor or facilitator invites girls to share their goals in pairs or in a large group circle. The mentor or facilitator models positive feedback, support, and reinforcement and encourages girls to do likewise.

Snack Break

Activity 3: Linking Values, Goals, and Relationships

The mentor or facilitator lists the five most important values on a flip chart or blackboard. On the left side, she lists values and lists her long-term and short-term goals on the right side. Then she invites girls to do the same.

The mentor or facilitator can help girls link values and goals by first posing the following questions.

- What are your most important values? How would we know these are your values? What do they look like?
- What is your goal for next week? What are some of your goals for one year from now? Long-term goals?
- What have you done in the past two to three days that would show us these are your short-term and/or long-term goals?
- How do these steps toward your goals reflect your values?

To help girls take ownership and recognition of their goals:

- How would we know that she is achieving her goal over the next week?
- What would we notice?

To help girls make connections among their values, goals, and their dating relationships, ask:

- How might goals relate to where we are in our lives?
- What might goals have to do with our dating relationships?
- Who gets to plan what happens in your relationship?
- Who in your life will support you in achieving your goals? How? How will you let these people (or person) know about your goals?

In pairs or small groups, the mentor or facilitator invites girls to talk about the relationships among their values, goals, and relationships.

Closing

The mentor or facilitator leads the closing reflection by asking:

- What was it like to hear other people talk about their values and goals?
- What did you learn about yourself?
- Has anything changed since you started coming to the group?
- How might our discussions relate to how you are in a relationship?

The mentor or facilitator expresses any appreciations for individuals or the group. Girls can also be asked to express appreciation once they are comfortable in the group. The mentor or facilitator reminds girls to revisit goals each day and report back next week and to use their journals.

Question Box

See Session 1.

Assessment

See Session 1.

Session 6: Communication and Choice

Group discussion focuses on encouraging and supporting girls in asserting themselves—both in what they want and what they do not want. Girls will learn a variety of skills and strategies that will help them deal with unsafe and challenging situations in sexual and relationship decision making. As girls become more in touch with their values and goals, they can make more conscious choices about their sexuality, including delaying activity or ensuring they are protected physically and emotionally.

The mentor or facilitator will

- lead girls to revisit and revise goal-setting ideas,
- introduce principles and practices of sexual and relationship decision making, and
- lead girls to revisit the mantra.

The participants will

- practice clear messages—saying no (or yes), and
- describe and apply principles of sexual and relationship decision making.

Procedure, Process, and Activities

Free Expression

See Session 1.

Question Box

Address questions from Session 5.

Review: Goals and Values

The mentor or facilitator invites girls to share the successes and challenges of their goal-setting experiences, and to make revisions to their goals based on these experiences, and model supportive behavior. Group members provide support to each other by celebrating small changes that have been achieved (i.e., exercising, cutting back on smoking or drinking alcohol, etc.). They are also encouraged to set steps toward their goals for the upcoming week (or longer as appropriate).

Activity 1: Tie Goal-Setting to Choices about Sexual Activity and Relationships

- How would someone know if you were ready for sex?
- How do you know someone else is ready for sex?

Responses will generally lead into some of the many myths, assumptions, and misinterpretations we make about people, such as

- how they dress,
- how they act,
- whether someone has had sex before, and
- when girls say no, they mean yes.

The mentor or facilitator can expand the discussion by posing questions, such as

- If a girl were dressed in a sexy way, would you think she wanted sex?
- If a girl went to a guy's house knowing no one was home …?

- If a girl was flirting with a guy . . .?
- If she had sex with him before, is it okay to assume . . .?
- Do you think guys are different from girls when it comes to being ready for sex? How?

Snack Break

Activity 2: Refusal Skills: Describe, Demonstrate, Practice

The mentor or facilitator reviews the *saying no* role playing scenarios from Session 4 and invites new scenarios from the group. The mentor or facilitator then leads a discussion about change, self-awareness, assertion, mixed messages, and so on.

The mentor or facilitator leads development of a scenario on practicing saying no to sex. The mentor or facilitator leads discussion using some or all the following debriefing questions.

- How do you know what you really want?
- Why do people have sex?
- Are some reasons to say no or yes better than others?
- Is it okay to change your mind?
- Why do people say yes to sexual activity when they don't want to?
- Are there times girls feel they are expected to be sexual, even if they aren't interested?

Review Mantra

The mentor or facilitator reviews the mantras as recorded on flip chart paper.

- Take care of ourselves and each other.
- Don't have sex if we are not ready.
- When in doubt, run!
- Use condoms every time.
- Abstinence is still the safest choice.

Closing

The mentor or facilitator leads a short closing (in the circle format) as previously described.

Question Box

See Session 1.

Assessment

See Session 1.

Session 7: Notions of Power

Through discussion and awareness activities, girls will examine notions of authentic and false power in relationships.

The mentor or facilitator will

- invite girls to revisit and redefine personal goals, and
- help girls identify personal meaning about power in relationships.

The participants will

- gain information on the difference between authentic and false power in relationships.

Materials and Resources Required

In addition to the usual materials, use a copy of the abuse wheel in the brochure *How Can I Help: A Practical Guide on Adolescent Dating Abuse* by Banister (2006; also available from http://www.youth.society.uvic.ca/resources/abusepamphlet/abuse_nonFN_June2006.pdf).

Procedure, Process, and Activities

Free Expression

See Session 1.

Question Box

Address questions from Session 6.

Review: Goals and Values

Girls are invited to share the successes and challenges of their goal-setting experiences and to make revisions based on these experiences. Group members are encouraged to provide support by celebrating small changes that have been achieved (i.e., exercising, cutting back on smoking or drinking alcohol, etc.) and to encourage further success with goal setting. Tie goal-setting in with choices about sexual activity and relationships.

Activity 1: What Is Power?

On a flip chart at the front of the room, write: What is Power? or Power is . . . Invite group members to provide answers or ideas in response to this question. It is important not to comment or censor, but prompt girls to clarify their statements (i.e., ask what is meant by strength or control, etc.). Post this sheet at the front of the room.

On a second flip chart write *Power Chart.* Draw a line down the center of the paper. Write *Power* on one side and *Non-Power* on the other. Ask who has power over whom in this society. Answers can reflect how girls as well as the broader society view different groups. Try to generate a list that shows how people can be on both sides of the chart, depending on what the context is (adapted from Wolfe, Wekerle, Gough, Reitzel-Jaffe, Grasley, et al., 1996). Avoid sweeping generalizations by providing inclusive understandings of relationships. The flip chart papers can be kept and posted on the wall in subsequent sessions.

Debriefing Questions

- Where do you see yourself on the chart? (Explain)
- Where are you? On the power side? The non-power side?

- When do you feel powerless?
- How does this connect with your dating relationships?

Snack Break

Activity 2: Power Lecture

The facilitator or mentor provides a brief lecture about power using the following guidelines.

- Power is the ability to accomplish a task; it is having the capacity to choose what will happen.
- Explain different types of power. Power can come in many forms. For adolescents, power is usually relational or positional (based on popularity, such as social standing or status, money, talent or appearance).
- Physical power is based on group numbers, size, or strength (Wolfe et al., 1996).
- Other types of power are based on the following.
  - Information: how much information holds and/or the ability to access it.
  - Connection: the means to connect with influential people.
  - Resources: the ability to access money, education, people, technology.
- Brainstorm the differences between authentic (inner) and false power.

Power is not inherently a bad thing. There is a difference between having authentic (i.e., personal or inner) power and having false power (over someone) or feeling as if someone has power over us. The term *power over* implies an abuse of power; someone is using the power they have (relational, physical, etc.) to force us do what they want. The abuse of power is a key element of relationship violence.

Activity 3: Illustrating Power

In pairs, have girls search through magazines, select and discuss pictures that reflect authentic inner power and power imbalances (power over situations). Girls regroup into a larger group format prepared to show and discuss pictures.

The mentor or facilitator leads further discussion by posing a few questions, such as:

- What's going on in the picture? What did you notice?
- How do you see power played out in the picture?
- What would it look like if the roles were reversed?
- How would this particular picture look if it were more balanced?
- Does this (or how does this) relate to your relationship?

Closing

- The mentor or facilitator encourages reflection by posing questions (see the previous session)
- Journal reminder
- Goal-setting reminder

Question Box

See Session 1.

Session 8: Authentic Power

In this session, group members will be introduced to the concept of authentic and false power in relationships and to the abuse of power.

The mentor or facilitator will

- help the girls differentiate between authentic power and false power,
- help girls appreciate their own power or authentic voice, and
- help girls consider their personal rights in relationships.

Materials and Resources Required

- Necklace materials—beads, pendants, string, and so forth.

Procedure, Process, and Activities

Free Expression

See Session 1.

Question Box

Address questions from Session 7.

Activity 1: What Is Violence?

The girls are asked to think about and write their response to the question What is violence? They can brainstorm in pairs or in their journals. Discuss their ideas.

Have the definition of violence written on a separate flip chart and look at it after the brainstorming.

Mini-Lecture: Defining Relationship Violence

Violence is any attempt to control or dominate another person. Review the discussion of authentic (inner) and false power (power over) from Session 7. Authentic power comes from inside (inner power). False power is stolen; it comes from other people and is usually about hurting or humiliating others (power over . . .).

- When you look at your answers to What is violence?, can you see examples of false power? What does it look like?
- How have you seen authentic power used? What does it look like?
- How do you notice these two forms of power in your life right now?

Review: Authentic Power

Authentic power comes from inside (inner power). False power is stolen.

Questions

Following are sample questions that relate this session to sexuality and relationships.

- How does authentic power relate to our sexuality and relationships?
- What would it feel like to make choices based on authentic power?

Activity 2: Creating a Necklace: Representing Authentic Power

Provide materials for girls to create a necklace, such as a bead or pendant on a leather string or whatever materials can be made available within the intervention budget. Each girl creates her own necklace that is intended to represent her authentic voice (Banister & Begoray, 2004). A concrete object, such as a necklace, can help girls associate with using their authentic voice.

Discussion

Following completion of the necklace, the mentor or facilitator asks:

- How might the necklace represent your authentic power?
- When have you felt a genuine sense of authentic power (like helping someone)? What took place?

Homework

Remind the girls to observe people who they perceive as having authentic power. Note how these people convey their authentic power. Also, ask the girls to note what they experience in the presence of someone with authentic power.

Closing

See Session 1.

Question Box

See Session 1.

Session 9: Relationship Violence

Through discussion, the girls will learn to define relationship violence. They will have the opportunity to reflect upon the process of leaving a relationship that is considered violent.

The mentor or facilitator will

- introduce the girls to aspects of power and control in relationships, and
- review authentic and false power to appreciate their own power.

The participants will

- consider and connect with their personal rights, and
- consider and listen to a guest speaker speak about her process of leaving an abusive relationship.

Procedure, Process, and Activities

Free Expression

See Session 1.

Review: Group Principles

It is important to reiterate the group principles and bounds of confidentiality to remind the girls that they have a choice about what they wish to share.

Question Box

Address questions from Session 8.

Activity 1: Authentic Power

Have the girls write out what they noticed about their authentic power during the week. How might the necklace have helped?

Activity 2: Components of Power and Control in Relationships

Provide the girls with a blank circle to create their own power and control wheel with just the spokes (creating 6 or 7 sections of a pie). Explain what the sections represent and have them brainstorm ideas about behaviors that would qualify for each type of abusive power in Appendix B. The facilitator and mentor could role play interactions showing different kinds of abuse to illustrate this for the girls (particularly more subtle forms).

Invite the girls to draw pictures (or write words, thoughts, experiences, etc.) that represent different pie sections.

Using the handout as a template (Appendix B), draw a circle on a flip chart (or have photocopies available) and divide it up into the pie chart sections for the girls to create a group power and control wheel. Write the headings of each section in the pie but leave the rest blank (i.e., peer pressure, emotional abuse, threats, control, bossing you around, etc.).

Brainstorm the different behaviors the girls have seen for each type of abusive power and write them in each section. This will paint a picture of what abuse looks like. Often, particularly with emotional abuse, behaviors are so normalized that girls may not see them as abusive. Facilitators may have to help the girls with some of the areas.

Discussion

Discuss the ways in which people use power over others in relationships. It is important for the mentor or facilitator to talk about how normal many of these behaviors are—in our lives, in media, even in certain ethnic or religious communities. While it is important to be sensitive to cultural differences, it is also important to discuss where values and beliefs about gender and power come from.

Make the connection between the power and control wheel and the discussion about authentic power. People who use the tactics on the wheel are using power over or false power. By using fear and intimidation, they are trying to control another person. People with authentic or inner power do not need to resort to these tactics; they are able to respectfully assert their needs without hurting others.

Activity 3: Guest Speaker

Note: It is important to prepare the girls for a guest for this session a few sessions prior. The guest needs to be chosen carefully. She needs to be someone who, over time, has developed self-confidence and connected with her authentic power. She will be focusing on the process of leaving the relationship and her steps to connect with her authentic power rather than the abusive relationship itself.

Explain to the girls that the guest is joining the group to share her process of leaving a relationship that was abusive. Explain that the guest will share her process of moving into healthier relationships.

Prior to the guest speaker arriving, ask the girls to write out a question on a card that they can then read to the guest—or have the facilitator read the question. This is less intimidating than asking the question themselves.

Closing and Reflection

See Session 1.

Question Box

See Session 1.

Session 10: Sexually Transmitted Infections (STIs)

In this session, group members continue to explore healthy sexuality by understanding the nature of sexually transmitted infections (STIs), including types and symptoms, modes of transmission, and disease prevention.

The mentor or facilitator leads girls to revisit and revise goal-setting ideas by

- helping girls understand the nature and characteristics of STIs,
- helping girls understand the risks of unprotected sexual activity, and
- helping girls understand how to protect themselves from STIs.

Materials and Resources Required

In addition to the usual materials, a handout "What You Need to Know about STD" (Health Canada, 2002) can be ordered or downloaded from http://www.phac-aspc.gc.ca/publicat/std-mts/.

Procedure, Process, and Activities

Free Expression

See Session 1.

Check-In

See Session 3.

Question Box

Address questions from Session 9.

Review: Goals and Values

The mentor or facilitator invites girls to share the successes and challenges of their goal-setting experiences and to make revisions based on these experiences. Group members are encouraged to provide support by celebrating small changes that have been achieved and to encourage further success with goal setting. The mentor or facilitator connects goal setting to choices about sexual activity and relationships.

STI Trivia

The mentor or facilitator introduces the topic of sexually transmitted infections by asking the group questions such as:

- What can you tell me about sexually transmitted infections (STIs)?
- What have you heard about STIs?
- What do you know about STIs?

The mentor or facilitator continues to assess the knowledge level of the group and teach some basic concepts by incorporating a game of trivia. Girls can create game cards with a question on one side and the answer on the other side. Once everyone has contributed two or more questions, teams can be formed. Cards can be mixed, and the questions asked with teams gaining points for correct answers.

Snack Break

Mini-Lecture: Modes of Transmission

The mentor or facilitator provides the following information orally or with the use of a visual containing key points.

When both partners want and are prepared for sexual activity, it can be an enjoyable, wonderful thing. Sexual expression can feel great, physically and emotionally. But healthy sexual activity means that partners take care of themselves and each other by taking responsibility for their emotional and physical health. Sex can be risky; many infections can be spread through many kinds of sexual contact—not just sexual intercourse. In Canada, the highest rates of and increases in STIs are in people ages 15 to 24. STIs can lead to infertility, cancer, or even death (Health Canada, 2002).

People who are infected with an STI often have few or no symptoms. That means they may not know they have an STI. Partners need to be responsible for their own health and the health of others. We know that talking about sex can feel weird or uncomfortable—even adults can have a hard time with it. But communication is an important part of taking care of oneself and creating healthy sexuality and healthy relationships.

What is a Sexually Transmitted Infection (STI)?

The term sexually transmitted infection (STI) covers many types of diseases. Basically, there are two main types of STIs, bacterial (caused by bacteria) and viral (caused by a virus). The main difference between them is that bacterial infections are curable with antibiotics and viral infections are not—the symptoms can be managed but the disease stays in the body. It is important to know that even curable STIs often have no symptoms so they can go unrecognized for long periods of time. If they are not treated, even curable STIs can result in long-term health problems for both men and women (Sexuality Information and Education Council of the United States [SIECUS], 2006).

Many STIs can be transmitted by oral sex as well—either fellatio (a "blow job") or cunnilingus ("going down on")—although some are more easily passed than others. These include:

- Human papillomavirus (HPV) (viral)
- Herpes simplex virus (viral)
- Hepatitis B (viral)
- Gonorrhea (bacterial)
- Syphilis (bacterial)
- Chlamydia (bacterial)
- Chancroid (bacterial) (Edwards & Carne, 1998)

HIV can be passed through oral sex; but saliva tends to inactivate the HIV virus, so this form of transmission is relatively rare (P. Hitchcock, Sexually Transmitted Diseases Branch, National Institute of Allergy and Infectious Diseases, Bethesda, MD, personal communication, August 21, 2000; http://www.agi-usa.org/pubs/journals/3229800.html#14).

STIs can be spread in different ways:

- through intercourse (oral, anal, vaginal) because the bacteria or viruses travel in semen, vaginal fluids, and blood,
- through saliva (or spit) if there is even a tiny cut in or around your mouth,
- through direct contact with an infected area,
- through infected blood on needles and syringes, and
- by infected women to their babies during pregnancy, childbirth, or breastfeeding.

It is possible to catch some STIs more than once and to have more than one STI at a time.

An HIV-positive person who also has another STI increases the chance of giving HIV to his or her partner. A person who has an STI but doesn't have HIV has an increased chance of getting HIV from an HIV-positive partner (Health Canada, 2002).

Symptoms of STIs include:

- Different or heavier discharge from the vagina
- A burning feeling when urinating (peeing)
- Sores, particularly in the genital or anal areas
- Itchy feeling around the sex organs or anus
- Appearance of a rash
- Swollen glands in the groin
- Discharge from the penis

Remember, lots of people have *no* symptoms at all (Health Canada, 2002).

Bacterial Infections

Bacteria are not all bad. We have many healthy bacteria in our bodies, including healthy bacteria in the vagina. These bacteria help the body to work properly. The mentor or facilitator can bring a carton of yogurt to the group to show how bacteria can be helpful. Bacterial STIs are not healthy. They are dangerous and very sneaky. These so-called bad bacteria can live in our bodies, and we may not even know it. A quick, painless test can tell us if we have an STI. Remember—bacterial STIs can be beaten with antibiotics, but even they can be very damaging if they are not stopped.

Bacterial infections include:

- Chlamydia
- Gonorrhea
- Syphilis

Viral Infections

Many common infections, such as colds, are caused by viruses and eventually go away; but some viruses stay in the body where they can change shape and multiply. Viral STIs can be managed with drugs but they are not curable. They stay in the body; sometimes they hide, and sometimes they appear in what we see as symptoms such as lesions on the face or body. Viral STIs can be passed from one person to another even when they are not visible, that is, they are lying dormant. Viral infections include:

- Human Papillomavirus (HPV)
- Genital Herpes
- Hepatitis B
- Human Immunodeficiency Virus (HIV) and AutoImmune Deficiency Syndrome (AIDS)

Other STIs

Some STIs are caused by microscopic creatures called protozoa (trichomoniasis) and other organisms (crabs or pubic lice and scabies). These STIs are curable with antibiotics or topical creams and lotions (SIECUS, 2006).

Debriefing Activity

The mentor or facilitator directs girls to draw their versions of STI figures (e.g., depicting the bad virus as a nasty, evil character with moustache, black clothes, etc.). The mentor or facilitator reinforces the message of using condoms—*every time.* (Remind girls of the mantra.) A teen's greatest chance of getting an infection happens by having unprotected sexual activity. Inform the group that at the next session they will receive a condom demonstration.

Closing

The mentor or facilitator closes as usual. Give each girl a copy of the handout "What You Need to Know about STDs."

Question Box

See Session 1.

Assessment

See Session 1.

Session 11: Anger

Through discussion and role play, group members explore healthy and destructive manifestations of anger and how choice and responsibility can alter, lessen, or heighten angry situations. Girls are socialized to push feelings of anger, resentment, or hostility underground and often use relational weapons such as ignoring, rejection, social isolation, threats, and rumors, to assert their power over each other. Relationships often become a catalyst for girls' anger. This session will provide tools for them to deal more effectively with their feelings.

The mentor or facilitator will

- lead girls to revisit and revise goal-setting ideas,
- define anger,
- lead girls to understand differences between angry feelings and actions,
- lead girls to examine the link between anger and the abuse of power, and
- help girls to explore relationship violence.

The participants will

- work on goal setting,
- understand anger and the difference between feelings and actions,
- explore the link between anger and the abuse of power, and
- understand relationship violence.

Procedure, Process, and Activities

Free Expression

See Session 1.

Check-In

See Session 3.

Question Box

Address questions from Session 10.

Review: Goals and Values

The mentor or facilitator reviews power discussion from Session 7 (five minutes) by asking girls to recall main points.

Activity 1: What Is Anger?

The mentor or facilitator asks the group:

- What is anger?
- How do you know someone is angry?
- How does angry behavior make you feel?
- How do you respond when you are with someone who is angry?

The mentor or facilitator writes responses on a flip chart at the front of the room. Ideas are probed for further meaning or clarification but are not censored. For example, if a girl suggests that control or violence represent anger, ask her in what way(s), what this looks like, or what she means by these terms. As much as possible, use girls' exact words.

Activity 2: Expressing Anger

The mentor or facilitator generates a discussion on anger making the following statement.

Anger is a signal that something is wrong—it tells us to pay attention! Anger is not necessarily a bad thing; a healthy expression of anger can be a powerful and energizing force to create change. Anger about our bad habits might make us seek new ways to behave. On the other hand, unhealthy ways of expressing anger are usually destructive to oneself and others. They may be effective in the short-term, but eventually can destroy relationships.

The mentor or facilitator leads a brainstorming session on healthy versus unhealthy ways to express anger. Write responses on flip chart paper in two columns.

Next, the mentor or facilitator leads a further discussion by asking some of the following questions.

- What makes you angry?
- What do you think makes other people angry?
- What happens to you when you get angry?
- Where do you feel it?
- What do you do when you get angry?
- Do you act out (on others) or act in (on yourself)? Or both?

The mentor or facilitator shares the following information orally or on flip chart paper.

In relationships, anger is often about power but there are also a variety of other reasons for anger. Some reasons include:

- Wanting to control a situation or another person's behavior
- Avoiding responsibility by blaming someone else
- Responding with anger as a habit
- Seeking an anger high (a rush or high associated with violence)
- Responding to a threat
- Blocking other emotions (fear, sadness, guilt, shame), thus, anger becomes a secondary emotion (e.g., we feel fear and respond with anger)

Snack Break

Activity 3: Anger Role Play

Role play is an effective way to involve girls in low-risk, practice situations. They can try out new behaviors and personas, which they can use in the future in highly emotional and high-risk situations, such as dealing with an angry partner. (For more information, see Banister and Begoray, 2004.)

To get the girls thinking about how anger and power play out in their relationships, the mentor or facilitator on her own or with a more extroverted other acts out an anger scenario for the group to discuss (use the following sample scenario or let the girls think of their own). Girls are then invited to practice and present anger scenarios through role play. The mentor or facilitator encourages the girls to create real-life situations. If an example is needed, the mentor or facilitator could introduce the following scenario.

Jenny and Kevin are out on a date, standing outside waiting to go to a movie on a Tuesday night. A group of Jenny's friends are standing in line behind them and start talking to her. Kevin gets quiet and moody. Kevin says, "Let's get going—I'm tired of waiting in line." Jenny wants to stay but she is afraid to say anything because he may yell at her as he has in the past. She is upset and wants to talk.

Make time for as many girls to be in the scenario as possible. After the role playing is completed, the mentor or facilitator asks the following debriefing questions. It is important not to focus too much on any one girl's relationship challenges so that everyone gets a chance to participate. This discussion will take time. The mentor or facilitator may need to remain late or arrange other opportunities to talk individually with any girls who need to debrief and do not want to talk in the group.

- What might the angry person be thinking or feeling?
- What values and or attitudes are causing him (her) those feelings?
- What is underlying the anger person's words and actions? What is he (she) feeling deep inside?
- How could this scene be played out in a different way that might work for both people?
- How do these scenarios relate to the power imbalances we discussed earlier?
- Who is responsible for the actions that were taken?

Closing

The mentor or facilitator leads reflection by asking:

- What are you noticing about yourself?
- What did you learn today?
- What stood out for you today? Or how was today for you?
- What (if anything) has changed for you since you started coming to the group?
- How do activities relate to how you are in relationships?

The mentor or facilitator and/or participants express appreciations or acknowledgments and offer reminders about journal and goal setting.

Question Box

See Session 1.

Assessment

See Session 1.

Session 12: Assertion

Assertion is one of the most effective communication skills. As girls become more in touch with their values, goals, and healthy choices, they need to be empowered by learning ways to make themselves heard. This session explores how our responses to challenging situations can either resolve or exacerbate a conflict situation. Activities focus on empowering oneself through assertive, rather than passive or aggressive, behavior. Participants have a clear understanding of these different ways to respond—particularly in relationship situations.

The mentor or facilitator will

- lead girls to revisit and revise goal-setting ideas,
- define assertion, aggression, and passivity,
- help girls to explore the difference between assertive, aggressive, and passive behavior, and
- help girls to understand the link between assertion and empowerment.

The participants will

- learn the differences between assertive, passive, and aggressive behaviors,
- develop and practice assertion skills, and
- examine the link between assertion and empowerment.

Materials and Resources Required

In addition to the usual materials, healthy and unhealthy anger chart, and role-play scenarios (from Session 10), three empty chairs and labels (passive, aggressive, assertive).

Procedure, Process, and Activities

Free Expression

See Session 1.

Check-In

See Session 3.

Question Box

Address questions from Session 11.

Review: Goals and Values

Girls are invited by the mentor or facilitator to share the successes and challenges of their goal-setting experiences and to make revisions based on these experiences.

Review: Power and Anger

The mentor or facilitator leads a discussion on the concept of choice and responsibility using the following statement.

> We can't make someone behave in a certain way if they are angry with us (i.e., if they choose to hit us, we didn't raise their hand for them). It is okay to feel angry; what we do with the feeling is a matter of choice. Sometimes, what we choose to do is *not* okay.

No matter what the situation is, we always have choices about how we behave in response. We can choose to respond rather than react. Our behavior is our choice and a boyfriend's or girlfriend's behavior is *his* or *her* choice. We are never responsible for someone who chooses violence or abuse as a way of acting out their anger. For example, we do not make someone hit us through our behavior.

Application

The mentor or facilitator uses the healthy and unhealthy anger chart and role play scenarios (from Session 10). They lead a discussion about the choices in each scenario and review which choices are okay (not abusive) and which are not okay (violent or abusive). (For more information, see Wolfe et al., 1996.)

Defining Assertion

The mentor or facilitator defines the meaning of assertion using the following information provided orally or on chart paper.

- Assertion is the ability to say what you think and feel without putting down or threatening someone else. When we assert ourselves, we speak only for ourselves and allow the other person to speak for him or herself. Assertion allows us to listen to the other person's point of view without feeling like we have to agree with it or change to suit it.
- There are various choices we have to communicate what our needs are in relationships:
  - assertion is about choice and inner (or authentic) power or strength,
  - aggression is about power over someone, and
  - passivity appears as a lack of power.

Three-Chair Role Play

The mentor or facilitator sets up three chairs in the front of the room with a label on each chair (passive, aggressive, or assertive) and draws a behavior/feeling chart on the flip chart as in Figure 3.1.

	Passive	Aggressive	Assertive
Behavior			
Feelings			

Figure 3.1 Three-Chair Role Play Behavior/Feeling Chart

The mentor or facilitator explains to the group that each chair represents a different response to a challenging or a conflict situation. The mentor or facilitator will act differently (using language, body language, and other relevant behaviors) depending on which chair she is sitting in to demonstrate each response. Scenarios for response will be posed by the mentor or facilitator or by another group member. The girls will observe as the mentor or facilitator acts out each role—passive, aggressive, or assertive. The mentor or facilitator appoints a recorder to fill in the chart.

The mentor or facilitator then moves from chair to chair, acting out responses. After each chair, the mentor or facilitator asks the girls which behaviors (facial expression, voice, eye contact, language) and feelings they notice by asking the following questions.

- When I'm in this chair, what do you notice about my behavior and body language?
- What might I be feeling in this chair? How might I be feeling about myself?
- How can you tell I'm aggressive (passive, assertive)?

The recorder notes these in the appropriate categories on the chart (see Figure 3.2)

The mentor or facilitator informs the group that after the break they will have the opportunity to try on the different behaviors in a role play. Girls are encouraged to come up with different scenarios (individually or in small groups) during the break.

Snack Break

Extended Role Play

Group members are given time to practice and present the different communication responses through role play, with a focus on learning assertive behavior techniques. The mentor or facilitator will need to assess the willingness of group members to participate and assume a role in a scenario as necessary to model responses and encourage participation.

The mentor or facilitator leads a discussion on the three-chair activity by asking the following questions.

- What might these people be thinking or feeling? How do you know?
- What happened when she responded aggressively? passively?
- How could this scene be played out in a different way that might work for both people? What would it look like if she responded assertively?
- How do these responses relate to the power imbalances we discussed earlier?
- Who is responsible for the actions that were taken in these scenarios?

	Passive	Aggressive	Assertive
Behavior	Quiet, no eye contact, fidgeting	Standing, clenched fists, yelling	Good posture, even voice, calm
Feelings	Bad about self, walked over, afraid	Fear, bad, powerful, embarrassed afterward	True to self, nervous, good about self

Figure 3.2 Example of Completed Three-Chair Role Play Behavior/Feeling Chart

Closing

The mentor or facilitator leads reflection by asking the questions as described in previous sessions and reminds them of journal writing.

Question Box

See Session 1.

Assessment

See Session 1.

Session 13: What Next?

This final session provides group members with a review of important concepts related to healthy sexuality and relationships. Opportunities are also provided for girls to maintain connection, awareness, and responsible action once the program is complete.

The mentor or facilitator will

- lead girls to revisit and revise goal-setting ideas,
- review program concepts,
- help girls to visualize a special place for support, and
- assist girls to create a resource card for future reference.

The participants will

- review program concepts and ask questions,
- learn to visualize a special place for support, and
- create a resource card for future reference.

Materials and Resources Required

- Worksheet: Assertion
- Reference Web sites—see "A Special Place" activity here in Session 13
- Resource cards, design materials
- Laminating machine (if possible)

Procedure, Process, and Activities

Free Expression

See Session 1.

Check-In

See Session 3.

Question Box

Address questions from Session 12.

Review: Goals and Values

Girls are invited by the mentor or facilitator to share the successes and challenges of their goal-setting experiences and to make revisions based on these experiences. Group members are encouraged to provide support by celebrating small changes that have been achieved and to encourage further success with goal setting. The mentor or facilitator connects goal setting to choices about healthy sexuality and relationships.

Review: Assertion

The mentor or facilitator reviews the concept of choice and responsibility using the following statement.

> We can't change someone else's behavior but we can change our response to that behavior. When we change what we do, the relationship may change as well. Assertion

79

is a respectful and powerful way to maintain our rights and responsibilities while not hurting someone else. Our intent is not to overpower someone or give up our rights when we behave assertively.

Activity 1: A Special Place

The mentor or facilitator refers to Andrea Johnson's Web sites that provide information and facilitation notes for this activity and the Girls Speak Out program. These resources provide strategies for girls to access when examining future challenges relating to sexuality and relationships (see http://www.girlsspeakout.org/).

The mentor or facilitator leads girls to identify and visualize their own special place (actual, perhaps a corner of their house, or virtual, a place they can see only in their mind's eye) that they can go to at any time when relationships or life become a struggle. Girls can draw, sketch, or write about this special place in their journals for future reference.

Activity 2: Resource Cards

The mentor or facilitator brings in recipe cards, brochures collected from school counseling office or local health clinics, and copies of the local phonebook. Introduce the activity of creating a youth resource card. Working with the whole group, have pairs of girls discover names of organizations and contact information that they can post on a whiteboard or on flip chart paper. After 10 minutes, stop the activity and categorize the resources under headings such as: "Where Do I Go to . . . ," for example, get birth control advice, get a vaccination, talk to someone when I'm depressed, and so on. Some schools and libraries offer laminating services for low cost that will preserve cards for future use.

Review: Mantra

The mentor or facilitator leads the final review of the mantra: Take care of ourselves and each other. . . . When complete, ask girls if there is anything they would like to add to the mantra for themselves. Share or record privately in journals.

Closing

The mentor or facilitator leads reflection by asking the following questions.

- What have you noticed about yourself throughout this program?
- What stood out for you? What did you enjoy the most?
- If you had some advice to give girls in a group like this, what would you tell them?
- What (if anything) has changed for you since you started coming to the group? What do you still want to change (if anything)?
- How will you use what you have learned in your current and future relationships?

The mentor or facilitator will express appreciations and acknowledgments to each girl and to the group as a whole. She will then direct girls to take their journals home with them and encourage them to keep using them. Finally, she will remind the girls to keep setting and meeting goals.

Assessment: Session and Program

As usual, the mentor or facilitator needs to permits record their observations of the successes and challenges of the session and program. If time permits, girls should also be involved in writing comments to guide future mentors and facilitators to improve the program.

References

Ackard, D. M., Neumark-Sztainer, D., & Hannan, P. (2003). Dating violence among a nationally representative sample of adolescent girls and boys. *Journal of Gender Specific Medicine, 6*(3), 39–48.

Banister, E. (2006). *How can I help: A practical guide on adolescent dating abuse.* Retrieved October 19, 2006, from http://www.youth.society.uvic.ca/resources/abuse pamphlet/abuse_nonFN_June2006.pdf

Banister, E., & Begoray, D. L. (2004). Beyond talking groups: Strategies for improving adolescent health education. *Health Care for Women International, 25*(5), 481–488.

Banister, E. & Daly, K. (2006). Walking a fine line: Negotiating dual roles in a study with adolescent girls. In B. Leadbeater, E. Banister, C. Benoit, M. Jansson, A. Marshall, & T. Riecken (Eds.), *Research ethics in community-based and participatory action research with children, adolescents, and youth* (pp. 157–174). Toronto, ON: University of Toronto Press.

Banister, E., & Leadbeater, B. (2007). To stay or leave: How do mentoring groups support healthy dating relationships in high-risk girls? In B. Leadbeater & N. Way (Eds.), *Urban girls revisited: Building strengths* (pp. 121–141). New York: New York University Press.

Banister, E., Jakubec, S., & Stein, J. (2003). "Like, what am I supposed to do?": Power, politics, and public health concerns in adolescent women's dating relationships. *Canadian Journal of Nursing Research, 35*(2), 16–33.

Centers for Disease Control. (2004). *Youth risk behavior surveillance: United States.* Retrieved June 25, 2005, from http://www.cdc.gov/mmwr/PDF/SS/SS5302.pdf

Christians, C. G. (2000). Ethics and politics in qualitative research. In N. K. Denzin & Y. S. Lincoln (Eds.), *Handbook of qualitative research* (2nd ed., pp. 133–155). Thousand Oaks, CA: Sage.

Compian, L., Gowen, L. K., & Hayward, C. (2004). Peripubertal girls' romantic and platonic involvement with boys: Association with body image and depression symptoms. *Journal of Research on Adolescence, 14*(1), 23–47.

Downey, G., Bonica, C., & Rincon, C. (1999). Rejection sensitivity and adolescent romantic relationships. In W. Furman, B. B. Brown, & C. Feiring (Eds.), *The development of romantic relationships in adolescence* (pp. 148–174). Cambridge, UK: Cambridge University Press.

Edwards, S., & Carne, C. (1998). Oral sex and the transmission of viral STIs. *Sexually Transmitted Infections, 74*(1), 6–10.

Health Canada. (2002). *Women and sexual and reproductive health.* Retrieved June 25, 2005, from http://www.hc-sc.gc.ca/english/women/facts_issues/facts_sexual.htm

Hutchinson, M. K. (1998). Something to talk about: Sexual risk communication between young women and their partners. *Journal of Gynecologic and Neonatal Nursing, 27*(2), 127–133.

King, A. J. C., Boyce, W. F., & King, M. A. (1999). *Trends in the health of Canadian youth.* Ottawa: Health Canada.

Pastor, J., McCormick, J., & Fine, M. (1996). Makin' homes: An urban girl thing. In B. J. R. Leadbeater & N. Way (Eds.), *Urban girls: Resisting stereotypes, creating identities* (pp. 15–34). New York: New York University Press.

Rhodes, J. E., & Roffman, J. G. (2002). Relationship-based interventions: The impact of mentoring and apprenticeship on youth development. In R. M. Lerner, F. Jacobs, & D. Wertlieb (Eds.), *Handbook of applied developmental science: Promoting positive child, adolescent, and family development through research, policies and programs.* Thousand Oaks, CA: Sage.

Sexuality Information and Education Council of the United States. (2006). *Fact sheet: The truth about STDs.* Retrieved October 22, 2006, from http://65.36.238.42/pubs/fact/fact0019.html

Taylor-Seehafer, M., & Rew, L. (2000). Risky sexual behavior among adolescent women. *Journal of the Society of Pediatric Nurses, 5*(1), 15–25.

U.S. Department of Justice. (1997). *National crime victimization survey.* Washington, DC: Bureau of Justice Statistics, Author.

Villarruel, A. M., Sweet-Jemmott, L. S., Howard, M., Taylor, L., & Bush, E. (1998). HIV prevention and adolescent peer educators. *Journal of the Association of Nurses in AIDS Care, 9*(5), 61–72.

Walker, G., & Freedman, M. (1996). Social change one on one: The new mentoring movement. *The American Prospect, 27,* 75–81.

Wolfe, D. A., Wekerle, C., Gough, R., Reitzel-Jaffe, D., Grasley, C., Pittman, A., et al. (1996). *The youth relationship manual: A group approach with adolescents for the prevention of woman abuse and the promotion of healthy relationships.* Thousand Oaks, CA: Sage.

Appendix A: Your Personal Rights

- The right to act in ways that promote your dignity and self-respect as long as others' rights are not violated in the process
- The right to be treated with respect
- The right to say No without feeling guilty
- The right to take time to slow down and think
- The right to change your mind
- The right to ask for what you want
- The right to do less than you are capable of doing
- The right to ask for information
- The right to make mistakes and accept responsibility
- The right to feel good about yourself

Appendix B: Components of Power and Control in Relationships

Peer Pressure

- Spreading nasty rumors
- Telling or threatening to tell people your secrets
- Making you feel like a loser if you don't go along with things

Anger and Emotional Abuse

- Making you feel bad about yourself
- Name-calling: fat, slut, frigid, whore, and so on
- Playing mind games
- Making you feel guilty

Bossing You Around

- Treating you like a servant, giving orders
- Making all the decisions
- Acting like king of the castle

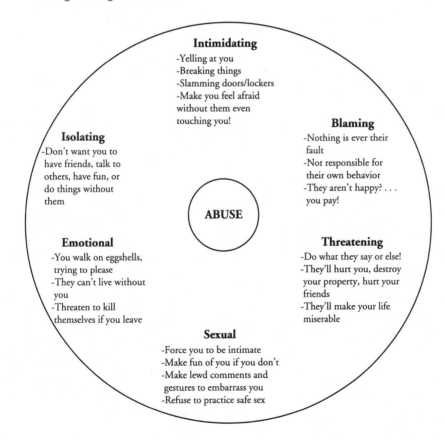

Figure 3.3 Love Doesn't Have to Hurt Teens Web site. Adapted from www.apa.org/pi/pii/teen/.

Scaring You or Threats

- Smashing or wrecking stuff
- Hurting or threatening to hurt pets
- Showing guns, knives, or other weapons
- Threatening to leave, to commit suicide, or to report you to the police
- Making you do illegal things

Pressure or Force to Get Sex

- Not taking No for an answer
- Making you feel like you owe sex for any reason
- Getting you pregnant
- Threatening to take your kids away
- Getting you drunk or drugged to get sex

Control and Isolation

- Controlling what you do, who you see, talk with, what you read, or where you go
- Calling you all the time on your cell to keep track of you
- Keeping you away from others or saying they are jealous

Chapter 4

An Evidence-Based HIV Prevention Intervention for African American Female Adolescents: *SiHLE*

Gina M. Wingood, ScD, MPH, and Ralph J. DiClemente, PhD

RATIONALE FOR DEVELOPING THE SiHLE HIV INTERVENTION

The risk of acquiring a sexually transmitted disease (STD), including human immunodeficiency virus (HIV), is one of the most significant and immediate risks to the health and well-being of adolescents. While there has been marked progress in the development of HIV prevention interventions for adolescents, programs designed specifically for females, and more specifically for African American females, have lagged behind that of other at-risk adolescent populations. Thus, the goal of this chapter is to provide a detailed description of an HIV prevention intervention specially tailored for African American adolescent females that has been demonstrated to be efficacious for this understudied and underserved at-risk population.

In an attempt to address this health disparity, as well as to attend to some of the limitations in previous intervention studies, our research team recently developed and evaluated a theory-guided, culturally

appropriate, and gender-tailored sexual risk reduction program for African American female adolescents, ages 14–18, called SiHLE (Sistas Informing, Healing, Living and Empowering). SiHLE was conceptualized by Ralph DiClemente and Gina Wingood and is a modified version of an established and efficacious HIV intervention specifically for African American woman (18–29 years of age) that has been defined by the CDC as an evidence-based HIV prevention intervention for African American female adolescents (Lyles, Kay, Crepaz, Herbst, Passin, et al., 2007).

THE EVIDENCE FOR USING SiHLE: EFFECTS OF THE INTERVENTION

To assess the effectiveness of the SiHLE HIV intervention on reducing risk associated behaviors, data collection occurred at baseline (i.e., before the participants were randomly assigned to either the SiHLE intervention or a time-equivalent general health promotion comparison condition), as well as 6 and 12 months after participating in either the SiHLE or general health promotion intervention. At each assessment data were obtained from four sources. First, participants completed a self-administered questionnaire assessing sociodemographics and psychosocial mediators of HIV-preventive behaviors. Subsequently, a trained African American female interviewer administered an interview assessing sexual behaviors. Next, the interviewer assessed participants' ability to correctly apply condoms using a direct observation of skills assessment protocol. Finally, participants provided two self-collected vaginal swab specimens that were analyzed for the presence of three sexually transmitted diseases; chlamydia, trichomonasis, and gonorrhea.

Relative to participants in the general health promotion condition, participants in the SiHLE intervention condition were more likely to report using condoms consistently in the 30 days preceding the 6-month assessment (Intervention = 75.3% vs. Comparison = 58.2%), and at the 12-month assessment (Intervention = 73.3% vs. Comparison = 56.5%). Likewise, participants in the SiHLE intervention were more likely to report using condoms consistently during the six months prior to the 6-month assessment (Intervention = 61.3% versus Comparison = 42.6%), and the 12-month assessment (Intervention = 58.1% versus Comparison = 45.3%). Additionally, participants in the SiHLE intervention were more likely to report using a condom at last vaginal sexual intercourse, less likely to self-report a pregnancy, and less likely to report having a new male sex partner in the 30 days prior to the follow-up assessments. Importantly, this was the first intervention to demonstrate effectiveness in reducing new chlamydia infections in the SiHLE intervention group participants over the entire 12-month follow-up period (see DiClemente, Wingood, Harrington, Lang, Davies, et al., [2004] for a detailed description of the findings).

The SiHLE intervention also had strong effects on empirically and theoretically derived psychosocial mediators of HIV-preventive behaviors. In general, participants in the SiHLE intervention reported fewer perceived partner-related barriers to condom use, more favorable attitudes towards using condoms, more frequent discussions with male sex partners about HIV prevention, higher condom use self-efficacy scores, higher HIV prevention knowledge scores, and demonstrated greater proficiency in using condoms at the 6- and the 12-month assessments, and over the entire 12-month period.

While other studies have shown that self-reported sexual risk behaviors can be reduced in adolescents, this is the first trial demonstrating that an HIV intervention can result in substantial reductions in sexual risk behaviors, including the acquisition of a new male sex partner, and markedly enhance theoretically important mediators and skills associated with HIV preventive behaviors among sexually experienced African American adolescent females. Given that STDs, particularly chlamydia, are prevalent among adolescents (Weinstock, Berman, & Cates, 2004), and facilitate HIV transmission (Fleming & Wasserheit, 1999; Wasserheit, 1992), even small reductions in incidence could result in considerable reductions in treatment costs as well as sizeable reductions in HIV morbidity (Bozzette et al., 2001) and their associated treatment costs (Chesson, Blandford, Gift, Tao, & Irwin, 2000) This is particularly important in light of findings from mathematical modeling studies suggesting that reductions in incident chlamydia infections may be one of the most promising surrogate markers for HIV incidence in prevention trials (Pinkerton & Layde, 2002).

INTRODUCTION TO THE SiHLE HIV INTERVENTION

The study was conducted from September 1995 to August 2002. From December 1996 through April 1999, recruiters screened 1,130 African American adolescent females seeking services at four community health agencies. Of these, 609 (53.9%) met eligibility criteria. Eligibility criteria included being an African American female, 14–18 years of age, reporting vaginal intercourse in the preceding six months, and providing written informed consent (parental consent was waived). Of those not eligible, nearly 93% were not sexually experienced. Thus, 522 adolescents agreed to participate in the study, completed baseline assessments, and were randomized to study conditions. Participants were compensated $25 for travel and childcare to attend intervention sessions and complete assessments. The University of Alabama at Birmingham Institutional Review Board approved the study protocol prior to implementation.

The study design was a randomized controlled trial. Participants were randomly assigned, using a computer generated algorithm, to either the HIV intervention (SiHLE) or a general health promotion condition. The

HIV intervention consisted of four, four-hour interactive group sessions, implemented over consecutive Saturdays. Each session averaged 10–12 participants, and was implemented by a trained African American female health educator and two African American female peer educators cofacilitated each condition. Peer educators were instrumental in modeling skills and creating group norms supportive of HIV prevention. To reduce the likelihood that the effects of the HIV prevention could be attributed to group interaction or Hawthorne effects participants randomized to the general health promotion condition also received four, four-hour interactive group sessions, two sessions emphasizing nutrition and two sessions emphasizing exercise, administered on consecutive Saturdays. Given the focus of this chapter, the content and activities of the general health promotion condition will not be discussed further.

THE TREATMENT MANUAL

The aim of SiHLE was to reduce the risk of HIV and STDs among sexually active African American adolescent females (DiClemente et al., 2004). Social cognitive theory (SCT) (Bandura, 1994), and the theory of gender and power (Wingood & DiClemente, 2000) were complementary theoretical frameworks guiding the design and implementation of the SiHLE intervention. Social cognitive theory addresses both the psychosocial dynamics facilitating health behavior and the methods of promoting behavior change. Applying the gender-relevant theoretical framework of the theory of gender and power was critical as it highlights HIV-related social processes prevalent in the lives of African American female adolescents such as: having older male sex partners, having violent dating partners, being stereotyped by the media, perceiving society as having a limited regard of African American teens, engaging in serial monogamy, experiencing peer pressure, and communicating nonassertively about safer sex. Ultimately, by creating an intervention for adolescent females grounded in both SCT and the theory of gender and power we hoped to more fully address the processes that specifically impede young women's adoption of risk-promoting behaviors while teaching them multidimensional strategies to protect themselves from acquiring STDs and HIV (see Table 4.1 for details on how the theories were applied to the intervention).

By using theory mapping, intervention activities associated with constructs articulated in SCT and the theory of gender and power were designed to address the social realities that are more prevalent among

TABLE 4.1 Mapping of theory to the SiHLE intervention sessions

	Social cognitive theory	Theory of gender and power
Session 1	• Provide an opportunity for goal setting • Reinforce health promoting thoughts and actions in the group	• Address and challenge the societal norms that dictate appropriate emotional and sexual behavior for females • Address factors that place women at an economic disadvantage
Session 2	• Provide knowledge on condom use and correct misconceptions of risk-reduction practices • Discuss positive outcomes of reducing risky sexual behavior • Reinforce previous sessions message through discussion, problem solving and decision making • Promote norms supportive of reducing risky sexual behavior	• Reaffirm personal self-worth and pride as it relates to gender and ethnicity
Session 3	• Enhance emotional coping responses by practicing communication skills in arousing situations • Enhance self-efficacy through role plays • Promote mastery through skills learning activities • Provide opportunities for decision making and problem solving	• Create an atmosphere of normality surrounding women taking control over sexual health
Session 4	• Enhance coping during emotional arousing situations • Consider multiple avenues to reduce risky sexual behavior	• Breakdown societal and institutional structures that creates a power imbalance in relationships

African American adolescents. To be effective, HIV prevention programs must be behavior specific and teach adolescents about safe and risky sexual practices as well as the outcomes associated with each practice. Effective programs must also teach adolescents critical skills such as goal setting, recognizing stimuli that trigger unsafe behaviors, reinforcing positive behaviors, and effective communication skills, that are vital for relationship formation and negotiating safer sex (Bandura, 1992). Thus, all sessions were designed to be engaging with liberal use of interactive games, music, role plays, and open discussions in an effort to be deemed effective intervention activities. Additionally, the thematic focus of the intervention, "Stay Safe for Yourself, Your Family, and Your Community," was designed to promote a sense of solidarity and ethnic pride among participants, and may have inspired them to modify risk behaviors for altruistic motives; by enhancing their health they were also enhancing the health of their family and the broader African American community. Unlike many HIV/STD prevention interventions that focus only on cognitive decision making and social and technical competency skills, SiHLE also focused on developing relational skills and amplifying intrinsic motivation (altruism, pride, self-esteem, perceived value, and importance in the community) and mobilizing extrinsic motivators (peer normative influences from the group, modeling by the peer educator) to create an environment that enhanced adolescents' likelihood of adopting and, as important, sustaining preventive behaviors after participation in the intervention. In the following treatment manual, we describe, albeit briefly, each of the four sessions of SiHLE.

Session 1

The first session, titled "My Sistas ... My Girls," began with an icebreaker activity, which consisted of a fun game, to allow the group to become acquainted with one another. This activity was followed by providing vital information about the program, introducing the young ladies to the SiHLE motto, and establishing group ground rules. The goal of the first session was to foster sisterhood among young women through activities that promote discussion about African American adolescent topics. Throughout the session, the young women were encouraged to begin developing positive relationships within the group. It was important for the young women to feel a sense of camaraderie with each other as well as with the health educator and peer educator to help make the program a success. Working from the gender-relevant theoretical framework of the theory of gender and power the activities in session were created to highlight HIV-related social processes prevalent in the lives of African American female adolescents. Through the examination of poetry written by African American women, discussion of challenges and joys of being an African American female, exposure to artwork from African American women, identifying African American role models, and prioritizing personal values participants were empowered to raise their expectations of what it is to be a woman cognizant of her sexuality regardless of how society may view them. Also following from the theory of gender and power, other activities in the first session, such as stressing the importance of completing educational requirements, developing career goals, and writing effective professional resumes, were designed to be economically empowering. Table 4.2 provides a detailed overview of the specific activities employed in Session 1.

One activity that demonstrates how the message of sisterhood and self-pride was articulated and promoted in Session 1 is Activity F, "A Room Full of Sisters."

A Room Full of Sisters (an excerpt) by Mona Lake Jones

A room full of sisters, like jewels in a crown
Vanilla, cinnamon, and dark chocolate brown ...
Now picture yourself in the midst of this glory
As I describe the sisters who are part of this story.
They were wearing purples, royal blues, and all shades of reds
Some had elegant hats on their heads
With sparkling eyes and shiny lips
They moved through the room swaying their hips
Speaking with smiles on their African faces
Their joy and laughter filled all the spaces.
They were fashionable and stylish in what they were wearing;
   beautiful sisters all, who were loving and caring ...
You see it's not about how these sisters appeared;
   their beauty was in the values they revered.

Peer Educator

Did Mona Lake Jones "reveal her pride in being a Black woman in this poem? If so, how?
   Mona Lake Jones described Black women's outer beauty.
   What were some descriptive phrases she used to describe Black women's outer beauty?
      "... like jewels in a crown"
      "... wearing purples, royal blues, and all shades of reds"

"...with sparkling eyes and shiny lips"
How did she describe Black women's inner beauty?
"...Their beauty was in the values they revered"
"...loving and caring"

Table 4.2
Themes and Activities in Session 1

	Theme	Description
Session 1 **My Sistas ... My Girls**		
Activity A	Greeting and Icebreaker	Allows the group to introduce themselves to each person in the group by participating in a fun activity.
Activity B	SiHLE Program Introduction	Discusses the name of the program and the objectives of the program.
Activity C	Who are SiHLE Sistas?	Introduces the SiHLE concept and fosters a sense of sisterhood.
Activity D	The SiHLE Pact	Discusses the importance of young ladies participating in the workshops as an important step in their learning how to be a SiHLE Sista. Also covers the SiHLE motto.
Activity E	Young, Black, & Female	Encourages the SiHLE Sistas to think of positive characteristics that describe young Black women by allowing the Sistas the opportunity to assert their self-worth and pride.
Activity F	A Room Full of Sisters	Encourages the SiHLE Sistas to further discuss pride among young Black women by describing the many shades of beauty that are so common among Black women.
Activity G	Strong Black Women	Encourages the SiHLE Sistas to recognize the importance of African American women as role models by identifying important women in their life and by learning about African American women important in shaping our history.
Activity H	A Taste of Culture	Teaches the SiHLE Sistas about African American culture by making their own pictures using African American prints.
Activity I	Values—What Matters Most?	Encourages the SiHLE Sistas to recognize their personal values and to assist them in understanding why it is important to first consider their personal values before they make a decision.
Activity J	Thought Works	Promotes the participant's identification of their goals and dreams.

Session 2

The goal of the second session, titled "It's My Body," was to introduce the young women to the risks related to STDs, especially HIV, and what this can mean to them. This workshop began with a review of the young women's values, goals, and dreams. Additionally, the girls were provided information about STDs and HIV, including a discussion of behaviors that put them at risk for the diseases, and how the diseases can affect their goals and dreams. Subsequently, correct condom skills were introduced as a means of lowering STD risk. The workshop ends with a review of STD/HIV information. The majority of activities in this session focused on defining and discussing facts evolved around AIDS, STDs, and HIV prevention strategies, the discussion of situations and behaviors that may increase women's HIV risk (douching, having older partners, gang involvement, and sexually degrading media exposures). This information was imperative in providing adolescents with the knowledge to prevent infection. Table 4.3 provides a detailed overview of the specific activities employed in Session 2.

Table 4.3
Themes and Activities in Session 2

	Theme	Description
Session 2: **"It's My Body"**		
Activity A	Greetings and Icebreaker	Greets participants and reinforces group bonds.
Activity B	Motto	Recites and reinforces the SiHLE motto.
Activity C	Call Me Black Woman	Reinforces the concept that SiHLE Sistas are beautiful women with a strong rich heritage by reading and discussing poetry written by an African American artist.
Activity D	Share Your Thoughtworks	Reviews the SiHLE sistas personal values and future goals and reinforce their importance in decision making.
Activity E	SiHLE Sistas Are Special!	Reinforces and reexamines concepts taught in Session 1.
Activity F	Speaking of STDs...	Teaches SiHLE sistas about STDs and how having an STD affects pregnancy.
Activity G	Card Swap Game	Illustrates to the SiHLE sistas how HIV is spread by heterosexual contact and injection drug use.
Activity H	HIV/AIDS: What Every SiHLE Woman Should Know	Educates the SiHLE sistas about what AIDS is, myths about AIDS, and how to protect yourself from AIDS.
Activity I	R U at Risk?	Informs the SiHLE sistas about sexual behaviors that reduce their chance of getting STDs, including HIV.
Activity J	Consider This . . . The Penetrating Question	Evaluates how getting an STD including HIV could change the SiHLE sistas values and goals.
Activity K	Takin' Care of You!	Introduces the concept of responsibility by having women state how they care for themselves.
Activity L	Introducing OPRaH	Refines women's knowledge of HIV/STD prevention.
Activity M	SiHLE Jeopardy	Refines women's knowledge about HIV/STD transmission and prevention.

One activity that exemplifies how the message of protecting ones self from STDs and HIV was integrated into Session 2 is Activity L, "Introducing OPRaH."

Peer Educator

OPRaH consists of four simple steps: Open, Pinch, Roll, and Hold!

O = Open the package and remove rolled condom without twisting, biting, or using your fingernails. This could damage the condom and allow fluid to leak out.

P = Pinch the tip of the condom to squeeze the air out, leaving 1/4 to 1/2 inch extra space at the top.

R = Roll condom down on penis as soon as the penis is hard, before you start to make love.

a = and after sex is over . . .

H = Hold the condom at the rim or base while partner pulls out after ejaculation but before the penis goes soft. You could lose protection if the condom comes off inside you.

Session 3

The third session, titled "SiHLE Skills," addressed resisting partner pressures to engage in unsafe sex. Often, it is difficult for young women to make healthy choices about sex when they are not assertive during sexual encounters especially if their partner plays the dominant role in those encounters. Young women must assertively convey their sexual intentions and possess the skills to negotiate safer sex to make choices for a healthier lifestyle. While males and females are both responsible for safer sex, the responsibility often falls on the female partner, because males do not always practice safer sex and young women bear the disproportionate burden of adverse health outcomes. Previous sessions focused on the fact that females can protect themselves from engaging in unsafe sex. However, this session provided the young women with the skills to properly use condoms and refuse risky sex. Through role plays women also learned how to eroticize condom use to develop their positive attitudes towards using condoms and enhance their male partner's acceptance of condom use. The group facilitators were especially crucial in this session as they created a norm as it relates to females putting condoms on their male partners. Additionally, this activity led into a group discussion on how a woman's ability to apply a condom tends to reduce their perceived barrier to utilizing condoms for HIV/STD prevention. Role plays were also used to model assertive communication. These role plays were designed as a hierarchical gradient, first in nonsexual scenarios and then in progressively more sexual situations. As the women actively participated in role plays focusing on assertive communication they were able to increase their communicative self-efficacy as well as develop new strategies for handling emotions that often accompany difficult conversations with romantic partners. Facilitators provided positive reinforcing feedback for role plays that used assertive communication and corrective feedback for role plays that did not utilize assertive communication. They also provided positive reinforcing feedback for demonstrations of correct condom use. Table 4.4 provides a detailed overview of the specific activities employed in Session 3.

One activity that is highly representative of the strong emphasis on skill development throughout Session 3 is Activity I, "Talking the Talk."

Peer Educator

Scenario: Andre and Tijuana.

Tijuana has been attending a woman's group called SiHLE. She has learned a lot about being a strong black woman who has a right to realize her dreams and goals. She has learned an important way to stay healthy—a simple way to prevent STDs, HIV, and unplanned pregnancy. She has made the decision to use condoms every time they have sex.

Role play Tijuana's talk with Andre. Make sure that you use an assertive style of communication. Pay particular attention to both your body language and your verbal language. Make sure they are clear, consistent, and unambiguous.

Table 4.4
Themes and Activities in Session 3

	Theme	Description
Session 3: **"SiHLE Skills"**		
Activity A	Greeting and Icebreaker	Greet one another, reinforce the message of timeliness and enhance group bonds.
Activity B	Motto	Reads and reinforces the SiHLE motto.
Activity C	Phenomenal Woman	Refines the SiHLE sistas sense of beauty, self-worth and pride.
Activity D	Luv and Kisses	Enhances the SiHLE sistas knowledge about what sexual behaviors place women at risk for HIV/STD infection.
Activity E	What's in it For You	Increases the SiHLE sistas knowledge about HIV/STD prevention.
Activity F	Why Don't People Use Condoms?	Introduces the SiHLE sistas to some common reasons why young women don't use condoms and to reintroduce the concept of sexual responsibility for using condoms.
Activity G	KISS: Keep it Simple Sista!	Teaches the SiHLE sistas a model to assist them in asking their sex partner(s) to use condoms.
Activity H	Three Ways to Say It	Teaches the SiHLE sistas to distinguish between passive, assertive, and aggressive communication styles.
Activity I	Talking the Talk	Teaches the SiHLE sistas the difference among passive, aggressive, and assertive communication styles by having them model in sexual scenarios, both verbally and through body language, these communication styles.
Activity J	OPRaH "Rehearsal"	Teaches the SiHLE sistas the steps for proper condom use.
Activity K	Alcohol and Sex: Not a Good Mix	Teaches the SiHLE sistas the importance of avoiding alcohol prior to and during sex.
Activity L	Condom Consumer Report	Teaches the SiHLE sistas the importance of examining the condom for safety, personal appeal, and ease of application.
Activity M	Thought Works Assignment	Reviews the concepts taught in today's session.

Session 4

The fourth session, titled "Relationship and Power," was designed to encourage women to take ownership of their bodies by informing them that their partner's decisions and choices regarding their bodies should be second to their own decision and choice. The session commenced by distinguishing healthy from unhealthy relationships and defining the words *abuse* and *respect*. Adolescents were taught that the lack of recognition by other people is viewed as disrespectful and abusive. Subsequently, adolescents were taught coping skills to more effectively handle a verbally abusive or physically abusive partner. Participants were also taught coping skills to more effectively handle abuse that may occur as a consequence of introducing HIV/STD prevention practices (i.e., condom use) into the relationship. The majority of activities in Session 4 were designed to address and breakdown the power imbalance often present in sexual heterosexual dyadic relationships. Defining healthy and unhealthy relationships, discussing local community resources for participants who are in unhealthy relationships, and explaining the relationship between having an unhealthy partner, HIV/STD risk taking, and HIV/STD acquisition were all activities employed which enabled the participants to act on or to change their own relationships. Table 4.5 provides a detailed overview of the specific activities employed in Session 4.

One activity that exemplifies the emphasis on relationships and power in Session 4 is Activity E, "What Do Healthy and Unhealthy Relationships Look Like?"

Peer Educator

When you are in a healthy relationship, it is easier to negotiate with your male partner to use a condom *every* time you have sex. Let's look at why this is true.

First, let's talk about what a healthy relationship is. A group of SiHLE women like you were asked to describe a healthy relationship. The following characteristics and attributes are what they identified as important in a healthy relationship.

Power is balanced
No one has an unfair advantage over the other
Communication is good
Both partners talk and listen
Respect is real
For oneself and one another
Trust is strong
Feeling safe both physically and emotionally with one another

When you are in an unhealthy relationship, it is more difficult to negotiate with your male partner to use a condom *every* time you have sex. Let's look at why this is true. First, let's talk about and describe an unhealthy relationship.

Power is not balanced
One partner has an unfair advantage over the other
Communication is not good
Neither partner listens or talks to each other
Respect is not real
For oneself and one another
Trust is not strong
Not feeling safe both, physically and emotionally, with one another

---

Table 4.5
Themes and Activities in Session 4

	Theme	Description
Session 4: "Relationship and Power"		
Activity A	Greeting	Greet one another, reinforce and practice assertive communication skills.
Activity B	Motto	Reads and reinforces the SiHLE motto.
Activity C	Poem: Still I Rise	Enhances the self-confidence and pride among the SiHLE sistas by reciting poetry written by African American women.
Activity D	What Have We Learned?	Refines the women's knowledge about HIV/STD transmission and prevention.
Activity E	What Do Healthy and Unhealthy Relationships Look Like?	Discusses the influence of power, communication, respect, and trust on relationships.
Activity F	Pieces and Parts	Raises women's awareness about healthy and unhealthy relationships.
Activity G	What Does Abuse Look Like?	Increases women's knowledge about verbal, emotional, physical, and sexual abuse.
Activity H	The Power Pie	Discusses how imbalances of power within a relationship can make it difficult to practice safer sex.
Activity I	Your Options	Discusses a woman's options for safety and counseling if she is concerned about her relationship.
Activity J	Your Time to Shine	Refines and enhances the women's safer sex knowledge and safer relationship knowledge and skills by conducting role reversal activities.
Activity K	Graduation	Acknowledges appreciation of the SiHLE sistas for participating in the SiHLE program by giving them certificates of empowerment and having a graduation exercise.

CONCLUSIONS

This chapter has highlighted the public health problem created by increased rates of STDs and HIV in adolescents, especially in African American adolescent females. This disproportionate burden necessitates the urgent design and implementation of gender-tailored and culturally tailored STD/HIV risk-reduction interventions specifically targeting this particularly vulnerable subpopulation of adolescents. Thus, the main focus of the current chapter was to provide a detailed description of, to our knowledge, the only demonstrated effective HIV intervention specifically designed for sexually active African American adolescent females.

Several characteristics of the SiHLE program may have attributed to the efficacy of the intervention in reducing risk-associated behaviors in African American adolescent females. First, the utilization of SCT, which provided a theoretical framework for developing the skills training components of the SiHLE intervention, in addition to the theory of gender in power, which was employed to address the role of contextual and sociocultural variables such as gender, class, and ethnicity and their influence on adolescent females sexual behavior, was a successful combination that broadened the scope of the intervention beyond the individual.

Related to this, the efficacy of the SiHLE intervention may be attributable partly to the gender-tailored and culturally appropriate framework that highlighted the underlying social processes, such as the dyadic nature of sexual interactions and relationship power and emotional commitment that may promote and reinforce risk behaviors. Conceptualizing HIV prevention within the broader context of a healthy relationship also marshaled new intervention strategies and offered new options for creating STD/HIV preventive behavior change. Additionally, the thematic focus of the intervention, "Stay Safe for Yourself, Your Family, and Your Community," was designed to promote a sense of solidarity and ethnic pride among participants and may have inspired them to modify risk behaviors for altruistic motives; by enhancing their health they were also enhancing the health of their family and the broader African American community.

Finally, the role of the facilitator is vital to the overall success of the program, and ultimately the young ladies making healthy changes in their lives. Therefore, having the SiHLE intervention implemented by a trained and experienced African American female health educator and African American female peer educators as cofacilitators was likely a factor contributing to the efficacy of the intervention. Employing health educators and peer educators matched to the participants' gender and race was instrumental in modeling social and technical competency skills, and creating a group norm supportive of HIV/STD prevention.

In the current era of HIV prevention, there is a need to prioritize designing STD/HIV prevention programs for adolescents that are developmentally, culturally, and gender appropriate. As the SiHLE intervention illustrates, it is possible to develop programs that address contextual factors or conditions that confer significant vulnerability for young women's risk of HIV/STD (i.e., age, ethnicity, and risk behaviors). Encouragingly, empirical data suggests that the greater the specificity between the HIV prevention intervention and the contextual factors prevalent among a target population, the greater the likelihood the program will be effective in reducing HIV risk (Wingood & DiClemente, 2006). Combining the three aforementioned features (theoretical frameworks that expand the scope of the intervention to include broader contextual and social variables, specificity of content tailored to the gender and culture of the participants, and employing trained, matched-to-sample health educators to implement the intervention) in the SiHLE intervention optimally enhanced the specificity between the HIV intervention and directly addressed, through diverse learning strategies, contextual factors that enhanced participants' risk for STDs and HIV. Undoubtedly, this targeted and tailored approach significantly contributed to the overall success of the SiHLE intervention.

In conclusion, as the need for effective STD/HIV risk-reduction interventions for adolescents remains high, we as clinicians, practitioners, and prevention researchers working with America's youth need to continue to strive to meet the needs of the population we serve. As suggested by this chapter, acknowledging that adolescents are not a homogeneous group, but rather a heterogeneous population, is a critical first step in designing effective risk-reduction interventions tailored for diverse at-risk adolescent subgroups.

References

Bandura, A. (1992). A social cognitive approach to the exercise of control over AIDS infection. In

R. J. DiClemente (Ed.), *Adolescents and AIDS: A generation in jeopardy* (pp. 89–116). Newbury Park, CA: Sage.

Bandura, A. (1994). Social cognitive theory and exercise of control over HIV infections. In R. J. DiClemente & J. Petersons (Eds.), *Preventing AIDS: Theories and methods of behavioral interventions* (pp. 25–29). New York: Plenum Publishing.

Bozzette, S. A., Joyce, G., McCaffrey, D. F., Leibowitz, A. A., Morton, S. C., Berry, S. H., et al. (2001). Expenditures for the care of HIV-infected patients in the era of highly active antiretroviral therapy. *New England Journal of Medicine*, 344(11), 817–823.

Chesson, H. W., Blandford, J. M., Gift, T. L., Tao, G., & Irwin, K. L. (2000). The estimated direct medical cost of sexually transmitted diseases among American youth, 2000. *Perspectives on Sexual and Reproductive Health*, 36, 11–19.

DiClemente, R. J., Wingood, G. M., Harrington, K. F., Lang, D. F., Davies, S. L., Hook, E. W., et al. (2004). Efficacy of an HIV prevention intervention for African American adolescent girls: A randomized controlled trial. *Journal of the American Medical Association*, 292(2), 171–179.

Fleming, D. T., & Wasserheit, J. N. (1999). From epidemiological synergy to public health policy and practice: The contribution of other sexually transmitted diseases to sexual transmission of HIV infection. *Sexually Transmitted Infections*, 75, 3–17.

Lyles C., Kay L., Crepaz N., Herbst J., Passin W., Kim A., et al. (2007). Best-evidence Interventions: Findings from a systematic review of HIV behavioral interventions for US populations at high risk, 2000–2004. *American Journal of Public Health*, 97, 133–143.

Pinkerton, S. D., & Layde, P. M. (2002). Using sexually transmitted disease incidence as a surrogate marker for HIV incidence in prevention trial. *Sexually Transmitted Diseases*, 29, 298–307.

Wasserheit, J. N. (1992). Epidemiological synergy: Interrelationship between human immunodeficiency virus infection and other sexually transmitted diseases. *Sexually Transmitted Diseases*, 19, 61–77.

Weinstock, H., Berman, S., & Cates, W. (2004). Sexually transmitted diseases in American youth: Incidence and prevalence estimates. *Perspectives on Sexual and Reproductive Health*, 36, 6–10.

Wingood, G. M. & DiClemente, R. J. (2000). Application of the theory of gender and power to examine HIV related exposures, risk factors and effective interventions for women. *Health Education and Behavior*, 27, 313–347.

Wingood, G. M., & DiClemente, R. J. (2006). Enhancing diffusion of HIV interventions: Development of a suite of effective HIV prevention programs for women. *AIDS Education and Prevention*, 18, 161–170.

Chapter 5

Social Skills Training: A Treatment Manual

Craig Winston LeCroy

Social skills training (SST) is being increasingly used as a treatment method in working with children and adolescents. Teaching young people social skills is a direct method of influencing how that young person is likely to interact with others in the future. The goal is to teach people the skills needed to sustain social interactions that will lead to positive outcomes. The strategy of social skills training is straightforward: identify the skills needed and select a method to teach those skills (LeCroy, 2002). This structured training approach is characterized by learning skills through practice. Their are various methods for the practice to occur. Typically, young people are taught skills through the use of role play practice with feedback from group members and the group leader. However, skills can also be learned through observing models, reviewing video tapes, reading stories that model the skills, playing games that emphasize the skills, and many other methods.

The preferred method of teaching young people social skills is in the group setting. For attention deficit/hyperactivity (ADHD) children Hinshaw (2005) insists group-based treatment is the preferred mode. Social skills are interpersonal social behaviors and the group provides a natural environment in which to learn such skills. Group training is particularly effective because of the following.

- Participants benefit from the opportunity to interact with others. This means there are interactions that would not occur in individual training.
- Groups provide greater feedback to individuals. This includes both positive feedback and encouragement about practicing the skills and negative feedback about how to make the skills appear more realistic or acceptable to others.
- Groups provide more motivation for young people to learn the skills. Young people prefer to interact with each other while learning social skills. Because they enjoy such interactions the group is more motivating than individual treatment would be.

- By having a group of people to practice with, better learning takes place. This is because participants can practice the skills with different people and learn to respond to the unique qualities of the individuals.

There are clearly good reasons to teach social skills in the group, however, social skills training is a valid model for work with individuals as well. And it is noteworthy that in some contexts where youth are exposed to similar acting-out youths the intervention may promote deviant behavior (Dishion, McCord, & Poulin, 1999). More research is needed to tease out under what conditions group-based SST is effective. This manual will provide a group treatment model so adaptations will need to be made when working with individuals. Also, being an effective group leader will be critical to the success of a social skills training group. This manual does not address the group skills needed for leading successful groups. For more information about group treatment and group leadership skills see Rose (1998).

SOCIAL SKILLS FOR WHO?

Human service practitioners have found that social skills training is an appropriate method for helping many different young people with different problems.

During adolescence many skills are needed by *all* young people, not just those in trouble. Many practitioners have used social skills training programs for prevention as well as treatment. For prevention, all young people can be offered a generic program of social skills training or young people identified as at-risk can be offered a specialized social skills training program. More troubled youth with specific difficulties can be thought of as having a deficit in certain skills and can be taught these skills to remedy their deficits.

Young people in today's society face many difficult demands. Many of these demands require needed social skills. For example, friendship is important to many young people, yet, some young people have a difficult time starting and maintaining conversations. Also, as young people move into dating a more complex set of social demands may require advanced social skills. What do you do in a situation where your boyfriend or girlfriend begins to pressure you into sexual relationships you aren't comfortable with? Or more simply, what are the skills needed to get along

better with friends, teachers, parents, and siblings? As a young person gets older there will be more demands on their abilities to resolve conflict and negotiate with others. Without such skills interpersonal relationships will suffer and the young person may develop undesirable alternatives such as aggression or withdrawal. Social skills training can be helpful in each of these situations.

Through social skills training young people acquire more control and direction over their lives. It is a method that enhances their locus of control. By experiencing that they can go out and have an effect on their world they develop a greater sense of self esteem. Too often young people become discouraged because they believe they cannot be effective in their environment. Social skills training can help change that.

Social skills training programs are administered in various settings. Often school is where social skills training takes place as it affords access to young people. Social skills programs are often a part of the regular school day, held as an after school activity, or held in the evenings. Some social skills programs are implemented over the noon hour. In addition to schools many social skills training programs become a regular part of a treatment protocol. For example, at residential treatment centers there will often be group time set aside for social skills training. Or day treatment programs may include a period of time for skills training. Young people may be court referred to a group social skills training program. Voluntary groups can also be formed, for example, in housing projects, or at community based agencies.

EVALUATION AND RESEARCH ON SOCIAL SKILLS TRAINING

Research has documented that the capacity to use problem solving for social and interpersonal problems is an important aspect of adaptive functioning. Indeed, deficits in problem-solving abilities and social skills are related to both dysfunctional difficulties and clinical disorders. For example, problem-solving and social skills deficits are related to delinquent behaviors (Kazdin, 2003), depression (Lewinsohn & Gotlib, 1995), and coping with stress (Compas, Benson, Boyer, Hicks, & Konik, 2002; Compas, Connor-Smith, Saltzman, Thomsen, & Wadsworth, 2001). Without social skills children and adolescents are more likely to experience friendship difficulties, inappropriately expressed emotions, and an inability to resist peer pressure (LeCroy, 2006). Problem solving and social skills training are widely used interventions that focus on either learning how to generate and use more effective solutions to situational conflicts or learning the skills needed to respond effectively to situational conflicts. Sometimes these interventions are used separately and sometimes they are combined, for example, when problem solving is conceived of as an accessory social skill as in the current program. Problem solving is a cognitive behavioral strategy that teaches thought processes to help children and adolescents confront difficult interactions. Social skills training is a behavioral strategy that teaches new behaviors or skills for addressing difficult situations.

The social skills training program presented here was based on research conducted by LeCroy and Rose (1986). In this study seventh grade middle school students were randomly assigned to one of four experimental groups: social skills training, problem solving training, combined model, or a placebo control group. The combined model of both social skills training and problem solving showed the greatest benefit on multiple measures of outcome. All three intervention groups out performed the placebo control group.

Social skills training is used in both prevention and intervention programs. In prevention programs, social skills programs might focus on friendship skills (Frankel, 2005), pregnancy, HIV prevention (St Lawrence, Jefferson, Alleyne, & Brasfield, 1995), or substance use and prevention (LeCroy & Mann, 2004). Some programs are more general and attempt to promote competencies that are likely to reduce risky behavior. Social skills training is often the treatment of choice for children with emotional and behavioral disorders (Gresham, Cook, & Crews, , 2004). Often in clinical settings social skills groups will be established to meet a variety of needs of individual children. Regardless of the many clinical problems being experienced by such children most need to learn more adaptive social skills to get along better with peers. This observation has led to a number of programs that use social skills training as one aspect of a more comprehensive treatment.

In a study comparing a placebo treatment and SST focused on anger management, Hinshaw, Buhrmester, and Heller (1989) reported reduced aggressive behavior when SST was combined with a pharmacological intervention. In a subsequent chapter Hinshaw (2005) concludes: "combinations of psychosocial and pharma-

cological treatments may yield optimal performance of critical social skills" (p. 367). In a similar study, Kazdin, Siegel, and Bass (1992) compared problem solving skills training, parent management training, and problem solving skills training together with parent management training for children with antisocial behavior. Posttreatment and one-year follow-up assessments showed that the combination of problem solving and parent management training obtained better outcomes than either of the treatments delivered alone.

Many outcome studies have documented reasonable benefit from social skills training programs. A challenge is that the overall thrust of social skills training is embedded in many other treatments or combined with treatments such that the separate effectiveness of social skills training is difficult to decipher. Interestingly, in a meta-analysis of social skills programs, Quinn and colleagues (1998) found very modest effects. For all group studies the effect size was .20—the participant was better off than only 58% of the participants receiving no training. Gresham, Van, and Cook (2006) note that this conclusion may be due to studies that were included with insufficient intervention exposure to remediate long-standing social skill deficits. These researchers found stronger effects when students were exposed to intensive (60 hour) social skills training. Furthermore, in meta-analyses of social skills training with students with, or at risk for, emotional and behavior disorders, social skills training produced results that showed a 64% improvement rate relative to control subjects.

In a more comprehensive study, Tobler and colleagues (2000) examined child and adolescent outcome studies over 20 years. Programs were classified as noninteractive or interactive and interactive programs obtained stronger effects. In particular, high intensity interactive programs with 16 or more hours of curriculum had greater impact than low intensity (six hours or less). Greater benefits were also found for programs that included life skills models, refusal skills, goal setting, assertiveness, communication, and coping strategies. All of which are key ingredients of social skills training programs. Similar results were found by Wilson, Gottfredson, and Najaka (2001) who reported that social competency programs using cognitive behavioral methods were effective in reducing dropout rates, nonattendance, substance use, and conduct programs. On the basis of this research, Zins, Weissberg, Wang, and Walberg (2002) make a compelling case for the relationship between programs that promote psychosocial functioning and improved school attitudes, behavior, and performance.

In conclusion, social skills training programs have shown good effects in many studies and appear to be best suited for children with emotional and behavioral disorders. Social skills training programs are also ideal for targeted prevention programs. Further, social skills training is an ideal intervention when used to supplement other treatments, especially when the goal is obtaining meaningful social relationships with peers.

GENERAL CONSIDERATIONS IN CONDUCTING THE SOCIAL SKILLS TRAINING GROUP

Who to Include in the Group

Because social skills training is a broad based teaching method that is individualized for each group member, you will find that most young people can benefit from this type of group. Therefore, soliciting volunteers is one method of recruitment depending on the goals and purpose of your particular program. However, it may be necessary to limit participation to a certain number of young people. In this case you will want to institute a procedure where you can identify the young people who are likely to benefit the most from the program. Depending on your situation this could be done by (1) administering assessment devises, (2) conducting pregroup interviews, (3) designing a referral system for teachers or other professionals to refer directly to the group, or (4) selecting young people who meet certain risk criteria. Discuss with other professionals in your area what would be the best and most practical method for obtaining young people to participate in the social skills group.

Group Composition

Factors influencing group composition include how well the young people know each other in the group, how heterogeneous the group is, and how large the group is. Too much familiarity with one another can lead to problems with control. It is recommended that not too many good friends be involved in the same group. Heterogeneous groups appear to work well—some age variation (three to four years), gender mix, and cultural and ethnic mix create an interesting group for everyone involved.

PRACTICAL CONSIDERATIONS

One of the most important practical considerations is how big to make the group. Social skills groups are best when kept to approximately 6 to 10 members. It is important for every member to be able to practice skills during the group—so it can't get too large. Groups tend to function better when there are two group leaders, especially if the group is up to 10 members. Because participants practice different skills every week, it is important to find a desirable and easily accessible meeting place. Convenience is important since getting to the group should occur without any barriers. These same considerations apply with regard to how to schedule the group. Most social skills groups meet on a weekly or biweekly basis for about 1 to 2.5 hours. Groups can be longer if an activity is incorporated into the structure of the group (e.g., a 30-minute basketball game).

SCREENING AND INTAKE CONSIDERATIONS

All young people who are interested in the program should be screened individually to assess their potential to benefit from the group. Additionally, it may be desirable to hold a meeting for parents. During the screening the group leader can interview the young person to assess their social skills. Also, if desired pretreatment assessment instruments can be administered (see Fischer & Corcoran [2006] for examples). This meeting is seen as the working contract between the group leader and participant. In order to reach a mutual agreement the leader can describe the nature and goals of the group and the young person can describe how they think they may benefit from the group. Establishing appropriate expectations concerning the group should be an important goal during this time. For example, the leader may want to review and provide handouts describing the skills to be learned, the methods used, and the program rules for being in the group. A group contract can be written and signed by the participating young person.

SOCIAL SKILLS TAUGHT

A careful review of the literature, previous social skills programs, and extensive experience led to the selection of 11 social skills that are believed to be critical to the promotion of positive interactions with others. These skills provide a broad representation of skill areas but do not significantly overlap each other. Of course, depending on the clients being served, some skills may need to be added and other deleted. However, the format is well specified and makes it easy for practitioners to expand and contract the social skills program to meet their unique needs. The social skills program consists of the eleven units.

Social Skills Training Units

Unit 1: Creating Positive Interactions
Unit 2: Getting to Know Others: Starting Conversations
Unit 3: Making Requests: Getting More of What You Want
Unit 4: Expressing Your Feelings Directly
Unit 5: Getting Out: How to Say "No"
Unit 6: Asserting Your Rights: Tell it Like it Is
Unit 7: Identifying How Others Feel: The Art of Empathy
Unit 8: Dealing with Those in Authority: Staying out of Trouble
Unit 9: Responsible Decision Making: Think about It
Unit 10: Learning to Negotiate: Conflict Resolution
Unit 11: When You're in Need: Asking for Help

Unit 1: Creating Positive Interactions

Introduction and Overview

Today we are going to learn about how to create more positive interactions with others. One easy way to do this is to give another person a compliment or say something nice about the person. By giving someone a compliment you are creating a positive interaction. The other person will feel better about you and you will feel better about yourself. Just as you like to hear nice things about yourself, other people in your life such as friends, parents and teachers, like to hear nice things about themselves. In creating positive interactions it is important to learn how to both give and receive compliments. Many people have a difficult time receiving a compliment because they become embarrassed (gosh, are they talking about me?) or they can't accept it so they reject it (I'm really not that good of a baseball player). By receiving a compliment, you are letting the person who gave you the compliment know that you like what that person is saying. If we practice this skill it will be easy for you to give others compliments but we must remember that any compliments we give have to be true or sincere (don't say, "I really like those shoes" when you really think they are ugly). Think about what you really like about another person before you give them a compliment.

Discussion Questions

Why is it important to learn the skill of giving and receiving compliments?
   Encourage the group to realize the following points.

   1. Learning to give compliments can help you have more positive interactions with others because you are saying something nice about the other person. Also, this may encourage the other person to give you a compliment later.
   2. Learning to give compliments will let other people know what it is you like about them or why you think they are nice.
   3. If you give a person a compliment when they do something for you, they are more likely to do other things for you.

Looking at Examples

Describe a situation where you recently used the skill of giving and receiving a compliment.
   Conduct a role play where the skill was *not* used appropriately to generate a discussion about why the skill is important (this will be especially important with the skill of receiving the compliment).
   Examine the situation according to the following questions.

   1. What was the setting where this occurred?
   2. Who was present?
   3. What was the statement used to give the person a compliment?
   4. Was the statement a compliment (positive, encouraging positive interactions)?
   5. Was the compliment true or sincere?
   6. What was the outcome of the compliment?
   7. How did you feel afterward?

Have the group present their own examples.

Model the Skill

Although it is easy to learn how to give good compliments, many of us do not use this skill as much as we should. Therefore, it is important to practice so you will feel more comfortable giving and receiving compliments. By practicing it a lot we will be more likely to give compliments. I'll start by doing a role play to model how to give a compliment.

Giving Compliments

Modeling Situation: When you arrive a school today you see that your friend has just gotten a new hair cut—one that is much different than this friend had before. You like the change and decide to give a compliment to your friend.

YOU: *Hey, I really like your new hair cut. It really looks good on you.*

PEER: *Well thanks, I'm still getting use to it.*

YOU: *Well, I think it looks great!*

Skill Review

Let's look at what skills were demonstrated in this role play. The model was successful in using the following skills.

1. Looked the person in the eye and used good body language (smiled, was positive with an enthusiastic tone of voice).
2. Used an "I" statement.
3. Gave a clear and specific compliment to the other person.
4. Followed up the compliment with another statement that reinforced the previous compliment.

Receiving Compliments

It is also important to practice the skill of receiving compliments. Remember the goal here is to accept the compliment.

Modeling Situation: You worked very hard on a social science report that was due last week. Your teacher has graded the reports and you go to see her to pick up your report.

TEACHER: *I really liked your social science report. You did an excellent job.*

YOU: *Thank you! I really enjoyed doing the report and I spent a lot of time on it.*

TEACHER: *Well, it certainly shows.*

YOU: *Thanks, I really learned a lot from this report.*

Skill Review

In this role play, what specific skills needed to receive a complement were demonstrated?

Encourage the group to identify the following skills.

1. Looked the person in the eye and used good body language (smiled while accepting the compliment).
2. Said thank you right away and did so in a manner that showed pride not embarrassment (Oh, gee, I guess so, thanks) or overconfidence (I always do good on reports).
3. Followed up the first comment with a second thanks.

Practice Opportunities

Each group member should practice *both* giving and receiving compliments during the group session. First, practice giving compliments, then using some of the same situations, practice receiving compliments. Select one team to observe the nonverbal skills and another team to observe the verbal skills.

Situation 1. Compliment your parents on a dinner that you really enjoyed.
    You would say:
Situation 2. Compliment a friend who you really enjoy doing things with.
    You would say:
Situation 3. Compliment a friend or parent on how they look.
    You would say:
Situation 4. Compliment someone who did a good job playing a team sport with you
    (basketball, football, softball).
Situation 5. Compliment a friend who shared a problem that he or she had
    with you.

Extra Assignments

1. In the group practice giving compliments by having each member of the group give the person on their right a genuine compliment. The compliment doesn't have to be personal but does need to be sincere. The person receiving the compliment can practice skills at receiving compliments.
2. During the week, make a point to give four different people compliments. In your diary keep track of who you gave a compliment to, what you said, what they said, and how you felt. Bring your diaries to the group next week for discussion.

Unit 2: Getting to Know Others: Starting Conversations

Introduction and Overview

Getting to know other people is an important skill that we all need to learn. For some people this is easy but for others it is more difficult. To be successful in life one important skill is getting to know others by starting conversations. This can be important because you may need information that the other person needs and so you must get to know that person in order to ask about the information. For example, lets say you need some information about how difficult it is to get accepted on the soccer team. If you didn't know anybody who was on the soccer team, you'd have to get to know them in order to find out about how difficult it might be. Also, you could get other important information like how much time it takes, whether you think it might be fun, and so forth. There are three parts to a conversation that require skills. The first is *starting* a conversation, the second is *keeping the conversation going,* and the last part is *ending the conversation.*

Discussion Questions

Why do we need to learn skills for getting to know others?
   Encourage the group to realize the following points.

1. Learning how to get to know others can help you meet new people and make new friends.
2. Learning how to get to know others can help you feel comfortable in a variety of situations (e.g., parties, introducing yourself to someone you don't know, etc.).
3. Learning how to get to know others can help you get to know your friends better.
4. Learning how to get to know others can help you get information from other people that you may want.
5. Learning how to get to know others can help you share things about yourself so that you develop stronger friendships.

Looking at Examples

Describe a situation where you recently used the skill of starting a conversation.
   Conduct a role play where the skill was *not* used appropriately to generate a discussion about why the skill is important (show what happens where a person does not know how to start, maintain, or end a conversation).
   Examine the situation according to the following questions.

1. What was the setting where this occurred?
2. Who was present?
3. What was the statement used to start the conversation?
4. How was the conversation maintained?
5. How did the conversation end?
6. What was the outcome of the conversation?
7. How did you feel afterward?

Have the group present their own examples.

Model the Skill

Starting, maintaining, and ending a conversation can be a complex set of skills. I will model each aspect of starting a conversation. Closely observe how I model each separate part of the conversation.

Modeling Situation: You would like to get to know a new person that has recently moved to your neighborhood. You go outside and see this person walking toward you on the sidewalk by your house.

YOU: *Hi, I'm _____. Hey, aren't you new around here?*

PEER: *Yes, we moved just about a month ago from California.*

YOU: *What was it like to live through an earthquake?*

PEER: *Well, lots of times you can't tell they happened, but once I was eating breakfast and everything on the table started to shake.*

YOU: *Wow! That must have been scary.*

PEER: *Well, you get use to them after awhile.*

YOU: *What kind of sports do you like to play?*

PEER: *I was on the soccer team at my old school.*

YOU: *Great, I'm just learning to play soccer but I love it. Hey, I've got to get going to meet a friend, nice to meet you, let's practice some soccer sometime.*

PEER: *Okay, see you later.*

Skill Review

Let's look closely at this role play to see what skills the model demonstrated about how to get to know someone. What skills did the model show?

Encourage the group to generate the following list of skills.

1. Looked the person in the eye and had good body language (showed interest and enthusiasm).
2. Greeted the person by saying his name and asking a question.
3. Asked an open-ended question about the person.
4. Made a statement to follow up on the person's response.
5. Asked another open-ended question about the person.
6. Made another statement about the conversation.
7. Ended the conversation by letting the person know he had to leave. Made a plan to get together again.

The three skills used in conversations were demonstrated by:

1. Started the conversation by saying his name and using a question as an open opportunity to talk with the person.
2. Kept the conversation going by making statements about the conversation and asking additional open-ended questions.
3. Ended the conversation by stating clearly that he had to leave and made a plan to get together in the future.

It may be helpful to review with the group the difference between an open-ended and a close-ended question. A set of close-ended questions can be presented to the group and they can rephrase them as open-ended questions. Some close-ended questions you can use include the following.

1. Are you a new student here?
2. Do you like to play basketball?

3. Do you like art class?
4. Do you go home after school?
5. Did you read that book for English class?

Practice Opportunities

Each group member should practice the skill at least once during the group. Use the following situations or have the group generate situations that they would like to practice.

Situation 1. Starting a conversation with a friend's parent you don't know very well.

Situation 2. Starting a conversation with someone you sit next to in school but haven't gotten to know.

Situation 3. Talking with your coach after a practice about how you are doing.

Situation 4. Talking with a student at a photography show to find out how they took a picture.

Situation 5. Talking with an uncle that has come to visit that you do not know very well.

Situation 6. Joining a conversation with several friends who have been discussing a particular class in school.

Extra Assignments

1. Play 10 questions where everyone in the group must think of 10 open-ended questions to ask another person in the group. You may need to practice with the group how to distinguish open- versus close-ended questions.
2. Select someone you do not know very well and start a conversation with them. In your diary, record your thoughts about what happened and how it went.
3. Carefully observe two people having a conversation and record what you think they did well to make the conversation go better and record what you think they didn't do well to keep the conversation going.
4. Use the situations on starting conversations to also practice conversations with the opposite sex. Set up the role plays so that it is a boy–girl interaction. Have the group members discuss the differences encountered when the interactions are of mixed gender. Also, give the group members an assignment of starting a conversation with someone of the opposite sex with whom they would like to get to know better.

Unit 3: Making Requests:
Getting More of What You Want

Introduction and Overview

If we learn to make requests of others we will be able to get along better with others and to get more of what we want. We all have to make requests of other people. Sometimes those requests aren't easy and sometimes we don't say them in the most appropriate manner. For example, after a difficult math class you may want to ask another person in your class some questions about how to do some homework. This would be an example of making requests of others. As you can see, this can be a critical skill—if you can ask for and receive help you will get more of what you want (in this case help on your homework). Because making requests of others involves asking people for favors you must do it in a polite and appropriate manner. What would happen if you simply said, "Hey, you need to help me with this homework assignment, I don't understand it." This type of demand may lead the other person to say to you, "Forget it, I don't have to help you do anything." So as you can see learning how to make requests also includes how to do it in a polite and appropriate manner.

Discussion Questions

In your own words, why is it important to learn how to make requests of others?
   Encourage the group to realize the following points.

1. Learning to make requests will help you get more of what you want because you will be asking for it directly.
2. Learning to make requests will help you feel more in control of your life because you will be taking charge of more things.
3. Learning to make requests will help you get along better with others when you do it in a polite and appropriate manner.

Looking at Examples

Describe a situation from your own life where you had to use the skill of making requests. Or give an example where you could have used this skill but didn't. Point out the consequences of not using this skill.
   Examine the situation according to the following questions.

1. What was the setting where this occurred?
2. Who was present?
3. What was the statement used to make the request?
4. How was the request made in an appropriate and polite manner?
5. What was the outcome of making the request?
6. How did you feel afterward?

Have the group present their own examples

Model the Skill

Making requests is not always that hard to do although it is important to do so in a nice manner.

Your friend refers to you as "big toes" and you'd rather be called by your real name or by a different nickname.

PEER: *Hey, big toes, did you get out of class early?*

YOU: *I know you use nicknames for everyone—and most people like it, but I'd like you to call me by another name.*

PEER: *Well, I didn't know it bothered you. I guess I can call you by your name but big toes really fits you.*

YOU: *There's just something about big toes that I don't like—maybe you could come up with something different that I would like.*

PEER: *That's cool.*

YOU: *Thanks.*

Skill Review

Let's examine how this skill was used in the role play. The model demonstrated the following:

1. Looked the person in the eye and used good body language.
2. Made a clear, direct request of the other person.
3. Used an "I" statement, if appropriate.
4. Showed appreciation, if the request was accepted, by thanking the person.

Practice Opportunity

Each member should practice the skill at least once during the group session. Select group members to evaluate each individual's performance according to the skill steps.

Situation 1: You forgot your lunch money and want to ask a friend if you can borrow some money from him or her.

Situation 2: You have been working very hard on a paper for your science class. When you get your paper back you were disappointed that you received a C grade. You want to ask the teacher to please review your paper again because you feel it deserves a better grade than a C.

Situation 3: Your friend has been teasing you a lot about your girl- or boyfriend. You want to ask him or her to please stop teasing you.

Situation 4: You get into a conflict with your parents and you believe they have not let you tell your side of the story. You want to ask them to please listen to your story.

Extra Assignments

1. Describe a situation in which you would like to make a request of another person. Try to think about an event from the last two weeks where you wish you would have used the skill of making requests. Write out a script of what you would say to the other person.
2. During the next week write down as many situations as you can think of where you either did make a request or could have made a request.
3. Ask group members to generate situations where a person needs to use the skill of making requests. Use these situations for continued role play practice or have group members write out responses of what they would say. Discuss the different responses of the group.

Unit 4: Expressing Your Feelings Directly

Introduction and Overview

An important skill for all of us to learn is how to express our feelings directly. Often, it is hard to directly state how you are feeling to another person. But if someone is doing something you don't like, it is important to let that person know how you are feeling. When we speak directly to others about our feelings we often avoid getting into fights or walking away with hurt feelings. When we express our feelings directly we often end up feeling better about ourselves. This is because expressing your feelings may help you cope better with your emotions. For example, if a friend does something that makes you really mad it is better to express your feelings to that person directly than to walk away angry. Sometimes people who express their feelings are called complainers; that is not likely when you use this skill in an appropriate manner and at the right time. It is important to use this skill when you want to make things better, not as a way of making others feel bad.

Discussion Questions

Why is it important to learn how to express our feelings directly to others?
   Encourage the group to realize the following points.

   1. Learning to express your feelings can help you avoid situations that could lead to trouble, such as fights.
   2. Learning to express your feelings can help you feel more in control of your life.
   3. Learning to express your feelings can help you get along better with others.
   4. Learning to express your feelings will help other people listen to what you have to say.

Looking at Examples

Describe a situation from your own life where you had to use the skill of expressing your feelings directly. Or give an example where you could have used this skill but you didn't. Point out the consequences of not using this skill.
   Examine the situation according to the following questions.

   1. What was the setting where this occurred?
   2. Who was present?
   3. What was the statement used to express your feelings?
   4. How did you express your feelings in a direct manner?
   5. What was the outcome of expressing your feelings?
   6. How did you feel afterward?

Have group members describe their own examples.

Model the Skill

We are taught to express our feelings in a direct manner so this can be difficult to do. I will do a role play to model how to express your feelings and then we can do our role play practice.
   Modeling Situation: You are working on a project with a friend and you make a mistake and your friend calls you stupid.

PEER: *You just messed it up! You are so stupid!*

YOU: *When you call me stupid it makes me really mad. Anyone can make a mistake.*

PEER: *I just say that all the time to people, I didn't mean to get you mad.*

YOU: *Well, it does make me mad, so please don't call me that.*

Skill Review

Let's look carefully at how this skill was used in this role play. The model demonstrated the following.

1. Looked the person in the eye and used good body language.
2. Stated feelings in a clear and direct manner.
3. Listened to what the other person had to say in response to you.
4. Stated how the other person can avoid the situation in the future.

Practice Opportunity

Each member of the group should practice the skill at least once during the group session. Select group members to evaluate the performance according the skills steps. The group may want to help the role player identify the appropriate feeling to express in the different situations.

The group can use examples of situations that were discussed previously or select from the following sample situations.

Situation 1. Your friend keeps changing the channel and you are interested in watching a specific TV show.

PEER: *I'm going to see what else is on.*

YOU:

PEER: *I didn't know you wanted to watch that show.*

Situation 2. Your teacher assigns you to work with two other class-mates on an art project. You have been working hard to get the project completed but your classmates are just sitting around talking.

PEER: *I thought that was a really great movie.*

YOU:

PEER: *Well, okay, we'll pitch in.*

Situation 3. You have gone to the movie with several of your friends. This is a movie you really wanted to see. During the movie your friends start talking loudly and you can't hear or concentrate on the movie.

PEER: *I can't believe your parents make you do that.*

YOU:

PEER: *Sorry, we'll be more quiet.*

Extra Assignments

1. The focus here has been on expressing feelings directly to others, however, this may be a good opportunity for young people to also learn how to respond when others are expressing feelings about them. It is difficult for young people to listen to others

tell them about their feelings—that others don't like what they are doing or that others are hurt by what we are saying. Group members can practice listening to others and thinking about what others are telling them.

2. Describe a situation where you would like to express your feelings more directly. Write out a script of what you would say to the other person. If you have an opportunity during the week to use this skill make a note of it and report back to the group.

3. It is important to help the group members learn how to recognize feelings. Have each member take home an assignment card that says at the top of it, "Feelings I Had This Week." Have them list the feeling and then describe the situation in which that feeling arose.

Unit 5: Getting Out:
How to Say "No"

Introduction and Overview

We often hear people talking about the importance of saying *no*. This is because we often end up doing things that we really don't want to do. We get talked into something or pressured to act a certain way. This skill is important when you are pressured into something *you don't want to be pressured into*. This is often one of the most difficult skills for us to learn. This is because we want to get along with our friends and at the same time we must refuse to get involved. Let's look at an example. What if a group of your friends all decided to cheat on an upcoming school test. If you *didn't* want to be involved you would have to say no to them. Of course, you don't want to hurt their feelings at the same time you don't want to be involved in the cheating. By learning to say no you will learn to have more control over your life. It will be easier for you to express your true feelings and may help you avoid trouble.

Discussion Questions

Why is it important to learn the skill of how to say *no*?
    Encourage the group to realize the following points.

1. Learning to say no can help you stay out of trouble.
2. Learning to say no will put you more in control of your life.
3. Learning to say no can help you feel better about yourself because you won't do something that you don't want to.
4. Learning to say no will help prevent others from taking advantage of you.

Looking at Examples

Describe a situation where you had to use the skill of saying no. Or give an example of where you wish you had been able to say no but you were pressured into doing something you really did not want to do. Another alternative is to do a role play where the skill was *not* used and then generate a discussion about why the skill is important.
    The group leader may wish to use an example from their own life to share with the group. Examine the situation according to the following.

1. What was the setting of the situation?
2. Who was present?
3. What was the statement that put pressure on the person?
4. How did you say no?
5. What was the outcome of your saying no? (did your friends react positively? negatively?)
6. How did you feel afterward?

Have the group present their own examples

Model the Skill

Saying no is not as easy as it looks. It takes a lot of practice and work to be good at this. I will do a role play to model how to say no and then we can all practice this skill.
    Modeling Situation: You agreed with your parents that you would be home at 9:30 tonight. It is now 9:00 and you are at a friend's house and he says,

PEER: *Hey, lets go to the mall, I know Tom and Blake will be there.*

YOU: *I'd like to go with you to meet them but I can't, I promised I'd be home by 9:30 tonight.*

PEER: *Come on they won't care if you are a little late.*

YOU: *No, I really can't do that. Let's plan to get together with them next week.*

PEER: *Well, okay, I guess I'll go without you.*

Skill Review

Let's look at what skills were demonstrated in this role play. The model did the following.

1. Looked the person in the eye and used good body language.
2. Said no clearly and early on.
3. Said no in a way that was polite.
4. Restated the no when continued pressure was applied.
5. Suggested an alternative activity.

Practice Opportunities

Have each group member practice the skill at least once during the group session. Select group members to evaluate the performance giving feedback on one of the five skill steps. This will help the group members focus their feedback and observe the role play more closely.

The group can use examples of situations that were discussed previously or select from the following sample situations.

Situation 1. A friend comes up to you at school and wants to borrow a magazine you just bought and want to read during your break.

PEER: *Hey, can I borrow that? I've been wanting to read that magazine.*

YOU:

PEER: *Let me read it now, you can read it when you get home.*

YOU:

Situation 2. Some friends decide to go to the record store and begin to talk about shoplifting some CDs. Everyone is expected to steal a CD. You decide you don't want to be involved in the stealing.

PEER 1: *Everyone take one CD when you are in there. It's easy, they never watch you, I took three CDs last week.*

YOU:

PEER 2: *We are all going to do this, come on we're all in this together.*

YOU:

PEER 3: *You're a jerk, let's go—leave him behind.*

Situation 3. One of your good friends calls you at home and wants to come over. You are really busy and have a lot of homework to finish before tomorrow.

PEER: *I'll be over in 1/2 hour.*

YOU:

PEER: *You're always doing homework, come on take a break, how about getting together for only an hour?*

YOU:

Extra Assignments

1. During the week keep track of situations where you need to say no. Pay attention to how difficult or easy it is for you. Prepare a situation for role plays next week.

2. Interview two people outside the group about situations they have faced where they had to say no. What was the situation? What did they do? Were they able to resist the pressure? What did they say? Do they think they could have handled the situation better, if so, how?

3. Have the group members get into pairs. Let the pairs create their own situations or have some already made up on index cards. Have one person make a demand of the other and instruct the other person to practice saying no loudly and clearly. Repeat this several times so each person is very familiar and comfortable with this exercise.

Unit 6: Asserting Your Rights: Tell it Like it Is

Introduction and Overview

Asserting your rights is an important skill to learn. We all have certain rights and we need to both identify and accept our own personal rights. Asserting your rights means letting people know you want to be treated fairly. To assert our rights effectively, we need to be able to know when we are being assertive as opposed to being aggressive or passive. Some people react to situations in different ways. For example, lets say someone borrows something from you without asking. You could react in one of three ways: you could be aggressive by demanding or physically taking the borrowed object from the person; you could be passive by deciding to just forget about it and not let the person know that it isn't right to borrow without asking; or you could be assertive by letting the person know that if they want to borrow things from you they need to ask you first.

Discussion Questions

Why do you think it is important to learn about asserting your rights?
   Encourage the group to realize the following points.

1. Learning to assert your rights can help you increase your own self respect. Because you are standing up for your own rights you can develop greater self-confidence about yourself.
2. Learning to assert your rights can help you get more of what you want. By being direct and honest about what you want you are more likely to be successful in getting what you want.
3. Learning to assert your rights can help you feel more control over yourself.
4. Learning to assert your rights can help you avoid situations where other people treat you unfairly.

Looking at Examples

Describe a situation from your own life where you had to use the skill of standing up for your rights. Or give an example where you could have been assertive but you weren't. Emphasize the consequences of not using assertiveness appropriately.
   Examine the situation according to the following questions.

1. What was the setting where this occurred?
2. Who was present?
3. What was the statement you used to stand up for your rights?
4. Was the statement assertive and not passive or aggressive?
5. Was the statement a direct, honest, and appropriate expression of your concerns and feelings?
6. What was the outcome of standing up for your rights?
7. How did you feel afterward?

Have the group present their own examples.

Model the Skill

Many of us are not comfortable standing up for our own rights. Lots of us are taught to not express our rights but instead to just react passively and do nothing. Some people learn to be aggressive but not assertive. I will do a role play to model how to stand up for your rights and then the group can do role plays to practice the skills.

Modeling Situation: One of your friends asked to borrow a favorite book of yours. You let the person borrow it but asked that they return it within two weeks. At the end of the two weeks you reminded the person to return the book but they still have not given it back to you.

PEER: *Hi! How are you today?*

YOU: *I'm fine. Would you please bring back that book I let you borrow? I'd like you to bring it back tomorrow.*

PEER: *I'm sorry. I keep forgetting.*

YOU: *Well, it is important to me to get it back so please remember. Why don't you write a note to yourself so you don't forget.*

PEER: *Ok. I'll do that right now.*

Skill Review

Let's examine how this skill was used in the role play. The model demonstrated the following.

1. Used good body language and looked the person in the eye.
2. Asserted rights in a direct, honest, and appropriate manner.
3. Asserted rights in a way that would not get the other person upset.
4. Listened to what the other person had to say in response to what was said.
5. Offered a suggestion to help deal with the situation.

This model was a good example of appropriate assertiveness but how is this different from an aggressive response and a passive response?

An aggressive response might be: "You're so dumb, why can't you remember to bring back my book!"

This is aggressive because it makes the other person feel upset and is likely to make them angry at you. A likely outcome is a fight with this person.

A passive response would be:

YOU: *Do you think you could bring back my book?*

PEER: *Well, I'd really like to keep it until the end of the school year.*

YOU: *Well, I guess that would be okay.*

This is passive because the person is not honest and direct about how they feel. They will probably end up angry at their friend and may end up angry at themselves for not standing up for their rights. It does nothing to resolve the situation.

Practice Opportunity

Each member needs to practice this skill once during the group session. Select group members to evaluate the performance using the skills discussed in the skill review. Make sure the performance includes a direct, honest, and clear response and that the other person is not upset by what is said.

Situation 1. A teacher asks you to come in from recess even though you have permission to stay outside from the teacher who is responsible for you at that time.

TEACHER: *Recess is over, you have to come in now.*

YOU:

Situation 2. A friend of yours has gotten in the habit of calling you names. You don't like it and it makes you feel bad.

PEER: *Come on Bozo, lets go outside.*

YOU:

Situation 3. You are waiting in line to see a movie that you really want to see. A group of five people cut in front of you in the line without going to the end of the line.

YOU:

Extra Assignments

1. During the group time have group members brainstorm the different rights that young people have. For example, I have the right to be treated with respect by not having others call me names. Have each member select one right and express to the group what that right is, "I have a right to . . . " Each member can discuss how comfortable he or she was with the exercise.
2. Have group members come up with a situation for asserting their rights. For each situation have them write down an assertive, aggressive, and passive response. Use these in the group to discuss the differences.
3. Have each group member describe one of the most difficult situations for them to stand up for their rights. Use these situations for role plays during group practice.

Unit 7: Identifying How Others Feel: The Art of Empathy

Introduction and Overview

The skill of empathy is a very important skill to learn. Empathy means being able to understand how another person feels—not just the surface feelings but the deep-down feelings the person has inside of them. If a teacher gets mad at your friend and she gets into trouble, how do you feel? If you feel bad for her, then you are using empathy. To express empathy you have to be able to feel what it is like to be another person. The skills do not come naturally, but you can learn how to be more empathic. In the situation described above you might say, "I'm sorry you got in trouble. You seem really upset over it." Sometimes people do not express their feelings but we can sense what they are feeling. To be able to sense another person's feeling is using the skill of empathy.

In learning how to be empathic we have to learn how to identify others' feelings. Once we can do this, we can express to the other person that we understand how he or she feels. When we use the skill of empathy our friends feel like we really understand them and we can help them feel better about themselves. People like to feel understood; using empathy can help others feel this way.

Discussion Questions

Why is it important to learn the skill of empathy? Encourage the group to identify the following points:

1. Learning to use empathy can help you understand and get along with others better.
2. Learning to use empathy can help others feel better because they know that someone understands them.
3. Learning to use empathy can help you feel better because you helped someone else by understanding them.
4. Learning to use empathy can help you get to know another person better because you have shared feelings with them.

Looking at Examples

Describe a situation where you recently used the skill of empathy. Conduct a role play where the skill was *not* used appropriately to generate a discussion about why the skill is important (show what happens when one person ignores another person's feelings). Examine the situation by answering the following questions:

1. What was the setting where this occurred?
2. Who was present?
3. Did you listen carefully to what the other person said?
4. What were the other person's feelings?
5. Why was the person feeling this way?
6. What empathic statement was made to the other person?

Have the group present their own examples.

Model the Skill

Learning the skill of empathy takes practice, because it is hard to learn how to identify what another person is feeling. I will do another role play to provide an example.

Modeling Situation 1

PEER: *My parents have been fighting a lot and now they are going to get a divorce.*

YOU: *I'm really sorry. This must be hard on you. I know I'd be really upset.*

PEER: *Well, I'm just going to have to learn how to deal with it but, man, I really want to live with both of them.*

Modeling Situation 2

Not all feelings are sad. Empathy can also be used for happy feelings. Suppose your friend is a good speller and she has been studying hard to do well on the big spelling test coming up. She wins and is very happy.

PEER: *Guess what? I won! I beat everybody on the spelling test.*

YOU: *Go You! I knew you could do it. I was really rooting for you. I'm happy for you.*

Skill Review

Let's look at this role play to see what skills the model demonstrated about how to show empathy for someone. What skills did the model show? Encourage the group to generate the following list of skills:

1. Looked the person in the eye and had good body language.
2. Listened carefully to the other person's situation or problem.
3. Identified the other person's feelings.
4. Identified a reason for the person's feelings.
5. Stated an empathic response.

Practice Opportunity

Each group member should practice the empathy skill at least once during the group meeting. Use the following situations to have the group itself generate situations that they would like to practice.

Situation 1. Your friend plays on the basketball team and he made it all the way to finals. Last night the team lost. He comes up to you in the hall and is looking sad.

Situation 2. Your friend really wants to have the lead role in the school play. She has been practicing every day for the rehearsal. Yesterday was the competition for the role. When she sees you she says, "I can't believe it—I got the lead role!"

Situation 3. A friend of yours got into a big fight with another kid at school. This is someone your friend really likes and now she is mad at her. She says to you, "I know she really hates me now. I'm never going to be able to work this out."

Situation 4. Your friend runs up to you in the hall. She looks really happy. She says "Guess what? My parents are taking me to Disney World for my Birthday!"

Extra Assignments

1. Read a story to the group and have the group members identify the feelings that the different characters were experiencing. Discuss how one could use skills of empathy in the story.
2. Act out a play that includes expression of a lot of different feelings. Use the play as a modeling experience to coach the group members about how to be empathic.
3. Develop a work sheet that includes different statements from different people (friends, teachers, parents, and so forth). Have group members practice identifying the feelings involved in each situation.
4. Ask each group member to write down an experience he or she had in which he or she either used empathy skills or could have used them. Have them write down the situation, feelings, and what was said. Use these for group discussion.

Unit 8: Dealing with Those in Authority: Staying out of Trouble

Introduction and Overview

Growing up we all have to deal with others who are in a position of authority—people who are responsible for us, like teachers, bosses, parents, group leaders, coaches, police, and so forth. Sometimes it is difficult to deal with those who have authority over us. However, these people often ask for your respect and want to get along with you. As a result, sometimes we have to treat those in authority differently than we treat our friends. Learning how to deal with those in authority is important if you want to avoid arguments and stay out of trouble. If a teacher asks you, "Why aren't you in your class, recess is over?" and you snap back, "I'll get to class—when I want to," you could get into even more trouble. It is also important to realize that how we say something can sometimes get us in trouble.

Discussion Questions

Let's examine why it is important to learn skills involved with dealing with those in authority. Encourage the group to mention the following points.

1. Learning to deal with authority can help you get along better with adults.
2. Learning to deal with authority can help you avoid problems caused by an inappropriate response.
3. Learning to deal with authority will show others that you are mature and they may give you more responsibility in the future.
4. Learning to deal with authority will increase the likelihood of more positive interactions.

Looking at Examples

Describe a situation from your own life where you had to use the skill of dealing with authority. It is helpful if the group understands that even adults must deal with those in authority. Also, give an example where you could have used this skill but you didn't. Point out the consequences of not using this skill.

Examine the situation according to the following questions.

1. What was the setting where this occurred?
2. Who was present?
3. How did you listen to the person in authority?
4. Did you apologize to the person, if necessary?
5. Did you ask for suggestions, if appropriate?
6. How did you feel afterward?

Have the group present their own examples.

Model the Skill

Dealing with those in authority can be difficult for many people. As children we have to learn to deal with parents but as adults we must also learn to deal with bosses. When we are trying to do the right thing it is often difficult to accept what someone in authority has to say to us. I will do a role play to model how to deal with those in authority and then the group can practice these skills.

Modeling Situation: You went to spend the afternoon with some friends but agreed to be home by 4:00 because the family had planned to go to dinner with some friends. You lost track of time and did not get home until 4:45.

PARENT: *You were suppose to be home by 4:00—you're 45 minutes late! You're going to lose weekend privileges for two weeks.*

YOU: *I'm sorry I was late. I know you were counting on my being home at 4:00, I'm sorry I let you down. I should have paid more attention to what time it was but I didn't.*

PARENT: *That's right, you let me down! You are going to have to learn how to be more responsible.*

YOU: *I know I am. Maybe you can help me come up with some ways that will help me remember better.*

Skill Review

An examination of the skills used in this role play show that the model demonstrated the following.

1. Looked the person in the eye and used good body language.
2. Listened attentively to what the person had to say.
3. Apologized directly to the person.
4. Took responsibility for their behavior.
5. Offered a suggestion to avoid the difficulty in the future.

Practice Opportunity

Each member should practice the skill at least once during the group session. Select group members to evaluate the performance according to the skill steps described in the skill review.

Situation 1. You arrive late for class because you were talking to someone.

TEACHER: *You were late for class and I expect you to be here on time.*

YOU:

Situation 2. Your boss asks you to do something and you forget exactly what he wanted you to do. When he comes by to check your work he informs you that you have done it all wrong.

BOSS: *That's not the way I asked you to do it.*

YOU:

Situation 3. A teacher catches you throwing something at another person during class.

TEACHER: *You know that there is no throwing anything in the classroom.*

YOU:

Extra Assignments

1. Change the role plays so that the person in authority displays considerable anger. Discuss with the group how these types of situations may call for different skills.
2. Ask group members to record any situation they encounter where they have to deal with someone in authority—either successfully or unsuccessfully. Use the situations for group discussion and role plays.

Unit 9: Responsible Decision Making: Think about It

Introduction and Overview

In this unit we are going to learn about how to make decisions. All of us have to make decisions—everyday. But often we don't make the best decision and as a result the outcome isn't always positive. The focus in learning decision making is making *responsible* decisions. To do this you have to think about the decision and evaluate both the positive and negative outcomes or consequences involved in the decision. What happens a lot is that we simply make a decision without *thinking* about what the decision means for us. Making responsible decisions is a skill like the other skills we have been learning. However, it is different in that it is a thinking skill—not a skill that involves other people. Once you've made a decision then you might need some of the skills we've been learning to act on that decision. An example might be: Your friends have planned a party that you really want to go to and your mom asked you to stay home that night because some old friends you haven't seen in a long time are coming over. You have to decide what to do in this situation. Should you go to the party or should you stay home to visit with the company? No matter what you decide there is a consequence to each. In order to make the best, most responsible decision you need to think about what the alternative choices are, what the positive and negative outcomes might be, and decide on a plan.

Discussion Questions

Why is it important to learn how to make decisions?
    Encourage the group to discuss the following points.

1. Learning to make decisions can help you make better, more effective decisions.
2. Learning to make decisions can help you think about situations and choices more carefully without jumping to the first idea that comes up.
3. Learning to make decisions can help you prepare for future decisions that will be difficult, like what job or career to get.
4. Learning to make decisions can help you feel better about the choices you do make because you will have carefully thought about them.

Looking at Examples

Describe a recent situation where you had to make a difficult decision. Share with the group how you went about thinking about the choices you had, how you considered the consequences both positive and negative, and what choice you made and finally how you acted on that choice. If possible, explain how you may have arrived at a different conclusion if you had not carefully used decision making skills. Also, share with the group a situation where you didn't use good decision making skills and the consequences that followed.
    Examine the decision making situation using the following questions.

1. What was the setting where this occurred?
2. Who, if anybody, was present?
3. What process did you use to make the decision?
    a. generating alternative choices
    b. describing the positive and negative outcomes of each choice

    c. choosing one or a combination of choices

    d. acting on the decision

  4. How did you feel afterward?

Have group members describe an example from their own life.

Model the Skill

Because this is a thinking skill, I'll model for you the thinking process that you go through when using responsible decision making.

Modeling Situation: It's the beginning of the school year and you are interested in being involved in two after school activities but they occur at the same time. You want to be involved in basketball but you are also interested in the computer club. Most of your friends are in basketball and it would probably be more fun. Your parents are pushing you to be involved in the computer club, especially since they just bought you a new computer.

1. Generate alternative choices.
   a. You could sign up for basketball.
   b. You could sign up for the computer club.
   c. You could do one this year and the other next year.
   d. You could look into a different basketball or computer club option—one not connected with school but with the YMCA.
2. Describe the positive and negative outcomes of each choice.
   a. This would be the most fun because more of your friends are involved in basketball but your parents would be disappointed because they want you to learn more about computers.
   b. This would please your parents but wouldn't be as much fun, however, you do have a few friends in the computer club.
   c. This would be sort of a compromise. You could do the computer club but then let your parents know that next year you want to hold out for basketball.
   d. This sounds good because you might get to do both but it wouldn't be much fun since it doesn't involve any of your school friends. Also, you'd have to find transportation so it might not really be feasible.
3. Choose one or a combination of choices.
   a. You decide on choice C because it gives you the most options. You will please your parents and make use of the new computer they bought you (that you wanted). It will still be fun since there are a few friends of yours in the computer club. You will plan to attend the basketball games and still be involved with the other friends. Still, it makes clear to your parents that you really want to play basketball and that you will probably do that next year.
4. Act on the decision.
   a. You make a plan to sit down with your parents and discuss your decision and how you arrived at the decision. You ask them for their support in your decision. You sign up for the computer club. You discuss your decision with your basketball friends.

Skill Review

Review the steps involved in responsible decision making. In this example the model demonstrated the following skills.

1. Generating as many alternatives as possible.
2. Examining each alternative or choice for positive and negative outcomes.
3. Deciding on one or a combination of choices.
4. Developing a plan to act on the decision.

Practice Opportunity

Each member should practice the skill at least once during the group decision. Have the members think out the decision making process aloud so others can examine and evaluate the skills being used.

The group may want to use examples shared by the group or they may want to select from the following sample of situations.

Situation 1. Two different people have asked you to go to the game with them. One person is a good friend that you like and want to keep and the other person is someone new that doesn't know many people and you want to get to know them better. You think they probably wouldn't like each other that much.

Situation 2. You are out with two of your friends who decide they want to soap someone's car windows. You like these friends a lot and don't want to offend them but also do not want to get into trouble.

Situation 3. Your parents ask you to stay home Saturday afternoon because they are expecting a delivery. The delivery person calls and says he can't come today. Your friend calls you and invites you over. Your parents expect you to be home but now there is no reason you really have to.

Situation 4. You are trying to do well in your math class. Last week you got sick with the flu and missed several days of classes. You have a midterm exam coming up and want to do well but are afraid you might not understand some of the material that was covered when you were sick.

Extra Assignments

1. Use some problem situations to practice with the group decision-making skills. Present the problem and work with the group to generate alternatives, think of consequences and plan a course of action. Encourage the group for creative thinking and their abilities to examine consequences.

2. Make a game out of the process. Present a problem situation and see if each group member can generate two different alternative choices. Or divide the group in half and have teams independently work through a problem.

3. Have each group member identify a problem situation where they had to use decision-making skills. Have them describe the process and evaluate their performance in using responsible decision making. Or have the person discuss a time when they made a bad decision and how that decision could have been better.

Unit 10: Learning to Negotiate: Conflict Resolution

Introduction and Overview

We all have to face conflict situations in our lives. Everyday we come into contact with different people—our friends at schools, our teachers, our parents, our aunts and uncles—and as a result we don't always get along with everybody as well as we would like. When we don't it is usually because of a conflict. A conflict may be a misunderstanding about something, a disagreement about something, or a different viewpoint about something. The important thing about a conflict is that the people involved are not happy with what is going on. Let me give you some examples. A conflict might be between friends about whether to invite another friend along on a planned trip. A conflict with parents might be about how late you can stay up on weekend nights. A conflict with a teacher might be about whether the homework you turned in is acceptable for the assignment. As you can see there are a lot of ways you can get into conflicts! Therefore, it is important to learn ways to resolve the conflict—we do this through negotiation. That means learning to comprise and talk it out when you have a conflict. This is better than getting mad at the other person because of the conflict. When this happens you both get mad and an argument or even a fight could happen. You could just not deal with the conflict but it does not just go away. So the best thing to do is to learn *conflict resolution* skills that include learning to negotiate or compromise. That means making suggestions to the other person about how to solve the conflict and working with the person to reach an acceptable solution for all people involved.

Discussion Questions

Why is it important to learn how to negotiate with other people?
   Encourage the group members to recognize the following points.

   1. Learning to negotiate can help you get along better with other people since you can solve conflicts.
   2. Learning to negotiate can help you understand other people better since you have to listen to the other person's viewpoint.
   3. Learning to negotiate can help you get more of what you want in a situation since you can reach a compromise with the other person.
   4. Learning to negotiate can help you earn the respect of the other person or keep your friendship with the other person since you are working together to solve the problem.

Looking at Examples

Describe a situation from your own life where you had to use the skill of negotiation. Or give an example where you could have used this skill but you didn't. Point out the consequences of not using this skill.
   Examine the situation according to the following questions.

   1. What was the setting where this occurred?
   2. Who was present?
   3. What was the statement used to begin the negotiation?
   4. Did you offer an alternative solution?
   5. Was an alternative solution offered by the other person?

6. Did both people try to reach a compromise?
7. Was a compromise accepted or did both people agree that, although they tried to compromise, no clear solution is available at this time?

Have group members describe their own examples.

Model the Skill

We all have conflicts with other people so we need to be good at negotiating with them to solve those conflicts. There are a couple of things to remember to be able to use negotiation successfully. First, think about some solutions before you attempt to solve the problem and second, remember to stay calm and not get angry or mad when trying to negotiate. I will do a role play to model how to negotiate and solve a conflict with another person.

Modeling Situation: A new television show has started this fall and you really want to watch it. Your sister has been watching another show that comes on at the same time as the show you want to watch.

YOU: *Can we discuss our plans for watching TV?*

SISTER: *Sure.*

YOU: *You know that show that you always watch at 7:00 p.m.? Well, there's a new show on at the same time that all my friends watch and they say its really great. I'd like to be able to watch that new show. Do you have any ideas about how we can solve this conflict?*

SISTER: *Well, we've been watching the other show and I really like that show, so I'm not sure what to do.*

YOU: *What do you think about us taking turns? I could watch my show one week and you could watch your show the next week.*

SISTER: *Well then I would miss half the shows!*

YOU: *I know, but that seems fair—and we both get to see part of our shows. Maybe, we could also ask Mom for another TV.*

SISTER: *Sure! That would be great. I guess for now we can take turns.*

YOU: *Thanks for helping solve this problem.*

Skill Review

Let's look carefully at how this skill was used in this role play. The model demonstrated the following.

1. Looked the other person in the eye and used good body language.
2. Asked to speak with the person about the conflict.
3. Explained the conflict in a clear and relaxed manner.
4. Listened to the other person's ideas for possible solutions.
5. Proposed a compromise by offering a solution.
6. Thanked the person for working out the conflict.

Practice Opportunity

Each member should practice the skill at least once during the group session. Select group members to evaluate the performance according the previous skill steps. The group may want to help the role player think of different solutions to propose prior to doing the role play.

The group can use examples of situations that were discussed previously or select from the following situations.

Situation 1. You would like to be able to stay out later on weekends. You have had the same curfew for over a year and you're older now and most of your friends can stay out later.

YOU: *(Ask to speak with the parent about the problem.)*

PARENT: *Sure.*

YOU: *(Present the conflict.)*

PARENT: *Just because other kids stay out later that doesn't make it right.*

YOU: *(Ask for suggestions to solve the conflict.)*

PARENT: *I don't think that's possible.*

YOU: *(Propose a compromise, negotiate a solution.)*

PARENT: *Well, I'll think about it.*

YOU: *(Thank parent for listening.)*

Situation 2. You are discussing your plans for the weekend with your best friend. You have already invited another friend to go with you on Saturday night. However, your best friend doesn't really like this person and says that he does not want to go if the other person is going to go with you.

YOU: *(Ask to speak with your friend about the problem.)*

FRIEND: *Okay.*

YOU: *(Present the conflict.)*

FRIEND: *I don't really like that guy.*

YOU: *(Ask for suggestions to solve the conflict.)*

FRIEND: *Well, I don't know, I was just planning on us going.*

YOU: *(Propose a compromise, negotiate a solution.)*

FRIEND: *Well, I'll give that a try.*

YOU: *(Thank friend for listening.)*

Situation 3. You are playing a new game of basketball that you learned in school with two friends. A conflict starts because each of you have a different understanding of what the rules are.

YOU: *(Ask to speak with your friend about the problem.)*

FRIEND: *Okay.*

YOU: *(Present the conflict.)*

FRIEND: *Well, that's the way I remember learning it.*

YOU: *(Ask for suggestions to solve the conflict.)*

FRIEND: *I am sure that's the way it's played.*

YOU: *(Propose a compromise, negotiate a solution.)*

FRIEND: *Well, we can try that for now, until we ask the teacher.*

YOU: *(Thank friend for listening.)*

Extra Assignments

1. Present a number of conflicts to the group or as a homework assignment. Have participants practice brain storming solutions to the various conflicts. Point out that arriving at a solution will be easier if you are good at thinking up different alternative choices as solutions.
2. As a homework assignment have each group member recall a conflict that could have been solved with conflict resolution skills. Have each person write out the situation, what happened, and what the result was. Now have each person go back

over the situation and write out a script for how they could have used conflict resolution skills. .

3. Have each member write a story about conflict resolution. Have them fantasize a conflict, describe what happened and then continue the story with how the conflict was resolved using negotiation skills.

4. Develop a series of conflict situations as stories about interesting people and circumstances. Use guided imagery as you describe how the person in the story resolved their conflict through their use of negotiation skills.

Unit 11: When You're in Need: Asking for Help

Introduction and Overview

Today we are going to learn about what to do when you need help. All of us face different difficulties that are sometimes too much for us to handle alone. When this happens we need to ask for help, although it may not be easy to do so. This can be a critical skill because you may be dealing with a problem that is serious and needs to be brought to another person's attention. For example, some kids get really down on themselves even to the point of wanting to commit suicide, other kids get abused or physically punished to the point of bruises, or kids may end up addicted to drugs. In all of these situations, you need to ask for help. Other situations may not be as serious but you still may need to ask for help. For example, you may just be feeling lonely and want someone to talk with or you may be having a conflict with your parents and may want to discuss it with someone else. As you can see, knowing who to talk to and how to ask for help can be an important skill to learn.

Discussion Questions

Why do we need to learn skills for asking for help?
   Encourage the group members to recognize the following points.

   1. Learning to ask for help can assist you in dealing with serious problems that may be too much for you to handle.
   2. Learning to ask for help can assist you in feeling better about yourself.
   3. Learning to ask for help can assist you in feeling more in control of your circumstance.
   4. Learning to ask for help will lead to respect from others because you asked for help when you needed it.

Looking at Examples

Describe a situation from your own life where you had to ask for help (if it is not too personal), or describe a situation from someone you know who had to ask for help.
   Examine the situation according to the following questions.

   1. What is the setting where this occurred?
   2. Why is there a need to ask for help?
   3. What kinds of help are needed?
   4. Who are some people you could see to get help?
   5. Who should you see to get help?
   6. How would you describe your problem to the person helping you?
   7. How do you think you would feel afterward?

Have the group present their own examples.

Model the Skill

Asking for help and knowing what kind of help to get can be difficult. I will model how to ask for help. However, most of what I model will be what you need to think to yourself so I will just be thinking out loud.

Modeling Situation 1: Your parents have been fighting and it has gotten really bad the last six months. Finally, they told you that they were going to get a divorce and you have been afraid this was going to happen. You are very upset and have been crying for several days. You just can't get it off your mind.

YOU: *I need to ask for help—I'm really feeling upset. I've been upset before but now I just can't keep from crying and I can't stop thinking about their divorce. I'm not doing well at school either because I just can't concentrate. I could use some help with this problem.*

YOU: *I could get help from a number of people. I could talk with my friend, I could talk to my teacher, I could call that kids help line, I could see a school counselor, and I could talk with my aunt.*

YOU: *I think I'll see a school counselor because they deal with those kinds of problems. But today if I'm still feeling bad when I go home I'm going to also call that kid's line, just to talk with someone.*

YOU: *(You make an appointment to see a school counselor and when you go to your appointment you describe your situation.) I'm really upset because my mom and dad are getting a divorce.*

Modeling Situation 2: You and a couple of friends start goofing off during P.E. class and the teacher gets really mad and starts yelling at you, calling you names and tells you to go to his office. When you get there he starts yelling at you again and then says he's going to spank you. He gets out a wooden paddle and makes you bend over and really spanks you hard.

YOU: *He really hurt me with that spanking—I can't even sit down. I think what he did was wrong. We weren't really doing anything that bad and he just lost his temper and took it out on us. Also, I heard that kids weren't suppose to get spanked anymore. I know they suspend kids from school but spanking them isn't right.*

YOU: *I need to ask for help—what he did wasn't right and I should tell somebody so this doesn't happen again or so it doesn't happen to somebody else.*

YOU: *I could ask for help from my other friends, my home room teacher, the school counselor, or my parents.*

YOU: *I think I should talk with my parents first. I'll tell them what happened and see what they think. I might also mention it to a school counselor but I'm not sure they can help me with this.*

YOU: *(When your parents get home from work you tell them you need to discuss something with them.) Something happened to me in school today and I just wanted you to know about it. We were goofing off in class and the teacher got really mad at us—so mad he yelled at us and gave us a spanking. But it really hurt—I can't even sit down because he hit me so hard. I just don't think this was fair—we weren't doing anything that bad, he just lost his temper and took it out on us.*

Modeling Situation 3: You and your best friend get into a really big fight. She is not talking to you anymore. You feel really bad about this because you really like her and you want to be friends again.

YOU: *I really like her and I don't think we should stay mad at each other. This isn't helping anybody. I've tried to talk with her and she won't speak to me. I feel hurt and at the end of my rope.*

YOU: *I need to ask for help—we haven't been able to solve this problem and she won't talk to me. I'm feeling more upset each day.*

YOU: *I could discuss this with another friend of mine, my teacher, my parents or go see the school counselor.*

YOU: *I think I should talk with my mom first. She knows her and she might have some ideas about what I can do.*

YOU: *(After getting home from school you tell your mom you need some help.) Mom, I need your help. I'm really upset because my best friend and I had a fight and she won't talk with me. I just don't know what to do.*

Skill Review

Let's look closely at this role play and see what skills the model demonstrated about how to ask for help. What guidelines did the model use in thinking about this situation?

Encourage the group members to generate the following guidelines.

1. Why is there a need to ask for help?
2. What kinds of help are needed?
3. Who are some people you could see to get help?
4. Who should you see to get help?
5. How would you describe your problem to the person helping you?

Practice Opportunity

Let's practice how you might prepare yourself to ask for help. Using the following situations, think out loud how you would use the skills of asking for help.

Situation 1. You are having a difficult time in one of your classes. On the last test you got a D. You really want to do better. How would you ask for help in this situation?

Situation 2. Your parents got in a really big fight last night and your mom left and hasn't come home. You are very upset and want someone to talk to. How would you ask for help in this situation?

Situation 3. You feel very shy and have a hard time meeting people. Also, there are some kids at school that make fun of you because you are shy and don't know what to say at times. Having your school mates pick on you is really getting to you. How would you ask for help in this situation?

Situation 4. Your friend is very down on himself. He has been getting more and more depressed. Lately he has been talking about making life easier by not being around. You are afraid he is serious about committing suicide. How would you ask for help in this situation?

Extra Assignments

1. Write a story about someone that was having a difficult life and needed help. Describe how that person got help. Have each person share their story with the group.
2. Present a number of situations to the group where a person needed to ask for help. Have the group brainstorm who they would ask for help and discuss why that would be the best person to choose.
3. Ask each group member to share an example of someone that they knew who should have asked for help to solve a problem. Discuss how they could have received help by asking for it.

References

Compas, B. E., Benson, M., Boyer, M., Hicks, T. V., & Konik, B. (2002). Problem-solving and problem-solving therapies. In M. Rutter & E. Taylor (Eds.), *Child and adolescent psychiatry* (4th ed., pp. 938–948). Boston: Blackwell Science.

Compas, B. E., Connor-Smith, J. K., Saltzman, H., Thomsen, A. H., & Wadsworth, M. E. (2001). Coping with stress during childhood and adolescence: Progress, problems and potential. *Psychological Bulletin, 127*, 87–127.

Dishion, T. J., McCord, J., & Poulin, F. (1999). When interventions harm: Peer groups and problem behavior. *American Psychologist, 54*, 755–765.

Fischer, J., & Corcoran, K. (2006). *Measures for clinical practice and research: A sourcebook two-volume set.* New York: Oxford University Press.

Frankel, F. D. (2005). Parent-assisted children's friendship training. In E. D. Hibbs & P. S. Jensen (Eds.), *Psychosocial treatments for child and adolescent disorders.* Washington DC: American Psychological Association.

Gresham, F. M., Cook, C. R., & Crews, S. D. (2004). Social skills training for children and youth with emotional and behavioral disorders: Validity considerations for future directions. *Behavior Disorders, 30*, 32–46.

Gresham, F. M., Van, M. B., & Cook, C. R. (2006). Social skills training for teaching replacement behaviors: Remediating acquisition deficits in at-risk students. *Behavior Disorders, 31*, 363–377.

Hinshaw, S. P. (2005). Enhancing social competence in children with attention-deficit/hyperactivity disorder: Challenges for the new millennium. In E. D. Hibbs & P. S. Jensen (Eds.), *Psychosocial treatments for child and adolescent disorders: Empirically based strategies for clinical practice* (2nd ed.). Washington DC: American Psychological Association.

Hinshaw, S. P., Buhrmester, D., & Heller, T. (1989). Anger control in response to verbal provocation: Effects of stimulant medication for boys with ADHD. *Journal of Abnormal Child Psychology, 17*, 393–407.

Kazdin, A. E. (2003). Problem solving skill training and parent management training for conduct disorder. In. A. E. Kazdin & J. R. Weisz (Eds.), *Evidence-based psychotherapy for children and adolescents.* New York: Guilford Publications.

Kazdin, A. E., Siegel, T. C., & Bass, D. (1992). Cognitive problem-solving skills training and parent management training in the treatment of antisocial behavior in children. *Journal of Consulting and Clinical Psychology, 60*, 733–747.

LeCroy, C. W. (2002). Child therapy and social skills. In A. R. Roberts & G. J. Greene (Eds.), *Social work desk reference* (pp.406–412). New York: Oxford University Press.

LeCroy, C. W. (2006). Designing and facilitating groups with children. In C. Franklin, M. B. Harris, & Paula Allen-Meares (Eds.), *The school services sourcebook: A guide for school based professionals* (pp. 595–602). New York: Oxford University Press.

LeCroy, C. W., & Mann, J. (2004). Preventing substance abuse among youth: Universal, selected and targeted interventions. In L. A. Rapp-Paglicci, C. N. Dulmus, & J. S. Wodarski (Eds.), *Handbook of preventive interventions for children and adolescents* (pp. 198–226). Hobokin, NJ: John Wiley.

LeCroy, C. W., & Rose, S. D. (1986). Evaluation of preventive interventions for enhancing social competence in adolescents. *Social Work Research and Abstracts, 22*, 8–17.

Lewinsohn, P. M., & Gotlib, I. H. (1995). Behavioral theory and treatment of depression. In E. E. Beckam & W. R. Leber (Eds.), *Handbook of depression* (pp. 352–375). New York: Guilford Press.

Quinn, M. M., Kavale, K. A., Mathur, S. R., Rutherford, R. B., & Forness, S. R. (1998). Meta-analysis of social skills interventions for students with emotional and behavioral disorders. *Journal of Emotional and Behavioral Disorders, 7*, 54–64.

Rose, S. D., (1998). *Group therapy with troubled youth: A cognitive-behavioral interactive approach.* Thousand Oaks, CA: Sage Publications.

St Lawrence, J. S., Jefferson, K. W., Alleyne, E., & Brasfield, T. L. (1995). Comparison of education versus behavioral skills training interventions in lowering sexual HIV-Risk behaviour of substance-dependent adolescents. *Journal of Consulting and Clinical Psychology, 63*, 154–157.

Tobler, N. S., Roona, M. R., Ochshorn, P., Marshall, D. G., Streke, A. V., & Stackpole, K. M. (2000). School-based adolescent drug prevention programs: 1998 meta-analysis. *Journal of Primary Prevention, 20*, 275–337.

Wilson, D. B., Gottfredson, D. C., & Najaka, S. S. (2001). School-based prevention of problem behaviors: A meta-analysis. *Journal of Quantitative Criminology, 17*, 247–272.

Zins, J. E., Weissberg, R. P., Wang, M. C., & Walberg, H. J. (2002). *Building school success through social and emotional learning.* New York: Teachers College Press.

Part II

Treatment Manuals for
Social Problems

Chapter 6

TAME: Teen Anger Management Education

Eva L. Feindler, PhD, and Meghann Gerber, MA

THE DEVELOPMENT OF ANGER MANAGEMENT TRAINING

The antisocial behavior of children and adolescents presents a significant challenge to the clinical community. Although the rate of youth arrests for violent and aggressive crimes appears to be dropping during the past decade, the prevalence of conduct disorder among children and adolescents remains high, which indicates that maladaptive aggression continues to be a significant problem (Connor, 2002; Snyder & Sickmund, 2006). Furthermore, aggressive and antisocial behavior problems appear to be stable over time if left untreated (Kazdin, 1995). Although a number of direct and indirect factors are theorized to contribute to the etiology of aggressive behavior and conduct problems (for a brief review see Nelson, Finch, & Ghee, 2005), the cognitive-behavioral model focuses on the cognitive processes that play a significant role in the generation of anger and the sometimes aggressive responses to provocation.

Novaco's (1975) cognitive-behavioral conceptualization of anger and anger management problems functions as the basis for the anger management procedures described by Feindler and her colleagues (Feindler, 1987, 1990, 1995; Feindler & Ovens, 1998; Feindler, Marriott, & Iwata, 1984; Feindler, Ecton, Kingsley, & Dubey, 1986). Based on Meichenbaum's (1975) stress inoculation model, Novaco (1975) identifies anger as a stress reaction with three response components: cognitive, physiological, and behavioral. The cognitive component is characterized by one's perception of social stimuli and provocation cues in the social context, by one's interpretation of these stimuli, by one's attributions concerning causality and/or responsibility, and by one's evaluation of oneself and the situation. This component represents a significant area for intervention with aggressive adolescents as their perceptions and attitudes serve to prompt most behavioral responses to provocation.

Research on the social and cognitive processing in aggressive youth indicates that distorted interpretations, attributional biases, and deficiencies in problem solving can all influence the selection of aggressive behavior responses (Crick & Dodge, 1994; Lochman & Dodge, 1994). Furthermore, cognitive processing patterns are likely to become more rigid over time, and as such the maladaptive aggressive behaviors prompted by dysfunctional cognitions will be maintained (Crick & Dodge, 1994; Harvey, Fletcher, & French, 2001).

In addition to cognitive deficits and distortions, aggressive adolescents display high states of emotional and physiological arousal. One of the many contributions to the field of cognitive-behavioral treatment made by dialectical behavior therapy is the emphasis on emotion dysregulation and its impact on impulsive behaviors (Linehan, 1993a). Indeed, many youth presenting for treatment suffer from various aspects of emotion dysregulation (Keenan, 2000). Children and adolescents who have problems with impulsive aggressive behaviors seem unable to cope with the lower levels of the affective experience of anger in a prosocial or constructive way. The irritability or annoyance that results from goal-blocking or mild interpersonal conflict often gives way to intensified anger and explosive rage.

Given the highly charged nature of these youth and the difficulties prompted by their behaviors, the need for treatment is clear; the format for such treatment, however, has been the focus of some debate. There have been concerns in recent years that group treatment for youth with antisocial behavior problems may have an iatrogenic effect, thus resulting in an increase rather than a decrease of such behaviors among group participants (e.g., Arnold & Hughes, 1999; Dishion, McCord, & Poulin, 1999). In an empirical review of studies that asserted such claims and a subsequent meta-analysis of 66 treatment studies, 53% of which contained a group component, Weiss and colleagues (2005) found little evidence supporting previous claims to this effect. The results of the meta-analysis, concluded that studies in which there were group components actually had a smaller chance of producing a negative effect size. In addition, in their empirical review of the literature, Weiss and colleagues point to a number of problematic assumptions made by previous authors, including the assertion that increases in group participants' antisocial behavior while in treatment are likely due to group treatment involvement rather than circumstances occurring outside of the treatment setting. Thus, further research may be needed, but current evidence does not warrant a rejection of group treatment for youth with antisocial behavior problems.

This chapter will present a complete anger management intervention designed for a group of aggressive adolescents. Particular attention will be paid to awareness of emotional arousal, cognitive deficits and distortions that have been identified, and treatment strategies that directly target misattributions, misperceptions, and poor problem-solving ability. Anger management strategies designed to effect change in the physiological and behavioral components will also be described in this detailed chapter. Further, recommendations for assessment and implementation of the group intervention and for clinical issues in the areas of generalization enhancement, diagnostic decision making, and group process will be made.

A GENERAL DESCRIPTION OF ANGER MANAGEMENT TRAINING

Based on the premise that adolescents who lose control over their anger do so because of particular cognitive and behavioral skill deficits, Feindler and her colleagues (Feindler & Guttman, 1994; Feindler & Ovens, 1998; Feindler et al., 1984; Feindler et al., 1986) developed an anger management program for youth. The current enhanced anger management intervention (Feindler & Weisner, 2005), focuses on the control of emotional and impulse responding, as well as on the appropriate expression of anger in an assertive and rational manner, by teaching arousal-management skills and cognitive strategies designed to promote the enhancement and generalization of self-control skills. As the adolescent builds a repertoire of skills, he or she begins to experience greater satisfaction from effective communication in interpersonal conflicts, and as a result suffers less from the punishing and isolating consequences of aggressive responding.

The enhanced anger management program uses a self-regulatory coping skills approach with special emphasis on the cognitive components of anger. Adolescents are taught to recognize, moderate, regulate, and prevent anger and its often accompanying aggressive component and to implement problem-solving actions in response to interpersonal provocation. In addition, elements of dialectical behavior therapy (DBT) emotion regulation strategies and interpersonal effectiveness skills (Linehan, 1993b) are included to enhance adolescents' ability to build awareness of emotional arousal and increase prosocial behavior options in the face of interpersonal conflict. Behavior change, in specific terms of reduced physiological arousal, aggressive responding, and negative anger sustaining attributions and self-statements, is the desired outcome of the intervention program.

Whether administered on an individual client basis or to a group of adolescents, the intervention program consists of interrelated training strategies and therapeutic goals designed to help youth achieve self-regulatory skills. Throughout, youth are educated about (1) interaction among cognitive, emotional, physiological, and behavioral components of their anger experience; (2) the adaptive and maladaptive functions of their anger; (3) the situational triggers that provoke their anger; (4) the concept of choice and self-responsibility in their responses to provocations; and (5) the importance of appropriate verbal expression of affect.

INTRODUCTION TO THE TREATMENT PROTOCOL

Cognitive-behavioral anger management training is generally presented as a didactic program in which skills development is emphasized. The three main components—arousal management, cognitive restructuring, and prosocial skills—correspond to the hypothesized deficiencies and distortions in social information processing and emotion regulation implicated in the development of anger outbursts and aggressive behavior patterns. For each component a specific set of skills or strategies are presented in an educational format, modeled, rehearsed through repeated role play provocation scenes and then applied to the natural environment through homework exercises. Each session provides practice of newly acquired strategies as well as graduated exposure to more intense anger triggers. The program is designed to teach the adolescent to assess each anger provocation and to implement the most effective responses from his or her repertoire of anger management skills (Feindler et al., 1986). The general emphasis on interpersonal problem solving and assertive communication of anger arousal is designed to provide optional responses and prevent the automatic aggressive response.

Prior to implementation of the following 10 session treatment protocol, a number of clinical issues need to be addressed. First, clinical assessment designed to conceptualize the youth's anger disorder must be completed in order to determine the appropriateness of this cognitive behavior therapy (CBT) anger management approach. An examination of the psychological profile and behavioral history of the aggressive adolescent should indicate that deficiencies in arousal management, impulse control, and prosocial responses to interpersonal provocation exist. Other factors to consider on interview and screening include psychiatric diagnosis, level of cognitive functioning, emotional maturity, group readiness, and motivation for treatment are discussed fully elsewhere (Feindler & Baker, 2004).

There are a number of structured assessment methods that may be considered to further delineate the adolescent's anger management difficulties. There are a number of easy to administer self-report inventories that are appropriate for this population and that will help to evaluate treatment effectiveness using pretest and posttest assessment. These include the 41-item Adolescent Anger Rating Scale (Burney, 2001), the 29-item Aggression Questionnaire (Buss & Perry, 1992), the 30-item Children's Inventory of Anger (Nelson & Finch, 2000), the 54-item How I Think Questionnaire (Gibbs, Barriga, & Potter, 2001), the 20-item Normative Beliefs About Aggression Scale (Huseman & Guerra, 1997), and finally the 54-item Multidimensional School Anger Inventory (Smith, Furlong, Bates, & Laughlin, 1998). Given possible response bias and social desireability elements inherent in self-report assessment, clinical investigators are encouraged to use additional data collection methods such as direct observation; ratings by parents, teachers, and staff; analogue role play methods; and self-monitoring. A detailed review of assessment methods and issues can be found in Feindler (1990) and Feindler and Baker (2004).

Once a group of adolescents who may benefit from anger management skills training have been identified, there are some additional clinical issues to consider. Foremost is the need for motivational support for program implementation. The anger management philosophy should fit within the treatment or educational context and necessary resources provided. The following represents a set of typical questions asked by those planning to implement a program.

Issues to Consider When Planning Anger Management Interventions for Adolescents

How long should the sessions be? Given that young people typically have short attention spans, sessions should last no more than 45 minutes, so a maximum amount of material can be digested. However, sessions can be extended for mature adolescents and in groups that form a cohesive bond.

How long a period should elapse between sessions? There should be approximately one week or less between sessions. This will give the students time to process the information they have learned and practice their new skills. However, with less mature or frequently disruptive adolescents, sessions might need to occur more than once per week. School and residential environments offer opportunities for more frequent sessions.

Should there be a co-therapist? Yes. Having two therapists to lead a group can be very helpful. First, the two therapists can role play provoking incidents together for the students. Second, having two therapists attending to the actions of the students is valuable when providing feedback and assessing progress. Third, the therapists can take turns introducing the content and in-group exercises, and monitoring in-group behavior.

Should both therapists be the same sex? If possible, it would be useful to have therapists of opposite genders co-lead groups. This will increase diversity and the members of the group can witness both a male and female acting in a controlled manner and negotiating differences between them.

How many adolescents should be in a group? Approximately eight adolescents per group. With this size group each adolescent does not feel too conspicuous and yet a feeling of intimacy and openness can develop among the group members. Also, in a group this size there will be fewer distractions between group members. Some group activities are designed for two teams to compete and thus at least six group members are necessary.

What's better, same-sex or mixed-sex groups? Same-sex groups are better when initially teaching anger management. Adolescents may attend better when they are not distracted by members of the opposite sex. However, given that in abusive relationships, management of anger is often a problem, ideally after the students have gone through the program in same-sex groups, review groups could be implemented as mixed-sex groups.

Can staff members who may continue to run this type of training program at the residence sit in on the session? Yes, but it is not advised to have more adults than adolescents in a group. For a group of eight adolescents with two therapists no more than two staff members should sit in at a time. Also, if at all possible, the same staff members should sit in on every group. The reasons for this are twofold. First, it would help to maintain consistency for the adolescents in the group. Second, if the staff members are participating to learn how to implement this type of program, they should see it through from start to finish. Additional staff from the adolescents' environment might serve as cues for more controlled responses to provocation in natural settings.

Would it be useful to use video equipment? Yes. It would be particularly helpful if other staff members will be learning the anger management techniques. This way, when staff watch the video, they can see the skills being taught and watch the students implement the techniques in the exercise portion of the treatment. However, if the group coleaders determine that video equipment will distract the group members, it should not be used. Further, videotapes of group sessions allow for the examination of treatment fidelity, an important component of program evaluation.

What should the leader do about noncompliance to in-group tasks and to homework assignments? First, explore the reasons for noncompliance and clear up any possible misunderstandings concerning requirements or rationale for assignment completion. Then remind students about the contingency that he or she will not be able to participate as an actor in role play situations and he or she will not be given reinforcers unless compliance is achieved. This may effect his or her chances of participating in a lottery at the end of the program. Finally, if the student continues to be oppositional, the leader maintains the option of dismissing him or her from the group.

Are there any adolescents who would definitely not benefit from anger management training? Yes. Adolescents experiencing extreme depression and/or suicidal thoughts may not have the motivation to participate. Also, adolescents who are currently abusing substances will not benefit from the program because the substances reduce their motivation and dampen their cognitive functioning. Finally, adolescents with thought disorders or delusions will be unable to glean much from the program because they will have difficulty understanding the cognitive restructuring components. These issues would need to be addressed prior to the adolescent's involvement in anger management training.

What about using individual therapy concurrently with group anger management training? This would not pose a problem as long as there is consistency between what the individual youth is expected to accomplish in his or her individual therapy and the skills being taught in anger management treatment. However, theoretical orientation between both treatment modalities needs to be compatible.

What ages should group members be? This program was initially designed for adolescents, with group members between the ages of 13 and 18. However, the treatment program's pace and content can be scaled down for children of younger ages.

Is it acceptable for all the group members to know each other or be in the same classroom or living unit? Yes. A benefit to having the students know each other is that they can monitor each other's behavior in the natural environment. As the students implement the techniques outside of the training setting, their peers can reinforce and give feedback regarding how effectively the anger control skills were used. One cautionary note: in-group role plays are less likely to be of a hypothetical nature and may be more volatile and carry over to other situations in the natural setting.

Is there any optimal setting for this type of skills training program? It would be optimal to hold the group training sessions in a number of different settings (e.g., a classroom, a residence hall lounge). In this way generalization would be increased because the students would be practicing their skills in different surroundings. The anger management program can be integrated into a variety of different settings as well.

Are closed- versus open-ended groups more effective? Certainly closed-ended groups are desirable as all members will be learning all the same content in the sequenced fashion the program is designed. However, with many cases in many situations, students may leave the program prematurely or be assigned to the program because of spontaneous administrative decisions. New students should be oriented and taught skills already learned by group members who have been in the program from the beginning.

How can treatment fidelity be assured? Each session should have a checklist of all activities and skills taught. After session completion, leaders should go through this checklist to ensure that all content was covered. Sessions can also be videotaped so that this review can be completed by a supervisor.

Should parents and other family members be involved in the anger management program? In many cases, parents, other family members, as well as staff members could greatly benefit by learning anger management skills themselves. Often, this is not practical to have a concurrent group. However, all adults involved with the youth participating in the program should have a preprogram orientation concerning which skills will be taught and should be invited to the wrap-up session to hear how the youth have learned to manage their anger and aggressive behavior.

Session 1: Group Orientation

A. Introductions
1. Introduce coleaders and have each group member introduce him or herself.
2. Discuss confidentiality and its limits.
3. Introduce the rationale of the program.
    a. To teach new skills that will enable the students to control their anger in provocative situations and decrease both overt and covert aggression as a response to anger.
    b. To increase the students' personal power by learning the skills necessary to communicate their needs and desires effectively.
4. Review rules of the program.
    a. Describe role plays and introduce need for participation.
    b. Discuss participation in group discussions.
    c. If applicable, discuss use of a points system where a special prize is awarded to the persons with the highest point totals for appropriate behaviors during group meetings.

B. Introduce emotions
1. Explain basic information about the nature of emotions and moods.
2. Discuss how every culture gives names to emotions and that when people are able to describe and name an emotion, they understand it better and are better able to manage it.
3. Explain the steps in naming emotions.
    a. Recognize when you are feeling an emotion
    b. Describe the emotion by considering
        • the provoking stimulus or event
        • the interpretation of the event (i.e., thoughts and beliefs)
        • physiological sensations
        • body language (i.e., face and posture)
        • verbal communication of the emotion
        • actions or behaviors taken in response to the emotion
4. Introduce the emotion of anger as main focus of group. Generate a discussion of how anger might be defined. Talk about variations in frequency and intensity.
5. Exercises.
    a. Think about angry situations and try to describe what happens. Write on the board the physical and other cues students notice when they get angry.
    b. Have students name different intensities or variations of anger (e.g., hatred, frustration) and place them on a thermometer continuum from warm to boiling.
    c. Introduce a brief relaxation technique, "Take Three." Taking three slow, deep breaths can help students maintain a controlled response to anger provocations. Give students examples of athletes (e.g., figure skaters, gymnasts, baseball players) who visibly use a few deep breaths before attempting some event. Remind students about their physiological cues, for example, muscle tension in the neck, lower back, or shoulders, or heart palpitations. Other cues include fist clenching, cursing, or gritting of the teeth. Explain that deep breathing will function to reduce physiological tension, refocus attention away from

external provoking stimuli to their internal control, and provide a time delay before making a choice of how to respond.

d.   Have the students think about a situation in which they were very angry. Students may need to be prompted with questions such as "Think, for a moment, of the last time someone really got you steamed," or "Can you remember the last time you were in a situation when you wanted to hit someone who was really pushing your buttons?" Have students enumerate what physiological and other cues they noticed. Write these cues on the board.

e.   Model for the students how, when they first notice that they are beginning to get angry, they should stop and remind themselves to relax and take one or two deep breaths.

f.   Have the students provoke each other. For example, one student might say to another, "Just get out of my face." Ask them to say "relax" aloud and take the deep breaths. In this way the leader can determine if the students understand this procedure.

g.   Have the students practice diaphragmatic breathing. Tell them to imagine they have a balloon in their stomachs and they have to blow it up without moving any other part of their bodies. Check to make sure they are not lifting and tensing their shoulders.

C.   Introduce the Hassle Log
1.   Hand out Hassle Logs (see Table 6.1) to students and ask various students to read the separate items in the log aloud.
2.   Run through an example of a hypothetical conflict with students to demonstrate how to fill out the Hassle Log.
3.   Give the rationale for using a Hassle Log. It is a self-monitoring device that will provide each student with an accurate picture of how he or she handled conflict situations during the week. It is a device for students to learn what sets them off. It provides an opportunity to report situations that were different and that were handled well. Finally, it provides scripts for in-session role play. Explain to each student the contingency: if they complete the Hassle Log appropriately, then it will be used as a script for role plays.

Table 6.1
Hassle Log

Hassle Log

Name:_____ Date:_____ Time:_____
Where were you? ___Home ___School ___Outside ___Car/Bus ___Other
What happened: ___Teased ___Told to do something ___Someone stole from me
 ___Someone started a fight with me ___I did something wrong
 ___Other _____
Who was that somebody? ___Friend ___Sibling ___Another student ___Parent
 ___Teacher ___Another adult ___Therapist/Counselor
 ___Other _____ _____
What did you do: ___Hit back ___Ran away ___Yelled ___Cried ___Ignored
 ___Broke something ___Was restrained ___Told adult
 ___Walked away calmly ___Talked it out ___Told friend
How did you handle yourself: ___Poorly ___Not so well ___OK ___Good ___Great
How angry were you: ___Burning mad ___Really angry ___Moderately angry
 ___Mildly angry ___Not angry at all

Notes: _____

D. Summary and conclusion
1. Explain Hassle Log requirements. Review mechanics of completing Hassle Logs. Students may be able to earn points that can be exchanged for reinforcers. Also, they can participate as actors in role plays.
2. Tell the students to fill in their Hassle Logs, and to record examples of their use of the deep breathing technique during a conflict situation.

Session 2: Self-Assessment of Anger and the ABCs of Behavior

A. Collect and review Hassle Logs and homework assignments. Students who did not comply will not earn session points if applicable, and will not be permitted to be actors in role plays. Further, explain to the noncomplying student that he or she is a member of the group and in order to learn the skills being taught he or she needs to complete the homework assignments.

B. Recap. Always review what was covered in the previous session and field any questions about skill implementation. For this session, review the brief relaxation techniques and ask students if they had any difficulty implementing this strategy in the past week. For example, the relaxation technique may not have been effective if the student continued to focus his or her attention on the provocative stimuli instead of on the deep breaths he or she was taking.

C. Introduce self-assessment of anger and the concept of ABCs (that is, antecedents, actual behavior, consequences). Hand out the ABCs Worksheet (see Table 6.2) so the students can visualize what is discussed.
    1. Provoking Stimulus. Start with, "What gets you angry?" Discuss situational variables and setting events in terms of what is going on in the environment (overt [outside] activating events) and physiological states of fatigue, hunger, and so on (covert [inside] activating events).
    2. Introduce the idea of triggers (anger provoking activating events). In this discussion, focus on the beginning of the anger/aggression sequence.
        a. Direct triggers. These are direct aversive provocations by another person, which may be verbal (being told what to do) or nonverbal (a kick, push, obscene gesture, or the like).

Table 6.2
ABCs Worksheet

ABCs Worksheet
Instructions: Write a statement about an event that you were in or observed recently. Just tell a short story version.

_____	_____	_____
_____	_____	_____
_____	_____	_____
_____	_____	_____

In the box below write in as many of the ABCs as you can about the incident.

Action or Hassle Event	Behavior/Belief	Consequences
Indirect trigger:	Cognitive/Thinking:	Positive:
_____	_____	_____
_____	_____	_____
_____	_____	_____
Direct trigger:	Physiological/Body:	Negative:
_____	_____	_____
_____	_____	_____
_____	_____	_____

b.   Indirect triggers. These aversive stimuli include the misperception or misattri-
bution of events such as feeling blamed or feeling like someone is disapprov-
ing. Most of these events involve a faulty appraisal of what is going on, such
as "He put me on restriction because he doesn't like me." Help students to
identify different ways of interpreting provoking incidents.

3.   Actual behavior/reaction. Ask, "How do you know when you are angry?" Focus
on the cognitive or physiological covert (inside) or overt (outside) cues that
occur.
   a.   Negative statements to self (e.g., "I'm an idiot," or directed at others, "I want to
   kick him in the face").
   b.   Physiological cues (e.g., muscle tension, rigid posture, angry stare, butterflies in
   stomach, tense facial muscles, etc.).

4.   Consequences. Inquire, "What happened to you as a result of not controlling
your anger? Did you get in trouble?" There may also be positive consequences of
temper loss in that the individual may feel personal satisfaction or achieve some
desired goal or object.

D.   Exercises:

1.   The Trigger Finger. Break into two teams of equal number. Ask the students to see
which team can come up with the longer list of activating events or triggers that
typically result in angry reactions. Each team has five minutes.

2.   Model how direct triggers and indirect triggers (misattributions or misperceptions) can heighten a conflict. Then have students provoke each other. The student
being provoked should relate the cognitive self-statements he or she generated in
response to provocative activating event.

3.   Going to the Head. Form two teams. Team A states a physiological cue and Team
B must identify a verbal overt (outside) or cognitive covert (inside) cue. If both
members give plausible cues, then a member of Team B must come up with a
cognitive cue this time, and a member of Team A with a physiological cue. If one
team member cannot respond, the other team has the chance to steal a point by
coming up with a cue. For example, a member of Team A states that a physiological cue is "getting hot" and a member of Team B says a cognitive cue is "I'm going
to kill him." These are both correct answers. Now a member from Team A must
state a cognitive cue, such as "She better not take another step toward me." And
a member from Team B must state a physiological cue, for example, "Heart palpitations." Again both teams are correct. Team A continues by stating a physiological cue and Team B offers a cognitive cue. This time Team A incorrectly identifies
physiological cue as "I'm going to smash him," so Team B has a chance to steal a
point. Team B does this by stating both a correct cognitive cue, since Team A was
wrong, and stating the physiological cue, which is what they were supposed to
identify.

4.   Working as teams again, the students now compete to develop the longest list
of positive and negative consequences for the provoker. The leader supplies a vignette of a provocative situation.
   a.   Trainers demonstrate role play of a provocative event (e.g., thinking that
   a peer or adult is lying with regard to something promised to the adolescent). Demonstrate the identification of activating events, behaviors, and
   consequences.
   b.   Ask two group members to role play a provocative event of their choice or
   one supplied by leaders. Have the actors and other members from the group
   identify activating events, behaviors, and consequences.

E. Summary and conclusion
   1. Review ABCs
   2. Hand out ABCs worksheet and assign the analyses of two incidents. Also, hand out additional Hassle Logs to complete. Hassle Logs will be used for role play scripts.

Session 3: Refuting Aggressive Beliefs

A. Collect and review Hassle Logs and homework assignments. Discuss any anger provoking scenarios.

B. Recap last session.

C. Introduce interpretation of events
   1. Explain that most events do not automatically cause emotions. Instead, the emotion is caused by the person's interpretation of the event or how the person thinks about the event.
      a. For example, Maria doesn't like Susan or Jenny. Susan gets very angry with Maria for not liking her, but Jenny just gets afraid. Why would they have two different emotions from the fact the Maria doesn't like them? Susan gets mad because she is thinking how much she has done for Maria, and that therefore, Maria should appreciate it and like her. Meanwhile, Jenny becomes afraid because she thinks that if Maria doesn't like her after all she has done for Maria, then maybe no one will like her.

D. Refuting aggressive beliefs
   1. Explain that sometimes we have beliefs about why people act in certain ways toward us. These beliefs lead to thoughts that another person is acting aggressively or nonaggressively.
   2. Explain there are both aggressive and nonaggressive ways to interpret situations. For example, an aggressive belief would be, "If someone looks at me differently or acts differently toward me, maybe he is having a bad day."
   3. Explain that interpreting situations in nonaggressive ways will help control anger responses.

E. Exercises
   1. Brainstorm and list all the attributions the group makes about why people act in certain ways or do things. For example, ask the group to write down reasons someone might have passed them in the hall and said some derogatory statement (e.g., bitch) as they passed by. The students will probably generate a list of aggressive beliefs regarding what happened, such as, "She did it on purpose," or "She wants to start something with me," and so on.
   2. Brainstorm and list all the alternative nonaggressive explanations for the examples in Part 1. For example, "She wasn't talking about me," or "She was having a bad day." Generate alternative and nonaggressive attributions.
   3. Have the group discuss whether the nonaggressive interpretations are or are not plausible interpretations.

F. Summary and conclusion
   1. Review differences between aggressive and nonaggressive beliefs or interpretations of situations.
   2. Hand out additional Hassle Logs for completion during the week.

Session 4: Assertion and Relationship Techniques

A. Collect and review Hassle Logs and homework assignments.

B. Recap previous session.

C. Introduce objectives effectiveness (adapted from Linehan [1993b]).
   1. Explain that being effective in a relationships means getting what you want or need from another person, that is, achieving a goal or objective in the course of an interaction with someone else. This includes making sure your own rights are respected, asking someone to do something in a way that increases the chance that they will do it, and resolving conflicts so that they don't worsen or continue.

D. Introduce skills to enhance objectives effectiveness. Start with the DEAR MAN objective effectiveness skills used in dialectical behavior therapy (Linehan, 1993b). Explain that DEAR MAN stands for
   1. *Describe.* State the facts about a situation without being judgmental. For example, one can be objective by saying, "This is the third time this week you have borrowed my MP3 player," rather than, "You are such a leech! You need to get your own MP3 player."
   2. *Express.* Communicate your feelings, thoughts and opinions about the situation. Don't assume that someone else knows what you believe or how you feel. Expressing yourself clearly can prevent others from misunderstanding you. For example, you might say, "I would love to share my candy with you, but I only have a few left and I promised them to Anna, so I can't give you one." This prevents someone from assuming you aren't sharing because you don't like her, or because you are selfish.
   3. *Assert.* Clearly say what you're asking for or what you are saying no to. Again, don't assume people will know what you mean without clearly stating it. Remember to say what you want or need, but not what others should do. Saying "Hey, can I borrow your MP3 player?" is much more effective than saying, "Are you using your MP3 player?" "No." "Oh, I just wanted to know," and then getting angry because the other person did not let you borrow it.
   4. *Reinforce.* When someone does give you what you have asked for, or responded to you in a positive way, it's important to reward him or her. *Rewarding* usually means saying positive things back to the person, or by describing the positive effect his or her actions have on you. You can sometimes reinforce others before they respond to you and include it in your request. For example, "I will be able to get my work done faster if you let me listen to your MP3 player, and then I will be able to help you study for the test sooner," or "I would really appreciate it if you would help me put this stuff away."
   5. (stay) *Mindful.* This is about keeping your attention on your goals for the interaction, and not allowing yourself to get sidetracked or distracted onto something else. Techniques for staying focused on your goal will be presented and include broken record, ignoring, and escalating assertion.
   6. *Appear confident.* Present yourself in such a way that communicates you are effective, assertive, and your requests deserve respect. Think about posture, eye contact, and how you might use your voice. How would these aspects be differ-

ent from someone who appears arrogant? How effective is someone who always appears shy?

7. Negotiate. This is about adjusting your request or offering to do something in exchange in order to solve the problem or resolve the conflict. You can also turn it around and include the other person by asking him or her to generate a solution by asking, "How should we solve this problem?"

8. Other techniques for achieving objectives.
   a. Broken record. This response involves calmly expressing yourself over and over. This technique is effective when students can prevent the conversation from becoming loud or aggressive and instead focus on the repetition and persistence.
   b. Ignoring. This technique is useful for keeping focus on your objective and not letting the other person determine the direction of the interaction. When the other person is attacking or making threats, ignoring it will keep the student on track, whereas responding to it will give the other person control of the conversation. Using broken record and ignoring together can be very effective for not allowing oneself to be diverted from one's goal.
   c. Empathic assertion. This is a form of assertion that involves sensitive listening on the student's part to the other person's feeling state. This method is particularly useful when dealing with authority figures who are angry. For example, if a staff member complains, "This room is a mess. I can't believe you guys are such slobs! Start cleaning immediately," the student who learns how to use empathic assertion might answer, "I know you're upset with the mess, but we just got back from the rec room and haven't had time to clean up yet." Discuss how the staff member in this situation would have felt better because his or her feelings were heard.
   d. Escalating assertion. This is a sequence of responses that increases in assertiveness in order to obtain a desired outcome. Begin with a minimal assertive response and escalate to final contract option in which a threat to the other person for noncompliance to original demand is presented. For example: (1) "Please return my MP3 player"; (2) "I asked you to return my MP3 player"; (3) "I want my MP3 player now"; (4) "If you don't give me my MP3 player now, I will go tell the staff and they will come and get my MP3 player for me."
   e. Fogging. This is a technique used to short-circuit an aggressive verbal conflict by confusing the provoker. The individual being provoked should appear to agree with the provoker, but not really agree. For example, the provoker might say, "You are stupid," and the target student might reply, "I know you think I'm stupid." Explain to group members that such an agreement does not indicate truth, but rather a way to turn things into a joke. Students can also use their description skills to state plainly (and nonjudgmentally) what is happening rather than responding to the aggression. For example, a student might respond to repeated verbal attacks by saying, "you keep telling me insults and I keep ignoring them."

E. Exercise
   1. Ask for volunteers to role play the following situations using the listed techniques.
      a. Please describe to a staff member how you deserve to get the bathroom pass first because you have been waiting the longest and you have not been able to use the bathroom all day.
      b. A person wants to close the window in the room because it is cold, but you are hot, by expressing your feelings or opinions clearly, ask the person to leave the window open.

c. Directly assert your wish to eat an apple that your friend does not seem to be eating.

d. Reinforce someone for letting you use his or her MP3 player.

e. Stay mindful when asking someone to leave you alone by ignoring them when they are teasing you about your hair, then your shoes, and then your shirt.

f. Stay mindful when asking someone to stop talking about your friend by using broken record when they keep saying different bad things about her.

g. Appear confident when telling someone you are not going to let them cheat off your paper during the test next period.

h. Negotiate with someone in order to get him or her to help you study for an exam.

F. Introduce relationship effectiveness. Part of being effective means maintaining or improving a relationship while trying to get what you want or need. Relationship effectiveness also requires students to contrast and balance immediate goals with long-term relationship objectives. Students can be asked, "Is it possible to both get what you need from someone and have that person feel good about giving it to you?"

G. Introduce the relationship effectiveness skills used in dialectical behavior therapy represented by the acronym GIVE (Linehan, 1993b). Explain that GIVE stands for

1. (be) Gentle. Pose the question, "Do you respond to others better when they attack, threaten and judge you or when they approach you in a polite and considerate manner?" This skill is not only about avoiding overtly harsh tactics, but also refraining from implicit judgment about what others *should* do.

2. (act) *Interested.* People will respond more positively to you if they believe that you are interested in where they are coming from. Give the other person the chance to speak about his or her opinion, and listen to what he or she has to say.

3. Validate. Communicate that you recognize the other person's position, difference of opinion, or feelings about the situation. This can be as simple as saying, "I know you have to study for a test tomorrow, so I will make this brief . . ."

4. (use an) *Easy* manner. This skill is about trying to be upbeat or lighthearted to get someone to work with you on your request. Using an easy manner can be contrasted with putting someone in a hard place, pushing him or her around, or using guilt trips.

H. Summary and conclusion

1. Discuss with students when to use assertive responses rather than withdrawal or aggressive responses. Assertion is optimal when the adolescent is certain of his or her rights in a situation and when there is a high probability of a nonaggressive, successful outcome to the problem situation.

    It is not a good idea to use an assertive response when the individual is not clear about his or her rights (e.g., the student is not sure if the MP3 player another person has belongs to him or her or not). An assertion technique also should not be used if there is a good chance that it will lead to further aggression or harm.

2. Assign more Hassle Logs for homework. In addition, ask the students to write down at least two incidents when they use one or more of the assertion techniques, DEAR MAN, or GIVE sequences.

Session 5: Self-Instruction Training

A. Collect and review Hassle Logs and homework assignment.

B. Recap previous session.

C. Introduce self-instruction training.
    1. Define *reminders* as things we say to ourselves to guide our behavior or to get us to remember certain things. Ask group members to think of specific things they say to remind themselves to bring certain items to class, and so on.
    2. Give examples of situations where reminders can be used in pressure situations, such as at the foul line during a very close basketball game.
    3. Describe how students can implement reminders by recognizing that they are getting angry and then stopping themselves by pausing, kicking back, looking away for a moment, and saying to themselves, "stay calm." The key components to this sequence are: Stop, Press the Pause Button, Kickback, and Remind.
    4. Describe how reminders can also be helpful in situations in which the student has to try to stay calm. Reminders or internal self-control statements are key ingredients of increased personal power. Thinking before acting gives students control over their anger arousal and helps them determine their choice in response to provocation.

D. Application of reminders procedure: transitioning from overt (outside) to covert (inside) reminders.
    1. Model the use of overt (outside) reminders and role play a situation in which one student is cursing out another who is emitting audible reminders in order to ignore these behavior. Suggest the use of reminders instead of reacting to the direct provocation.
    2. Fully describe the substitution procedure, whereby a youth has a choice after recognizing the activating anger trigger. She or he can either react in an angry or aggressive way, which may lead to receipt of negative consequences, or she or he can emit covert (inside) reminders to remain calm and uninvolved in the conflict situation. Emphasize the personal power inherent in not responding to anger provocation.
        a. Demonstrate use of covert (inside) reminders, and review rational for maintaining this level of self-control.
        b. Emphasize the idea that the timing of reminders is critical. Provide examples of someone who uses reminders before any actual provocation (too soon) and after she or he has received a punishment for explosive behaviors (too late).
        c. Discuss candidly with the students situations in which they would be unwilling or unlikely to ignore a direct provocation.

E. Exercises
    1. Have the group members generate a list of reminders that they use in those highly charged situations. Write them on the blackboard. Examples include: Slow down, Take it easy, Take a deep breath, Cook it, Chill out, and Ignore this.
    2. It's Hot in the Middle. Have students choose the best reminders and write them on index cards. Shuffle the cards and have the students sit in a circle with one

student in the middle. Have other students provoke him or her and have the student being provoked practice aloud using the reminder on the index card, and any others she or he might generate.

F. Summary and conclusion
    1. Review the concept of reminders and the effective use of reminders.
    2. Provide more Hassle Logs. Ask students to write down two incidents in which they practice using reminders.

Session 6: Thinking Ahead

A.   Collect and review Hassle Logs and homework assignments. Have the students give one another feedback on how hassles were managed. This will model the use of direct peer social reinforcement for improved anger control outside the therapy room.

B.   Recap prior sessions (include deep breathing, ABCs, assertion techniques, etc.).

C.   Introduce "Thinking Ahead" procedure as another self-control technique to use in conflict or anger-provoking situations.

   1.   Define thinking ahead as using problem solving and self-instructions to estimate future negative consequences for possible current aggressive responses to a conflict situation. For example, "If I slap her in the face, I will get restriction and not be able to go home this weekend," or "If I slap her in the face, I'll get suspended from school and have to go to summer school," or "If I start a rumor about her, she might start one about me that will embarrass me."

   2.   Explain thinking ahead procedure by stressing the importance of using future negative consequences as a reminder to not get involved in acting-out behaviors, and discuss the relevance of appropriate timing when using the thinking ahead procedure.

   3.   Define covert (inside) and overt (outside) consequences of aggressive behavior.
      a.   Covert (inside) examples: people not liking you, people not trusting you, losing your friends, or being burdened by the reputation of acting out so everyone assumes you were involved in any given conflict.
      b.   Overt (outside) examples: having your privileges removed or being placed in a more restricted environment.

   4.   Explain to students that they should remind themselves of negative consequences, stop the possible misbehavior and substitute an alternative behavior such as deep breaths, assertion techniques, or reminders. This process underscores the principle of *thinking before acting*.

D.   Exercises:

   1.   Have the students break into teams and develop a list of covert (inside) and overt (outside), short-term and long-term, internal and external punishing consequences for aggressive behavior (e.g., hitting another student, talking back to a teacher). Have them order the list hierarchically from the least punishing consequence to the most punishing consequence.

   2.   Have the group sit in a circle and have them provoke each other. During the provocation, have them use the thinking ahead procedure by saying aloud the statement "If I (misbehave) now, then I will (future consequences)."

   3.   Have two students role play a provoking event from their Hassle Log. During the role play have them identify the course of action they would normally have taken for the audience. Then have them remind themselves aloud what the negative consequences would be for such an action. Have them substitute an alternative behavior (e.g., assertion, reminders), and have them identify which alternative behavior they are using. Have the actor and group discuss the positive consequences of the alternative behavior.

E. Summary and conclusion
    1. Review thinking ahead procedure. Have students identify negative consequences that might occur in the future that they can use to control their present behavior. Also, discuss the future positive consequences for achieving better anger control (e.g., more privileges).
    2. Hand out more Hassle Logs. Also ask the students to implement the thinking ahead procedure and write about its effectiveness.

Session 7: Problem Solving Training

A. Collect and review Hassle Logs and homework assignments.

B. Recap previous session.

C. Introduce "Problem-Solving Training." This is the process used to make a choice between anger control alternatives. Emphasize that the following questions cannot be generated unless the student is able to recognize that she or he is angry, stop, pause, and think. Present the following sequences to students on a board and review each step, giving examples from the Hassle Logs the group presented during the session.

   1. Problem definition. *What is the hassle?* Identify the activating stimuli, including provoking stimulus, situational variables, and internal anger cues. Combine all of these components into a clear definition. For example, if accused of stealing money from another student, the problem definition is that the innocent student is getting angry (heart palpitations, burning cheeks), because she or he has been accused unfairly of stealing.

   2. Generation of alternative solutions. *What are my options?* ("What can I do?") This phase requires individuals to brainstorm all of the possible responses to the problem situation. The process of brainstorming precludes the evaluation or critique of any responses generated until a later time.

   3. Consequence evaluation. *What is my penalty?* ("What will happen if . . . ?") Using methods similar to those incorporated in the thinking ahead procedure, identify positive and negative consequences for each response. These consequences should be overt (outside) and covert (inside), and long and short term.

   4. Choosing a solution. *What action will I take?* ("What will I do?") This phase involves rank ordering all solutions generated according to the desirability/undesirability or severity of the consequences enumerated previously. The solution that optimizes positive consequences, minimizes negative consequences, and solves the presenting problem is the one to implement first.

   5. Define *self-evaluation* as a method of providing oneself with feedback on how a conflict situation was handled. Self-evaluation responses are reminders that occur *after* a conflict situation to provide the individual with immediate feedback on behavior and feelings during the conflict. Thus, they can be thought of as *after-reminders*. Discuss how positive and negative after-reminders might affect the behavior that preceded it. (This is a lesson on the process of self-reinforcement.)

   6. Feedback. *How did it work?* The final step in the problem solving procedure involves the evaluation of the solution based on its effectiveness in solving the problem. The use of after-reminders should also be prompted at this stage. If a chosen solution is not effective, then a second choice solution should be implemented.

D. Exercises

   1. Where there's a will, there's a way. Have the students generate solutions to a problem in which there are a few or no solutions. The vignette should not have an interpersonal component. For example, What should Susan do if she is stranded on a highway alone, 20 miles from civilization, and has no cell phone? Through this exercise the students will be able to differentiate between problems that really have few solutions and those where there are alternatives.

2. Using examples from students' Hassle Logs, have the students
   a. Identify the problem as a group.
   b. Break into teams and generate alternative solutions.
   c. Come back to the group and discuss positive and negative consequences of all the possible solutions generated by both groups.
   d. Choose a problem solution by majority vote.
   e. Help the students determine its effectiveness.

E. Summary and conclusion
   1. Review problem-solving sequence.
   2. Provide additional Hassle Logs and also ask the students to write down incidents in which they used this sequence to solve a problem.

Session 8: Bullying Prevention: Specific Problem-Solving Techniques

This session is adapted from Child Abuse Prevention Services (2003).

A. Collect and review Hassle Logs and homework assignments.

B. Introduce bullying prevention. Explain that many of the problems that will be covered in this session have to do less with the type of aggression talked about in previous sessions. This different type of aggression is often expressed in the way girls relate to one another. Students can be asked to take a moment and think, "Do students in your school belong to cliques? Are there leaders and followers in cliques? How does someone become part of a clique or get kicked out? Does being popular mean that someone is nice?"

    1. Exercise

        a. Ask the students to generate a list of the positive aspects of friendships between girls. Next, generate a list of things students have noticed that girls do to one another that are mean or disrespectful.

        b. Ask the students if they can think of reasons why girls can have really strong friendships and still do mean things to people who might be considered their friends. Why are some people unwilling to stand up to such treatment?

C. Distinguish between good and bad teasing.

    1. Friendly teasing. Explain that the purpose here is to be playful, to relate, and to join. This is different than an intention to do harm.

    2. Unfriendly teasing. Explain that the purpose in this type of teasing is to hurt or exclude someone. Unfriendly teasing is often used to put someone down.

D. Exercise

    1. Rumors. Read the following case example:

        Regina and Graciela are good friends and are a part of the same group of friends in their seventh grade class. Everyone agrees that Graciela is one of the prettiest girls in school. Lately Graciela has been getting a lot of attention from Richard, a popular eighth grader. Regina likes Richard, and begins spreading rumors about Graciela. Regina tells people that Graciela thinks she's better than everyone else, and even claims that there is a sexual relationship between Richard and Graciela.

        a. Generate a discussion with students by posing the following questions and writing down their responses on the board.

            i. What are the facts?

            ii. What might Graciela be feeling in this situation?

            iii. How do you think Regina is feeling?

            iv. Why is Regina behaving this way?

            v. If Regina and Graciela don't resolve this problem, what might Graciela learn from the experience?

E. Friendship inventory. Explain that every friendship has its ups and downs, but it can be difficult to decide when a friendship is worth saving. A friendship inventory is a series of questions students can ask themselves to help clarify difficult situations.

    1. What do you need from a friendship? What makes a good friend?

    2. What are your responsibilities in the friendship? What are your friend's responsibilities?

3. What would your friend have to do in order for you to decide to end the friendship? What would you have to do in order for your friend to decide to end the friendship with you?

4. What are the pros and cons of ending the friendship?

F. Talking it out. Ask students if they think it is possible for Regina and Graciela to work things out. Explain that oftentimes we choose not to try and talk things out because we are afraid of losing the friendship, or we fear that the other person will turn more people against us. In addition, these situations often involve feelings like jealousy, hurt, and lack of confidence, which can be very hard to admit to having. However, choosing to not work things out prevents us from having an honest relationship. Introduce the steps to talk out a conflict and use the case example above to illustrate.

1. Step one: Preparation
   a. Write down the facts of the situation, with all of the details (when it happened, who said what, etc.). Then write down how you felt during the incident, how you are feeling now, and what you want to happen.
   b. Write down what you want to say to the other person and practice in front of a mirror. Remember objectives and relationship effectiveness skills (DEAR MAN and GIVE) when deciding what to say. Pay attention to body posture, voice tone, and eye contact. You can also practice with a trusted adult and ask for feedback.

2. Step two: Confrontation
   a. Do not approach the other person in front of his or her friends. Choose a place and time in which you feel safe to talk. Ask for a private conversation or invite an adult to be present.

G. Exercise
   1. Have students practice by generating ideas about how Graciela might go about the preparation to confront Regina. Write responses on the board.
   2. Role play the confrontation. Have student observers offer feedback.

H. Apologizing
   1. Explain that apologizing can be a difficult skill to master, but it's very important for maintaining and improving relationships. Apologizing is a mature gesture, which requires that you recognize how you have negatively impacted someone else and take responsibility for your actions.
      a. How do you make an apology? Describe how an apology is only effective when
         • It's genuine, meaning there is a real understanding of the hurt caused and the person making the apology is sincere. Forced apologies are generally not effective.
         • The person making the apology speaks only about his or her actions, without adding any insults or excuses.

I. Exercise
   1. Have students role play Regina's apology to Graciela and have the observers offer feedback.

J. The power of words. Verbal aggression
   1. Ask students why they think certain words have so much power, like the words bitch or slut. Who gets called these words, and why?
   2. Ask students if they monitor or change their behavior in fear of being labeled with a powerful word. What behaviors would elicit these labels from others?

K. Introduce self-respect effectiveness (Linehan, 1993b). Explain that this is about keeping respect for yourself in your interactions with others. This includes respecting your own beliefs and values. Skills for self-respect include

1. Be fair to yourself and to others. Self-respect is not just about watching out for yourself, it is actually about being and acting like someone worthy of your respect. Not being fair or taking advantage of others makes it hard to respect yourself.
2. Remember your values and act accordingly. Don't do something that goes against what you believe just to obtain a short-term goal, like getting someone to like you. Maintain your integrity by sticking to your own moral code.
3. Be truthful with others. This means avoid lying and exaggerations. It may seem like lying occasionally is not a big deal, but over time you will come to see yourself as dishonest, and your goal is to be the person you want to respect.

   These skills foster self-respect, but it's good to remember that respect from others comes naturally when you have respect in yourself.

L. Summary and conclusion
1. Review bullying prevention skills.
2. Provide additional Hassle Logs. Also, ask the students to write down some incidents in which they practiced doing a friendship inventory, using techniques for talking out a problem, apologizing, or using self-respect effectiveness skills.

Session 9: Program Review

A. Collect and review Hassle Logs and homework assignments.

B. Program review. Before the session, write the name of each skill taught in the program on a separate index card. When the session begins, ask each student to select one index card at random. Give the students a few minutes to think about how to describe/define the strategy for using the skill card, how to demonstrate the strategy, and when is the best time/situation to implement the strategy. The students, using the outline above, will discuss the skill they chose with the group. Cards should include at least 10 skills (Take Three, Kickback, DEAR MAN, GIVE, Broken Record, Fogging, Reminders, Thinking Ahead, Problem Solving, ABCs, I-messages, Empathic Assertion, Escalating Assertion, Refuting Aggressive Beliefs). Review of each skill should include the following.

1. Deep breaths. Remind students about their physiological cues and how the deep breathing technique can be used to reduce tension and stress, redirect their attention away from external provoking stimuli to internal control, and provide a time delay before making a choice how to respond.

2. Concept of ABCs.
    a. Activating events are provoking stimuli. Overt (outside) activating events are situational variables in one's environment that provoke anger. Covert (inside) activating events are physiological states, such as fatigue.
    b. Triggers are provoking stimuli. Direct triggers are direct aversive provocations by another person. These may occur in verbal or nonverbal form. Indirect triggers are the adolescent's misinterpretation or misattribution of events, the result of a faulty appraisal system. Indirect triggers may also include observed injustice or unfairness.
    c. Faulty reminders or beliefs need to be replaced with statements directing the student to let go of personalized anger and look at other ways to view the situation less aggressively.
    d. Behavior is the individual's actual reaction to the provoking stimuli, which can involve a variety of cognitive, physiological, covert (inside), and/or overt (outside) responses.
    e. Consequences are events that happen as a result of controlling or not controlling anger. Consequences can either be rewarding or punishing.

3. Assertion techniques include objective and relationship effectiveness skills (DEAR MAN, GIVE, Broken Record, Ignoring, Fogging).

4. Reminders are things we say to ourselves (overtly and covertly) to guide our behavior or to help us to remember certain things.

5. The thinking ahead procedure is another type of reminder that utilizes problem solving and self-instruction to estimate future negative consequences for current misbehavior to a conflict situation.

6. Problem solving
    a. What is the hassle? (problem)
    b. What are my options? ("What can I do?")
    c. What are the penalties? ("What will happen if . . . ?")
    d. What action will I take? ("What will I do?")
    e. Feedback ("How did it work?")

C. Discuss situational and personal elements that would help the student determine which strategy to use.

    1. Introduce barbs. A *barb* is a provocation statement made directly to the target adolescent in situations other than the actual training one. The adolescent is issued a warning first: "I'm going to barb you." Then the barb is delivered, (e.g., "why were you watching TV when your privileges have been revoked?"). The person giving the barb notes the adolescence's response and gives both positive and constructive feedback. Gradually the barbs should more closely approximate realistic inquires made by staff members, parents or others in their environment. If possible, these barbs should also be delivered by carefully selected others in more natural environments. These challenges should occur spontaneously with graduated intensity.

        a. The leader should barb the students at this point so they get used to the procedure. Because this is phase one, all of the barbs should start with a warning.

        b. Role plays can also be done in which group members barb one another. Those members watching can identify which anger management skills were exhibited.

    2. Ask students to describe in detail several conflict situations that have occurred. Ask them to describe the various anger management techniques they used during the provocations. Another option is to have the students role play several scenes using the anger management skills they have learned. Pass a hat filled with the index cards that identify the various anger management techniques. Whatever technique is selected, the student has to try to use that skill in his or her role play. Other students observing have to guess which technique(s) are being implemented.

D. In closing

    1. Provide students with feedback on

        a. His or her cooperation during the program

        b. His or her performance during the exercises and role plays

        c. His or her enthusiasm and/or interest in various components of the program

        d. His or her motivation for change; being on time, completing homework assignments and Hassle Logs, and so on

        e. Observable changes in behavior, including any anecdotal observations from another person involved with students

    2. Let the student know what you have learned by participating in the group and tell the student that you enjoyed working with him or her.

    3. Ask each group member to review his or her participation. Have each of them give self-evaluative praise statements regarding their participation and improvement in anger management. Prompt students to reinforce observed changes in each other.

    4. Prepare students for situations in which their newly acquired anger management skills may not work out as they hope or expect. Leaders can role play failed scenarios in order to prepare group members for future frustrations.

    5. Plan for a follow-up or booster session.

E. Administer post-test questionnaires if applicable.

Session 10: Follow-up/Booster Session

A. Collect and review any additional Hassle Logs completed since the end of the formal program.

B. Program review. Before the session, write the name of each skill taught in the program on a blackboard. When the session begins asks each student to pick a skill and (1) describe/define the strategy; (2) demonstrate the strategy; and (3) discuss when is the best time/situation to implement the strategy.

   The skills taught include
   1. Deep breaths
   2. Concept of ABCs
      a. Antecedents
      b. Triggers
      c. Faulty reminders
      d. Behavior
      e. Consequences
   3. Assertion techniques and DEAR MAN and GIVE
   4. Reminders
   5. Thinking ahead
   6. Self-evaluation statements
   7. Problem solving
      a. What is the problem?
      b. What can I do?
      c. What will happen if . . .?
      d. What will I do?
      e. How did it work?
   8. Ask students to describe in detail several conflict situations that have occurred. Ask them to describe the various anger control techniques they used during the provocations.

C. In Closing:
   1. Provide students with feedback on
      a. His or her cooperation during the program.
      b. His or her performance during exercises and roles.
      c. His or her enthusiasm and/or interest in various components of the program.
      d. His or her motivation for change; being on time, completing homework assignments and Hassle Logs, and so on.
      e. Observable changes in behavior, including any anecdotal observations from other persons involved with the student.
   2. Ask students to give one another feedback in terms of positive change.
   3. Let the student know what you have learned by participating in the group and tell the student that you enjoyed working with him or her.
   4. Ask each group member to review his or her participation and any change since the program ended. Have each of them give self-evaluative praise statements regarding their participation and improvement in anger control. Prompt students to reinforce observed changes in each other.

5. Generalization and maintenance. Through group discussion review situations/events in which anger management led to a positive outcome. Also review situations in which their newly learned skills did not lead to a positive outcome. Brainstorm alternative responses.

6. Wrap-up. Thank students for coming and ask them to be a mentor to a friend who might benefit from learning anger management skills.

FUTURE CONSIDERATIONS FOR ANGER
MANAGEMENT INTERVENTIONS

Research has demonstrated sufficiently that anger management training results in specific emotional and behavioral changes in youth. According to the meta-analyses completed by Beck and Fernandez (1998) in which 25 of the 35 studies included children and adolescents, those receiving CBT treatment were better off than 76% of untreated subjects. However, few studies have examined long-term generalization and maintenance of behavior change and many studies suffer from assessment and methodological flaws (Feindler & Baker, 2004).

Anger management interventions are often complex packages of specific components delivered across several modalities. The five main components—arousal reduction, cognitive change, behavioral skills development, moral reasoning, and appropriate anger expression—can be provided in at least six different ways: (1) individual therapy; (2) group skills training; (3) family anger management; (4) dyadic anger managements, that is, with siblings; (5) parent-only anger management; and (6) classroom anger management education. To date, few research studies have compared treatment components across these modalities in terms of treatment efficacy and efficiency. The optional client-treatment match remains unclear and requires comprehensive assessment and comparative analyses. Further, most anger management interventions implemented in school or residential facilities are embedded within a behavior management system used to ensure the safety of all in congregate care. How these two programs interface and how they can complement one another to ensure generalization and maintenance of behavior change has yet to be explored. Similarly, the role of corollary interventions such as parent or staff training designed to enhance the outcomes of youth anger management needs examination.

Much recent research on the development of anger and aggression patterns in children and adolescents has focused on the various manifestations of aggression and the demarcation of subtypes. Although confusion in terms of diagnostic formulations continues (see Kassinove, 1995), future developments in youth anger management protocols should consider some of these subtypes. Distinctions between proactive and reactive aggression (Hubbard, Dodge, Cillessen, Coie, & Schwartz, 2001; Dodge, Lochman, Harnisch, Mates, & Petit, 1997) indicate that reactive aggression is related to the nature of the dyadic relationship and is characterized by heightened emotional arousal and hostile attribution bias. Distinctions between overt and relational aggression (Crick & Bigbee, 1998; Putallay & Bierman, 2004) highlight some interesting gender differences in manifestations of anger and aggression and indicates differences in social status of those who bully others and those who are victims of bullying (Griffin & Gross, 2004). Frick and his colleagues (2003) have suggested that certain youth who manifest conduct disorders and aggressive behavior patterns have identifiable callous and unemotional traits which clearly portend a poor treatment outcome. And finally, Tangney and colleagues (1996) have explored shame reactions of children and adolescents. Their research suggests that certain youth develop *shame-proneness*, which is associated with increased anger levels, suspiciousness, tendency to blame others, and indirect expressions of aggression. Since each of these subtypes of angry and aggressive youth presents a different clinical picture as well as a developmental history, we might hypothesize that different mechanisms operate in their anger difficulties. Hubbard and colleagues (Hubbard, McAuliffe, Rubin, & Morrow, 2007; Hubbard et al., 2001) suggest that if practitioners adopt a differentiated approach to treatment in order to target specific correlates, treatment efficacy might be enhanced. The matching of specific anger management strategies to the subtype of anger/aggression disorder would seem to be the direction for the future.

In summary, clinicians and researchers are encouraged to expand and explore the issues raised in the context of the available anger management treatment technology. Reviews of treatment outcome (Feindler & Baker, 2004; Feindler & Weisner, 2005) indicate that many youth across a variety of clinical, educational and detention settings will benefit from anger management. However, assessment issues remain a concern since the majority of evidence published to support treatment efficacy have relied on verbal report of youth and/or ratings by others, methods often influenced by subjectivity. Few studies have reported change in actual rates and intensities of aggressive behavior as directly observed or as recorded in a reliable and continuous fashion. The impact of youth anger and aggression outside of the treatment room remains a crucial aspect and requires continued emphasis.

References

Arnold, M. E., & Hughes, J. N. (1999). First do no harm: Adverse effects of grouping deviant youth for skills training. *Journal of School Psychology, 37*, 99–115.

Beck, R., & Fernandez, E. (1998). Cognitive behavioral therapy in the treatment of anger: A meta-analyses. *Cognitive Therapy and Research, 22*, 63–74.

Burney, D. M. (2001). *AARS: Adolescent anger rating scale: Professional manual.* Odessa, FL: Psychological Assessment Resources, Inc.

Buss, A. H., & Perry, M. (1992). The aggression questionnaire. *Journal of Personality and Social Psychology, 63*, 452–459.

Child Abuse Prevention Services. (2003). *What's up? Girl talk: A bully prevention workshop for girls.* Unpublished manuscript.

Connor, D. F. (2002). *Aggression and antisocial behavior in children and adolescents: Research and treatment.* New York: Guilford.

Crick, N. R., & Bigbee, M. A. (1998). Relational and overt forms of peer victimization: A multi-informant approach. *Journal of Consulting and Clinical Psychology, 66*, 337–347.

Crick, N. R., & Dodge, K. A. (1994). A review and reformulation of social information processing mechanisms in children's social adjustment. *Psychological Bulletin, 115*, 74–101.

Dishion, T. J., McCord, J., & Poulin, F. (1999). When interventions harm: Peer groups and problem behavior. *American Psychologist, 54*, 755–764.

Dodge, K. A., Lochman, J. E., Harnisch, J. D., Mates, J. E., & Petit, G. (1997). Reactive and proactive aggression in school children and psychiatrically impaired, chronically assaultive youth. *Journal of Abnormal Psychology, 106*, 37–51.

Feindler, E. L. (1987). Clinical issues and recommendations in adolescent anger control training. *Journal of Child and Adolescent Psychotherapy, 4*, 267–274.

Feindler, E. L. (1990). Cognitive strategies in anger control interventions for children and adolescents. In P. C. Kendall (Ed.), *Child and adolescent therapy: Cognitive-behavioral procedures* (pp. 66–97). New York: Guilford.

Feindler, E. L. (1995). An ideal treatment package for children and adolescents with anger disorders. In H. Kassinove (Ed.), *Anger disorders: Diagnosis, definition and treatment* (pp. 173–195). Washington, DC: Taylor & Francis.

Feindler, E. L., & Baker, K. (2004). Current issues in anger management interventions with youth. In A. P. Goldstein, R. Nensen, B. Daleflod, & M. Kalt (Eds.), *New perspectives on aggression replacement training: Practice, research and application* (pp. 31–50). New York: Wiley & Sons.

Feindler, E. L., Ecton, R. B., Kingsley, D., & Dubey, D. R. (1986). Group anger-control training for institutionalized psychiatric male adolescents. *Behavior Therapy, 17*, 109–123.

Feindler, E. L., & Guttman, J. (1994). Cognitive-behavioral anger control training. In C. W. LeCroy (Ed.), *Handbook of child and adolescent treatment manuals* (pp. 170–199). New York: The Free Press.

Feindler, E. L., Marriott, S. A., & Iwata, M. (1984). Group anger control training for junior high school delinquents. *Cognitive Therapy and Research, 8*, 299–311.

Feindler, E. L., & Ovens, D. (1998). *Treatment manual: Cognitive-behavioral group anger management for youth.* Unpublished manuscript.

Feindler, E. L., & Weisner, S. (2005). Youth anger management treatments for school violence prevention. In S. R. Jimerson & M. J. Furlong (Eds.), *Handbook of school violence and school safety: From research to practice* (pp. 353–363). Mahwah, NJ: Lawrence Erlbaum.

Frick, P. J., Cornell, A. H., Bodin, S. D., Dave, H. A., Barry, C. T., & Loney, B. R. (2003). Callous-unemotional traits and development pathways to severe conduct problems. *Developmental Psychology, 39*, 246–260.

Gibbs, J. D., Barriga, A. Q., & Potter, B. (2001). *How I think (HIT) questionnaire.* Champaign, IL: Research Press.

Griffin, R. S., & Gross, A. M. (2004). Childhood bullying: Current empirical findings and future directions for research, *Aggressive and Violent Behavior, 9*, 379–400.

Harvey, R. J., Fletcher, J., & French, D. J. (2001). Social reasoning—a source of influence on aggression. *Clinical Psychology Review, 21*, 447–469.

Hubbard, J. A., Dodge, K. A., Cillessen, A. H. N., Coie, J. D., & Schwartz, D. (2001). The dyadic nature of social information processing in boys' reactive and proactive aggression. *Journal of Personality and Social Psychology, 80*, 268–280.

Hubbard, J. A., McAuliffe, M. D., Rubin, R., & Morrow, M. T. (2007). The anger aggression relation in violent children and adolescents. In T. A. Cavell & K. T. Malcolm (Eds.), *Anger, aggression and interventions for interpersonal violence* (pp. 267–280). Mahwah, NJ: Lawrence Erlbaum.

Huesman, L. R., & Guerra, N. G. (1997). Children's normative beliefs about aggression and aggressive behavior. *Journal of Personality and Social Psychology, 72*, 408–419.

Kassinove, H. (Ed.). (1995). *Anger disorders: Definition, diagnosis, and treatment.* Washington, DC: Taylor & Francis.

Kazdin, A. E. (1995). *Conduct disorder in childhood and adolescence* (2nd ed.). Thousand Oaks, CA: Sage.

Keenan, K. (2000). Emotion dysregulation as a risk factor for child psychopathology. *Clinical Psychology: Science and Practice, 7*, 418–434.

Linehan, M. M. (1993a). *Cognitive-behavioral treatment of borderline personality disorder.* New York: Guilford.

Linehan, M. M. (1993b). *Skills training manual for treating borderline personality disorder.* New York: Guilford.

Lochman, J., & Dodge, K. A. (1994). Social-cognitive processes of severely violent, moderately aggressive and non-aggressive boys. *Journal of Consulting and Clinical Psychology, 62*, 366–374.

Meichenbaum, D. (1975). A self-instructional approach to stress management: A proposal for stress inoculation training. In C. Speilberger & I. Sarason (Eds.), *Stress and anxiety* (Vol. 2). New York: Wiley & Sons.

Nelson, W. M., III, & Finch, A. J., Jr. (2000). *Children's inventory of anger (CHIA) manual*. Los Angeles: Western Psychological Services.

Nelson, W. M., III, Finch, A. J., Jr., & Ghee, A. C. (2005). Anger management with children and adolescents: Cognitive behavioral therapy. In P. C. Kendall (Ed.), *Child and adolescent therapy: Cognitive-behavioral procedures* (3rd ed., pp. 114–165). New York: Guilford.

Novaco, R. W. (1975). *Anger control: The development and evaluation of an experimental treatment*. Lexington, MA: D.C. Heath & Co.

Putallay, M., & Bierman, K. (Eds.). (2004). *Aggressions, antisocial behavior and violence among girls*. New York: Guilford.

Smith, D. C., Furlong, M., Bates, M., & Laughlin, J. (1998). Development of the multidimensional school anger inventory for males. *Psychology in the Schools, 35*, 1–15.

Snyder, H. N., & Sickmund, M. (2006). *Juvenile offenders and victims: 2006 national report*. Washington, DC: U.S. Department of Justice, Office of Justice Programs, Office of Juvenile Justice and Delinquency Prevention.

Tangney, J. P., Wagner, P. E., Hill-Barlow, D., Marschall, D. E., & Gramzow, R. (1996). Relation of shame and guilt to constructive vs. destructive responses to anger across the lifespan. *Journal of Personality and Social Psychology, 70*, 797–809.

Weiss, B., Caron, A., Ball, S., Tapp, J., Johnson, M., & Weisz, J. R. (2005). Iatrogenic effects of group treatment for antisocial youth. *Journal of Consulting and Clinical Psychology, 73*, 1036–1044.

Chapter 7

TALK: Teens and Adults Learning to Communicate

Patricia Lester, MD, Mary Jane Rotheram-Borus, PhD, Carla Elia, PhD, Amy Elkavich, MA, and Eric Rice, PhD

There are more than one million people living with HIV/AIDS in the United States, many of whom are living longer with the aid of antiretrovirals and medical treatment (Kaiser Family Foundation, 2006). The transition of HIV/AIDS from an illness that primarily affects men who have sex with men (MSM) and intravenous drug users (IDU) to a chronic illness that disproportionately affects ethnic minority communities suggests a shift in our preventive intervention paradigm.

Using individual intervention models in the context of today's HIV/AIDS pandemic may not serve well in reaching prevention and treatment goals (Repetti, Taylor, & Seeman, 2002). People with HIV (PWH) now have longer life spans, increasing the opportunity to parent children. Furthermore, as one of our most

basic social structures, families often serve as primary support and caretakers when a family member is ill. Families require intervention programs designed not only to improve overall health and reduce transmission, but also to decrease the rates of infection for future generations. Child behaviors often reflect the routines and habits of their parents and they are at risk of imitating behaviors that may increase their chances of infection (Doherty, 1992). Therefore, it is essential to focus on the family and not only the individual when designing a prevention and treatment program (Rotheram-Borus, Flannery, Rice, & Lester, 2005).

In 1993, we began a randomized, controlled intervention trial called Project TALK (Teens and Adults Learning to Communicate). This family-based intervention was developed from a cognitive behavioral, skills training model (Rotheram-Borus, Lee, Gwadz, & Draimin, 2001; Rotheram-Borus et al., 2003; Rotheram-Borus, Lee, Lin, & Lester, 2004; Jemmott & Jemmott, 2000). From 307 PWH, 413 adolescents

Special thanks to the TALK facilitators who revised and updated the manuals: Sara Green, Connie Jackson, Talia Mandel. The authors also wish to thank Lisa Flook and Lynwood Lord.

were eligible for participation in the study (average n per family = 1.5, SD = 0.7, range 1–5). Families (PWH and all their adolescent children) were randomly assigned to the coping skills intervention condition (n = 153 PWH, n = 206 adolescents) or the control condition (n = 154 PWH, n = 207 adolescents). Intervention facilitators were provided with an extensive, detailed manual outlining each session's goals and activities (Rotheram-Borus et al., 2001).

The intervention was delivered in three modules. Module 1 of the intervention addressed challenges faced by the PWH during eight sessions and was only attended by parents. Three issues were addressed: (1) parents' negative emotions related to their serostatus; (2) reducing their own problem behaviors that impacted their ability to parent well; and (3) making decisions about disclosure of HIV status to their children.

The intervention's long-term goal was to improve children's adjustment, therefore, Module 2 included both parents and adolescents (if the parent had disclosed their serostatus). Parents were encouraged to make custody plans (Rotheram-Borus, Lester, Wang, & Shen, 2004) and were counseled on strategies to parent and monitor their children's behavior while ill. The program aimed to decrease adolescent's problem behaviors, emotional distress, and teenage pregnancy, negative outcomes previously associated with chronic parental illnesses (Romer et al., 2002). If parents died, the young people and their new parental guardians were invited to a third module for eight sessions focused on establishing positive relationships with the guardian and setting new life goals.

There were significant benefits for the families over four years (Rotheram-Borus et al., 2003). Parents decreased their problem behaviors and emotional distress for two years and were less likely to relapse into substance abuse or to be drug dependent over four years. Their adolescent children reported fewer problem behaviors and less emotional distress over two years, and were less likely to have babies and more likely to have positive coping styles at four years. While there was relapse in problem behaviors from two to four years following the intervention, adolescents' conduct problems and parents' problem behaviors tended to be lower in the intervention condition over four years compared to the control condition.

Six years after intervention, the adolescents in the intervention condition demonstrated a positive effect in several major tasks of young adulthood, including greater school enrollment, higher rates of employment, less welfare payments, and lower rates of early childbearing, all domains that have a high societal cost (Rotheram-Borus, Lee, et al., 2004). In addition, many years after daughters and their PWH received the family-based, skill-focused intervention, the grandchildren of PWH demonstrated significantly fewer behavioral symptoms and tended to have better cognitive outcomes and more enriched home environments than grandchildren in families coping with HIV who did not receive an intervention. Although these results were unexpected when the intervention was designed, they demonstrate the importance of providing interventions to families living with parental HIV.

A central challenge of preventive interventions for HIV/AIDS is adaptation. As treatments have improved and life expectancies have increased, families are confronted with new medical, social, and psychological stressors. Challenges faced by families affected by PLH today focus around the physical and emotional challenges of chronic illness, transmission behaviors for the PLH who continue to be sexually active, family conflict, imitative transmission behaviors of adolescents, substance abuse, and effective parenting practices. Intervention adaptation must also address contextual issues caused by geographic, immigration, cultural, linguistic, and practical differences in populations. The TALK intervention has evolved to meet changing needs of families affected by HIV/AIDS.

The most recent iteration of the TALK intervention is designed to meet the changing needs of a pandemic with intergenerational consequences. The family-based intervention has 16 sessions (12 parent only, 12 youth only, and 4 joint parent-youth sessions) and is delivered in 3 modules: (1) Healthy emotions; (2) Healthy living; (3) Family relationships. The adapted intervention retains core components, including (1) framing the impact of HIV/AIDS for families; (2) providing health-specific information; (3) skill building, including emotional regulation, problem solving, assertive communication, and skill building; (4) building social supports; and (5) addressing environmental barriers.

Framing the impact of HIV/AIDS begins at the time of intake, when the parent with HIV establishes a timeline for diagnosis and other family events since that time. This helps the participant frame the experience, and enables the facilitator to appreciate and normalize some of the family's experiences of diagnosis and illness. Early in the intervention the participant defines a *life project*, which also provides the participant with long-term goals in the context of HIV illness.

Social support building, when paired with SMART problem solving, helps participants make the positive decisions necessary to end destructive, unsupportive relationships. Assertiveness training increases successful communication and promotes internal strength in decisions made to preserve and promote overall health. These principles are the underlying foundation of the TALK intervention and are consistently employed by the facilitators throughout the intervention.

Role plays and group activities provide safe and engaging situations to begin practicing these principles in small groups. Some activities are central to the intervention and are used throughout the sessions. For example, the feeling thermometer is implemented as both an individual and group emotional regulation skill that participants use to label and regulate their emotions (Figure 7.1). Once introduced, participants use it to make connections among feelings, thoughts and behaviors, replacing unhealthy behavior and cognitions

with more adaptive ones. Similarly, other core skills, including problem solving, assertive communication, and goal setting are introduced and used throughout the intervention sessions. Goal setting skills promote self-efficacy and promote successful long-term responsibility concerning overall health and mental health.

In addition to role plays and activities, key group intervention techniques are used, including positive reinforcement, verbal praise, and tokens. Tokens are provided for use in every session and are meant to offer encouragement, promote interaction, and give positive feedback by both the facilitator and the participants. Facilitators are also trained to observe and identify nonverbal communication and promote verbal expression of thoughts and feelings. In this way, everyone is involved and each participant has a role.

Participants are taught the importance of both verbal and non-verbal communication, and the role that body language can play in effective assertive communication. Body language and facial expression are also discussed as possible ways of communicating unwanted behaviors or conflict with what is being said during role-plays and throughout the intervention. Facilitators are provided with suggestions on how to help participants who lack social skills take an active role within the group.

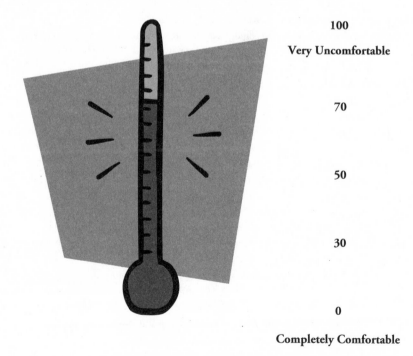

100

Very Uncomfortable

70

50

30

0

Completely Comfortable

FIGURE 7.1 The Feeling Thermometer.

Reframing is a concept introduced to help participants be more positive and seek positive solutions to potentially difficult or risky situations. By removing blame from a situation, facilitators help participants find confidence in their decision to say no, rather than guilt or shame. Reframing allows participants to uncover the intent of behavior and simplify problem solving. Reframing may also provide sufficient distance between parents and siblings to allow for a reduction of personal attachments and identification with a problem.

General clinical principles followed throughout the intervention are concerned with what shapes individual and family behavior. Shaping behavior involves knowing that a better learning experience will more likely lead to repeating it; and the longer the period of time between bad experiences, the more likely a good experience is bound to be repeated. Intervention design respects the iterative nature of behavior change, wherein effective change occurs in incremental steps, successively approaching the desired outcome.

It is important to highlight the notion of mutual dependence within families. As interdependent units, decisions impact both the individual and the family as a unit. The family unit is part of a larger community in which they receive both economic and social support. Decisions impacting the family may often be a product of the community and social environment they live and work in. Happier, better-adjusted families tend to influence behavior through reward giving rather than punishment. Social and behavioral problems often arise in families that have unclear role assignments and punishment as the chosen method of behavior change. Families function well if individual roles are clearly articulated and adults accept responsibility as caregivers.

The parent and joint sessions (parent and adolescent) for the TALK intervention are included below. Adolescent sessions parallel the parent version of the manual, and are not included due to space limitations, but may be obtained by contacting the authors (Dr. Lester or Dr. Rice). The overall principles and tools discussed in this introduction are explained in great detail prior to the intervention to ensure frequent use and adequate instruction during each of the sessions.

In closing, it is essential to continually assess intervention accuracy as it pertains to participant effectiveness. This specific intervention has gone through several edits and adaptations as the target population evolved. Cultural references and social norms were updated to retain maximum relevance and participant recognition. As the needs of those diagnosed with HIV/AIDS change, so too should the interventions designed to serve them.

References

Doherty, W. J. (1992). Linkages between family theories and primary health. In R. J. Sawa (Ed.), *Family Health Care* (pp. 30–39). Newbury Park, CA: Sage.

Jemmott, J. B., III, & Jemmott, L. S. (2000). HIV risk reduction behavioral interventions with heterosexual adolescents. *AIDS, 14*(Suppl 2), S40–S52.

Kaiser Family Foundation. (2006). People living with HIV/AIDS (adults and children). Retrieved March 1, 2007, from http://globalhealthfacts.org/topic.jsp?i=1&srt=2#table

Repetti, R. L., Taylor, S. E., & Seeman, T. E. (2002). Risky families: Family social environments and the mental and physical health of offspring. *Psychological Bulletin, 128*(2), 330–366.

Romer, G., Barkman, C., Schulte-Markwort, M., Thomalla, G., & Riedesser, P. (2002). Children of somatically ill parents: A methodological review. *Clinical Child Psychology and Psychiatry, 7*(1), 17–38.

Rotheram-Borus, M. J., Flannery, D., Rice, E., & Lester, P. (2005). Families living with HIV. *AIDS Care, 17*(8), 978–987.

Rotheram-Borus, M. J., Lee, M. B., Gwadz, M., & Draimin, B. (2001). An intervention for parents with AIDS and their adolescent children. *American Journal of Public Health, 91*, 1294–1302.

Rotheram-Borus, M. J., Lee, M., Lin, Y. Y., & Lester, P. (2004). Six year intervention outcomes for adolescent children of parents with HIV. *Archives of Pediatrics and Adolescent Medicine, 158*, 742–748.

Rotheram-Borus, M. J., Lester, P., Wang, P. W., & Shen, Q. (2004). Custody plans among parents living with human immunodeficiency virus infection. *Archives of Pediatrics and Adolescent Medicine, 158*, 327–332.

Rotheram-Borus, M. J., Lee, M., Leonard, N., Lin, Y. Y., Franzke, L., Turner, E., et al. (2003). Four-year behavioral outcomes of an intervention for parents living with HIV and their adolescent children. *AIDS, 17*(8), 1217–1225.

Module 1: Mental Health

Feeling, Thinking, Doing
Life Goals/Projects
Stress Management
Thinking and Acting SMART
Creating a Positive Environment at Home

Mom Session #1: Feeling, Thinking, Doing

Outcome and Skills

Outcome: Participants will be able to better identify and regulate their feelings, thoughts and behaviors.

Skill 1: Participants will identify uncomfortable situations surrounding HIV or an event from last week.

Skill 2: Participants will rate their comfort level on the feeling thermometer.

Skill 3: Participants will apply the FTD framework to events in their lives.

Agenda/Timeline (Total time: 105 min.)

Check-In (30 min.)

Introductions
Introduce tokens
Goals of the workshop
Group rules
Review of this session

Skills-Building (50 min.)

Increase ability to regulate feelings through:

Practicing FTD
Using feeling thermometer
Identifying uncomfortable/difficult situations

Relaxation Exercise (10 min.)

Wrap-Up and Goal Setting (15 min.)

Review goal for the week
Make one positive statement about oneself
Identify one gain made through the session
Preview next session and encourage attendance

Preparation/Materials

Post on the Wall Ahead of Time

FTD Poster
Feeling thermometer poster

Write on Flipchart Ahead of Time

Goals of group

Today's topic/goals for the session
Group rules
FTD triangle
Feeling thermometer chart

Other Materials Needed

Tokens
Goal cards
Pens

Handouts

Relaxation exercise
Feeling thermometer chart
FTD card
Feeling thermometer card
Goal cards

Check-In (30 min.)

Introductions

Welcome
First names
Participants identify one area of strength

> One good thing about themselves (as a parent or as a person)

Introduce tokens

Distribute

Distribute tokens

> We will be using these tokens throughout the sessions. Each of us will have a set at the beginning of each group. They are tokens of appreciation and help us be in touch with what we like.
> Whenever someone says or does something that makes you feel good, give them a token as a way of recognizing that you liked what they did or said.
> For instance, it can be when you feel proud of someone or you feel that you admire them. It can be a smile or the way someone listens to you.

Directions

Model use of tokens throughout the session

> When I notice something I like, I'll give a token (i.e., you just looked me in the eyes and that makes me feel like you are really listening to me; or you asked me a question which makes me feel like you care about what we are talking about.)
> Have any of you already noticed anything about anyone in the group that you like?

Goals of the Workshops: Why we are here

Write on flipchart ahead of time (in lay terms).

Overarching goals:

> Help you take better care of yourself
> Help you take better care of your children.

Sub goals:

Improve how you cope with stressful life situations
(i.e., daily routines: physical health, sadness and worry, parenting, relationships, etc.).
Increase the number of positive feelings, thoughts and behaviors.
(i.e., Learn to feel, think and act more positively about today, tomorrow, yourself and the people around you.)
Improve positive relationships with family, children, and yourself.
(i.e., better ways of communicating, resolving conflict, balancing personal and child needs, etc.)

Directions

Elicit other goals that participants may have.
Add goals generated by participants on flipchart.

Each of you may have other goals that you would also like for us to talk about.
Having goals gives us a powerful reason to want to take care of ourselves in order to make our dreams come true.
Having goals is also a great thing to model for your children so that they can learn to set goals for themselves. You can also teach them how to plan to accomplish their goals.

Don't Forget: Point out commonalities.

Group Rules

Generate group rules

It is important for you to feel safe in the group and to feel good about coming here.
What could be some rules or expectations that we can have that will help you feel comfortable about being HIV positive and being here?

Write group rules on flipchart and maintain throughout sessions

---

Don't Forget: It is important for the women to own the group rules. Therefore, allow them to generate the group rules so that it is individualized for the particular group. However, make sure to elicit the following rules:

Confidentiality among group members
Don't come high
Arrive 10 minutes before the group begins
Respect for individual differences
Stick to workshop content
Provide equal time

Directions

Remind participants that the group rules are intended to create a safe and supportive environment. Therefore, if a participant does not respect the group rules, the facilitator or other group members may ask the participant to leave the group for that day.

Review today's topic and goal for session

Write on flipchart ahead of time:

Pay more attention to:

1. How we feel
2. What we think
3. How we act in different situations

Write on flipchart ahead of time:

Connecting Feeling, Thinking and Doing (Triangle)

Skills-Building (50 min.)

FTD

Skill: Increase ability to regulate emotions by:

Applying FTD to a situation that makes participants feel uncomfortable
Connecting physiological responses, thoughts, and actions

Distribute

Distribute and review FTD.

F refers to feelings. Feelings are body reactions you have to a situation. For example, if you are feeling angry, where do you feel it in your body?

T refers to thoughts. Thoughts are things you say to yourself. For example, if you have to go on a job interview, you might say to yourself I am smart, I can do this, or you might say, "I am going to throw up," or you might say, "Why is that teacher so hard?"

D refers to what you actually do, to behaviors. For example, if you have an argument with your partner, you might yell, call a friend, slam doors, write in a journal, cry, leave, or take time to calm down.

Directions

Use a scenario to demonstrate FTD

If a teacher calls you about your child doing something disruptive in the class, what do you feel, where do you feel it, what goes through your head, what do you do?

Don't Forget: Normalize that we often do not pay attention to our thoughts as they are automatic.
Point out that FTD is typically a habit.

Feeling Thermometer

Skill: Increase ability to regulate emotions by becoming aware of the level of comfort and discomfort.

Distribute

Distribute and review Feeling Thermometer card

	Situation	Body Reaction	Thoughts	Action
00				
0				
0				
0				
0				

Directions

Discuss that the Feeling Thermometer will be applied throughout sessions to help participants become more aware of what situations make them feel comfortable and uncomfortable.

The goal is to teach members to identify emotional or physiological responses to different feeling thermometer ratings.

Sometimes people completely shut down; they feel they are at 0; they split what they feel and what they think and do; they miss the signs for 20, 40, 60…; they jump to 100; there are subtle cues at 20, 40, 60; We will try to figure out these cues.

Don't Forget: Throughout group, check-in with members about their thermometer rating; If their rating is lower, ask them what helped to lower it; Praise them for being able to lower their discomfort.

Identify uncomfortable situations

Skill: Increase ability to regulate emotions by becoming aware of triggers: Difficult situations

What is a situation in the past month that made you feel uncomfortable (100)? They may relate to being HIV+ or any situation that may have occurred in the past week.

Don't Forget: The goal of this exercise is to help participants learn more about themselves and their patterns.

We cannot regulate our emotions until we can anticipate and be aware of how we feel; Once we have identified our triggers (i.e., types of situations that are difficult for us), we can learn tools (i.e., relaxation, positive self-talk) to self-regulate (i.e., how to cope with a situation of high discomfort or anxiety).

Directions

Connect situation to feeling thermometer

When you are feeling 100, where do you feel it in your body?

Feeling Thermometer Chart

Skill: Increase ability to regulate emotions by becoming aware of the connection between feelings, thoughts, and behavior.

We want you to know your own pattern of feeling, thinking and acting.

We begin to learn our individual habits or profiles.

We each have different situations where we are at a 0 or a 60.

For example, where are you if you have to speak to your child's teacher; where are you when you have to tell your child that she is grounded; etc.

We want to learn to know what our feelings are and how to manage them.

Directions

Write Feeling Thermometer Chart on flipchart

Thermometer Reading	Situation	Body Reaction	Thoughts	Action

Complete chart on flipchart based on group's responses to identified situations.

Possible situations

When the doctor first told you that you were HIV positive

Telling people about HIV status

Going to the doctors and adhering to medication regimen

Family's reaction to HIV

Feeling like you have no control over your health

Refusing unprotected sex with a long-term partner

Distribute Feeling Thermometer Chart

Distribute

Distribute Feeling thermometer chart.

Ask participants to complete their charts with recent situations, allow enough time for participants to complete at least 2–3 examples at different Feeling Thermometer levels.

Relaxation Exercise (10 min.)

Before we end this exercise, I want to do one more thing. I want you think about a situation that would cause you a high degree of discomfort.

Now, let's do a relaxation exercise.

Relaxation Sequence: On the Beach

Get yourself in a comfortable position. PAUSE

Observe your breathing. PAUSE

Now breathe out deeply three times.

One PAUSE

Two PAUSE

Three PAUSE

Close your eyes if you wish as we take a little journey.

You are in a little house by the beach. PAUSE

You open the door to the deck, and, before you can even step outside, the sun greets you warmly.

See how blue the sky is. PAUSE

Just a few wispy clouds.

Smell the tangy salt air. PAUSE

Feel the breeze gently passing over the skin on your arms. PAUSE

You walk to the edge of the deck and step down into the fine white sand.

Feel the warm sand between your toes. PAUSE

You hear the surf breaking and the sea gulls crying.

See the waves slowly rolling on the shore. PAUSE

You walk on the soft sand, moving closer to the ocean, and spread your towel.

You sit watching the soothing rhythm of the sea.

In and out PAUSE

In and out PAUSE

In and out PAUSE

You lie there on the empty beach.

Feel the sun on your face. PAUSE

On your shoulders. PAUSE

On your stomach. PAUSE

On your arms. PAUSE

On your legs. PAUSE

On your feet. PAUSE

Your whole body becomes one with the sun, waves, sand and sky.

See the gulls gliding without effort, nodding on the breeze as if they were asleep. PAUSE

See the gulls gracefully swoop and bank and turn. PAUSE

Feel the breeze blowing softly, cooling and cleansing you.

You seem to sink into the sand.

Feel your breath becoming deep and slow. PAUSE

Feel your heartbeat—regular, an easy rhythm, strong. PAUSE

You rest. PAUSE

You rest a little longer. PAUSE

Slowly you sit up. PAUSE

You see a little purple shell carved by the sea so that it seems to have magical writing on it.

Put it in your pocket.

You stand up. PAUSE

Walk slowly back to the beach house. PAUSE

The sand covers your feet and you dig with your toes.

You are almost at the step to the deck.

Step up. PAUSE

You look back at the ocean feeling so refreshed.

So peaceful. Open the door to the house and go in.

THE END

Following the relaxation exercise:

Where are you on the Feeling Thermometer right now?

Throughout the sessions, we will learn different ways that can help us feel better in stressful situations.

Relaxation can be a helpful way of dealing with negative feelings or when you're feeling uncomfortable.

Don't Forget: A relaxation exercise, especially one that involves closing the eyes may trigger anxiety for some participants; therefore, you may want to end group with eliciting some examples of comfortable situations.

Skip eliciting comfortable situations if at the end of the relaxation exercise, group members report being at a comfortable feeling thermometer rating.

Wrap-Up and Goal Setting (10 min.)

Review goal for the week: Completion of Feeling Thermometer chart

Have each participant make one positive statement about herself OR share one positive thing she liked about the group.

Connect session to positive outcomes for the children of the women

How may today's discussion improve the lives of your children and/or your relationship with your children?

Preview next session and encourage attendance.

Mom Session #2: Life Goals/Projects

Outcome and Skills

Outcomes: Participant will identify a life project.

Skill 1: Participant will apply a goal-setting strategy to identify an important life project.

Skill 2: Participant will use a problem-solving technique to identify and address potential obstacles.

Agenda/Timeline (Total time: 90 min.)

Check-In (25 min.)

Review last week's goal.
Preview of this session.

Skills-Building (50 min.)

Review goal-setting steps.
Introduce life project.
Identify a life project.

Activity (10–15 min.)

Ring Toss

Wrap-Up and Goal Setting (15 min.)

Set a small short-term weekly goal related to life project.
Review life projects and weekly goals.
Make one positive statement about oneself.
Preview next session and encourage attendance.

Materials

FTD poster
Feeling thermometer poster
Goal setting poster

Group rules
Tokens
Weekly goal card
Small laminated goal cards
Flipcharts
Pens

Handouts

Feeling thermometer chart
Goal cards
"My life goals"

Post on Wall Ahead of Time

FTD poster
Feeling thermometer poster
Goal setting poster
Group rules

Write on Flipchart Ahead of Time

Today's topic/goals for the session
Life projects

Check-In (25 min.)

Discuss goal set at previous session

Review feeling thermometer chart completed during the last week.

What were some of the situations that you put on your chart?
Which situations were at a 20, 60, 80?

Directions

Write Feeling thermometer chart on flipchart and utilize as a way of reviewing
met goals. This may facilitate participants' understanding of FTD and the feeling
thermometer.

Don't Forget: Emphasize and participants have choices about how they feel.

Reflect on the relationship between FTD and participants (i.e., so you were at an 80
and told yourself that you are a failure and then ate a bag of potato chips and felt even
worse afterwards).

Praise participants for completing the chart.

Look for situations where participants may have applied a calming technique to reduce
their discomfort level.

Look for patterns where the participant was able to make positive self-statements which
may have helped in reducing her level of discomfort.

Directions

Discuss unaccomplished goals:

Identify barrier to accomplishing goal

Problem-solve barrier to accomplishing goal i.e. What got in your way of accomplishing your goal?

State the problem/potential obstacles (one sentence)
Make a goal (Realistic and Specific) (One sentence)
Actions–Make a list of all the possible actions you could take and evaluate the pros and cons of each option
Reach a decision about which action you want to try
Try it and review it

Don't Forget: SMART is made explicit in the next section on Stress Management. Therefore, at this point facilitator takes the lead on problem-solving SMART.

Review today's topic and plan for session

Write on flipchart ahead of time (in lay terms).

Goal setting

Develop strategies for setting a goal.

Life Projects

Discuss what a life project is.
Identify a life project.
Link goal setting skills with life project: Help you move towards achieving your life project by identifying small goals or steps that you can make towards your life project.

Skills-Building (50 min.)

Review Steps to Goal Setting

Skill: Increased ability to practice goal setting.
We are going to start out talking about some strategies for setting goals.
First, let's talk about how you feel when you set a goal and accomplish it.

Elicit participants' feedback (i.e., feel motivated, excited, think I can do anything).

What happens when you set a goal and you don't accomplish it?

Elicit participants' feedback (i.e., feel discouraged, embarrassed, give up)

These are the reasons why today we are going to spend some time, talking about how to set a goal that we will actually accomplish.

Directions

Refer to Goal Setting Poster

A goal is most helpful if it is:

Stated in *one sentence.*
Realistic (can reasonably expect to complete between sessions)
Clear (participant understands exactly what steps must be taken to complete the goal)
Not too easy and not too hard (30–50 on the feeling thermometer; goal should be challenging, but not impossible)

Clear end point (measurable, participant should know when the goal has been accomplished)

What do you want more of (stated in a positive term)

Activity

"Ring Toss" game

Intention/Purpose: After discussing TALK strategies for setting goals, introduce Ring Toss as a way to demonstrate the necessity of setting goals that are not too hard and not too easy so that they will be able to complete the goal with success. Also explain how some big goals/Life Project (a 20 foot toss) require many small goals (3 foot toss) in order to complete them. I.e. getting a job may be the 20 foot toss/big goal/life project. A 3 foot toss might be buying a newspaper and looking at the classified ads or calling to make an appointment with your case manager to talk about jobs. (NOTE: first step would be calling to make the appointment rather than having the goal be "Talk to my case manager." The case manager might not be in the office when the person calls or may not be able to see the participant for a week.) When discussing Life Projects and having participants identify their Life Projects, you can refer to them as 20 or 25 foot tosses, maybe even 100 foot toss depending on the project. This will help participants clarify the differences between various goals and see how there might be several small goals they can take to reach their Life Project.

Supplies/Set-Up: Ring Toss game with 6 rings, 1 base, duct tape, permanent marker. Set up base at one end of room, measure 3 feet from base (can estimate distance) and put a piece of duct tape down to mark 3 feet, write 3 on the tape. From 3 foot mark, measure another 3 feet and put a piece of tape down, write 6 on the tape. Continue as far as you can, till about 20 or 25 feet. Make sure path is clear for the toss and that participants can stand behind last marker.

Directions: Give each participant a ring or two depending on size of group. Allow them to try the game from whatever distance they want. Tell them simply that their goal is to get the ring on the base. Hopefully participants will try from far distances first. Ask each participant where they are going to start. As the game continues, reinforce that the goal is to get the ring on the base and allow participants to attempt from any distance. They will probably choose closer markers until going for the 3 foot toss. In the last round make sure everyone tries from the 3 foot mark and gets the ring on the base.

Notes to Facilitator: Activity should be fun and lively. Facilitator should clap and cheer for all attempts and get group to support each other in a similar way. If facilitator is enthusiastic, participants will feel comfortable "playing"—something many of them might not have done for some time!

Group Discussion: When group returns to seats, open discussion for their ideas about how the activity relates to setting goals. Emphasize that they all completed their goal—getting the ring on the base—when they tried their toss from the 3 foot mark and that this relates to how we set and complete our goals in real life.

Distribute

Distribute goal setting card.

It is important to keep these strategies and steps in mind. When setting the goal, as they will increase the likelihood of achieving our goals.

We will refer to these goal setting steps throughout every session. There will be many opportunities to practice these steps.

Directions

Elicit a goal from the participants in order to practice the goal setting steps.

Repeat this one or two times in order to ensure that the goal setting steps are clear.

If participants are unable to identify the goal use the below examples to illustrate goal setting.

For example, what might be difficult about having the goal of winning a million dollars in a lottery?

Generate feedback from participants.
If needed, assist participants in seeing that this is not a realistic goal.

What might be difficult about having the goal of being a good person?

Generate feedback from participants.
If needed, assist participants in seeing that this is not a goal with clear steps or an end point.

What about having the goal of getting a degree in an area that you've always been interested in?

Generate feedback from participants.
This will likely be a realistic goal once the participant has engaged in problem-solving potential barriers (i.e., obtaining financial aid, securing childcare, securing transportation, etc.)

Introduce Life Projects

We are now going to talk about some of the life projects that you may have for yourself.
As a woman and a mother, you probably spend a lot of time taking care of others. This is an opportunity to focus on yourself and think about what is important to you.
We may have set goals for ourselves but haven't had the chance to work on them because life happens: We get married. We have children.
Many people living with HIV have put these goals on hold because they have focused on their health and rightly so. The Life Project is a way for you to shift some attention back to goals for yourself.
There are some good reasons why we want you to take some time and think about what is important to you and what your life projects are. Why do you think life projects are important to have?

Elicit the group members' feedback. Include the following:

1. First, people with goals are usually more interested in taking care of themselves.
2. Second, your families are naturally worried about what is going to happen to you. If you have goals, they will worry less.
3. Life projects give us meaning and purpose to our lives.
4. Keeping your eye on your most important goals helps you make small and big decisions that will help you get closer to your life projects.
5. Life projects give you motivation when times are difficult or when you do not feel motivated.
6. Life projects are also important because they model for your children the importance of setting goals and working towards them.

What are life projects?
A life project can be any dream that you ever had for yourself.
You can find them in daydreams, in what you think about when you are alone, in what you talk to your closest friend about.
It can be something that you always wanted to do but weren't able to maybe because of different obstacles that came your way.
It may also be something that you started but then got sidetracked and were not able to accomplish.

I want to emphasize that what is important to one person won't be important to someone else.

Each person's life project should be accepted as valuable.

Examples of Life Projects:

"To get a training certificate"

"To learn English"

"To learn to play a music instrument"

"To become a teacher"

Identify Life Projects

Skill: Increased ability to set a realistic life project.

Facilitate each member in identifying a life project.

Distribute

Distribute "My Life Project" Worksheet

There are different types of projects and dreams people have; examples include: education, work, romance/marriage, friends, achievements, feeling good about yourself.

I want you to write in your life projects.

You can make new categories or use some of the categories on the sheet.

You don't have to show your life project sheet to anyone.

My Life Project Goals

Instructions: under each category write your life project goals. You can have more than one goal under a category.

Education (examples: Get my GED; Get my B.A. or A.A. degree; Get a training certificate)

Work (examples: keep one job for a long time, work near home, or work as a nurse):

Relationship With Others

Family (example: talk to my child without yelling at her/him):

Partner (example: find a partner who accepts my HIV, be with a partner who does not hit me or verbally put me down):

Friends (examples: spend more time with my friends, or find friends similar to me):

Achievements (examples: learn to drive or play an instrument):

Feeling Good About Myself (examples: exercise, eat healthy, relaxation, volunteer):

Directions

Remind members that a life project can be related to any area in a person's life: that is, physical health, children, relationships, career, education, and so on.

Allow 5–10 minutes for filling out life projects

Now get with someone else in the room and share the life project you are comfortable talking about.

Allow five minutes for sharing.

Split up the pairs so that each participant can share their life project with the group.

Pick your most important life project and tell the group what it is. Make sure it is something you are really interested in because we will talk about this topic more as we go along.

It should also be something that you can work towards while we're participating in these workshops. It does NOT have to be completed by the time that the workshops end.

Encourage group members to generate ideas for those who may have difficulty identifying a life project.

Ask questions so that you can have a clear picture of each participant's life project.

Look for common life projects/themes among participants: Attempt to link up these participants in conversation.

Identify barriers to goals.

If time avails, problem-solve barriers to the life project. A participant may initially engage in brainstorming and identify 2–3 possible life projects; Evaluate these options in order for the participant to select the one life project with the most advantages for them or the one that is the most meaningful or realistic for them to work on.

Praise participants for their life projects.

Write each member's life projects on the flipchart: Keep this for future sessions.

Return the flipchart sheet with life projects to each session hereafter and post on the wall.

Write each member's life project for yourself so that you can reference to their weekly goal and check-in with member's progress on a weekly basis.

The life project should be referenced to throughout the intervention. This can be done in a number of ways. For example:

1. During the check-in, conduct a quick general follow-up with the participants (i.e., Is everyone keeping their life project goal in mind and working towards it?)
2. Some of the life project may not entail weekly small goals. For instance, if one member's life project is to get her A.A. degree, she may need to wait 3 weeks for the date of registration. Therefore, there is no need for a weekly check-in. You can do a quick reminder (i.e., we can't wait to hear how it goes when you go to registration next week) and then move on to the next participant.
3. If the weekly session (i.e., healthy physical habits) ties in with the life project (lose 20 pounds in one year), reference to the life project during the session.

Wrap-Up and Goal Setting (5 min.)

Goal Setting Surrounding Life Project

Don't Forget: Engage in goal setting ONLY if each participant has managed to identify a life project; If this has not been accomplished, use the remainder of the session to help each participant identify a life project.

Display great excitement and enthusiasm as you remind members that you and the rest of the group will be looking forward to hearing how each member's progress with their goal went.

Don't Forget: Have the above components of goal setting in mind as participants set their goals in order to optimize their ability to achieve their goal. However, remember that they were just introduced to goal setting steps in today's session and will have the remainder of the workshops to practice these steps. Therefore, the facilitator may take the lead in helping participants set realistic goals.

Make sure that each participant leaves with a meaningful goal. This will give them something to look forward to and want to return to the group and report about.

Identify a short-term goal (for the week) that is related to the life project.

> We are going to link the goal setting steps that we reviewed in the beginning of the session with your life projects.
>
> What this means is that you can begin to make small weekly goals that will help you reach your life projects. These small goals are small steps that you can take towards your bigger life project.
>
> What is a small step that you can take between now and next week towards your life project?

Review goals and distribute goal card.

> The goal of the week may either be the short-term goal related to life project or identifying a life project (for those who were unable to accomplish this in session).

Make one positive statement about oneself or say one thing you learned from today's group

Preview next session and encourage attendance.

Mom Session #3: Stress Management

Outcome and Skills

Outcomes: Participants will be able to appropriately apply coping strategies to identified personal stressors.

Skill 1: Participants will identify current stressors and coping strategies.

Skill 2: Participants will apply FTD and SMART as coping strategies to deal with unchangeable and/or changeable stressors.

Outcomes: Participant will be able to apply strategies in remaining calm, especially in high pressure situations.

Skill 1: Participant will practice imagery, deep breathing, and progressive muscle relaxation.

Agenda/Timeline (Total time: 90 min.)

Check-In (25 min.)

Review last week's goal
Preview of this session

Skills-Building (55 min.)

Identify current stressors
Practice imagery
Identify current coping strategies
FTD as means of coping with stressors
SMART as means of coping with stressors
Apply problem-solving to an identified stressor
Practice deep breathing
Rest, relaxation, and sleep
Goal setting related to identified stressors and Life Projects
Practice progressive muscle relaxation

Wrap-Up and Goal Setting (10 min.)

Review goals
Connect weekly goals to life projects
Make one positive statement about oneself
Preview next session and encourage attendance

Materials

FTD poster
Feeling thermometer poster
SMART poster
Goal setting poster
Group rules
Participant life projects
Tokens
Goal card
Flipcharts
Pens

Handouts

Goal card
SMART cards
Imagery
Deep breathing
Progressive muscle relaxation

Post on the Wall Ahead of Time

FTD poster
Feeling thermometer poster
Goal setting poster
SMART poster
Group rules
Participant life projects

Write on Flipchart Ahead of Time

Today's topic/goals for the session

Check-In (25 min.)

Discuss goal set at last session

Life project goal *and* goal related to last week's session topic.

Don't Forget: The life project goal should be posted on the wall and referenced to throughout the intervention. This can be done in a number of ways. For example:

During the check-in, conduct a quick general follow-up with the participants (i.e., is everyone keeping their life project goal in mind and working towards it?)

During the check-in, conduct a more specific follow-up asking members for their progress with their goals.

Some of the life project goals may not entail weekly small goals. If so, there is no need for a weekly check-in. You can do a quick reminder and then move on to the next participant.

Identify barrier to accomplishing goal

Don't Forget: Make sure that original goal was realistic. Use this as an opportunity to emphasize the importance of setting realistic goals in order to optimize success.

Review today's topic and plan for session

Write on flipchart ahead of time (in lay terms):

How to cope with stressors

How are you currently dealing with your stressors?
What strategies can you use in different situations to reduce your stress?
What strategies can you use to help you stay calm, especially in high pressure situations?

Skills-Building (55 min.)

Identify current stressors and relate to feeling thermometer

What are some recent situations that have happened with your friends, partner, children, family members that have put you at an 80–100?

Don't Forget: Each participant identifies at least one current stressor.

Directions

Write stressors on flipchart.

Strategy for Remaining Calm: Imagery

It can be stressful to think about our stressors the way we just spent some time identifying individual stressors. So right now, we are going to practice a strategy that can help us remain calm.
There are many skills that can be used to help us to remain calm and to be good decision-makers, even in high-pressure situations.
The same skills can help reduce feelings of stress. The first one is imagery.
The idea behind the use of imagery in reducing your stress and how uncomfortable you may feel is that you can use your imagination to enjoy a situation that is very relaxing.
The more intensely you imagine the situation, the more relaxing the experience will be.
You simply imagine a place that you think of as safe and peaceful.
You can use all of your senses to imagine it. For example, if you want to imagine being at the beach, you might think of the sounds of birds, the smell of the beach, the taste of salty water, and the warmth of the sun.

Directions

Practice Imagery

Get yourself in a comfortable position.
You might want to close your eyes, but you don't have to. (PAUSE)
I want you to think of a place that is familiar and comfortable for you.

A place where it is safe, comfortable, and peaceful. (PAUSE)

Have you got it?

Now, really picture that place.

Notice the colors there. (PAUSE)

Notice the smells there. (PAUSE)

Hear the sounds there. (PAUSE)

Feel that special place on your fingertips. (PAUSE)

See yourself there—feeling good, feeling calm, feeling at peace. (PAUSE)

Let yourself really sink into that special place. (LONG PAUSE)

Now, take a deep breath, and, if your eyes are closed, keep them closed a minute more.

Now I want you to think of your favorite flower. (PAUSE)

See that flower as a bud—not yet open.

See it begin to open. (PAUSE)

See it open a little more. (PAUSE) Look at the colors.

Now it is half way open. (PAUSE) The colors are becoming brighter.

Look at how beautiful the flower has become. (PAUSE)

It's fully open! (PAUSE)

Okay, come back into the room now.

You might want to yawn and stretch. (PAUSE)

Okay, how was that for you?

You can also use imagery to practice something that makes you nervous to do.

This is a technique frequently used by top athletes, who practice in their minds before a big game.

Identify current coping strategies for handling stressors

Directions

Categorize coping strategies based on FTD.

List may include exercise, social support network, relaxation techniques, writing, walking, reading, watching TV.

Emphasize the importance of *Rest, Relaxation and Sleep*

Some people do not realize that it is healthy to get enough rest and relaxation, and unhealthy not to rest each day.

Most people need at least nine hours of sleep a night; some need more and some need less.

If we don't get enough sleep, our energy and concentration go down and we do not function well or make good decisions.

What types of things do you find relaxing or restful?

Relaxation habits may include: walking, reading, writing, or watching TV, etc.

How many of you get about 8 hours of sleep?

Don't Forget: Emphasize and praise participants' strengths in coping with challenging and stressful situations.

This is an opportunity for participants to connect and learn from each other.

Discuss FTD as a coping strategy

A little while ago, we practiced imagery as one way of helping us cope with our stressors.

We can cope with different stressors by:

Feeling different (i.e., working on bringing our feeling thermometer to a more comfortable state by using a relaxation exercise),

Thinking different (i.e., having more positive thoughts or positive self-talk).

Activity:

We can't change our situations, but we can change the ways we think about them. In this activity we think we see one thing and then realize there are other ways to see it. We can choose to have our minds be more flexible about what we perceive to be going on in our lives.

Acting different (i.e., brainstorming different choices and picking the best one).

Thinking differently

Sometimes you can't change the situation, but you can make the most out of it.

For instance, you are not able to change the fact that you are HIV+.

However, you can cope with the diagnosis by changing your thoughts about it (i.e., reminding yourself that you can still have goals and hopes, that you want to live a long life because of your children, or that medications and healthy habits can help you stay well).

Acting different

Sometimes you can change the situation if you use your SMART problem-solving.

For instance, if you are stressed because your partner is hesitant about using a condom, there may be actual steps that you can take to cope with or change the situation (i.e., talk to him assertively about wanting him to use a condom, think about whether you want to continue being intimate with him, consider using a female condom for protection, etc.)

Introduce SMART as a coping strategy

We've talked about "acting differently" as a way of coping with stressors.

So let's talk about the different choices that we have in situations and how we can go about making the best choice.

Directions

Review smart chart

Don't Forget: Make above problem-solving steps explicit for participant and review throughout session each time there is an opportunity for problem solving.

Distribute

Distribute smart cards

Apply problem solving to identified stressors

1. State the stressor
2. Make a goal (Realistic and Specific); (one sentence)
3. Actions—Make a list of all the possible actions you could take and evaluate the pros and cons of each option
4. Reach a decision about which action you want to try
5. Try it and review it

Don't Forget: In step 3, discourage members from criticizing the options; Stress that at this step, we are trying to generate as many options as possible.

In generating options/actions, encourage participants to reflect on strategies they've used in the past that have been effective.

Encourage members to generate option/solutions.

Apply problem solving to as many identified stressors as time avails.

Strategy for remaining calm: Deep breathing

We have worked hard coming up with ways of coping with your stressors. So now we will try to relax by practicing another strategy that can help us remain calm in stressful situations.

All you have to do is take a number of deep, slow breaths and relax your body further with each breath. That's all there is to it!

Directions

Practice

Get yourself in a comfortable position. (PAUSE)

Pay attention to your breathing.

Don't try to change your breathing. Just pay attention to it. (PAUSE)

Become aware of your breathing out and your breathing in. (PAUSE)

Breathe in and pause. Breathe out and pause.

Breathe in and pause. Breathe out and pause.

Breathe in and pause. Breathe out and pause.

Now just pay attention to breathing out.

If you wish to close your eyes, that is fine.

Breathe out three times.

Out (PAUSE)

Out (PAUSE)

Out (PAUSE)

Feel your breath like a gate swinging back and forth in the breeze. (PAUSE)

Again three times.

Out (PAUSE)

Out (PAUSE)

Out (PAUSE)

Let all the tension go out with your breath. (PAUSE)

Feel the tension flowing out of your body and mind. (PAUSE)

Feel the calm—the peace—filling your body. (LONG PAUSE)

Okay, how was that for you?

Strategy for remaining calm: Progressive muscle relaxation

Before we end today, we will practice one last relaxation strategy.

This is especially good for those of you that tense your muscles when you feel stressed.

If you get headaches a lot, it might be from tense muscles

The idea behind Progressive Muscle Relaxation is that you tense up a group of muscles and then relax them. You do the same thing through your whole body, one area at a time.

By tensing your muscles before you relax them, you will find that you are able to relax your muscles more than would be the case if you tried to relax your muscles directly.

Directions

Practice

Get yourself in a comfortable position. (PAUSE)

Now make a tight fist with your right hand.

Feel the tension in your hand.
Open your hand and let the tension fly away.
Let's get rid of the tension in your body.
Now, tighten the muscles in your face. (PAUSE)
Do you feel tension? (PAUSE)
Sigh deeply and let it go.
Now, tighten the muscles in your shoulders. (PAUSE)
Sigh deeply and let it go.
Now, tighten the muscles in your arms. (PAUSE)
Sigh deeply and let it go.
Now, tighten the muscles in both of your hands and fingers. (PAUSE)
Sigh deeply and let it go.
Now, tighten the muscles in your stomach. (PAUSE)
Sigh deeply and let it go.
Now, tighten the muscles in your thighs. (PAUSE)
Sigh deeply and let it go.
Now, tighten the muscles in your feet and toes. (PAUSE)
Sigh deeply and let it go.
If you feel any remaining tension in your body, tighten those muscles (PAUSE)
Now sigh deeply and let it go.

Wrap-Up and Goal Setting (10 min.)

Goal Setting

Skill: Setting a goal related to an identified stressor.

Don't Forget: Each participant should set one goal that can be accomplished by next week's session.
    Participants may use the goal identified during the problem-solving exercise as their goal for the week.

Identify a goal related to a stressor AND a goal related to life project.

1. State goal in one sentence.
2. Realistic (can reasonably expect to complete between sessions)
3. Clear (participant understands exactly what steps must be taken to complete the goal)
4. Not too easy and not too hard (30–50 on the feeling thermometer; goal should be challenging, but not impossible)
5. Clear end point (measurable, participant should know when the goal has been accomplished)
6. What do you want more of (stated in a positive term)

Distribute goal card to help participants remember their weekly goal.
Make one positive statement about oneself.
Preview next session and encourage attendance.

Wrap Up Exercise #1

Imagery (this can be printed out and used as a handout)

Get yourself in a comfortable position.
You might want to close your eyes, but you don't have to. (PAUSE)

I want you to think of a place that is familiar and comfortable for you.
A place where it is safe, comfortable, and peaceful. (PAUSE)
Have you got it?
Now, really picture that place.
Notice the colors there. (PAUSE)
Notice the smells there. (PAUSE)
Hear the sounds there. (PAUSE)
Feel that special place on your fingertips. (PAUSE)
See yourself there—feeling good, feeling calm, feeling at peace. (PAUSE)
Let yourself really sink into that special place. (LONG PAUSE)
Now, take a deep breath, and, if your eyes are closed, keep them closed a minute more.
Now I want you to think of your favorite flower. (PAUSE)
See that flower as a bud—not yet open.
See it begin to open. (PAUSE)
See it open a little more. (PAUSE) Look at the colors.
Now it is half way open. (PAUSE) The colors are becoming brighter.
Look at how beautiful the flower has become. (PAUSE)
It's fully open! (PAUSE)
Okay, come back into the room now.
You might want to yawn and stretch. (PAUSE)

Deep Breathing (this can be printed and used as a handout)

Get yourself in a comfortable position. (PAUSE)
Pay attention to your breathing.
Don't try to change your breathing. Just pay attention to it. (PAUSE)
Become aware of your breathing out and your breathing in. (PAUSE)
Breathe in and pause. Breathe out and pause.
Breathe in and pause. Breathe out and pause.
Breathe in and pause. Breathe out and pause.
Now just pay attention to breathing out.
If you wish to close your eyes, that is fine.
Breathe out three times.
Out (PAUSE)
Out (PAUSE)
Out (PAUSE)
Feel your breath like a gate swinging back and forth in the breeze. (PAUSE)
Again three times.
Out (PAUSE)
Out (PAUSE)
Out (PAUSE)
Let all the tension go out with your breath. (PAUSE)
Feel the tension flowing out of your body and mind. (PAUSE)
Feel the calm—the peace—filling your body. (LONG PAUSE)

Progressive Muscle Relaxation (this can be printed and used as a handout)

Get yourself in a comfortable position. (PAUSE)
Now make a tight fist with your right hand.
Feel the tension in your hand.
Open your hand and let the tension fly away.
Let's get rid of the tension in your body.
Now, tighten the muscles in your face. (PAUSE)

Do you feel tension? (PAUSE)
Sigh deeply and let it go.
Now, tighten the muscles in your shoulders. (PAUSE)
Sigh deeply and let it go.
Now, tighten the muscles in your arms. (PAUSE)
Sigh deeply and let it go.
Now, tighten the muscles in both of your hands and fingers. (PAUSE)
Sigh deeply and let it go.
Now, tighten the muscles in your stomach. (PAUSE)
Sigh deeply and let it go.
Now, tighten the muscles in your thighs. (PAUSE)
Sigh deeply and let it go.
Now, tighten the muscles in your feet and toes. (PAUSE)
Sigh deeply and let it go.
If you feel any remaining tension in your body, tighten those muscles (PAUSE)
Now sigh deeply and let it go.

Mom Session #4: Thinking and Acting SMART

Outcome and Skills

Outcomes: Participants will increase practice of SMART thinking and acting.
Skill 1: Participants will learn SMART thinking and acting strategies.
Skill 2: Participants will set goals for increased SMART thinking and acting.
Skill 3: Participants will set a short-term goal for the week related to SMART thinking and acting and use a problem-solving technique to identify and address potential obstacles to goal.

Agenda/Timeline (Total time: 95 min.)

Check-In (20 min.)

Review last week's goal
Preview of this session

Skills-Building (50 min.)

Increase practice of SMART thinking and acting by

Defining current thinking and acting habits
Identifying SMART thinking habits
Identifying SMART acting habits

Activity (5–10 min.)

Self-talk descriptions
Muscle testing activity

Problem-Solving (15 min.)

Set a goal related to thinking and acting SMART
Set a life project goal
Problem-solve barriers to accomplishing goal

Wrap-Up and Goal Setting (10 min.)

Review goals
Connect session to life projects

Make one positive statement about oneself
Preview next session and encourage attendance

Materials

FTD poster
Feeling thermometer poster
Goal setting poster
SMART poster
Group rules
Tokens
Weekly goal card
Small laminated goal cards
Flipcharts
Pens

Handout

Goals related to thinking and acting SMART

Post on Wall Ahead of Time

FTD poster
Feeling thermometer poster
Goal setting poster
SMART poster
Group rules
Participant life projects

Write on Flipchart Ahead of Time

Today's topic/goals for the session

Check-In (25 min.)

Discuss goals set at last session

Life project goal AND goal related to last week's session topic.
Identify barriers to unaccomplished goals
See Appendix A for How to Identify Barriers to Accomplishing Goal

Review today's topic and plan for session

Write on Flipchart Ahead of Time (in lay terms).

Thinking and Acting SMART

Increase awareness of your current habits: how you usually feel, think and act.
Identify and practice SMART habits for feelings, thinking and acting.
Learn SMART ways of coping with your feelings, thoughts and difficult situations.
Set goals for thinking and acting SMART.
Set a short-term goal for the week related to SMART thinking and acting and
problem-solve potential obstacles to goal.

Skills-Building (50 min.)

Provide rationale for thinking and acting SMART

Just as someone might get enough sleep, eat well and exercise to take care of their physical health, a person can also do things to take care of their emotional health.

When it comes to reaching your life projects, thinking and acting SMART is just as important as being physically healthy.

Emotional health and physical health affect each other.

When emotions run high, when you're at a 100 on the feeling thermometer, when discomfort is high, it is harder to make good decisions or to take appropriate actions.

When emotions run high, it is easy to over-react, exaggerate, or not think as clearly as usual.

It can be very helpful to reduce discomfort and manage your emotions before making decisions or taking action.

There are different things that you can do to help yourself be "more SMART" about the way you feel, think and act.

Today, we will focus on how you can think SMART.

Identify a recent difficult situation

What is something that happened this past week that made you uncomfortable? Your feeling thermometer was over a 60?

Assess F: What was your feeling thermometer rating and body reactions.

Assess T: When this situation happened, what thoughts went through your mind?

Assess D: What do you end up doing?

Don't Forget: Use difficult situations to demonstrate FTD and the impact of thoughts on our behaviors. These situations may be used to illustrate how our thoughts may lead to negative outcomes and therefore, the importance of learning ways to think SMART.

Provide examples of how a self-talk habit might impact comfort level

To get started, I would like you to use your Feeling Thermometer to rate your comfort level related to certain ways that you may usually think.

I will read a habit about how you might talk to yourself when you are about to take a test and you record what your comfort level would be.

The situations are:

1. You are about to go on an interview and you say to yourself, "I know what to say, and I am going to do really well on this interview."
2. You are about to go on an interview and you say to yourself, "*This is going to be super hard, and I might blow this interview.*"
3. You are about to go on an interview and you say to yourself, "If I don't do well on this interview and don't get this job, I will never be able to get a job."

Can you see how saying different things to yourself can change your feeling thermometer?

Who would probably do best on the interview?

Why?

So as you can see our thoughts end up affecting the way we feel and the actions that we take.

Activity

Self Talk Descriptions on flipchart

Positive/Negative Self-Talk

Intention/Purpose: This activity allows participants to name the positive and negative self-talk that might be going on for the "participant" stick figure on the flipchart. With this displacement, participants can more easily identify how this "person" might be talking to themselves under similar circumstances as the members of the group.

Supplies: On flipchart draw the following image.

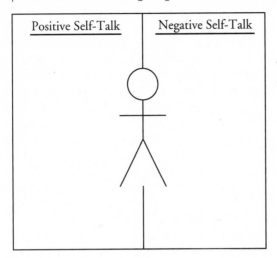

| Positive Self-Talk | Negative Self-Talk |

Figure 7.2

Directions: Tell participants that the "person" on the flipchart is in a similar situation as the participants. If this is a MOM group, then the person on the flipchart is an HIV+ woman with children. She may or may not have a partner, job, citizenship, etc. If this is a TEEN group, the teen has a mom who is HIV+, the person may or may not be HIV+ themselves, they are in school, have friends who may or may not know about their mom's status, may be sexually active, having an easy or challenging time in school, etc. Ask participants what they think would be going through this person's mind. What are they saying to themselves, positively and negatively? Hopefully participants will begin to give examples that they themselves have going on in their minds. The facilitator can ask, "If you were this person, what would you be saying to yourself?"

Group Discussion: This activity creates a visual of the amount of self-talk going on inside of participants. Allow participants to make connections between how we talk to ourselves affects how we think, feel and what we do (FTD Triangle). Ask how the self-talk on the chart affects the Feeling Thermometer of the "person" on the chart? What kinds of things affect how we talk to ourselves? How can we spend more time "talking to ourselves" in a positive way?

Activity

Muscle Testing

Intention/Purpose: This is an experiential activity to demonstrate how our thoughts and emotional health can affect us physiologically—that our bodies and physical health respond to our thoughts—both negative and positive. The hope is that participants will have an "ah-ha" moment about connecting the importance of thinking positively to maintaining good health. Many participants will have read or heard something about the power of the mind and our thoughts—this is a real-life experience of that power!

Set-Up: Ahead of time write on the flipchart the questions or phrases you will have participants say out loud during the activity:

"My name is…"
"I live in… (city)…"
"I hate myself, I am a terrible person."
"I love myself very much, I am a wonderful person."

Directions: Ask for a volunteer from the group, if none come forward choose someone who you think will be comfortable up in front of the group. Tell them that in a moment they will extend an arm straight out to the side at shoulder level. They will try to maintain their arm like that as you gently but firmly push down (using 2 fingers) on their arm. It is important that they try to resist you. Explain this to the volunteer and also the whole group since they will be doing the activity once the demo is over! Once you have explained what you are going to do and the volunteer understands, ask them to extend their arm and answer or say the four phrases, one at a time, as you try to push their arm down. Take your time with each phrase to try and push the arm down. Tell the group out loud what you are experiencing and noticing, as in, "her arm is still strong," "notice how her arm barely moved." Also check-in with the volunteer as to what they notice especially when they say phrase #4, confirm with the volunteer that their arm felt weaker when they were saying that they are a terrible person—you should have been able to push their arm down MORE than in the first three tries.

Thank the volunteer and then have the group pair up and try the activity on each other. Make sure each person, including the volunteer gets a chance to try both roles. Keep checking in with the "pushers" and "pushees" during the activity to make sure they are noticing a difference. After everyone has had a try return to seats.

Teens may want to try out more phrases, the difference between saying things that are true—"I'm 16 years old" and things that are false, "I live in Iceland." Allow participants to experiment until they feel complete and like they have totally experienced the activity.

Notes to Facilitator: Activity should be fun and lively. It is okay for participants to laugh and giggle. Make sure teen groups don't start hurting each other by resisting and pushing too hard! If a group seems to be having trouble "making it work" assist them by walking them through the process.

Group Discussion: When group returns to seats, open discussion for their experiences of the differences they noticed. It is easier to push down people's arms when they say phrase 3, they hate themselves and that they are terrible people, because it is a negative thought and is unsupportive—our negative thoughts weaken our bodies, self-esteem, and motivation to accomplish our goals. This can lead to a discussion about the importance of thinking SMART and more positively—especially since all the mom participants are living with a chronic illness that affects their healthy well-being.

Identify family patterns of thinking and acting

Sometimes we deal with situations in ways that we have learned from others.
For examples, we may believe that it is "fair" or "justified" for us to be treated in a certain
   way.
We may believe that it is ok for us to feel threatened or scared.
Can you think of patterns that you've seen in your family? Patterns that people have that
   make them feel bad or put their feeling thermometer at a 100?

Directions

Write responses on flipchart (Elicit responses from participants; If needed, use following examples.)

Possible Examples

Being negative
Inducing guilt
Doing too much
Trying to be perfect all the time
Always blaming yourself
Looking at the family patterns that you have come up with, which ones do you think you
   practice too? How may you be similar to the way your family thinks, feels and acts?
Which of your patterns of thinking and doing would you want to change?

Brainstorm examples of thinking SMART

Now that we know of some of your habits of thinking and acting that you would like to change, we will talk about what you can do to be "more SMART" about the way you think and act.

First, I would like for the group to brainstorm about what things you can do to be "more SMART" in what you say to yourself—the thoughts you allow yourself to have.

Directions

Post responses on the flipchart

Possible examples

Remind yourself of the positive things in your life
Not taking things too personally
Not catastrophizing (thinking it is the end of the world)
Positive self-talk
Catch yourself when you feel guilty
Catch yourself when you self-blame
It's ok to not be perfect all the time

Brainstorm examples of acting SMART

I would like for the group to brainstorm about what things you can do to act "more SMART" when your feeling thermometer is high.

Directions

Post responses on the flipchart

Possible examples

Exercising
Taking a walk
Writing
Reading
Getting enough sleep
Calling friends
Achieving a goal
Getting away from a negative relationship
Volunteering
Spending time with certain loved ones
Going to church

Identify uncomfortable situations and ways to think and act SMART

Distribute

Goals Related to Thinking and Acting SMART

How can I think and act SMART in an uncomfortable situation?

Directions: List up to three uncomfortable situations (FT = 80–100). Then, write some positive things that you can (1) *think* or say to yourself and (2) *do* that can bring your FT to a more comfortable rating (FT below 50).

Uncomfortable situation #1.

Different approaches

Think SMART:
Act SMART:

Think SMART:
Act SMART:

Think SMART:
Act SMART:

Uncomfortable situation #2.

Different approaches

Think SMART:
Act SMART:

Think SMART:
Act SMART:

Think SMART:
Act SMART:

Uncomfortable situation #3.

Different approaches

Think SMART:
Act SMART:

Think SMART:
Act SMART:

Think SMART:
Act SMART:

How can I think and act **SMART** in an uncomfortable situation?

Example

Uncomfortable situation #1: I'm leaving school/work at 5:00 P.M., and there is major traffic!

Different approaches

Think SMART: I am not going to stress over this.
Act SMART: Do a relaxation exercise (take a few deep breaths, progressive muscle relaxation).
Think SMART: I don't need to leave right at 5:00 P.M. I'm going to stick around and unwind.
Act SMART: Go to the gym. Take a walk. Hang out with a friend.
Think SMART: I need to leave right at 5:00 P.M., but traffic isn't going to get me down.
Act SMART: Listen to some music on the radio. Listen to a book on tape/CD.

Directions

Divide into pairs.

I am now going to handout a form you can use to write down some situations that make you feel really uncomfortable.
Then you write down, how you can think and/or act SMART in those situations.
They can be things we've listed on the board or other things you can think of for you.
Everyone is different.

Allow time for moms to complete their lists.

Wrap-Up and Goal Setting (15 min.)

Goal Setting

Identify a short-term goal (for the week) that is related to *thinking and acting SMART and a life project goal.*
The plan/goal should be:

State goal in one sentence.
Realistic (can reasonably expect to complete between sessions)
Clear (participant understands exactly what steps must be taken to complete the goal)
Not too easy and not too hard (30–50 on the feeling thermometer; goal should be challenging, but not impossible)
Clear end point (measurable, participant should know when the goal has been accomplished)
What do you want more of (stated in a positive term)

Make one positive statement about oneself.
Preview next session and encourage attendance.

Session #5, 1st Joint Session: Creating a Positive Environment at Home

Outcome and Skills

Outcomes: Teens and mothers will engage in behaviors to create a more positive atmosphere at home.
Skill 1: Teens and moms will create positive feelings and increase family cohesiveness by stating something each likes about the other and identifying family strengths.
Skill 2: Teens and moms will increase positive behavior in the family using social reinforcement and they will practice "catching someone doing something good."
Skill 3: Teens and moms will increase positive behavior in the family by increasing awareness of one another's life projects.
Skill 4: Teens and moms will set a short-term goal for the week and use a problem-solving technique to identify and address potential obstacles to goal.

Agenda/Timeline (Total time: 100 min.)

Check-In (15 min.)

Preview of this session
Create group rules for joint sessions

Skills-Building (60 min.)

Create a positive atmosphere at home by

Reminding each other of strengths ·
Practicing catching someone doing something good
Helping each other reach life projects

Problem-Solving (15 min.)

Make plan/goal for week
Engage in problem-solving exercise related to goal in order to optimize success and to plan for potential obstacles

Wrap-Up and Goal Setting (10 min.)

Connect session to life projects
Make one positive statement about oneself
Preview next session and encourage attendance

Materials

FTD poster
Feeling thermometer poster
Goal setting poster
SMART poster
Group rules
Tokens
Weekly goal card
Small laminated goal cards
Flipcharts
Pens

Post on Wall Ahead of Time

FTD poster
Feeling thermometer poster
Goal setting poster
SMART poster
Group rules generated by each of the group during individual sessions

Write on Flipchart Ahead of Time

Today's topic/goals for the session

Check-In (15 min.)

Review today's topic and plan for session

How can we create a positive atmosphere at home?

No matter how tough it can be at home sometimes, you have lots of strengths both as individuals and families. You can help to create a positive atmosphere at home if you:

Remind each other of your strengths: the things you like about each other; maybe things that you admire or are proud of.
Practice catching someone doing something good.
Help each other reach the life projects you set in our earlier workshops.
Help each other with weekly goal setting.

Ground rules for joint sessions

Generate group rules: Write on flipchart
Allow Moms and Teens to generate joint group rules. Write group rules on flipchart and keep for use with this group in future sessions.
Emphasize the following rules:

Confidentiality
Respect for similarities and differences
Stick to workshop content
Provide equal time

Review the importance of respect, including verbal or physical abuse.

I'll remind you if it seems a rule is being broken. Please remember that you might be asked to leave the session or the program if this gets to be a problem. It is important that everyone is safe and feels comfortable.

Skills-Building (60 min.)

Skill: Teens and moms will create positive feelings and increase family cohesiveness by: stating something each likes about the other, identifying family strengths, and discussing shared and differing values.

Feeling thermometer

Since this is the first session with teens and moms together, let's start with your feeling thermometer.
Where are your feeling thermometers right now?

Directions

Encourage discussion.
Allow up to ten minutes if needed for the group to discuss any anxiety or negative thoughts participants might have.
Validate feelings and use tokens to reward participation in discussion.
Remind group that showing up today is a positive and healthy behavior.

Introductions and one positive statement
Directions

Have each person introduce their family member by name and state one positive thing about the person.
Assist them, if needed, in stating the compliment positively and refraining from adding any qualifications or negatives.
Use tokens and praise.

I would like to go around the room and have each teenager introduce his or her mom to the group and say one positive thing about her, and I want each mother to introduce her teen to the group and say one positive thing about him or her.
Even if you are mad at your mom or teen right now, think of one positive to share with the group.
For example, "This is my son Ben and he is a great athlete."
To create a positive atmosphere at home it helps to let people know what you like about them.
We did it once just now, but saying what you like on a daily basis can make a difference.

Identifying family strengths

Now I would like mothers and teenagers to sit with someone who is not from your family unit. So teens should sit with one of the other moms and the moms should sit with other teens.
Your task is to identify your family strengths; good qualities about your family; things you like. You might think of ways you are proud of your family. Here are some examples:

"We stick together. If something happens to one of us, it happens to us all."
"We are survivors. No matter what happens we make it."

"We talk things over."

"We tolerate a lot of differences in the family."

Now take some time to come up with a list of your family strengths and then tell the other person about the strengths. You can help each other explain strengths in positive terms.

Directions

Encourage each participant to develop a list of strengths.
Allow about five minutes to complete the task.

OK. Let's go around and have each person tell us what he or she came up with.

Directions

Have each person share their strengths.
Give out tokens.

Catching someone doing something good

Skill: Teens and moms will increase positive behavior in the family using social reinforcement and they will practice "catching someone doing something good."

Another way to create a positive environment at home is to "catch someone doing something good."

Usually we think of catching someone doing something bad.

Did you know that the more we notice and mention the things people do, the more we increase the chances that they will do it again? So we want to pay the most attention to the good things they do rather than the bad things.

For example, *mother*, let's say you come in the kitchen and find that your teenager has done some of the dishes without being asked. If you want it to happen again in the future, it is helpful to notice that something good happened and to say so—"Hey, I really appreciate your doing the dishes!" It is not helpful to say, "How come you didn't do all of the dishes?"

Teenager, suppose you find that your mother has cooked your favorite dinner. You caught her doing something good. If you want her to do it again one day, you should say "Hey, mom, Thanks for cooking my favorite dinner." Don't say, "Wow, you sure made a mess in the kitchen!"

Let's practice "catching someone doing something good." We will try out catching someone doing something good.

The teenagers will go first. Ask your mother what she did yesterday, and as she tells you, let her know when you caught her doing something you liked.

Then we will reverse it, and the mother will ask what the teenager did yesterday and catch them doing something good.

Directions

Allow about three minutes for each interaction.

Don't Forget: Assist them, if needed, in stating the compliment positively and refraining from adding qualifications or negatives.
Use praise and tokens.

What was is like for you to practice "catch them being good"?
Was it hard or easy? Where are your feeling thermometers?

Directions

Encourage discussion.

Reward discussion.

Reward what worked for them and check out obstacles they experienced. How could they overcome the obstacles?

Identifying life projects

Skill: Teens and moms will increase positive behavior in the family by increasing awareness of one another's life projects.

Another way to create a positive environment at home is to help each other reach life projects.

For example, take a teen who really wants to graduate from high school. I am not suggesting that his mom do his homework assignments for him because that will not help him in the long run. However, it might help him if his mom makes sure his brothers don't go into his room while he is studying.

The first step in knowing how to help each other reach life projects is to know what each other's life projects are. Some of you already know the life projects of your family members, and some of you will be surprised to hear that you don't.

Each of you has come up with a life project during our individual sessions. You may have already shared this life project with each other.

Mom and teen share their life project with each other.

Now I would like mothers and teenagers to sit together in a family unit. You will have five minutes to find out from each other one *really important life project*—it would be helpful if you share with each other the goal that you've already come up with in group.

Mom and teen identify what they can each do to support the other in achieving the life project.

Next, take 10 minutes to ask each other for one thing that you can do to support each other in achieving your life project.

Allow 10 minutes; Assist as needed.

Go around the room and have each teen tell the group one life project that is really important to his or her mother.

Go around the room and have each mother briefly tell the group one life project that is really important to her teen.

Problem-Solving (15 min.)

Skills: Increased ability to set a goal that is realistic, clear, not too easy or too difficult and that has a clear end point; and increased ability to problem-solve in order to optimize success and to plan for potential obstacles.

Both mother and teen should identify a short-term goal (for the week) that is related to *creating a positive atmosphere at home (these may be linked OR separate goals).*

This will be homework for the week that we will ask you about next week. The plan/goal should be:

Realistic: can be completed between sessions

Clear: the exact steps are well understood

Not too easy or too hard: should be a surmountable challenge

Have a clear endpoint: it should be clear when goal has been achieved

Engage in problem-solving exercise related to goal in order to optimize success and to plan for potential obstacles.

State the problem/potential obstacles

Make a goal (Realistic and Specific)

Actions—Make a list of all the possible actions you could take and evaluate the pros and cons of each option

Reach a decision about which action you want to try

Try it and review it

Wrap-Up and Goal Setting (10 min.)

Make one positive statement about oneself.

Preview next session and encourage attendance.

Module 2: Healthy Living

Assertiveness
Social Support
Healthy Physical Habits
Dealing with HIV Diagnosis and Stress Responses
HIV Disclosure

Mom Session #6: Assertiveness

Outcome and Skills

Outcomes: Participants will increase assertive communication, related to negotiating safer practices and communicating with health care providers.

Skill 1: Participants will identify key components of assertive communication and incorporate them into a role-play.

Skill 2: Participants will identify and problem-solve potential barriers to assertiveness.

Agenda/Timeline (Total time: 95 min.)

Check-In (20 min.)

Review last week's goal
Preview of this session

Skills-Building (50 min.)

Increase skills related to negotiating safe sex practices by

Distinguishing between passive, assertive, and aggressive communication
Identifying key components of assertive communication
When should one be passive or aggressive
Role-play assertive communication with a partner
Role-play assertive communication with a medical care provider
Identify barriers to assertiveness
Problem-solving potential obstacles

Activity (10–15 min.)

Assertiveness role play game

Problem-solving (15 min.)

Set a goal related to thinking and acting SMART
Set a life project goal
Problem-solve barriers to accomplishing goal

Wrap-Up and Goal Setting (10 min.)

Review goals
Connect session to life projects
Make one positive statement about oneself
Preview next session and encourage attendance

Materials

FTD poster
Feeling thermometer poster
SMART poster
Goal setting poster
Assertiveness poster
Group rules
Participant life projects
Tokens
Goal card
Flipcharts
Pens

Post on the Wall Ahead of Time

FTD poster
Feeling thermometer poster
Goal setting poster
SMART poster
Group rules
Participant life projects

Write on Flipchart Ahead of Time

Today's topic/goals for the session

Check-In (20 min.)

Discuss goals set at last session

Life project goal *and* goal related to last week's session topic.

Identify barriers to unaccomplished goals

Review today's topic and plan for session

Write on flipchart ahead of time (in lay terms).

Assertiveness

> Identify key components of assertive communication: what it means to be assertive.
> Use components of assertive communication in a role-play related to sexual behavior and health care providers.
> Problem-solve difficult situations related to being assertive.
> Set an assertiveness goal.

Write on separate flipchart page ahead of time: Passive, assertive and aggressive (make three columns)

Write components of assertiveness on separate flipchart page

> 1. Use "I" statements (I would like this, I would not like that)
> 2. Say what you want respectfully
> 3. Pay attention to body language

Skills-Building (50 min.)

Identify one difficult situation

What is one difficult situation that happened this week related to your partner or with your medical provider? A situation that put you above a 60?

What was your feeling thermometer related to the situation? Where did you feel it in your body?

What did you end up doing? What was your response to the situation?

Don't Forget: Build a hierarchy of difficult situations:

For one mother, talking about condoms may be a comfortable task (30 on FT), talking to a partner about HIV may be more uncomfortable (50 on FT), and talking about the way she wants her partner to treat her daughter may be the most difficult (80 on FT).

These hierarchies will differ for each participant.

Point out commonalities.

Distinguish between passive, assertive, and aggressive communication

Elicit feedback from the group about what it means to be passive, assertive and aggressive.

Apply difficult situations identified by members to illustrate passive, assertive and aggressive communication.

For example: When you yelled at your partner, was that passive, assertive or aggressive?

Directions

Categorize feedback from the group in the 3 communication styles.

Facilitator demonstrates what it is like to be passive, assertive, or aggressive.

Helpful questions:

How can you tell when someone is being passive, assertive, or aggressive?

Where are your eyes?

How is your voice?

How about your body?

What other non-verbal behaviors (i.e., being in your space)?

Distribute

Assertiveness card

I Want It . . .

I	*Want It*	*. . .*
↓	↓	↓
"I" **Statements** **Do not blame** **Be respectful**	*Say **exactly** **what you want***	**Body** **Language** **Eye contact** **Personal space**

Don't Forget: Make sure the following components of assertive communication are highlighted:

Assertiveness means standing up for your own needs while also being concerned and respectful about the needs of the other person.

1. Use "I" statements (I would like this, I would not like that)
2. Say what you want respectfully
3. Pay attention to body language

Activity

Passive/Assertive/Aggressive Role Play Game

Intention/Purpose: To provide participants an opportunity to role play the different styles of communication and deepen understanding of the qualities and effectiveness of each style in a fun and interactive way.

Supplies: Pieces of paper labeled with each style of communication, 1 of each style for everyone in group. (Make sure pieces are same color and size so they all look the same.)

Directions: After identifying the components of the three styles of communication, tell group they are going to have an opportunity to role-play the three styles. If group is more than 4 people, divide group into 2 groups. While one group role-plays the other group will observe and watch for body language, tone of voice, words used, reactions in others. Explain to group that they are friends trying to decide where to go eat. You will give them each a communication style and they will "act" using that style within the role play situation. They should not show the style to the other members, so that the other people can guess what style they were trying to demonstrate. On the first round, only give participants passive and aggressive so that they can see examples of those two extremes. On the following rounds, hand out assertive roles to members whom you think understand well the definitions of assertive communication. After each round, have observing members, or members within the role play guess which style each person had. If people guess a style that the person did not have, talk about what they saw that made them think someone was using passive, assertive, etc. You can give different situations during each round. Do as many rounds as you think the group needs.

After giving group situations ask for 2 volunteers to be a mother and teen. Give them a simple and common family situation—you can even have them give the situation. First have both mom and teen use aggressive communication with each other as they try to resolve the situation. Once they finish talk about what the group saw and find out how the participants felt within their roles. Next use the same volunteers and situation but this time, mom and teen use assertive communication. Once they finish, talk about what was different, what group noticed, and how mom and teen each felt. If volunteers hit a standstill within the role-play, facilitator can intervene and take on one of the roles or suggest things that the mom or teen can say to make role-play more assertive.

Group Discussion: Have group discuss what they observed, what they were feeling, what they think was effective about each role-play. How does assertive communication work? What makes assertive communication different from passive and aggressive communication? How can we bring more assertive communication into our relationships with others, friends, family, children, parents?

Provide rationale for the use of assertive communication

Standing up for your own needs in a clear and respectful way will increase the chance you will get what you want.

Standing up for your own needs in a clear and respectful way will increase the chance you will stay safe and healthy and reach your life projects.

Are there times when one should be passive or aggressive?

Are there situations when it is appropriate to be passive?

Elicit a list from participants and write on the flipchart.

The following example may be used:

If someone is trying to steal money from you with a gun, it may be in your best interest to be passive.

Does being passive or aggressive work for the long run?

Some participants may feel that being passive or aggressive will work best in meeting their needs (i.e., "the only way to make a phone company listen is to yell at them"). Point out that while these strategies may work in the short run, they may not pay off if the participant wants to have a longer term relationship with the other person—such as their partner, friend or child.

The goal of this activity is to generate a discussion about the long-term consequences of being passive or aggressive (i.e., yelling at the receptionist may get her to listen to you the first time. What will happen during the next doctor visits? Will the receptionist accommodate you then?)

Are there times when you were passive or aggressive, and it did not work?
Were there consequences to you being passive or aggressive?

Directions

Elicit examples from group of real life situations where they would like to practice more assertive communication and then have participants role play examples with each other.

Have members stand up for the role play.
Help participants use "I" statements, be respectful, and pay attention to body language.
Facilitate brief discussion about experiences, problem-solving obstacles and emphasize comments related to increased feelings of efficacy or empowerment.
Praise Efforts

What was that like for you?
Where was your feeling thermometer?

Following role play:

What is your Feeling Thermometer?
What is one thing you liked, one thing you would do differently?
Was your behavior passive, assertive or aggressive?

Elicit feedback from the group regarding assigned observations.
Establish a positive model
Identify barriers to assertive communication in the role play.

Practice assertive communication in role-plays related to relationship with medical providers

Elicit a list of difficult situations (i.e., feeling thermometer over 60) related to medical care providers.
You may also use the situation ends identified in the beginning of the session.

Let's come up with some difficult situation ends with medical care providers. So that we can practice being assertive in getting your needs met in those situations.

Role play the situation.

Facilitator assumes the role of the provider.
Ask for a volunteer to be the patient.

Have members stand up for the role play.
Help participants use "I" statements, be respectful, and pay attention to body language.
Praise Efforts

> What was that like for you?
> Where was your feeling thermometer?
> Did you say no?

Facilitate brief discussion about experiences, problem-solving obstacles and emphasize comments related to increased feelings of efficacy or empowerment.

If the participants are unable to identify a situation, provide participants with the following scenario.

PATIENT: *You have not been taking one of your medications because you dislike the side effects.*

Your goal is to get your doctor to change your medication.

DOCTOR: *This patient has not been following your recommendations.*

Now, the patient says she has not been taking one of the medications.
It is very frustrating.
Your goal is to convince the patient about the importance of taking this normally very effective medication.

After five minutes, we will switch so the other person can practice.

Identify *barriers* to assertive communication related to partners, medical providers, and children

What would make it hard for you to be assertive with your partner, doctor or other care provider, and your children?

Examples of possible barriers with medical providers:

Being rushed
Feeling like you don't understand
Feeling like you are bothering the doctor

Identify *your rights* related to partners and medical providers

Directions

Write on board: Elicit from member; address the following if not mentioned.
Examples of rights with partners:

To control your body
To be treated fairly
To say no regardless of what he paid for, regardless of whether you had sex with him last week, and so on.

Examples of rights with medical providers:

To be treated fairly
To tell the professional what you think he or she should know about your situation history, symptoms (be specific), allergies, previous illness.
To make it clear if you want to be included when important decisions are being made about your care.

To understand: (i.e., asking professional to repeat the information)
To ask questions related to your health care provider

Problem-solve identified barriers

Problem-solve a few identified barriers in order to practice problem solving.

Wrap-Up and Goal Setting (15 min.)

Goal setting

Identify a short-term goal (for the week) that is related to *assertiveness* and *a life project goal*.

Don't Forget: The goal may also be related to assertiveness related to any healthy behaviors (i.e., asking a friend to not smoke in front of you; telling a friend that you would rather do activities with them that do not include drinking)

If a group member does not have a partner, the goal can be related to friends, family, or health care providers.

Review goals and distribute goal card if participants want to write down weekly goal.
Make one positive statement about oneself.
Preview next session and encourage attendance.

Mom Session #7: Social Support

Outcome and Skills

Outcomes: Enhanced social support building.
Skill 1: Participant will distinguish between negative versus positive sources of support.
Skill 2: Participant will identify sources of emotional, informational, and tangible support.
Skill 3: Participant will identify situations that require more support.
Skill 4: Problem-solve ways to increase positive support and/or decrease negative support.

Agenda/Timeline (Total time: 95 min.)

Check-in (20 min.)

Review last week's goal
Preview of this session, including how it relates to context of life projects

Skills (50 min.)

Increased ability to distinguish between positive and negative support
Increased ability to identify sources of emotional, informational and financial support

Brainstorming ways to increase positive support and/or decrease negative support
Practicing asking for better support

Activity (10 min.)

The Internet

Problem-solving (15 min.)

Goal setting surrounding social support building and/or life project
Problem-solve barriers to accomplishing goal.

Wrap-Up and Goal Setting (10 min.)

Review goals
Connect session to positive outcomes for the children of the women
Connect session to life projects
Make one positive statement about oneself
Preview next session and encourage attendance.

Materials

FTD poster
Feeling thermometer poster
SMART poster
Goal setting poster
Group rules
Participant life projects
Tokens
Goal card
Flipcharts
Pens

Handouts

Goal card
SMART actions in seeking support

Post on the Wall Ahead of Time

FTD poster
Feeling thermometer poster
Goal setting poster
SMART poster
Group rules
Participant life projects

Write on Flipchart Ahead of Time

Today's topic/goals for the session

Check-In (20 min.)

Discuss goals set at last session

Life project goal *and* goal related to last week's session topic.

Identify barriers to unaccomplished goals.

Review today's topic and plan for session

Write on flipchart ahead of time (in lay terms).

Social support

Who do you go to when you feel stress, down, or uncomfortable; when you need someone to listen to you, understand you and give you help.

Goals of this workshop

Definitions: Discuss the definitions of positive and negative social support.

Who: Identify who you go to for social support.

What: Identify situations in your life that require more positive support and/or less negative support.

How: Brainstorm ways to increase positive support and/or decrease negative support.

Practice: Practice asking for increase in positive social support and/or decrease in negative support.

Goal: Set a social support goal and problem-solve any potential barriers to accomplishing goal.

Skills Building (50 min.)

Positive Versus Negative Support

Skill: Increased ability to distinguish between positive and negative support.

The term *social support* means the people you go to when you feel stress, down, or uncomfortable; when you need someone to listen to you, understand you and give you help. The people that give you social support might include friends, family members, or professionals.

You are also a support *giver*. There are probably many people in your life that you give social support to when they need it.

Positive or helpful social support comes from those people who are interested in your healthy life projects; those who have your best interest at heart; Positive support increases your ability to make good choices and to feel better about yourself. This means that if you want to give positive support to others, it works best if you understand the life projects of the person you are trying to help.

Negative or unhelpful social support comes from those people who sidetrack you from accomplishing your goals; those who make you feel bad about yourself; those who get you in trouble (i.e., jail, drugs, etc.); they may actually make you feel more stressed.

It is possible that *one person can be a source of both positive and negative social support*. For example, maybe your best friend likes to go walking with you, which makes you more likely to get your exercise done. That is positive support. But, maybe the same friend tries to pressure you into having unprotected sex. That is negative support.

Sometimes people who give you positive social support help to decrease your feeling thermometer. An example might be a friend you talk to after having an argument with your child.

You might be surprised to hear that, in other situations, people who give you positive social support might increase your feeling thermometer. Examples include a friend who criticizes you for the way you are raising your kids.

Identify personal support network: Sources of emotional, informational and financial support

Sources of support may be friends, family members, service providers (i.e., case managers, agencies, shelters, support groups), health care providers (i.e., doctors, nurses), and other institutions (i.e., church).

Who do you go to when you need to talk to someone who you trust and feel like understands you?

Who do you go to when you need information on something (i.e., medication side effect, activities for children, support groups, schooling, employment, housing, etc.)?

Who do you go to when you need help with tangible things (i.e., bus tokens, rent, etc)?

As you can see, we often go to different people for different types of social support.

Identify comfort level before seeking support and after seeking support

Don't Forget: Relate to Feeling Thermometer

Social support building increases emotional regulation and coping with difficult life situations.

Positive sources of support will help you increase your comfort level in dealing with the situation; the goal is to identify support networks that help you regulate your emotions (i.e., you felt very uncomfortable (100) when a partner refused to wear a condom; after talking to a friend about how to negotiate safer sex, you felt more comfortable (20) about the situation).

Negative sources of support increase your discomfort level; You were stressed about your teen's acting out behavior (70); you talked to a friend who put the blame on you and judged your parenting style; you felt worse and more uncomfortable/aroused about the situation (100).

If a participant insists that she is comfortable with her lack of support, you may reframe it as a positive (i.e., how does she maintain her comfort level despite her lack of support, what other helpful tools does she have that the group can learn from).

Identify areas to increase positive support or decrease negative support

What situations would you like more support in?

What situations would you be more comfortable with if you had someone to share your thoughts and feelings with?

Can you think of a situation in your life that would be easier if you had more positive social support or less negative support?

When you think of this situation the way it is right now, how comfortable are you on your feeling thermometer?

If you were able to get more positive social support, how comfortable do you think you would be on your feeling thermometer?

Directions

Write responses on Flipchart (Elicit responses from participants; If needed, use below examples.)

Possible situations

How can I get my partner to help me remember my medical appointments?

How can I get my mother to stop blaming me for the way I parent my children?

How can I find out about section 8 housing?

How can I enroll in school and/or obtain job training?

Brainstorm ways to increase positive support or decrease negative support

Let's say you want to increase positive support and/or decrease negative support in this situation. How would you do it?

Directions

Write responses on Flipchart (Elicit responses from participants; If not mentioned, suggest the following.)

Incorporate SMART Actions in Seeking Support suggestions in discussion.

Increase Positive Support	Decrease Negative Support
Ask for help or for more help	Ask for less "help"
Ask for a specific type of help	Ask for different type of help
Negotiate for a win-win	Do not ask this person for help
Find a way to buy help (tutor, therapist, babysitter)	Avoid this person for this topic

Distribute

Distribute copies of SMART Actions in Seeking Support

Possible smart actions in seeking support

Before the conversation

Plan what you want to say ahead of time
Write it down
Use calming techniques to prepare
Wait until the other person is not rushed or distracted
Tell person you want to talk with them about something important.

During the conversation

Compliment other about something first; be positive; do not criticize; avoid putting down others' ideas and beliefs
Listen, repeat back what you are hearing, and ask questions to be sure you really understand both the thoughts *and* feelings of the other person
Share your thoughts *and* feelings about the situation
Use a soft voice, make good eye contact, watch body language
Be respectful
Use "I" statements
Try to propose a win-win situation
Respond well to an agreement for even part of what you wanted

---

Don't Forget: Following the discussion, distribute SMART Actions in Seeking Support handout. These actions should *not* be discussed in a didactic format. They should have been elicited from group members when eliciting ways to ask for positive support or decrease negative support.

Role play social support situation

Skills: Increased ability to establish positive support and/or reduce/eliminate negative support.

> Great, okay, let's practice now. I want you to practice talking with someone in your life about wanting better social support from him or her.
> You can be asking for support from a *family member*, like a parent or cousin; from a *professional*, like a teacher or doctor; or from a *friend*.
> Remember to use your *SMART steps* for problem-solving.
> Please pair up with one other person. Tell the person what you are going to practice so they know what role they should play. After five minutes of practice, we will switch so the other person can have a turn.

Directions

Have participants pair up and role play a situation. The situation may be one that they will use as their goal for the week. It will be most effective if each person has a specific situation in mind that they would like to work on during the week.

Walk around and ensure that the role plays are assertive and SMART actions are incorporated.

Activity

The Internet

Intention/Purpose: To provide a visual of the social support that exists in the participants' lives—to literally see networks of support.

Supplies: Ball of cotton yarn (easier texture than acrylic yarn) although any ball of string will work.

Directions: Tell group that they will be passing the ball of yarn between them as they each give an answer to questions about social support in their lives.

Only rules: hold on tight to your piece of string each time it's your turn and don't pass the string to the person next to you (won't make a web!).

Facilitator will ask a question and group will pass the yarn until everyone has answered that question. Facilitators can also participate in answering the questions. Keep activity going until there is a nice criss-cross of yarn in the center of the circle.

Possible questions

Name one person that supports you emotionally.
Who helps bring down your Feeling Thermometer?
Who catches you when you are thinking negatively about yourself?
Who can make you feel better when you are down?
Who supports you economically?
Who do you support?
Who makes you laugh?
Who can you go to when you need information about something?
Who can you count on to keep a secret?

Mom group only:

Who is your main support with your HIV diagnosis?
Who has helped you the most in dealing with your HIV?

Facilitators can adapt or add questions depending on the tone and openness of the group. Encourage members to be specific in who or what they name. It is ok for participants to name themselves, God, church, books, internet, music, etc as "members" of their social support networks.

Group Discussion: After completing the questions and while still holding the web, ask members what they see and what this web says to them about social support. Possible discussion is how we are all connected, how the group serves as social support, how we both give and receive support, how when we are well supported we are more available to support others (like our families) etc. Carefully wrap up ball of string!

Wrap-Up and Goal Setting (15 min.)

Goal Setting

Identify a short-term goal (for the week) that is related to *social support AND a life project goal.*

Review goals and distribute goal card if participants want to write down weekly goals.
Make one positive statement about oneself.
Preview next session and encourage attendance.

Mom Session #8: Healthy Physical Habits

Outcome and Skills

Outcomes: Participants will increase healthy physical routines.

Skill 1: Participants will identify goals for healthy routines, including improving medication adherence.

Skill 2: Participants will identify daily routines, reminder strategies, and social support that may support them reaching their goal.

Skill 3: Participants will problem-solve barriers to healthy physical routines.

Agenda/Timeline (Total time: 95 min.)

Check-In (20 min.)

Review last week's goal
Preview of this session

Skills Building (50 min.)

Identify healthy activities and relate to feeling thermometer and FTD
Identify group member's health routine
Identify barriers to healthy routine
Apply assertiveness and/or SMART problem solving to identify barriers
Identify goals for healthy routines
Use SMART to incorporate goals for healthy habits into daily routine
Identify areas to elicit support from the family in accomplishing healthy routines

Activity (5 min.)

Changing habits activity (hand/arm fold)

Problem-Solving (15 min.)

Goal setting surrounding healthy physical habits *and* life project goal
Problem-solve barriers to accomplishing goal

Wrap-Up and Goal Setting (10 min.)

Review weekly goal
Connect session to positive outcomes for the children of the women
Connect session to life projects
Make one positive statement about oneself
Preview next session

Materials

FTD poster
Feeling thermometer poster
SMART poster
Goal setting poster
Assertiveness poster
Group rules
Participant life projects
Tokens
Goal card
Flipcharts
Pens

Handouts

Goal card
My goals for healthy routines
My healthy routines

Post on the Wall Ahead of Time

FTD poster
Feeling thermometer poster
Goal setting poster
SMART poster
Assertiveness poster
Group rules
Participant life projects

Write on Flipchart Ahead of Time

Today's topic/goals for the session

Overall Reminders Throughout This Session

Don't Forget: Please review carefully prior to session.

The goal of the session

There is significant variability among members related to healthy physical habits. The goal is to determine *each member's unique profile* in taking care of their physical health.

The session begins with focusing on the positive: what are situations that participants feel good about when it comes to their health and what are the things that they are currently doing to take good care of their physical health.

This is followed by identifying areas related to their physical health that participants find challenging. This discussion intends to identify and manage challenges related to maintaining positive health behaviors, and to identify health related practices that participants may want to change.

Participants learn to: use coping skills and problem-solving ways to incorporate healthier physical habits into their daily routine.

The goal is to establish healthy physical habits, not necessarily to convince participants to take medication.

Being physically healthy may include: diet, exercise, sleep, medication, stress management, or maintaining appointments with doctors, and so on.

Participants may learn from each other about healthy physical habits.

The session is an opportunity for members to learn from each other about general healthy physical habits that may not necessarily relate to medication: what are they each doing to be physically healthy?

Participants who are currently not taking any medication may incorporate other healthy activities (i.e., exercise, drinking water, vitamins, sleep/rest) into their daily routine.

The session can be an opportunity for those who are not currently taking medication or who are inconsistent with their medication routines to learn from those who have well-established and effective medication routines and strategies.

There is variability related to medication adherence.

Please keep in mind that there may be significant variation among the group members in response to medication. It is important to address the unique needs of all participants regardless of their medication history.

Remember the following

Participants who are currently taking medication

Some feel comfortable with it; No or minimal side effects.
Some feel uncomfortable; Moderate to severe side effects.
Some have a medication plans that works for them and are consistent with their regimen.
Some are inconsistent with their medication adherence.

Participants who are no longer on medication

Some independently decided to stop taking their medication (i.e., side effects, emotional barriers—feels like it is an unpleasant reminder of illness, feeling like they didn't need the meds, etc.).
Some made a collaborative decision with their health care provider that it is in their best interest to not be on medications.

Participants who have never been on medications

Some independently made this decision.
Some made a collaborative decision with their health care provider.

How to keep participants engaged despite variability amongst group members

Engage participants who are currently medication adherent by problem-solving, and goal setting in relation to other aspects of physical health (i.e., diet, exercise, medical appointments, smoking, substance use, etc.).
For those who have no interest in taking medication, engage them by addressing other alternatives to maintaining healthy physical habits.
For those who may be curious or interested in learning more about medication, encourage them to elicit feedback from participants who are currently taking medication and have effective adherence strategies.

General reminders throughout session

Physical health concerns and medication adherence may be uncomfortable topics for many women. For some women, taking medications may feel like a stressful "reminder" of being HIV positive, and activate their worries about illness, death or prior stressful experiences with medical interventions or hospitalizations. If so, helping them to recognize their stress reactions and use positive coping skills (such as using FTD and relaxation exercises) may help them engage in their own health care habits more actively. Stress the impact of FTD on healthy physical habits.

One way to incorporate healthy physical habits into a daily routine is to use the SMART approach. For example, one barrier to taking meds is "forgetting." Brainstorming may involve identifying ways to "remember" (i.e., linking taking meds to a chain of existing behaviors—take meds after brushing teeth or before eating breakfast.)

Check-In (20 min.)

Discuss goals set at last session

During the check-in, conduct a quick general follow-up with the participants (i.e., is everyone keeping their life project goal in mind and working towards it?)

During the check-in, conduct a more specific follow up asking members for their progress with their goals.

Some of the life project goals may not entail weekly small goals. If so, there is no need for a weekly check-in. You can do a quick reminder and then move on to the next participant.

Life project goal *and* goal related to last week's session topic

Identify barriers to unaccomplished goals.

Review today's topic and plan for session

Write on flipchart ahead of time (in lay terms).

Become aware of how comfortable you feel about your physical health.
Discuss some of the things you are currently doing to stay physically healthy.
Identify the barriers or the things that get in the way of you keeping your healthy routine.
Figure out ways to overcome those barriers.
Learn ways to improve your physical health.

Skills Building (50 min.)

Identify healthy activities and relate to feeling thermometer and FTD

What is something that happened recently that made you feel good about your health? A situation that led you to be under 40?

Directions

Elicit situations from group members. If not mentioned, address the following.

Possible situations

1. Getting enough sleep.
2. Exercising.
3. Doctor telling you that your T-cell count has improved.
4. Friend telling you that "you look good."

Identify group member's health routine

What are you currently doing to help you stay healthy (i.e., medication, diet, exercise, sleep, etc.?)

Don't Forget: The goal is to determine each member's unique profile in taking care of their physical health.

Be careful not to give the impression that the session is attempting to convince members to take medication.

The goal is for members to establish and practice healthy physical habits, NOT necessarily for them to be medication adherent.

Identify barriers to maintaining healthy routine

Many of us find it hard to make it a high priority to take care of our physical health.
We are going to focus on how to overcome barriers to taking care of ourselves.
What is something that happened recently that got in the way of you maintaining your
healthy routine?

Directions

Elicit situations and barriers from group members. If not mentioned, address the following.

Possible situations

1. A friend asked you to go out drinking.
2. Your partner wanted to have unprotected sex.

3. Your kids wanted to eat fast food.

4. Your friend was smoking near you.

Apply assertiveness skills and/or SMART problem-solving to the identified barrier

I want us now to think of ways to overcome these barriers.

Select one or two barriers identified by the group and apply assertiveness skills and/or SMART problem-solving.

May apply assertiveness role-play to the identified situation.

Activity

Hand Folding/Arm Crossing Exercise

Intention/Purpose: To illustrate how uncomfortable it can be to change behavior that has become habitual but also to illustrate how easily the new positive behavior can become comfortable and habitual.

Supplies: Only the group and their hands and arms!

Directions: Ask group to fold their hands together, interlacing their fingers as they naturally would without thinking about it. Ask them to notice their fingers and hands and the sensation of having their hands folded this way. Then ask group to re-interlace their fingers with the opposite thumb on top and all the fingers changing position. Ask them to notice how it feels to cross their hands this way. Point out that this way is not bad or incorrect, but is new and feels strange. The other way feels comfortable because it is habitual, the new way feels strange because it is new. Point out that if they crossed their fingers in the new way for several days, it would probably start to feel less strange. Now have group cross their arms in front of their chests. Again have them notice how it feels, how comfortable and natural. Then have group re-cross their arms (sometimes this takes some work to get the arms in reverse!). Again have them notice how it feels and why it feels so strange. At the end participants can shake out their hands and arms to get rid of the weird feeling!

Group Discussion: Briefly allow group to talk about how bad health habits can become comfortable and how new positive healthy behavior can feel strange or even uncomfortable at first because it is new to us. As we practice our new positive behavior it will begin to replace the old habits.

Identify goals for healthy routines

You have each shared certain situations related to your health that you are uncomfortable with.

I would like each of you to spend five minutes completing the following handout.

Distribute

My goals for healthy routines.

This handout addresses some examples of different areas related to your health that you can focus on.

You may identify an area that is not listed in the handout.

Your goal may be something you have not done at all, haven't done for a while or something that you already do sometimes but would like to do more of or more consistently.

Please fill in as many as you like. You may have one goal or several.

Please make sure that your goals match the goal setting steps.

My goals for healthy routines

Instructions: Under each category write your goals for healthy routines. You can have more than one goal under a category or none. Be sure that your goals are realistic.

Diet (Food)

Exercise

Sleep/Rest/Relaxation

Appointments With Medical Care Providers

Medications

Substance Abuse (Smoking, Drugs, Alcohol)

Healthy/Safe Sexual Habits

Other:

From the above goals, which goal do I want to concentrate on for now:

Where in my routine can I incorporate my new goal:

Example:	**My Current Routine**	**My New Routine**
(Goal: More Exercise)	Turn off alarm	Turn off alarm
	Start coffee	Start coffee
	Shower	Do ten sit ups
	Make breakfast	Shower
		Make breakfast

Directions

Refer to goal setting poster.

Once everyone is done, I will ask each of you to share one that you would like to focus on for now and to start out with.

Directions

Walk around and assist participants in identifying realistic goals.

Once everyone is done, ask each participant to identify one goal.

The goals may be broad (i.e., exercise more). However, during discussion, assist participants in making a small, specific and concrete goal towards the larger long-term goal.

Write on flipchart each participant's identified goal for healthy physical habits.

Use SMART to incorporate goals for healthy habits into daily routine

What can you do to make sure you accomplish your goal?

Elicit feedback from group members related to each of the identified goals.

Encourage participants to generate alternatives for each other. They may share what they do to remember to maintain the healthy habits they have.

If not mentioned, suggest:

Incorporating goal into daily routines
Reminders
Getting support from others

Don't Forget: A detailed description follows regarding the 3 above suggestions. If time allows, distribute the healthy routines worksheet and have participants pair up and complete the worksheet.

If time does NOT allow, you may simply discuss where in their daily routine the participants may incorporate their goal and ask them to complete the healthy routine worksheet at home.

---

1. Incorporating goal into daily routines

   You may say:

   One of the big reasons people give for not following their goal for healthy routines is that they simply forget to do their goal.

   One of the ways to help remember your new goals for healthy physical habits is to connect doing the goal with other routines you normally do at that time of the day. This way it becomes part of an automatic process.

Distribute

Distribute and review healthy routine worksheet.

Directions

Explain that participants may have as many goals as they like for the topics on the worksheet.

Next ask them to identify the one goal that they would like to concentrate on for now and write it down.

Finally, identify where in their current routine, they can incorporate their newly identified goal.

Now can you think of a convenient place in your routine or chain of behaviors to add in the step, "take my meds?"

Ask participants to each complete the worksheet.
Ask a few participants to share their new routines.

2. Reminders

What kind of reminders can you use to help you remember your new goal?

Directions

Write on flipchart.
Elicit feedback from participants.

If not mentioned, address the following:
Ask someone else to remind you.
Alarms (clocks, watches, pagers, timers)
Notes to self (calendars, post-its)
Trigger objects (medication containers, large posted calendar)
Meals

3. Getting support from others

Who can support you in establishing or maintaining a specific healthy routine?

Directions

Elicit feedback from participants.
If not mentioned, address the following:

Informing a friend that you would rather exercise together than meet for drinks.
Refuse to allow anyone to smoke in your house.
Asking a friend to remind you of your doctor's appointment.
Asking your partner to remind you to take your medication.

Specifically, do you need any support from your children in accomplishing your health goals for your family?
Elicit feedback from participants.
If not mentioned, address the following:

Asking child to not beg for fast food every time you drive by a fast food location.
Asking teen to go for a walk with mom.

During our upcoming joint session, you can share these thoughts with your children and then ask them for help in these specific areas of support in working together as a family to stay healthy.

Don't Forget: Keep in mind that the intent of this exercise is to prepare moms for the joint session on healthy physical habits. Moms and teens will reunite during the joint session and identify areas that they would like each others' support in accomplishing a healthy family routine.

Wrap-Up and Goal Setting (15 min.)

Goal Setting

Identify a short-term goal (for the week) that is related to healthy physical habits goal addressed earlier *and a life project goal.*

Goals may be related to:

Medication adherence
Medical appointments
Diet
Exercise
Sleep/rest/relaxation
Social support related to physical health

Distribute goal card if participants want to write down weekly goal.
Make one positive statement about oneself.
Preview next session and encourage attendance

Mom Session #9: Dealing with HIV Diagnosis and Stress Responses

Outcome and Skills

Outcomes: Participants will reduce stress responses and improve positive coping related to HIV diagnosis.

Skill 1: Participant will identify normal stress responses to learning about HIV illness.

Skill 2: Participant will identify "traumatic stress reminders" related to illness and disclosure, and practice using coping skills to manage these reactions.

Agenda/Timeline (Total time: 95 min. for each part)

Check-in (20 min.)

Review last week's goal
Preview of this session

Skills (50 min.)

Identify stress responses related to learning about HIV illness
Identify and manage "traumatic stress reminders" related to HIV illness and disclosure
Share illness diagnosis/disclosure experiences in order to normalize reactions and reduce ongoing reactivity

Activity (5–10 min.)

Feeling thermometer measure of stress responses to HIV diagnosis

Problem-solving (15 min.)

Goal setting surrounding coping with HIV illness and life projects
Problem-solve barriers to accomplishing goal

Wrap-Up and Goal Setting (10 min.)

Review goal setting.
Connect session to positive outcomes for the children of the women
Connect session to life projects
Make one positive statement about oneself
Preview next session and encourage attendance

Materials

FTD poster
Feeling thermometer poster
SMART poster

Goal setting poster
Assertiveness poster
Group rules
Participant life projects
Relaxation handout (if needed)
Tokens
Goal card
Flipcharts
Pens

Handouts

Goal card
Remembering stressful events

Post on the Wall Ahead of Time

FTD poster
Feeling thermometer poster
Goal setting poster
SMART poster
Assertiveness poster
Group rules
Participant life projects

Write on Flipchart Ahead of Time

Today's topic/goals for the session

Throughout This Session

Don't Forget: Please review carefully prior to session.

The goals of this session include:

Illness diagnosis
To learn about normal stress reactions to HIV diagnosis in order to understand and normalize those reactions.
To share personal experiences regarding HIV diagnosis.
To better manage ongoing reactivity related to coping with HIV illness, particularly related to ongoing "traumatic stress reminders" related to illness and/or medical interventions.

Check-In (20 min.)

Discuss goals set at last session:

Life project goal *and* goal related to last week's session topic
Identify barriers to unaccomplished goals

Review today's topic and plan for session

Write on flipchart ahead of time (in lay terms)

Managing responses to HIV diagnosis
Provide information about typical reactions following stressful or traumatic events such as HIV diagnosis

Develop skills to recognize and manage "stressful reminders" of HIV diagnosis and/or medical intervention

Share individual experiences of learning about HIV diagnosis and link these to current stress reactions

Link these experiences to ongoing challenges related to illness coping and disclosure

Skills-Building (50 min.)

Make sure to

1. Normalize: People who have been through very stressful or traumatic experiences, such as learning they have a serious medical illness, a bad accident, or hurricanes/earthquakes—report experiencing similar reactions.
2. Validate: Given what they've experienced, these reactions make sense.
3. Provide information in a discussion format. Elicit experiences participant have had with stress reactions, and provide information around examples generated by the group.

Describe and discuss typical stress or traumatic reactions to very stressful experiences such as HIV diagnosis.

Explain that facilitator will first discuss some of the *common reactions that people have to very stressful or traumatic events*—like learning about HIV illness. These reactions are *common, understandable, and expectable*. In fact, we describe them as 'normal reactions to abnormally stressful events.' Although they are normal and expectable, they can create serious difficulties in people's day-to-day lives. Three kinds of reactions are common:

Intrusive reactions are ways in which the stressful experience comes back to mind even when you don't want it to:

Having upsetting memories of what happened come into your mind when you don't want them to.

Having nightmares about what happened.

Becoming upset or agitated when something reminds you of what happened, such as feeling very afraid, anxious, or nervous; or feeling sick to your stomach or feeling weakness in your muscles.

Avoidance and withdrawal reactions are things people do to keep themselves from experiencing these very upsetting intrusive reactions. They include:

Avoiding people, places, or situations that remind you of what happened.

Trying not to talk, think, or have feelings about the traumatic event.

Experiencing restricted emotions, even feeling numb, to protect against painful reactions to memories or reminders of what happened.

Feeling distant from friends and family and find it difficult to trust anyone.

Feeling different from other people, like no one really understands you.

Withdrawing from other people.

Losing interest in activities you used to enjoy.

Physical arousal reactions are physical changes that make the body react as if something bad is about to happen. These reactions include constantly being 'on the lookout' for danger, startling easily or being jumpy, irritability or having outbursts of anger, difficulty falling or staying asleep, and difficulty concentrating or paying attention.

Feeling irritable or on edge much of the time.

Getting angry easily.

Finding it difficult to pay attention in school, to concentrate on homework, or to remember things that you have read.
Having trouble sleeping.
Being jumpy or 'startling' easily.

Traumatic stress reminders

Describe and discuss information about traumatic experience reminders.

The goal is to define and describe traumatic stress reminders in concrete, personally relevant terms, and help participants understand how reminders elicit stress reactions discussed above.

Describe the concept of "Traumatic Stress Reminders": Traumatic stress symptoms tend to fluctuate in their intensity. For example, we can be feeling fine, and then something related to a past stressful experience—such as a person, a place, a sound, or even an emotion we're feeling—can remind us of what happened and bring up upsetting thoughts and feelings. Consider disclosure, medications, medical clinics, etc. as potential "reminders" of illness related stress responses.

Don't Forget: Make sure to provide information in a discussion format. Elicit experiences participants have had with reactions to traumatic reminders, and provide information around examples generated by the group. If an individual mentions current reactions, you may draw them out with questions such as: How often does this happen? How upsetting is this when it happens? Use FTD to describe reactions.

Directions

Using participant experiences as examples, discuss the following points

1. A reminder is something that brings up distressing memories or feelings related to a past stressful experience.

These reminders can be things *outside* of us, such as:

a person (a friend who you first disclosed to)
a place or a familiar sight (the medical clinic)
a specific time or date (anniversary of event)
a sound (sirens, loud noises)
a physical scar or disability
watching TV or listening to the radio (especially news or portrayals
    of the event)

Trauma reminders can also be things *inside* of us, such as:

bodily sensations (fast heartbeat or heavy breathing)
an emotion (feeling scared reminds me of other times I was very scared)

Have the individual share examples of their HIV diagnosis/illness reminders and the situations they might occur in. Be supportive. Help him/her focus in on the specific circumstances that trigger their response. Probe with questions such as following:

What are some of your most distressing reminders?
What kind of specific situations might you run into them?
How would you rank them on your feeling thermometer?
What thoughts might go along with them?
What have you done when you have these thoughts?

Activity

Feeling Thermometer measure of individual responses surrounding HIV diagnosis and HIV health maintenance

Stress Responses on the Feeling Thermometer

Intention/Purpose: To teach emotional regulation, a large visual Feeling Thermometer is used and participants are given the opportunity to record their levels of comfort to discomfort with various aspects of receiving and dealing with their HIV diagnoses and compare their responses and reactions to the responses of other members in the group.

Supplies: Flipchart with a large Feeling Thermometer; several different color markers; (optional—as many different color small post-it pads as there are members in the group).

Directions: Explain to group that they will have the opportunity to measure their Feeling Thermometer level in response to several aspects of their HIV diagnosis and living with HIV. Depending on the tone of the group, facilitator may write everything down on the flipchart OR each group member can have their own different color marker and the flipchart can be posted on the wall or the flipchart stand OR each member can have a different color post-it pad. IF members have their own markers or post-its, they will each come up and make a mark (stick a post-it or write their name) at the Feeling Thermometer level that best indicates the level of their reaction to the events or situations the facilitator lists. IF the facilitator is writing on the Feeling Thermometer, they will write participants' names next to the FT level that the member indicates. Facilitator should change marker color with each situation or event listed to help participants better see the differences of reactions among the group and with different situations. Below are listed several events, questions, situations and responses surrounding HIV diagnosis and living with HIV. Facilitator can use all or some depending on the group and can add events that may not be mentioned but seem relevant to the particular group.

Identify where you were on the feeling thermometer when:
You first found out that you were HIV+.
You told someone about your HIV for the first time.
You told your children that you are HIV+.
(for those who have not disclosed to children *or* anyone): When you think of disclosing
    your HIV status to your children or someone else.
You took your HIV medicine for the first time.
You take your HIV medicine now.
You go to your doctor's appointments.
You hear people talking about HIV or AIDS.
You come to group and talk about living with HIV.
Your children/family/friends ask you about HIV.
You first told a partner about your HIV status.
You experience side effects from the HIV medication.
You get your blood tested for cell counts.
Your feeling thermometer level today when you think about your HIV diagnosis.

Group Discussion: Briefly allow group to talk about the differences among the group in terms of different levels of reactions to the same events and situations. Point out the differences of Feeling Thermometer levels when they first found out about their HIV diagnosis and where they are today. What helped them lower their Feeling Thermometer OR for those who are still high—what are the barriers to lowering their Feeling Thermometer/what helps them lower their Feeling Thermometer/how does a high Feeling Thermometer get in the way with taking care of their health, etc. If there is someone in group who is consistently low on the Feeling Thermometer, invite the group to identify what it is that they think helps that person keep their

FT low. If there is someone in the group who is consistently high on the Feeling Thermometer, invite group to gently identify what it is they see in that person's personality that keeps them high on the FT.

Identify useful ways to handle reminders

1. Reducing Unnecessary Exposure

The first strategy has to do with limiting exposure to reminders and distressing situations in a commonsense fashion. It may also make sense to at least monitor the degree to which individuals visit settings or engage in activities that are really distressing for them if possible. This strategy for reducing unnecessary exposure, especially in the acute aftermath of a traumatic event, should be done in a conscious fashion so that it does not ultimately collude with traumatic avoidance. For example, it may be important to discuss that while participants cannot avoid health care settings entirely, it may be helpful to find a health care setting that does not act as a strong reminder for them.

2. Anticipating Exposure

A certain amount of exposure to reminder and distressing situations is unavoidable. As such, it may be appropriate to proactively plan for the exposure and resulting emotional reactions as well as provide appropriate forms of support. For example, if you know you have to go to the doctor, and that whenever you go near the clinic you experience stress reactions, it can help you plan for ways to manage those reactions (elicit social support, FTD, etc.)

3. Relaxation

Specific stress reduction and relaxation activities may be used prior to exposure to reminders or distressing situations in order to proactively manage levels of anxiety. Key techniques include abdominal breathing and progressive muscle relaxation. These will be presented later in this section and in subsequent sessions.

4. Building Resilience

Physical and emotional resilience can be increased through maintaining a healthy lifestyle which includes appropriate sleep, eating, and exercise routines.

5. Staying In-Touch and Active

It is very important to maintain your relationships and network of support. There is a tendency following traumatic stress (or loss) for people to become more isolated and less involved with fun or social activities. Maintaining contact with social supports and pursuing activities that you enjoy are good ways to manage stress reactions.

Dealing with HIV diagnosis: Sharing stories and feeling safe again

Directions

Ask each group member to tell their story about learning about HIV diagnosis/or illness related stressor.
Explain:

Sharing with others who love and care about you can do several things:

- It can promote a sense of safety as you are listened to while talking about something hard.
- It can also dissolve the hold a memory has had on you for a long time allowing yourself to be heard without everyone falling apart or feeling hurt beyond healing.
- It can provide information, support, forgiveness and a caring witness.

Wrap-up:

Compliment the participants on the hard work they did during the session.
Point out areas of strength and positive coping observed during sharing.

Don't Forget:
1. Make sure to compliment the participants on the hard work they did during the session, recognizing that it takes courage to share difficult experiences with others.
2. Use the Feeling Thermometer to help participants monitor their feelings during sharing of stories.
3. Point out areas of strength and positive coping observed during sharing by participant and group members.

Anticipating and Coping with Reminders about HIV

Completing the "Remembering Stressful Events Worksheet"

Directions

Have the mothers discuss how their story has caused them to have certain reminders and discuss what they have been.

Ask participants to write down a difficult memory related to their HIV diagnosis/medical treatment

Now ask them to complete the chart regarding reminders of this memory

Discuss how participants respond to reminders.

A key response, that is usually overlooked, is simply to be aware that the participant is having a reaction to a reminder. That way she can be prepared and plan for her reactions, and use her coping tools.

Wrap-Up and Goal Setting (15 min.)

Goal Setting

Identify a short-term goal (for the week) that is related to managing with HIV related stress reactions/reminders *and* a life project goal.

Review goals and distribute goal card if participants want to write down weekly goals.

Make one positive statement about oneself.

Preview next session and encourage attendance.

Mom Session #10: HIV Disclosure

Outcome and Skills

Outcomes: Participants will increase decision making skills regarding disclosure.

Skill 1: Participant will identify advantages and disadvantages of disclosing HIV status (to whom, when, and how).

Skill 2: Participant will practice disclosing to an identified person.

Skill 3: Social support building will be among group members and/or surrounding disclosure.

Agenda/Timeline (Total time: 95 min.)

Check-In (20 min.)

Review last week's goal
Preview of this session

Skills (50 min.)

Identify pros and cons of disclosing
Evaluate past positive and negative disclosure experiences
How to be SMART in telling someone about HIV
Role play/practice
Social support building

Problem-solving (15 min.)

Goal setting surrounding disclosure *and* life project goal
Problem-solve barriers to accomplishing goal

Wrap-Up and Goal Setting (10 min.)

Review goal setting
Connect session to positive outcomes for the children of the women
Connect session to life projects
Make one positive statement about oneself
Preview next session and encourage attendance

Materials

FTD poster
Feeling thermometer poster
SMART poster
Goal setting poster
Assertiveness poster
Group rules
Participant life projects
Relaxation handout (if needed)
Index cards of disclosure situations
Tokens
Goal card
Flipcharts
Pens

Handouts

Goal card
Guidelines for telling someone

Post on the Wall Ahead of Time

FTD poster
Feeling thermometer poster
Goal setting poster
SMART poster
Assertiveness poster
Group rules
Participant life projects

Today's topic/goals for the session
Pros and cons of disclosing
Before you tell and after you tell

Throughout This Session

Don't Forget: Please review carefully prior to session.

Illness Disclosure

Today's session does *not* intend to convince women to disclose or not to disclose. Instead, it is to help them figure out

1. is disclosing their HIV status to their benefit, and
2. if they make the decision to disclose, to help them decide to *whom, when, and how to disclose.*

Remember that there are situations when it is best for women and families to *not* disclose and it is important for women to learn how to evaluate such situations.

At some point, disclosure may come up for them and they can draw on the skills discussed in this session to help them prepare for the experience.

No guarantee that a well-thought out disclosure decision will lead to positive outcome

The session encourages women to identify the advantages and disadvantages of disclosing.

However, despite how well thought out a decision may be, there is no guarantee that the decision to disclose will lead to a positive outcome.

The skills of the session may be extended to other disclosures

The session is intended to increase effective decision making skills regarding disclosure of any personal, emotional, and/or private topic.

If the women do not wish to address disclosure of HIV status, you may engage them in discussing how to make decisions about disclosing other sensitive and private information.

Check-In (20 min.)

Discuss goals set at last session

Life project goal AND goal related to last week's session topic.
Identify barriers to unaccomplished Goals
See Appendix A for How to Identify Barriers to Accomplishing Goal

Review today's topic and plan for session

Write on Flipchart Ahead of Time (in lay terms).

To Disclose or to Not Disclose

Increase decision making skills regarding disclosure through:

Identifying pros and cons of disclosing HIV status
Deciding to who, when, how, what and where to disclose
Learning to identify and read cues/signs that lead to positive disclosure outcomes
Evaluating past disclosure experiences

The skills of this session can be used in other situations too

Past disclosure experiences and relate to FTD and feeling thermometer

Skill: Increased decision making surrounding disclosure through evaluation of factors that led to past positive versus negative disclosure experiences.

Identify the first person they told.

I want to hear from everyone about the first time you told someone that you are HIV positive.

What was your Feeling Thermometer when you told her?

What happened after you told?

Identify positive experiences: What DID go well?

To whom, when, and how?

Don't Forget: Stress what the women DID that led to a positive outcome (i.e., did they put a lot of thought in making the decision, did they look for certain signs, did they evaluate the pros and cons, did they practice what they wanted to say, etc.)

Identify negative experiences: What *did not* go well?

To whom, when, and how?

Don't Forget: Discuss what led to the negative outcome (i.e., did they not put a lot of thought in making the decision, did they not evaluate the pros and cons, did they not practice what they wanted to say, did the person they told respond in an unexpected way?)

Focus on what, if anything, the participant could have done differently to make the experience go better.

Participants who have never disclosed:

Where is your feeling thermometer when you think of disclosing?

Is there someone you have been thinking about disclosing to (to whom, when, how)?

What are the pros and cons of disclosing to this person?

What are their expectations about outcome (costs and benefits)?

Pros and cons of disclosure

Skill: Increased decision making surrounding disclosure through evaluation of pros and cons of disclosing.

Write on flipchart ahead of time: Pros and Cons of Disclosing

What can you gain from disclosing your HIV status and what can you lose?

Directions

Elicit feedback from participants. If not mentioned, make sure the following are addressed.

Pros of Telling

Gain positive support
Reduce loneliness, isolation and denial
Closer and more honest relationships
Allows children to share feelings more openly
Reduce burden of secrecy

Educate others

Plan for future together

Increased self-esteem (feeling good after disclosing)

Cons of Telling

Losing the person

Uncertainty about outcome

Person not keeping your secret

Stigma and rejection from family, friends, employers, housing

Discrimination and alienation

Leading to questions regarding risky drug use or sexual behaviors

Children and family being faced with discrimination

Don't Forget: Pros and cons may be generated as each member discusses her past disclosure experience.

Stress that you might want to pick and choose what information you tell others, depending on what you need and want. For example, there may be good reasons that you would decide to tell someone you have HIV or to decide not to tell someone.

Signs that can help in making a disclosure decision

Based on the positive experiences you have had surrounding disclosure, what are some things that you may want to consider as you decide to disclose to this person?

What cues can you look for (in the person or the situation) that can help you decide whether to disclose or not?

For disclosure situations that went well, how did you know that it would go well?

Directions

Write on flipchart. Elicit feedback from participants. If not mentioned, address the following:

Possible signs

Past behavior

Person's position (i.e., priest, counselor)

General attitudes towards HIV

How to be SMART in telling someone about your HIV status

Skill: Increased skill in effectively disclosing HIV status or any other personal and/or distressing information through practice and role play.

If you do make the decision to disclose to someone, what are some things to keep in mind, before you tell and after you tell?

Write on flipchart ahead of time:

Things to remember: (2 columns): (1) Before you tell and (2) After you tell.

Directions

Elicit feedback from participants. If not mentioned, make sure that all suggestions outlined in the handout "Guidelines for Telling Someone Distressing or Personal Information" are addressed.

Don't Forget: If needed, stress that we are not trying to tell the women to disclose but in case disclosure comes up in the future, we like them to be prepared as to how they would like to handle the situation.

"Guidelines for Telling Someone Distressing or Personal Information."

Guidelines for telling someone distressing or personal information

You have the *choice*:

To tell or not
To tell as much or as little as you wish
To share/show your emotions or not
To stop the conversation at any time

Before you tell:

Decide where, what, how and when you want to tell.
Decide if you will answer specific questions or not.
Decide if you want to share and show your feelings or not.
Practice what you plan to say.
Expect any kind of reaction and imagine ahead of time how you could cope with different responses.
If you feel panicky or nervous before talking to the person, you may:

Tell yourself, "stay cool."
Remember: "you can do it."
Remember: "it is frightening but you have gone through worse."
"take a few deep breaths."
Excuse yourself for a few minutes and try again a little later.
Go to the bathroom and get yourself back together

After you tell:

Find out what the other person is feeling or thinking.
Repeat back to them what you think they are feeling to be sure you understand and to show them you are listening.
End with a discussion of the next steps (if needed).
Remember that after the information sinks in, the person may have additional questions or areas to talk about.
Think about how you did; give yourself a pat on the shoulder; think about if and how you may wish to do things differently in the future.

Practice making a disclosure decision and role play

Elicit from a group of members, a list of persons who they are considering disclosing HIV status to. If the group members have difficulty identifying someone to disclose their HIV status to, they may also identify someone who they are considering disclosing something distressing or personal to.

Make a list on the flipchart of the identified persons.

Select and identify person from the list to practice making a disclosure decision and role play.

Instruct the group members to:

1. evaluate the pros and cons of disclosing,
2. identify their feeling thermometer rating,
3. use the "Guidelines for Telling Someone Distressing or Personal Information," and
4. role play the situation.

Role play:

Ask the players to keep in mind "The guidelines for telling someone"

Assign observation tasks to the audience (body language, tone of voice, use of the guidelines, etc.).

Following the role play, elicit feedback from the group:

Ask the players one thing they liked and one thing they would do differently.

Ask the remaining participants one thing they liked and one thing they would do differently.

Ask the observers for feedback on their observation task.

Use tokens, FTD, and Feeling Thermometer to facilitate discussion about their experiences during the role-play.

If there is time, conduct a second role play.

Social Support Building

Identify at least one person who you can reach out to for support when you are trying to:

1. Make a decision surrounding disclosure (*or*)

Don't Forget: Stress that this would be someone who would support them in evaluating the pros and cons of disclosing, putting thought into the decision, deciding to who, when, and how to disclose.

---

2. Disclose to someone.

Don't Forget: Stress that this would be someone who could be there for them once they decide to disclose to an identified individual.

Wrap-Up and Goal Setting (15 min.)

Goal Setting

Identify a short-term goal (for the week) that is related to *disclosure AND a life project goal.*

Review goals and distribute goal card.

Make one positive statement about oneself.

Preview next session and encourage attendance.

Module 3: Family Relationships

SMART Talking, Listening and Monitoring
Talking to Teens about Risky Behaviors
SMART Coping with Mom's HIV
Managing Teen Behaviors
A SMART Way to Disagree with Each Other
How Can We Be a Healthy Family?

Mom Session #11: Smart Talking, Listening, and Monitoring

Outcome and Skills

Outcomes: Participants will increase their ability to effectively talk and listen to the children in a SMART way.
Skill 1: Participants will increase knowledge of barriers to SMART talking and listening to children.
Skill 2: Participants will practice SMART talking and listening skills.
Skill 3: Participants will set a short-term goal for the week and use a problem-solving technique to identify and address potential obstacles to goal.
Outcomes: Participants will increase their ability to monitor their children.

Agenda/Timeline (Total time: 95 min.)

Check-In (20 min.)

Review last week's goal
Preview of this session

Skills-Building (50 min.)

Increase SMART talking and listening skills

> Identify comfort level related to parent-child discussions
> Understand SMART listening and talking
> Practice SMART talking and listening
> Identify barriers to SMART talking and listening

Problem-solving (15 min.)

Goal setting surrounding SMART talking and listening *and* life project goal
Problem-solve barriers to accomplishing goal

Wrap-Up and Goal Setting (10 min.)

Review goal setting
Connect session to positive outcomes for the children of the women
Connect session to life projects
Make one positive statement about oneself
Preview next session and encourage attendance

Materials

FTD poster
Feeling thermometer poster

SMART poster
Goal setting poster
Assertiveness poster
Group rules
Participant life projects
Relaxation handout (if needed)
Tokens
Goal card
Flipcharts
Pens

Handouts

Goal card
SMART talking and listening
Avoidant/blaming role play
SMART role play
Tips for monitoring

Post on the Wall Ahead of Time

FTD poster
Feeling thermometer poster
Goal setting poster
SMART poster
Assertiveness poster
Group rules
Participant life projects

Write on Flipchart Ahead of Time

Today's topic/goals for the session

Check-In (20 min.)

Discuss goals set at last session

Life project goal AND goal related to last week's session topic.
Identify barriers to unaccomplished Goals
See Appendix A for How to Identify Barriers to Accomplishing Goal

Review today's topic and plan for session

Write on Flipchart Ahead of Time (in lay terms).
Talking with and listening to your children.

Increase your ability to talk to your children in a way that makes you feel heard and understood.

Increase your awareness of your children's thoughts and feelings.

Increase your children's comfort and ability to talk to you about their thoughts and feelings.

Monitoring your children

Increase your ability to monitor your children: Keep track of your children.

Skills-Building (50 min.)

Identify comfort level related to parent-child discussions

What topics are uncomfortable to talk about with your children? Feeling Thermometer over 60?

Directions

Elicit feedback from participants. The following may be used to facilitate a discussion.

Possible topics

Mom's HIV
Will mom die?
How did mom get HIV?
Teen's risky behaviors
Teen behavioral problems at school or home
Mom being asked to baby sit all the time

What topics are comfortable to talk about? Feeling Thermometer under 50?

Directions

Elicit feedback from participants. The following may be used to facilitate a discussion.

Possible topics

Friendships
Teachers at school
Mom's employment
Shopping
Future goals
Being asked for a later curfew

Don't Forget: The goal is to support moms in identifying hierarchy of topics that are comfortable for them to address and listen to and ones which they may avoid or not discuss effectively due to high level of discomfort.

Moms' increased Feeling Thermometer may serve as a barrier to their ability to listen attentively to their child.

Moms will learn where their Feeling Thermometer needs to be for them to be most effective in talking and listening to their children.

Impact of FTD on SMART talking and listening: Barriers to SMART talking and listening

What gets in the way of being able to talk and listen to your children in a SMART way?

Don't Forget: Feeling Thermometer and distorted/negative thoughts serve as a barrier to listening and talking SMART.

Directions

Elicit feedback from moms. If not mentioned, address the following possible barriers:

Possible barriers

High Feeling Thermometer

The situation has been repeated many times

Mom feeling like the child does not listen

Being unsure of what is appropriate to say to your child

Worried that child will be frightened or angered by what you say

Worried that talking about one thing will lead to other questions that you are not prepared to answer

Feeling tired

Examples

When you are at a 80 in response to your teen asking you how you got HIV, what goes through your mind (i.e., I can't tell him, he'll feel angry or hurt if he knows the truth)? What do you end up doing (i.e., avoiding the discussion, making it short, not really answering teen's questions)?

Does the way you end up responding increase or decrease the likelihood that your child will approach you again to talk about something that is important to them?

When you are at a 100 because your teen broke her curfew, what goes through your mind (i.e., she does not care about how much I worry about her, she is irresponsible and selfish)? What do you end up doing (i.e., yell at her, tell her she will never be able to go out again).

Does the way you end up responding increase or decrease the likelihood that your child will listen to what you are saying?

Don't Forget: Emphasize that the choices we make lead to the same repeated arguments. Therefore, we can avoid the repeated arguments by making different choices.

Discuss the relationship between FTD on ability to talk to children and listen to what they have to say.

Relate previously discussed uncomfortable situations to FTD.

Feeling Thermometer and negative/distorted thoughts serve as a barrier to listening and talking SMART.

Listening to children in a SMART way

So we have talked about the way that your own feelings and thoughts may get in the way of you listening attentively to your children.

Now we will talk about how you can control the situation in a SMART way so that your feelings and thoughts don't dictate your actions. So that even though you are "angry" with your kid, you can still handle the situation in a SMART way.

How can you listen to your children in a way that encourages them to talk to you about their feelings, thoughts and questions?

What can you do to help your child feel like you understand them?

The teen sessions are helping your teen learn how to go about talking to you about what is on their mind.

Directions

Elicit feedback. Make sure the following are covered.

Write on flipchart: How to Talk and listen SMART

Distribute

Provide handout: SMART Talking and Listening

Smart Listening and Talking

State the problem

What is the fight about?

Listen: Don't be thinking of a response while the child is talking

Use "I" statements. Say how what the child does makes you feel. Do not blame.

State the problem in one sentence. Do not include old fights that have nothing to do with this conflict.

I.e., "She always wants to hang out with friends at the mall."

Make a goal (Realistic and Specific)

What is mom's goal?

> Consider what your feeling thermometer may be causing you to do: Are you wanting to avoid the conversation? Blame the teen?

What is teen's goal?

> Consider what the child is asking for: Is it information, reassurance or permission.

Joint goal?

> How can mom and teen come up with a goal that they can both accept and meets both of their needs?

Realistic?

Specific?

Win-win situation?

Actions—Make a list of all the possible actions you could take and evaluate the pros and cons of each option

Avoid nagging, criticizing, threatening or lecturing. This will push the person away.

Both mom and teen offer solutions.

After you have come up with all the solutions, together examine the advantages and disadvantages of each possible solution.

If you can't end up with one or two solutions that seem best, schedule another time to meet.

Reach a decision about which action you want to try

Joint decision where both of you agree with the solution.

Make sure that it is understood that each person is making a commitment to carry out the decision.

Be specific about the joint goal. (When do we start? What days? What do we need to start? How will we know that the other person is doing what they said they would?)

Try it and review it

Remember that sometimes solutions may need to be changed or modified.

Keep the door open for more communication if this is the case.

Evaluate the solution after a week, then two weeks, and so on.

Don't Forget: Do NOT read the handout. Elicit feedback from moms and generate a discussion and make sure the SMART steps in the handout are covered.

Practice SMART listening and talking: Role plays

Great, okay, let's practice now. We'll start with a script and then pair up for some additional practice.

Directions

Demonstrate role play.

Ask for two volunteers.

Assign observation tasks to the remaining group members based on discussed listening and talking steps.

Description of Role Play: Child: The goal of the child is to express her/his worry about mom's health and obtain reassurance that mom will feel better.

Mother: The goal of mother is to avoid the discussion because it raises her Feeling Thermometer.

Distribute

Distribute role play. ("Avoidance/Blaming")

Avoidance/Blaming Role Play

CHILD: *The goal of the child is to express her/his worry about mom's health and obtain reassurance that mom will feel better.*

MOTHER: *The goal of mother is to avoid the discussion because it raises her feeling thermometer.*

CHILD: *Mom, can I talk to you for a minute?*

MOM: *What is this about?*

CHILD: *I was wondering about your HIV. You've been sick for the past week. I'm really worried about you.*

MOM: *You are worried about me? If you're so worried, stop stressing me so much. Why don't you just go clean your room. You don't know anything about my health. I'm the one who worries about my health.*

CHILD: *Why do you have to get so angry. I'm just asking about your health.*

MOM: *I'm angry because you never do anything around the house. Did you do the dishes even once last week?*

CHILD: *Forget it. This is a waste of time (leaves room).*

Directions

Following role play, ask:

What is your Feeling Thermometer?
One thing you liked, one thing you did not like about the way you handled the conversation?
Elicit feedback from the observers.
What parts of SMART were used/missed?

Don't Forget: Make sure to address that mom's high Feeling Thermometer served as a barrier to her SMART listening and responding to her child. The child in this situation walked away not feeling heard or understood.

Description of Role Play: ("Using SMART")

CHILD: *The goal of the child is to express her/his worry about mom's health and obtain reassurance that mom will feel better.*

MOTHER: *The goal of mother is to help child feel like he/she is being heard and understood by mom.*

Distribute role play: ("Using SMART")

SMART Listening Role Play

CHILD: *Mom, can I talk to you for a minute?*

MON: *Can you wait until I'm done washing the dishes. (Few minutes later) Ok, what do you want to talk about?*

CHILD: *I was wondering about your HIV. You've been sick for the past week. Are you going to get better or are things getting worse?*

MOM: *What do you mean by "getting better"? Do you mean can I completely get rid of HIV so I won't ever be sick from it again?*

CHILD: *Yeah. You've been sick this past week.*

MOM: *You seem to be really worried about me and my health. Right now there is no cure for HIV so I can't completely get HIV out of my body. I can't promise that I'll always feel good. But I'm here for you now.*

Directions

Following role play, ask:

What is your Feeling Thermometer?
One thing you liked, one thing you did not like about the way you handled the conversation?
Elicit feedback from the observers.
What parts of SMART were used/missed?

Additional role plays: Pair up members.

I want you to practice talking with your child about something. You can pick something from this list on the flipchart or pick something that you plan to talk with them about.
Possible topics:

Your child asks you for money.
Your child asks you to let him/her go to a party.
Your child tells you she/he got a really bad grade in a class.
Your child tells you she/he got suspended from school.

Monitoring

We have spent today's session discussing ways to improve the way you talk to and listen to your children so that you can feel involved in your children's life.

One last strategy to discuss is monitoring. Monitoring is another way to be effective as parents by being involved in your children's lives.

It is hard to be SMART in the way you talk and listen to your children if you are not able to monitor *what they do, where they are at, and who they are with.*

While this is important at each stage of development, parents need to be especially concerned during adolescence, when their teens strive to gain greater freedom and independence.

Monitoring means making it a habit to keep track of your children, or to be sure that another person has this job when you can't do it. It means you or someone else being able to answer these four questions at all times: (1) *Who* is your teen with? (2) *Where* is he or she? (3) *What* is he or she doing? and (4) *When* will he or she be home?

The question is: How can you know the answers to the four questions without interviewing your teen each time he or she walks out the door?

Write on flipchart.

Elicit feedback from group members. Make sure the following are covered.

Talk with Your Teen
Manage Your Teen's Freedom
Set Clear Guidelines
Stay in Touch with Your Teen
Get Your Teen Involved in Adult-supervised Activities
Set a Good Example
Keep a Family Calendar
Talk with Your Teen's Teachers
Meet Your Teen's Friends

Distribute

Distribute handout on monitoring.

Tips for Monitoring

Talk with Your Teen: One way to find out things is to be an interested, active listener. Just by listening to the stories of your adolescent's day, you can show him that you genuinely care about what happens to him. It may only take 15 minutes a day of your undivided attention to learn about your adolescent's daily events. Listen carefully. What classes does she like? How are things going with his friends? What problems is she having? Building a positive relationship will help you monitor your teen's activities without seeming intrusive. This is the most important aspect of monitoring.

Manage Your Teen's Freedom: As teens learn how to manage increased freedom, parents need to monitor their progress. As they demonstrate responsibility at one level of freedom, parents can help them move to the next level by giving a little more freedom. For example, if your child always comes home by her curfew and asks to stay out later on weekends, you might feel comfortable letting her do this. However, if you find yourself calling around looking for her at her curfew time, she might not be ready for an increased level of responsibility.

Set Clear Guidelines: Even though they can handle more responsibility than younger children, teens still need some boundaries and limits. It is important that teens know exactly what is expected of them. After discussing the rules, you may even want to write them down to avoid disagreements over what was said.

Stay in Touch with Your Teen: If your children are supposed to be home at a certain time, plan to be home at the same time. If you can't be there, call to check on them or have a trusted friend or relative or neighbor check on them. Unsupervised children are less likely to get into trouble if parents keep in touch with them.

Get Your Teen Involved in Adult-supervised Activities: Find out what school and community resources are available. You might check into organized sports, youth organizations, or after-school programs. Make your home available and inviting to your teen and his or her friends. It is easier to keep track of your children when they are at home.

Set a Good Example: When you go out, let your children know where you are going, how long you'll be gone, and a number where they may reach you. This provides an excellent role model of considerate behavior.

Keep a Family Calendar: Have a space where all family members can write down their meetings, appointments, and activities. This helps family members keep track of one another; it also provides a form of communication.

Talk with Your Teen's Teachers: Find out how classes are going, and what problems your teen might be having.

Meet Your Teen's Friends: Much of your teen's behavior will be influenced by his or her friends. Teens who have a lot of unsupervised time on their hands are at risk for developing problem behaviors. Get to know your child's friends; better yet, get to know the parents of your child's friends.

Wrap-Up and Goal Setting (15 min.)

Goal Setting

Identify a short-term goal (for the week) that is related to one of the below topics:

1. talking and listening to your children in a SMART way
2. monitoring
3. life project

Review goals and distribute goal card.
Make one positive statement about oneself.
Preview next session and encourage attendance.

Mom Session #12 Talking to Teens about Risky Behaviors

Outcome and Skills

Outcomes: Increased ability to talk with teens about risk reduction.
Skill 1: Identify comfort level related to discussing risky behaviors with teens.
Skill 2: Identify barriers to communicating with teens regarding risky behaviors.
Skill 3: Problem-solve barriers to communication about risky behaviors.
Skill 4: Practice communication with teens about risky situations.

Agenda/Timeline (Total time: 95 min.)

Check-In (20 min.)

Review last week's goal.
Preview of this session.

Skills (50 min.)

Increased communication about risky behaviors through:

Identifying comfort level related to communicating about risky behaviors
Identifying barriers to communication
Problem-solving barriers to communication
Learning communication strategies
Role playing communication about risky situations

Activities (10 min.)

Condom demo and practice

Problem-Solving (15 min.)

Goal setting surrounding talking to teens about risky behaviors AND life project goal.
Problem-solve barriers to accomplishing goal.

Wrap-Up and Goal Setting (10 min.)

Review goals.
Connect session to life projects.
Make one positive statement about oneself.
Preview next session.

Materials

FTD Poster
Feeling Thermometer Poster
SMART Poster
Goal Setting Poster
Assertiveness Poster
Group Rules
Participant Life projects
Tokens
Goal Card
Flipcharts
Pens

Handouts

Goal Card
"Assertively Talking with Teens about Risk."
SMART Talking and Listening
Topics to Talk to Teens about
How to Talk to my Teen about HIV

Post on the Wall Ahead of Time

FTD Poster
Feeling Thermometer Poster
Goal Setting Poster
SMART Poster
Assertiveness Poster
Group Rules
Participant Life projects

Write on Flipchart Ahead of Time

Today's Topic/Goals for the Session

Check-In (20 min.)

Discuss goals set at last session

Life project goal AND goal related to last week's session topic.
Identify barriers to unaccomplished Goals
See Appendix A for How to Identify Barriers to Accomplishing Goal

Review today's topic and plan for session

Write on Flipchart Ahead of Time (in lay terms).
Goals of this workshop
Becoming aware of how comfortable you feel about talking to your children about risky behaviors: Behaviors that place them at risk for drug use, pregnancy, STDs and/or HIV.
Learning ways to improve the way you talk to your teens about risky behaviors.

Skills Building (50 min.)

Feeling Thermometer and FTD related to talking to teens about risky behaviors.
What situations related to talking about risk with your teens put you at a 100, 60, 20?

Don't Forget: Assist participants in developing a hierarchy of situations related to topics surrounding risk reduction and their comfort level with each situation.

Normalize that each participant will have different situations that they find comfortable versus uncomfortable related to talking to their children about risk reduction.

Remember that discomfort may contribute to mom's avoidance of discussing risk reduction with their children.

Emphasize situations that participants are comfortable talking to their children about: What helps them feel comfortable? This may be a good opportunity for modeling amongst group members.

If a participant states that talking to teens about risky behaviors is absolutely comfortable for her, ask participant to generate other topics/situations that may be uncomfortable to talk to teen about.

Directions

Elicit a list of situations from participants. If not mentioned, address the following scenarios to facilitate a development of a hierarchy.
Possible situations:

1. Talking to your teen about the importance of using condoms.
2. Talking to your teen about the risks related to alcohol or drugs.
3. Talking to your teen about how having a baby changes one's life.
4. Talking to your teen about how to be assertive about one's safety (related to sex and drugs).
5. Talking to your teen in detail about how HIV is transmitted.

Identify barriers to talking with teens regarding risky behaviors.

What makes it challenging to talk with your children about these topics?

Directions

Elicit feedback from participants.
If not mentioned, address the following.
Possible barriers:

Hard to decide how much to tell a child.
Worried that talking about HIV/drugs may raise questions about mother's history.
Worried that the discussion will raise questions that they are not prepared
    to answer.
Thinking that the child may get defensive and think that mother is accusing them.

Don't Forget: Relate to FTD and Feeling Thermometer.
Discomfort and negative/distorted thoughts may serve as barriers to talking with teens about difficult topics.

Problem-solve barriers through SMART

Assist participants in problem-solving barriers to talking with teens about difficult topics.

State the problem/potential obstacles

Make a goal (Realistic and Specific)

Actions—Make a list of all the possible actions you could take and evaluate the pros and cons of each option

Reach a decision about which action you want to try

Try it and review it

Don't Forget: Positive self talk, relaxation and seeking social support can be generated options.

How to communicate with teens about risky behaviors: Assertiveness and SMART

For those of you who had discussions with your teens about risky behaviors, *what helped your discussions to go well* (i.e., mom felt that the teen heard her, teen agreed to a healthy course of action, etc.)?

What do you think are some important things to keep in mind as you are about to have the discussion with your teens?

Directions

Write suggestions on flipchart.

Distribute

Handout on "Talking Assertively with Teens about Risk."

"Talking Assertively with Teens about Risk"

- If you are uncomfortable talking about sex, *share this feeling with your teen.* They are probably embarrassed or uncomfortable too. Sometimes it's easier to start the conversation based on something you have just seen together on TV.
- Inform your teen that *you want to talk about sex because it is your job* as a parent and because you are interested in his or her health. It isn't meant to be a message that you do not trust your teen; it is simply a normal part of life.
- Keep it an *open and honest discussion.* It will go better if it is NOT viewed as a lecture, criticism, punishment, or teasing.
- Try to *answer questions* you had at that age even if your teen doesn't ask them. Many teens are afraid to ask questions. Be as specific as possible, including information about how HIV is spread. It might help to think of what questions you had at that age. Remember, you don't have to know all the answers!
- Make this a *regular topic of discussion* so that it is easier for everyone.

Don't Forget: Tie in handout suggestions with suggestions made by the participants in the group.

If all suggestions have already been spontaneously discussed in the group, just review generally and give them the handout.

DO NOT facilitate this in a didactic format.

Remind participants of SMART talking and listening steps discussed in previous sessions. The steps that we talked about in our earlier session about SMART talking and listening to your children can be helpful when trying to talk to your teens about risky behaviors.

Distribute

SMART Talking and Listening and How to Talk to Teens about HIV

Smart Listening and Talking

State the problem

What do I want to talk about?

Listen: Don't be thinking of a response while the child is talking

Use "I" statements. Say how what the child does makes you feel. Do not blame.

State the topic in one sentence.

Make a goal (Realistic and Specific)

What is mom's goal?

> Consider what your feeling thermometer may be causing you to do: Are you wanting to avoid the conversation? Blame the teen?

What is teen's goal?

> Consider what the child is asking for: Is it information, reassurance or permission.

Joint goal?

> How can mom and teen come up with a goal that they can both accept and meets both of their needs?

Realistic?

Specific?

Win-win situation?

Actions—Make a list of all the possible actions you could take and evaluate the pros and cons of each option

Avoid nagging, criticizing, threatening or lecturing. This will push the person away.

Both mom and teen offer solutions.

After you have come up with all the solutions, together examine the advantages and disadvantages of each possible solution.

If you can't end up with one or two solutions that seem best, schedule another time to meet.

Reach a decision about which action you want to try

Joint decision where both of you agree with the solution.

Make sure that it is understood that each person is making a commitment to carry out the decision.

Be specific about the joint goal. (When do we start? What days? What do we need to start? How will we know that the other person is doing what they said they would?)

Try it and review it

Remember that sometimes solutions may need to be changed or modified.

Keep the door open for more communication if this is the case.

Evaluate the solution after a week, then two weeks, and so on.

How to Talk to Your Children about HIV

Talking with infants and toddlers (0–2 years): Infants and toddlers do not need to know the facts about HIV. By naming all the parts of their body, you are teaching them that their entire body is natural and healthy. ("This is your *arm*. This is your *elbow*. This is your *penis*. This is your *knee*.") By reacting calmly when they touch their genitals, you are teaching them that sexual feelings are normal and healthy. By holding them, hugging them, talking with them, and responding to their needs, you are laying the groundwork for trust and open discussions.

Talking with preschool children (3–4 years): Children at this age are learning about their bodies. They learn about their world through play. The best thing a parent can do at this age is to create a home where children will feel free to ask questions about their bodies, health, and sexuality. Children will then learn that sexuality is one of the things they can talk about in their homes.

Talking with young children (5–8 years): Children at this age understand more complex issues about health, disease, and sexuality. They may have questions or fears about HIV. They may have heard that people get HIV from being bad. They understand basic answers to questions based upon examples from their lives. If your child cuts her finger and blood appears, you have an excellent opportunity to explain how germs (things that make you sick) can get into the blood system from cuts. They need to know that they cannot get HIV from playing, studying, eating with, or talking with someone who is HIV+.

Talking with preteens (9–12 years): Because of the strong social pressures that start at this age, it is important that you talk about HIV/AIDS regardless of what you know about your children's sexual or drug experiences. Children at this age are concerned about their bodies, their looks, and what is "normal." For some, this time marks the start of dating, sexual experiences, and drug experimentation. During the changes of puberty, preteens are very curious about sex and need basic, accurate information. They need to know what is meant by sexual intercourse, homosexuality, and oral, anal, and vaginal sex. They need to know that sex has consequences, including pregnancy, diseases, and HIV infection. They need to know how HIV is transmitted, how it is *not* transmitted, and how to prevent transmission, including talking about condoms.

Talking with teens (13–19 years): You should tell your teenagers and preteens that the best way to prevent HIV infection is by not having any type of sexual intercourse or using any type of drugs. At the same time, you should share your values about sexual behaviors. Many parents want to tell their children to wait to have intercourse at least until they are no longer teenagers. But most children are not waiting. In fact, the majority of Americans have intercourse by their twentieth birthday. Therefore, most parents also want to make sure that their children can protect themselves against pregnancy, and sexually transmitted diseases, including HIV. You can talk to your teens about the full range of sexual behaviors that people find pleasurable. Many of these activities are "safer sex"—not transmitting HIV or causing pregnancy. They include kissing, handholding, caressing, masturbation, and other sexual behaviors that do not involve the exchange of body fluids. Social pressure to try sex and drugs are often very strong for teens. All young people must, therefore, know that:

Not having sexual intercourse (abstinence) is the best method for preventing HIV infection. It is also the best method for preventing other sexually transmitted diseases and pregnancy.

Teenagers that have intercourse must use *latex* condoms for each and every act of intercourse, including oral sex, anal sex, and vaginal sex. Condoms are very effective in preventing pregnancy and diseases. In fact, using a condom is 10,000 times safer than not using one.

Drugs and alcohol impair good decision-making and may suppress the immune system. Sharing needles of any kind puts people at risk for HIV. This includes using needles for injecting drugs, skin-popping, injecting steroids, piercing the ears and body, and tattooing.

Adapted from: How to Talk to Your Teens and Children about AIDS, available in Spanish, and Talking with Your Child about Sex. National PTA Web site. Challenges of Parenting Library (http://www.siecus.org/parent/talk/talk0001.html) copyright © 1996-2004, SIECUS/

Don't Forget: The handout on How to Talk to Teens about HIV does not need to be discussed. You may tell moms that this is a helpful handout for them to keep and review independently if they ever need some support in talking to their teen about HIV.

Identify topics to discuss with teens

If you can, each of you make a list of topics that you would like to talk to your teen about in regards to risky behaviors.

Distribute

Handout to write list of topics.

What I Want to Talk to my Child about When it Comes to Risky Behaviors:

1.

2.

3.

4.

5.

Role Play SMART Talking and Listening about Risk—Scripted

Great, okay, let's practice now. We'll start with a script and then pair up for some additional practice.

Directions

Ask for two volunteers.

Assign observation tasks to the remaining group members based on discussed listening and talking steps.

Distribute

Distribute role play. ("Avoidance/Blaming")

Talking to Teens about Risk—Avoid/Blame role play

MOM: *Honey, I brought these home for you from the clinic. (Hands daughter some condoms). Do you know what they are?*

DAUGHTER: *Please mom. Of course I do.*

MOM: *You do?! Well then you know how important it is to protect yourself if you're planning on having sex.*

DAUGHTER: *Yes, yes mom I know. Can we drop it?*

MOM: *Well, this is important. You shouldn't be having sex anyway. You're not old enough.*

DAUGHTER: *OK, can you please leave me alone mom. I know, I know.*

MOM: *No you don't know. Not until you're pregnant or have a disease. Then you'll really know.*

DAUGHTER: *Can we just drop it?*

MOM: *Fine, you can go to your room now. And later tonight I think we're gonna have to talk about your curfew . . .*

Directions

Following role play, ask:

What is your Feeling Thermometer?
One thing you liked, one thing you did not like about the way you handled the conversation?
Elicit feedback from the observers.
What parts of SMART were used/missed?

Great, okay, now let's practice having the same discussion in the SMART way; using our SMART talking and listening steps.

Directions

Ask for two volunteers.
Assign observation tasks to the remaining group members based on discussed listening and talking steps.

Distribute

Distribute role play. ("SMART")

Talking to Teens about Risk—SMART

MOM: *Honey, I brought these home for you from the clinic. (Hands daughter some condoms). Do you know what they are?*

DAUGHTER: *Please mom. Of course I do.*

MOM: *OK. So what do you know about using them?*

DAUGHTER: *Mom, do we have to talk about this?*

MOM: *Well, actually, yes we do. I know this can be a hard thing to talk about. It's uncomfortable for me too. But as a parent this is my job. I need to make sure you have all the information to protect yourself. Have you learned about this in school? Or from friends?*

DAUGHTER: *We learned in health class. And besides, I'm 15, of course I know these things. I have a boyfriend, mom.*

MOM: *I'm glad you feel like you are well informed. I can also be here to answer questions in the future. Having sex with someone is something you're going to have to decide when and whether it's right for you. I know it is sometimes embarrassing to ask me or hard to talk about, but if you have questions, I am open to talking about it with you.*

DAUGHTER: *Ok.*

MOM: *Do you have any questions about protection or using a condom?*

DAUGHTER: *No.*

MOM: *I know it sometimes seems like the "guy's" job to have the condom, but it is just as much the responsibility of the woman as the man to protect herself. You know condoms and protection are important for oral sex too. You can use what's called a dental dam for oral sex with a woman and if you like, I could always get you some from the clinic.*

DAUGHTER: *That's OK. I really feel like I know what I'm doing mom.*

MOM: *Ok, honey. Well just know that it's OK to talk about this stuff with me. Even though I worry about you and your safety, I don't want you to feel like you can't come talk to me if you have questions or are considering something, OK?*

DAUGHTER: *OK.*

Directions

Following role play, ask:

What is your Feeling Thermometer?
One thing you liked, one thing you did not like about the way you handled the conversation?
Elicit feedback from the observers.
What parts of SMART were used/missed?

Role Play SMART Talking and Listening about Risk—Unscripted

Pair up
Select a topic from your list and practice talking to your teen.
Keep in mind the SMART Talking and Listening steps

Walk around and provide assistance in ensuring that assertiveness strategies are practiced.

Tasks can be based on each of the communication steps (i.e., one person observe whether the mom is "listening"; is she understanding what the teen says, etc.)

Activity

Condom demonstration. Followed by participant's practicing putting condoms on penis/vagina models.

Intention/Purpose: To assist moms in feeling more comfortable talking about condoms with their teens and break through possible shame or embarrassment in handling condoms and demonstrating how they are used!

Supplies: Condoms; penis models; female condoms; vagina model; paper towels; wet wipes

Directions: Instruct group about how to properly put a condom on the penis model. Make sure to begin with checking the expiration date on the condom, making sure package does not have any holes, opening condom carefully so as not to tear it, taking out condom and grasping tip on the correct side, rolling condom down the penis model while grasping tip to keep air from entering, rolling condom all the way down the penis model. Make the point that after ejaculating, male will need to grasp base of condom and penis together and pull out penis while still erect to prevent condom from slipping off flaccid penis into partner! Condom should be removed, keeping semen in the condom, tie condom into a knot and throw into trash, do not flush down toilet.

After demonstrating, have group members each go through steps of putting a condom on the penis model.

Next have two members do a role-play of a mother and teen, mother explains to teen how to put on a condom, teen can ask questions they think a teen might have about safe sex and condom use. Even if moms don't think their teens would ask them to show them how to use a condom, explain that they have an opportunity to increase their comfort level discussing the topic of safe sex in this role-play. Allow other members in the group to assist role-playing members if they seem stuck, forget something or feel embarrassed.

Next demonstrate to group how to use female condom and the vagina model. Again have group check expiration date of condom, check for holes, and open carefully so as not to tear the condom. Female condom has two rings and one opening. Squeeze inner ring to insert into vagina model. Ring should sit behind pubic bone and over the cervix. Outer ring needs to remain outside the vaginal opening before, during and after intercourse. After ejaculation, grasp outer ring and twist it to close off condom, gently but firmly pull female condom out of the vagina and throw into trash—do not flush!

Next have members practice inserting female condom into vagina model. Role-play as desired.

Group Discussion: Briefly allow group to talk about their feelings about talking about safe sex and condom use within the group and with their teens. Discuss barriers to talking about safe sex and condom use.

Goal Setting and Wrap-Up

Goal Setting

Identify a short-term goal (for the week) that is related to talking to your teen about one topic related to risky behavior AND a life project goal.

Review goals and distribute goal card.

Make one positive statement about oneself.

Preview next session and encourage attendance.

Session #13, 2nd Joint Session: SMART Coping with Mom's HIV

Outcome and Skills

Outcomes: Teens and moms will increase communication regarding living with HIV.

Skill 1: Teens and moms will identify family rules and habits related to HIV disclosure.

Skill 2: Teens will practice sharing their thoughts and questions regarding mom's HIV with mom.

Skill 3: Moms will practice SMART listening and talking.

Skill 4: Teens and moms will set a short-term goal for the week and use a problem-solving technique to identify and address potential obstacles to goal.

Agenda/Timeline (Total time: 100 min.)

Check-In (15 min.)

Review last week's goal.

Preview of this session.

Skills-Building (60 min.)

Increase communication regarding living with HIV by:

Identifying family rules and habits related to HIV disclosure.

Practicing SMART listening and talking.

Helping each other reach life projects.

Goal Setting and Problem-Solving (15 min.)

Make plan/goal for week.

Engage in problem-solving exercise related to goal in order to optimize success and to plan for potential obstacles.

Wrap-Up (10 min.)

Connect session to life projects.

Make one positive statement about oneself.

Preview next session and encourage attendance.

Materials

FTD Poster

Feeling Thermometer Poster

Goal Setting Poster
SMART Poster
Assertiveness Poster
Group Rules
Tokens
Weekly Goal Card
Small Laminated Goal Cards
Flipcharts
Pens

Handouts

SMART Listening and Talking
What I Want to Talk to My Mom About Today

Post on Wall Ahead of Time

FTD Poster
Feeling Thermometer Poster
Goal Setting Poster
SMART Poster
Assertiveness Poster
Group rules generated by each of the group during individual sessions

Write on Flipchart Ahead of Time

Today's Topic/Goals for the Session

Check-In (15 min.)

Discuss goal set during last joint session

Life project goal AND goal related to last week's session topic.
Identify barriers to unaccomplished Goals
See Appendix A for How to Identify Barriers to Accomplishing Goal

Review today's topic and plan for session

Write on Flipchart Ahead of Time (in lay terms).
SMART Coping with HIV
Today we are going to talk about what it is like to live in a family in which someone has HIV.
We will:

Identify family rules and habits related to HIV disclosure.
Practice: Teens will practice sharing their thoughts and questions regarding mom's HIV
   with mom. Moms will practice SMART listening and talking.
Set a goal related to how to deal with mom's HIV.

Skills-Building (60 min.)

Skills: Teens and moms will increase communication regarding coping with HIV by identifying family rules and habits related to HIV disclosure and by practicing SMART listening and talking.

Why is it important for moms and teens to talk about mom's HIV?

Today we are going to work on increasing your ability to talk with each other about what it is like to live in your family with HIV.

Sometimes it is uncomfortable for moms and teens to have these types of talks, but it is important to have them because moms and teens who are able to talk about difficult topics are able to stay safer and have stronger relationships.

Conduct Feeling Thermometer Check

Knowing what the topic is for today, I want to start with a Feeling Thermometer check. How comfortable are you on the Feeling Thermometer?

Directions

If needed, address very high Feeling Thermometers by encouraging discussion or utilizing brief relaxation, otherwise proceed to the next step.

Family Rules of Disclosure

People with serious illnesses make different decisions about who to tell.

> Some people just talk about their illness with their doctor.
> Some people talk about their illness with everyone they know and even with strangers they meet.

I'd like us to spend a few minutes talking about how your family deals with this issue.
Does your family tell or not tell other people about mom having HIV?

Directions

Elicit feedback from the participants.
If needed, ask the following questions to facilitate a discussion.

How do you decide *who to tell?*
Who is allowed to tell and who isn't allowed to tell?
What do you tell and what do you decide not to tell?
How do you decide *when to tell?*
What is it like to tell?

Allow conversation to proceed for 30 minutes.
Reinforce choices and the idea that there are various ways to handle disclosure, all with pros and cons.

SMART Coping with HIV: Moms and teens group separately to prepare

For this next section, we are going to focus on talking about what it is like to cope with HIV in your own family.
For about ten minutes I want the mothers and teenagers to meet separately.

Directions

Have the mothers and teenagers meet in separate places.
A facilitator goes with each group.
Review the following preparation handouts with each small mom and teen group.

Mothers

Review goal of activity:
How to increase teens' ability and comfort in talking to mom about their thoughts and feelings.
Review and focus on the "Listening" part of SMART talking and listening.

This is a time for you to practice what you learned about increasing your children's comfort and ability to talk to you about their thoughts and feelings.

The teens have come up with something that they would like to talk to you about your HIV today.

Don't Forget: This exercise requires the facilitators' creativity to improvise and meet the needs of the group in managing the questions and answers.

The teens will be sharing a question or a thought about mom's HIV. Moms may respond to their own child and they may also respond to others' children as well.

The teen group facilitator may also ask moms questions anonymously in order to increase the teen's comfort level in asking their questions.

Distribute

SMART Listening and Talking

State the problem

What is the topic?
Be positive.
Tell the other person what feelings you have.

Make a goal (Realistic and Specific)

What is your goal? To hear what your teen is saying to you?
Consider what your feeling thermometer may be causing you to do: Are you wanting to avoid the conversation? Blame the teen?
What is teen's goal? Consider what the child is asking for: Is it information, reassurance or permission.
Joint goal? Closer relationship? How can mom and teen come up with a goal that they can both accept and meets both of their needs?
Realistic?
Specific?
Win-win situation?

Actions—Make a list of all the possible actions you could take and evaluate the pros and cons of each option

Avoid nagging, criticizing, threatening or lecturing. This will push the person away.
Both mom and teen offer solutions.
After you have come up with all the solutions, together examine the advantages and disadvantages of each possible solution ("Do you think this one would solve the problem?").
If you can't end up with one or two solutions that seem best, schedule another time to meet.

Reach a decision about which action you want to try

Joint decision where both of you agree with the solution.
Make sure that it is understood that each person is making a commitment to carry out the decision.
Be specific about the joint goal. Make sure that both people understand how the solution will be implemented. Raise questions about how to try out the solution. (When do we start? What days? What do we need to start? How will we know that the other person is doing what they said they would?)

Try it and review it

Remember that sometimes solutions may need to be changed or modified.
Keep the door open for more communication if this is the case.
Evaluate the solution after a week, then two weeks, and so on.

Your teen is being asked to think of one thing to tell you about how your HIV has impacted his or her life.

The goal is not to make you feel guilty, but to help you understand what it is like for them.

Your job is to listen to make sure you really understand what they are saying and feeling, and to let them know you understand.

Your teen is also being asked to come up with one question they have about your HIV.

You can decide if you want to answer the question or not, or if you want to think about it before deciding to answer it or not.

The important thing is to learn what type of questions your teen has about your HIV.

Again the focus is on listening and learning about your teen.

Listening will help them to feel more comfortable talking to you about your HIV.

Any questions? How comfortable are you on the feeling thermometer?

Directions

If needed, address very high Feeling Thermometers by encouraging discussion or utilizing brief relaxation, otherwise proceed to the next step.

Teens

Directions

If this session follows the individual teen session, "SMART Coping with Mom's HIV," the teens would have already selected the topic that they would like to address with their mom. In this case:

Review each teen's selected question or topic.
Assess teen's comfort level in addressing mom.
Assess whether any teens would prefer that the facilitator anonymously poses the teen
    questions to the mom's group.
Teens may also have the option of asking moms other teens' questions.
The goal of activity:
Think about how teens' life is impacted because of mom's HIV.

For example, some of you might have to take care of your mom sometimes. Some of you
    might have a strong emotion or worry because your mom has HIV.
Many families do not make the time to talk about these things. Many families find it un-
    comfortable to talk about these things.

Think of one way that your mom's HIV impacts you or your life that you are willing to share with her. It may be a question or just a thought about her HIV.

Maybe she doesn't know you are scared for her health when she skips her medications, or
    maybe you really want your mom to know that it really helps you when she asks your
    aunt to help out when she is sick.
Another example would be that you might wonder what the doctors are saying to her
    about her health, or you might wonder something about her medications.

Distribute

What I Want to Talk to My Mom about Today

One thing about my mom's HIV that affects me or my life:

One *question* I have for my mom about her HIV:

Allow 3–4 minutes for teens to write down what they want to share.

Write down one question and/or one thing you want to share with your mom about her HIV. This would be a question or a thought you are willing to ask her today. It can be the one thing you came up with during your individual session.

She may or may not answer the question, and that is okay, but it might be helpful for her to know what kinds of things you wonder about.

How comfortable are you on the Feeling Thermometer?

If needed, address very high Feeling Thermometers by encouraging discussion or utilizing brief relaxation, otherwise proceed to the next step.

SMART coping with HIV: Reunite moms and teens
Directions

Each teen tells mom one thing about her HIV.

I'd like each teen to tell his or her mother the one thing they wanted to say today. The moms will do their best to really understand what the teen is saying.

They might ask questions to be sure they really understand.

If teens are having difficulty telling mom one thing about her HIV, facilitator may take the lead and anonymously share some of the topics written by the teens or those listed here.

Common Questions Teens might have for their moms about their HIV

Who infected you/how did you get HIV?
Are you mad at the person who infected you?
What will happen to me if you get really sick one day?
Are you going to die?
Are you scared?
What is it like to take medicine?
When did you first tell me about your HIV?
Why don't you want to take your medicine?
Why don't you want to tell people about your HIV?
Who can I tell about your HIV?

Common ways that Teens' lives are affected by their mom's HIV

Sometimes I feel scared.
I am mad at the person who infected you.
I feel like I have more responsibility.
I feel closer to you.
I feel like I am keeping a big secret.

For mom groups without teens: provide list of questions and concerns from worksheet provided in Appendix A and allow mom's to respond. (Included at end of this session.)

Allow at least several minutes, but allow the talking to go on for ten minutes if it is productive.

How comfortable are you on the Feeling Thermometer?

If needed, address very high Feeling Thermometers by encouraging discussion or utilizing brief relaxation, otherwise proceed to the next step.

Each teen asks mom one thing about her HIV.

Now I'd like each teen to ask his or her mother the one question they wanted to ask today.

The moms will decide whether or not to answer the question. Either way is fine.

The most important part is for the moms to really understand what type of questions the teens have about her HIV.

If teens are having difficulty asking mom one question about her HIV, facilitator may take the lead and anonymously ask some of the questions written by the teens.

Allow at least several minutes, but allow the talking to go on for ten minutes if it is productive.

How comfortable are you on the Feeling Thermometer?

If needed, address very high Feeling Thermometers by encouraging discussion or utilizing brief relaxation, otherwise proceed to the next step.

If time allows, de-brief with the mom and teen group separately.

Wrap-Up and Goal Setting (15 min.)

Skills: Increased ability to set a goal that is realistic, clear, not too easy or too difficult and that has a clear end point; and increased ability to problem-solve in order to optimize success and to plan for potential obstacles.

Identify a short-term goal (for the week) that is related to coping with HIV in the family

Have each participant make one positive statement about herself OR share one positive thing she liked about the group.

Preview next session and encourage attendance.

Mom Session #14: Managing Teen Behaviors

Outcome and Skills

Outcomes: Increased ability to manage teen's problem behaviors.
Skill 1: Identify comfort level related to recent teen behaviors.
Skill 2: Learn strategies to manage their teen's problem behaviors.
Skill 3: Problem-solve barriers to managing teen's behaviors.
Skill 4: Practice managing teen's problem behaviors.
Skill 5: Build social support related to parenting.

Agenda/Timeline (Total time: 95 min.)

Check-In (20 min.)

Review last week's goal.
Preview of this session.

Skills (50 min.)

Increased ability to manage teen problem behaviors through:

Identifying comfort level related to recent teen behaviors.
Learning strategies to manage teen behaviors

Goal setting
Role play strategies to manage teen behaviors
Problem-solve barriers to managing teen behaviors
Social support building surrounding parenting

Problem-Solving (15 min.)

Goal setting surrounding managing teen behaviors AND life project goal.
Problem-solve barriers to accomplishing goal.

Wrap-Up and Goal Setting (10 min.)

Review goal setting.
Connect session to positive outcomes for the children of the women.
Connect session to life projects.
Make one positive statement about oneself.
Preview next session and encourage attendance

Materials

FTD Poster
Feeling Thermometer Poster
SMART Poster
Goal Setting Poster
Assertiveness Poster
Group Rules
Participant Life projects
Relaxation handout (if needed)
Tokens
Goal Card
Flipcharts
Pens

Handout

Strategies for Managing Difficult Teen Behaviors

Post on the Wall Ahead of Time

FTD Poster
Feeling Thermometer Poster
Goal Setting Poster
SMART Poster
Assertiveness Poster
Group Rules
Participant Life projects

Write on Flipchart Ahead of Time

Today's Topic/Goals for the Session

Check-In (20 min.)

Discuss goals set at last session

Life project goal AND goal related to last week's session topic.
Identify barriers to unaccomplished Goals
See Appendix A for How to Identify Barriers to Accomplishing Goal

Review today's topic and plan for session

Write on Flipchart Ahead of Time (in lay terms).
Goals of this workshop

Identify problem teen behaviors.
Increase ability to manage teen problem behaviors.
Increase social support surrounding parenting.

Skills Building (50 min.)

Feeling thermometer and teen behaviors

What is something that your teen has done recently that you were comfortable with (Feeling Thermometer 0–20)?

Don't Forget: Assist mothers in developing a hierarchy for teen behaviors that they are comfortable versus uncomfortable with.

Themes for hierarchy of behaviors may include:

Independence
Risky behaviors
Conflict/problem situation

Identify teen behaviors to change

Think of the *most recent* conflict you had with your teen. What was it about?
Where was your Feeling Thermometer?
What behavior was your child displaying that you want to see changed?
Be as specific as possible about the behavior. I.e., my son interrupts me when I am speaking, or my daughter eats her dinner in front of the TV instead of with the family.

Identify a goal related to the target behavior

What is it that you want your child to do more of?
Review goal setting

State goal in one sentence.
Realistic (can reasonably expect to complete between sessions)
Clear (participant understands exactly what steps must be taken to complete the goal)
Not too easy and not too hard (30–50 on the Feeling Thermometer; goal should be challenging, but not impossible)
Clear end point (measurable, participant should know when the goal has been accomplished)
What do you want more of (stated in a positive term)

Support participants in generating appropriate goals.

Don't Forget: Stress that it is helpful if parents set their child up for success. This means selecting a goal that is specific, realistic and not too easy or too hard.

Let's state your goal in a *positive way*. This means state what you want rather than what you don't want. So, for example, I would like my son to always wait his turn to speak, or I would like my daughter to eat dinner with the family every night.

We want to be sure that we set *goals that we are pretty sure our kids can achieve*. For example, it might be more realistic to restate the goals I've started to say: I would like my son to wait his turn to speak 50% of the time, or I would like my daughter to eat dinner with the family three nights per week.

In the first case, even though the eventual goal is for the son to refrain from interrupting, it is hard to break those habits. It would be a big change for him if he sometimes waited his turn.

In the second case, the daughter might want to have dinner with friends on the weekend and she might have basketball practice two nights a week during dinnertime. Three nights a week might be more realistic and give her some control.

Directions

Write each goal on the board.

Strategies for creating positive behavioral change

You now have each identified one thing that you want to see your child do more of. What kinds of techniques could be used to increase positive behavior in a teen?

Directions

Write ideas on flipchart.
Elicit feedback from participants. If not mentioned, address the following:

Praise positive behavior
Do not criticize while giving a compliment
Ignore negative/problem behavior
Attach consequence to problem behavior
Reward competing behavior

Don't Forget: Make sure that the following strategies are discussed and elicited from the mothers. Avoid conducting this in a didactic format.

Directions

Elicit below information from group members and generate a list on the flipchart.
Discuss at least 2 examples per suggestion.

1. Rewarding/praising positive behavior

"Catch them being good"

Examples: Let's say you catch your teen doing something you like and you thank them for it or do something nice for them as a way of thanking them. They will feel really good that you thanked them and that you were pleased. Because they like this feeling, you just increased the chances that they will do the positive behavior again. You also helped them feel good about themselves.

Let's say Beth picks up a shirt from the living room floor. You say "thanks for cleaning up Beth. I really appreciate it." Beth will now be more likely to pick her clothes in the living room.

Types of rewards

Verbal praise
Hugs/smiles
Extra privileges (i.e., staying out late, borrowing the car)
Rewarding activities (i.e., movies, having a friend over)
Tangible rewards (i.e., snacks, allowance, toys)

Rewarding the right behavior

Examples: How about this: How many of you have finally given up after your child has begged and begged you for something? If you give something to your child that he or she wants after they nag and beg you for a week, what behavior have you rewarded? What behavior is likely to go up in the future? And, how many of you enjoy it when your kids beg you for things? The idea here is to be careful about what behavior you are rewarding.

If you change your mind and decide to buy the shoes, you might consider linking it to another behavior. For example, you might say to your child that you will buy the shoes if she agrees to baby-sit for you on four Wednesday nights so you can go to a Church group. Now you are rewarding her for baby-sitting, not for begging.

2. Do not criticize while giving a compliment

Example: "Wow. I can't believe you actually cooked dinner; it's horrible when we have to eat junk food."

Do you enjoy the compliment less because of the criticism?

What to say instead? If your son cleaned the bathroom for the first time, but did a bad job, you might say "Wow. That is so nice that you cleaned the bathroom. Thank you." This is not the time to offer suggestions on how to do it better. You want him to feel good so he'll do it again. If he does a better job the next time, notice that too. "Wow, you did even a better job this time. The sink looks so clean."

3. Competing behavior

The idea is this: If you do not want your child to do something, one way to change the behavior is to allow them to do something else that competes with it. Or, you do something else that competes with it.

Example: If you don't like your son hanging out with kids who smoke on the corner after school, allow him to join a basketball team that practices after school (or do something else he really wants to do). He won't be able to hang out with the smokers and you won't have to argue with him about it all the time.

Or, if you don't like it that your daughter always nags you to make her a snack when she gets home from school even though she can do it herself, you might decide that you will walk your dog during this time each day so that you will not be around for her to nag.

Role play how to manage teen problem behaviors

Role play additional goals and parenting strategies if time is available.

Wrap-Up and Goal Setting (15 min.)

Goal Setting

Identify a short-term goal (for the week) that is related to managing teen behavior AND/OR Life Project.

Review goals and distribute goal card.

Make one positive statement about oneself.

Preview next session and encourage attendance.

Session #15, 3rd Joint Session: A SMART Way to Disagree with Each Other

Outcome and Skills

Outcomes: Teens and mothers will gain knowledge and utilize SMART to resolve arguments.

Skill 1: Teens and moms will increase knowledge about a SMART way to disagree.

Skill 2: Teens and moms will practice SMART.

Skill 3: Teens and moms will identify and problem-solve barriers to using SMART.

Skill 4: Teens and moms will set a short-term goal for the week and use a problem-solving technique to identify and address potential obstacles to goal.

Agenda/Timeline (Total time: 100 min.)

Check-In (15 min.)

Review last week's goal.
Preview of this session.

Skills-Building (60 min.)

Increase knowledge of and better utilize SMART skills by:

Practicing SMART.
Identifying barriers to SMART.
Problem-solve barriers to SMART.
Goal setting

Activity (10 min.)

Peanut butter and jelly exercise

Problem-Solving (15 min.)

Make plan/goal for week.
Engage in problem-solving exercise related to goal in order to optimize success and to plan for potential obstacles.

Wrap-Up and Goal Setting (10 min.)

Connect session to life projects.
Make one positive statement about oneself.
Preview next session and encourage attendance.

Materials

FTD Poster/Pens
Feeling Thermometer Poster
Goal Setting Poster
SMART Poster
Assertiveness Poster
Group Rules
Tokens
Weekly Goal Card
Small Laminated Goal Cards
Flipcharts
Peanut butter, jelly, bread, plastic knives

Handouts

SMART problem-solving guidelines
Power play role play script
SMART role play script
Additional role play scripts

Post on Wall Ahead of Time

FTD Poster
Feeling Thermometer Poster

Goal Setting Poster
SMART Poster
Assertiveness Poster
Group rules generated by each of the group during individual sessions

Write on Flipchart Ahead of Time

Today's Topic/Goals for the Session

Check-In (15 min.)

Review today's topic and plan for session

Conflict Resolution

Review a strategy: Review a helpful way to disagree with SMART.

Practice: Practice how to be SMART when you disagree with each other.

What gets in the way: Identify and problem-solve what might get in the way of you being SMART when you disagree with each other.

How does conflict relate to the different needs of teens and parents?

To start the process of learning how to resolve conflicts, it is important to recognize that *teenagers and mothers are coming from different places* for good reasons.

These *differences are normal* and often put teenagers and their mothers at odds.

Teenagers usually want to become independent, to have the freedom to make their own decisions. This normal developmental need helps them by preparing them for being on their own.

Mothers want to protect their teenagers from harm and do what they think is best for them.

Skills-Building (60 min.)

Skills: Teens and moms will increase knowledge about a SMART way to disagree, practice using SMART, identify barriers to using SMART, and brainstorm solutions.

State goal of SMART conflict resolution

Today we are going to work on a SMART way to resolving disagreements at home.

The goal is to use a SMART way to resolve disagreements so that teens and parents both end up feeling good about the outcome.

No one "wins" or "loses" at the expense of the other person.

You can learn to work together to search for a solution that may even be better than what each of you wanted in the first place and can strengthen your relationship.

Present common less effective conflict resolution strategies often employed

There are two ways parents often use to resolve conflict.

The first is for the parent to use his or *her authority and power.*

They might say, "I want you to come home by 7 P.M. because I am the parent and I told you to do it."

What is the parent's goal here? (being authoritative)

What impact does using this approach have on the teenager?

Directions

Elicit feedback from participants and record on flipchart. If not mentioned, address the following:

Sullenness
Resentment

Lying

Running away

No chance to practice making decisions—doesn't learn how to make them.

No sense of responsibility for decisions

What is the impact on the parent?

Elicit feedback from participants and record on flipchart. If not mentioned, address the following:

Feels pressured

Irritated

Stressed

The second approach to resolving conflicts is for the parent *to give in* and let the child have all the power. What does this lead to in the parent and teenager?

Elicit feedback from participants and record on flipchart. If not mentioned, address the following:

TEENAGER:	*Wild*
	Uncontrolled
	Impulsive
	Self-Centered
PARENT:	*Resentful*
	Failures

What Is the Best Way to Resolve Conflict? SMART

There is a third approach where both the parent and teenager win.

Distribute

"A SMART Way to Disagree"

State the problem

What is the fight about?

Listen: Don't be thinking of a response while the child is talking

Use "I" statements. Say how what the child does makes you feel. Do not blame.

State the problem in one sentence. Do not include old fights that have nothing to do with this conflict.

I.e., Kim always wants to hang out with friends at the mall.

Make a goal (Realistic and Specific)

What is mom's goal?

Consider what your feeling thermometer may be causing you to do: Are you wanting to avoid the conversation? Blame the teen?

What is teen's goal?

Consider what the child is asking for: Is it information, reassurance or permission?

Joint goal?

How can mom and teen come up with a goal that they can both accept and meets both of their needs?

Realistic?

Specific?

Win-win situation?

Actions—Make a list of all the possible actions you could take and evaluate the pros and cons of each option

Avoid nagging, criticizing, threatening or lecturing. This will push the person away.

Both mom and teen offer solutions.

After you have come up with all the solutions, together examine the advantages and disadvantages of each possible solution.

If you can't end up with one or two solutions that seem best, schedule another time to meet.

Reach a decision about which action you want to try

Joint decision where both of you agree with the solution.

Make sure that it is understood that each person is making a commitment to carry out the decision.

Be specific about the joint goal. (When do we start? What days? What do we need to start? How will we know that the other person is doing what they said they would?)

Try it and review it

Remember that sometimes solutions may need to be changed or modified.

Keep the door open for more communication if this is the case.

Evaluate the solution after a week, then two weeks, and so on.

Don't Forget: Avoid a didactic format. Elicit SMART from the participants so that they can "own" the approach.

Mention steps that may not have been generated by members.

Tie in participants' feedback and suggestions to SMART handout.

Practice Power Play Role Play

Now that we have reviewed the SMART approach, I need some volunteers to role-play in front of the group. Who will volunteer to play the parent and who will be the teenager?

Select volunteers to play daughter and mother (Power Role Play Script #1: See addendum).

If teenager wants to play the role of the parent, that is fine. Give them the role.

Read the background information aloud.

Background Information: Power Role Play #1

Mother: Your fifteen year old daughter has been wearing very sexy shirts to school. You told her before that you wanted her to stop, that her blouses were too low cut. She kept right on wearing them. You are afraid that she is sending the wrong messages to the boys in school. You don't want her to get a bad reputation or to encourage boys who will take advantage of her.

Daughter: Your mother has been on your back about the way you dress. She thinks you are showing too much skin. She doesn't understand that is the way girls dress nowadays. Your mother isn't living in the real world. She's back in the dark ages. If she took a look at any movie magazine, any fashion magazine, she would see how much women show.

Power Role Play Script #1

MOTHER: *Come in here, Chantall.*

DAUGHTER: *What do you want? I'm busy.*

MOTHER: *Come in here anyway. You can't keep wearing those blouses to school.*

DAUGHTER: *Not this again.*

MOTHER: *Do you want to look like a whore?*

DAUGHTER: *Don't talk to me.*

MOTHER: *With that blouse you can almost see down to your belly button.*

DAUGHTER: *No, you can't.*

MOTHER: *What are you doing—advertising something?*

DAUGHTER: *Leave me alone. Can I go now?*

MOTHER: *No, you can't. I'm telling you—no more low cut blouses to school. There's a right time to wear something like that, and school isn't it.*

DAUGHTER: *You can't stop me.*

MOTHER: *You would be surprised. If you wear a blouse like that again, I will take all of them away.*

DAUGHTER: *I'll get more.*

MOTHER: *I'll talk to your teacher, and if she tells me you wear something like that behind my back, you won't be going out of your room. I don't want you getting a bad reputation.*

DAUGHTER: *All you think of is your reputation. Don't you ever think of my being happy? You want me to lose all my friends? You should see the other girls.*

MOTHER: *I don't care about them. Let their mothers worry about them. You are my daughter, and I'm not letting you ruin your life.*

DAUGHTER: *Don't be so dramatic. Maybe you're just jealous.*

MOTHER: *Chantall, I've warned you about getting smart with me. It is finished. You can go now, and remember—No more low cut blouses.*

DAUGHTER: *Just wait and see.*

Directions

Divide the observers in half.
One half pays attention to the parent and the other half pay attention to the teenager.
Assign observation tasks.
Examples of what to watch follow:
You watch the . . .

facial expression
eye contact
gestures
voice
words used
posture
body tension

Start the role-play.
Have volunteers read Power Role Play.
They can either read the power-play script or make it up themselves.
Practice SMART: SMART Role Play #1 (see addendum for Script)
Now we will do it again using SMART. See if you notice differences.
Have volunteers role play the SMART approach.
They can either read the SMART script or make it up themselves.

Smart Role Play #1

MOTHER: *Chantall, are you busy?*

DAUGHTER: *No, what do you want?*

MOTHER: *I want to work on finding a solution to something that is bothering me—a solution that will be OK for both of us.*

DAUGHTER: *Sounds heavy.*

MOTHER: *You are so beautiful and I am normally very proud of the way you handle yourself. But, I feel very nervous when I see you wearing those low cut blouses to school because...*

DAUGHTER: *Not this again.*

MOTHER: *... because I am afraid you will attract some boy with one thing on his mind and he will take advantage of you.*

DAUGHTER: *What's that?*

MOTHER: *What's what?*

DAUGHTER: *The one thing on his mind?*

MOTHER: *Sex.*

DAUGHTER: *Don't you think I can handle it?*

MOTHER: *What do you mean?*

DAUGHTER: *I mean keep from getting hurt.*

MOTHER: *I don't know if you can handle it. I think at fifteen you are too young to try, but let's not get side-tracked. It's the low cut blouses that bother me because I don't want you to get a bad reputation or to send messages that you are available sexually.*

DAUGHTER: *Mom, all the girls show something. That doesn't mean they want sex with every guy they see. It's just the way we dress.*

MOTHER: *I'm uncomfortable with it. How do you feel?*

DAUGHTER: *It would make me miserable if I changed my way of dressing and then all my friends made fun of me and no boy ever looked at me again.*

MOTHER: *To lose your friends and be unattractive isn't something I want for you. What are some possible solutions that you can think of?*

DAUGHTER: *The only thing I can think of is to do what you say, and I don't want to do that.*

MOTHER: *Let's get some ideas out before we look at their advantages and disadvantages. One is to stop wearing the blouses to school.*

DAUGHTER: *I could hang out with kids who don't care about how they look.*

MOTHER: *What else?*

DAUGHTER: *I could wear some of my blouses only a couple days a week.*

MOTHER: *How do you like what this girl's got on in the magazine?*

DAUGHTER: *Oooooo! I like that. It only cost $200. You going to get it for me?*

MOTHER: *Not that one, but we could go shopping together.*

DAUGHTER: *So maybe getting some new clothes is a possible solution.*

MOTHER: *Clothes acceptable to both of us.*

DAUGHTER: *Sounds cool.*

MOTHER: *How do some of the other ideas sound?*

DAUGHTER: *Well, I don't want to find new friends. And cutting down on the number of times I wear a top isn't too terrible, if I had something else that was nice.*

MOTHER: *I don't want you to have to find a whole new group of friends. My preference is not to wear those blouses to school at all. I haven't got much money, but I'm willing to see what we can do buying some other tops you like.*

DAUGHTER: *And that you like.*

MOTHER: *I don't have to like them as long as they are not showing too much.*

DAUGHTER: *I have some money saved—maybe I could use a little of it on the clothes.*

MOTHER: *This makes me very happy.*

DAUGHTER: *We'll have to see what my friends think of my new style. Actually Karen doesn't wear stuff that is revealing.*

MOTHER: *Well, you're an attractive girl. We just have to find the clothes that suit you. So, we are going to try it. Right? We'll shop tomorrow, and you agree to wear something different on Monday.*

DAUGHTER: *Sounds worth trying.*

What differences did you see in the two approaches?
Encourage discussion, contrasting the Power approach and SMART.
Use the guidelines to make sure that all the possible differences are covered.
How do you think the mother and daughter felt in the different versions?
Focus on feelings and the difference that they make in the two scenes and in what will happen in the future.

Don't Forget: Emphasize the underlying assumptions about roles, responsibilities and rules: The impact of thoughts and feelings on actions.

Directions

Practice another SMART Role Play (#2)
Let's try another role-play. We want to try both a "Power" approach and a SMART approach to a conflict between a mother and her teen. Ask participants to generate Role Play #2 or use Role Play # 2 addendum.

Other Practice Scenes

Scene 1: The Boy Friend

Mother: You are very unhappy over your daughter's choice of boy friend—at least 10 years older, much too slick, doesn't work but has lots of money. A drug dealer? He gives your daughter expensive gifts. You think he is using her.

Teenager: You are dating an older man who seems to have everything: really cool, polite, takes you nice places and gives you expensive gifts. Your mother is against him. She thinks he's a drug dealer. He's been very good to you. It bothers you that your mother doesn't trust your judgment.

Scene 2: Sex

Mother: Your daughter started asking you questions about birth control. Pretty soon it became obvious that she is having sex with her boy friend. This really scares you. You don't want her to get pregnant or to get any diseases like HIV. The best thing for her is no sex at all. She is too young for sex.

Teenager: You asked your mother about birth control, thinking she would be pleased that you were taking care of yourself. She got all upset and started yelling at you about having sex. All your friends have sex. Your boy friend is very careful and uses a condom. You don't want to lose him. You know what you are doing.

Scene 3: Curfew

Mother: You think your 15 year old teenager should be in the apartment by 8 P.M. on week nights and by midnight on week ends. Your teenager doesn't agree. It irritates you he (she) won't do what you ask. Fifteen is too young to be out to all hours of the night. You are worried that something bad will happen.

Teenager: Your mother tells you that you have to be in by 8 P.M. on week nights and midnight on week ends. As far as you know, none of your friends have such restrictions. You can take care of yourself. All you are doing is hanging out with your friends. She is so strict.

Scene 4: Money

Mother: You give your teenager a little spending money, and your teenager has a part time job. All your teenager spends money on is tapes for the walkman. How can your teenager be so irresponsible? You think some of the money ought to go into savings for college, clothes, school supplies, lunch money.

Teenager: You got a part time job so that you could buy things you want. Now your mother is telling you how to spend your money. She should mind her own business. You spend your money on tapes for your walkman. It's your money.

Select volunteers to play teen and mother.

If a teenager wants to play the role of the parent, that is fine. Give them the role.

Divide the observers in half. One half pays attention to the parent and the other half pays attention to the teenager.

Assign observation tasks.

Examples of what to watch follow:

You watch the . . .

facial expression
eye contact
gestures
voice
words used
posture
body tension

Start the role-play.

Have the players begin. If neither one starts, prompt the mother to open the dialogue.

Stop the role play after a while for coaching and then continue it.

Let me stop you briefly for some coaching. Observers, I would like you to offer some helpful comments to the players. What did you see that you liked and what would you try differently?

After a few comments, offer any suggestions of your own and start the role play up again.

Let the role play go for about four more minutes.

Obtain feedback

Power Role Play #2

Mom's Goal: To get son to talk on cell phone less so that he does not go over his minutes and ring up a huge phone bill.

Son's goal: To continue to talk to his friends as much as he does and get his mom off his back about his phone use.

MOM: *Jose, we need to talk about your phone use.*

JOSE: *Mom, not this again!*

MOM: *This is ridiculous! I spent $30 extra dollars last month on the cell phone bill when you went over your minutes!*

JOSE: *You only give me 150 minutes a month on my phone! How am I supposed to talk to my friends with that? Max has 300 minutes, Donny has 500. It's so unfair.*

MOM: *Bringing home the grades you have gotten recently, you shouldn't be able to have a phone at all. This is a privilege you should earn! You have no appreciation for all the hard work I do just to pay the electricity around here. What do you think, money grows on trees?*

JOSE: *I work too mom! You act like I do nothing.*

MOM: *Well, you don't. When's the last time you helped me clean up around here? You don't deserve to have a cell phone at all if you can't learn to use it responsibly and stay within the allotted minutes. I am taking it away from you for 3 months. No cell phone at all. And on top of that, you will only be able to use the house phone from 3 to 7 at night.*

JOSE: *Fine! I'll just call Dad and tell him to buy me one. He at least understands me!*

MOM: *Go ahead and do it and you'll see what kind of privileges you get around here from now on.*

(JOSE STORMS OUT OF THE ROOM)

Smart Role Play #2

Mom's Goal: To get son to talk on cell phone less so that he does not go over his minutes and ring up large charges.

Son's goal: To continue to talk to his friends as much as he does.

MOM: *Jose, we need to talk about your phone use.*

JOSE: *Mom, not this again!*

MOM: *We need to come to some sort of agreement on this. I can't continue to pay an extra $30 a month because you are going over your minutes. Can we think of a way to avoid this?*

JOSE: *I don't mean to go over, I just feel like 150 minutes is not enough.*

MOM: *Well, I'm sorry you feel that way. I know it's important for you to talk to your friends and I know I ask you to call me if you're going to be late, but 150 minutes is all I can afford right now. So can we try to think of some solutions that work for both of us?*

JOSE: *I guess. I guess I could use some of my own money from work to pay the bill.*

MOM: *You could, but I know you like to save that money for things like movies and clothes.*

JOSE: *Yeah, I do.*

MOM: *Another option would be for you to use the home phone more when you are at home.*

JOSE: *But the home phone is in the kitchen or your room. Sometimes I want to talk privately.*

MOM: *I understand that. Maybe we could move the phone from my room into your room since I don't talk much.*

JOSE: *That would be cool. I think I could save a lot of minutes if I did that.*

MOM: *And all the local calls are free, so it shouldn't cost anymore.*

JOSE: *And what if I go over on my minutes still?*

MOM: *I don't know. What do you think would make sense?*

JOSE: *I guess then I could use some of my money from work.*

MOM: *OK. And if you do stay within the 150 minutes this month, maybe I could give you some extra money at the end of the month to add to your spending cash.*

JOSE: *Yeah, that'd be cool.*

MOM: *So what do you say? Should we try it out this month?*

JOSE: *Sounds OK to me.*

I want to start with the "mother" and "teenager." Tell us how you felt on your feeling thermometer and tell us one thing you did that you liked and one thing that you would do differently.

Now let's hear from the others. Tell us one thing that you liked about the way the mother and teenager did the role-plays and one thing you would do differently.

Activity

Peanut Butter and Jelly Sandwich Activity

Intention/Purpose: To illustrate the importance of clear communication and the differences of understanding and definitions of topics of discussion.

Supplies: Loaf of bread, jar of peanut butter, jar of jelly, knife, spoon, plate, table/tray/or chair to use as table, paper towels or napkins to clean up!

Directions: Bring out the sandwich supplies so group can see what you have. Ask for a volunteer to give directions about how to make a peanut butter and jelly sandwich. This volunteer will stand outside of the group with their back to the group so they can't see what you are doing as they give directions. Instruct them that they are NOT to turn around until you tell them to, no matter what they hear. Tell the volunteer that their job is to instruct you how to make a sandwich using all the supplies that you have shown them but that they cannot watch what you are doing.

FACILITATOR directions: Facilitator will follow directions *literally* and with some *exaggeration*. Facilitator's job is to NOT know how to make a sandwich and take the directions at face value. For example, when volunteer says open the bread, facilitator can rip open the bag, tear open the bag and the bread, etc. If volunteer says put some peanut butter on the bread, facilitator can put the entire, unopened jar on top of the loaf of bread, scoop out peanut butter with their hands or finger and put a big glop on the bread, etc.

When volunteer completes their directions, ask them if they are done and then tell them they can turn around. Show them the sandwich they instructed you to make. Praise volunteer for their willingness to volunteer and make sure group does not criticize volunteer. If there is time, ask for another volunteer who thinks they can give instructions. Again, follow instructions literally.

Group Discussion: Allow for discussion about how group sees activity relating to communication, dealing with conflict and negotiating within the family. Real life example might be that a mom might tell her kid to clean his/her room. Kid cleans room according to their definitions of clean—maybe everything under the bed, maybe only a path made on the floor, maybe everything organized into neat piles, etc. Mom comes back to check and says that the room is NOT clean and kid says the room IS clean. Mom's definitions of clean are vacuumed floor, emptied trash, clean sheets on bed, dirty clothes in hamper, etc. Mom and kid have different ideas of clean that did not get communicated—just like in sandwich exercise, open the bread meant two different things to the volunteer and the facilitator. How can we make sure that people understand us and that we understand other people?

At the conclusion of the activity:

How do you think this exercise relates to communication?

Facilitator can use the example of asking a child to clean their room, which to them, may mean a spotless room with clothes put away, vacuuming, cleaning under the bed etc. . . The child's definition may be to push all of the clothes under the bed to create space on the floor. This is similar to the peanut butter and jelly exercise, where putting the peanut butter on the bread can mean the WHOLE JAR of peanut butter if not clearly explained.

Identify barriers to using the SMART approach and brainstorm solutions

Sometimes parents and teens have attitudes that are obstacles to using the SMART procedure.

For example, parents might think that if they used it, they would always end up giving in to their kids.

Parents who typically use power may feel that parents should never "compromise."

Parents who usually give in may tell themselves, "Well, I will end up giving in anyway, so why go through the procedure."

Teenagers may think, "I am going to lose anyway, so why try to resolve the problem."

Teenagers may say that they will lose face if they "compromise."

I believe a solution that satisfies both the parent and the teenager is so much better than a forced one, that it will be worth trying the SMART steps.

Also when parent and teenager work together, they often find better solutions than the ones each person had before. Together there is a lot more creative wisdom that gets generated.

Wrap-Up and Goal Setting (15 min.)

Skills: Increased ability to set a goal that is realistic, clear, not too easy or too difficult and that has a clear end point; and increased ability to problem-solve in order to optimize success and to plan for potential obstacles.

Both teens and moms should set a short-term goal (for the week) that is related to a SMART way to disagree. For example, the goal may focus on an area of disagreement between the teen and mom they can work on together.

Make a positive statement about self or share something learned from group.

Preview next session and encourage attendance.

Session #16: How Can We Be a Healthy Family?

Outcome and Skills

Outcome: Teens and mothers will change a daily routine to improve the physical health of the family.

Skill 1: Teens and moms will identify unhealthy family habits related to physical health.

Skill 2: Teens and moms will practice joint SMART problem-solving to make a long-term healthy decision for the family.

Skill 3: Teens and moms will set a short-term goal for the week and use a problem-solving technique to identify and address potential obstacles to goal.

Agenda/Timeline (Total time: 145 min.)

Check-In (15 min.)

Preview of this session.
Create group rules for joint sessions

Skills-Building (60 min.)

Improve the physical health of the family by:

Identifying pros and cons of unhealthy physical habits.
Identify an unhealthy family habit.
Seek family support in accomplishing health goal.
Identify a family health goal.
Practicing joint SMART problem-solving to make a long-term healthy decision for the family.

Activity (45 min.)

Healthy/Unhealthy Collage Activity

Problem-Solving (15 min.)

Make plan/goal for week.
Engage in problem-solving exercise related to goal in order to optimize success and to plan for potential obstacles.

Wrap-Up and Goal Setting (10 min.)

Connect session to life projects.
Make one positive statement about oneself.
Preview next session and encourage attendance.

Materials

FTD Poster
Feeling Thermometer Poster
Goal Setting Poster
SMART Poster
Assertiveness Poster
Group Rules
Tokens
Weekly Goal Card
Small Laminated Goal Cards
Flipcharts
Pens

Post on Wall Ahead of Time

FTD Poster
Feeling Thermometer Poster
Goal Setting Poster
SMART Poster
Assertiveness Poster
Group rules generated by each of the group during individual sessions

Write on Flipchart Ahead of Time

Today's Topic/Goals for the Session

Check-In (15 min.)

Discuss goal set at last session

Life project goal AND goal related to last week's session topic.
Identify barriers to unaccomplished Goals
See Appendix A for How to Identify Barriers to Accomplishing Goal

Review today's topic and plan for session

Write on Flipchart Ahead of Time (in lay terms).
How Can We Be A Healthy Family?
Your family knows better than most the importance of physical health. Today you will be challenged to make one change at home to improve the health of your family.
We will:

Discuss unhealthy family habits.
Use SMART problem-solving to identify a healthy family goal and brainstorm some actions to take.
Decide the first step to take (short-term goal) towards the healthy family goal.

Skills-Building (60 min.)

Introductions and one reason why you want to be physically healthy

I would like to go around the room and have each teenager and mom introduce his or herself to the group and say one reason why you want to be physically healthy.
For example, "My name is Mary and I want to be healthy so I can win at track."
Good job. To stay healthy, it can help to remind yourself of the reasons why you want to be healthy.

Don't Forget: It may be uncomfortable for families to discuss sex, drugs and alcohol in a family session. Therefore, it may be more comfortable to address these areas in a general way (i.e., issues that "other" families may be dealing with versus asking participants to talk about substance abuse or risky sexual behaviors within their own family.

Unhealthy habits do not need to relate to the family in particular. They can be general unhealthy physical habits that any family may experience.

Identifying unhealthy family habits

Ask mother and teen pairs to sit together.

Ask pairs to create a list of unhealthy physical habits within their individual family.

Your task is to make a list of your unhealthy family habits related to *physical* health.

Here are some examples:

"We eat fast food several times per week."
"We love fried foods."
"We are couch potatoes—we hate to exercise."
"Most of us smoke cigarettes."
"We have a hard time getting to bed on time."

Directions

Allow about 10 minutes to complete the task.

Have each family share their unhealthy family habits.

Write unhealthy family habits on flipchart.

If you hear one that you forgot to add to your list, go ahead and add it on.

Identify areas to obtain support from family in establishing or maintaining healthy routines

Whenever we want to work on a goal, it is often helpful to have support in accomplishing what we have set out to do.

So let's spend some time talking about each of the goals that you came up with during your individual sessions about your healthy routine and figure out if there are ways that you can work together as a family on these routines.

Ask each mom and teen to share their goal with the group and what they would like from their family in accomplishing their goal.

If the members have difficulty in sharing their goal or asking for support, the facilitator or other group members may intervene in facilitating the process, or helping them to set joint goals.

Don't Forget: The intent of this activity is to create an opportunity for moms and teens to share the goals set during each individual healthy physical habits session and to develop a family plan to support each other in accomplishing the goals.

Identify a family health habit goal

In addition to each of your individual health goals, what health goal would you like to work on together as a family?

Assist group members to identify a joint health goal.

Don't Forget: The goal of this exercise is for families to identify an area that they would like to work together on as a family.

The goal is to support families in remembering that they have "choices" in any given situation about the way they are going to think and act.

It is important to apply SMART and generate the different options you have in any given situation in terms of how you are going to THINK and what you are going to DO and then pick the best option.

Activity

Healthy/Unhealthy Physical Habit Collage

The goal of this activity is to provide an opportunity for families to engage in a joint activity which will allow them to explore their view of healthy versus unhealthy through their own creative expression.

Separate into family dyads and allow approximately 30 minutes to make the collage.

Allow fifteen minutes to allow time for families to share their collages.

How Can We Be a Healthy Family?

Intention/Purpose: The goal of this activity is to provide an opportunity for families to engage in a joint activity which will allow them to explore their views of healthy vs. unhealthy physical habits through their own creative expression.

Supplies: magazines (at least 3–5 per participant; of varying topics so that both teens and moms will find images that express their views); poster board, scissors; glue sticks; markers

Directions: Give each mom and teen dyad a piece of poster board, scissors and glue and explain that they will be finding images of healthy and unhealthy physical habits in the magazines and cutting them out and gluing them onto the poster board. Sometimes families divide the poster in half with healthy on one side and unhealthy on the other OR just make groupings of different habits—like food, exercise, relaxation, etc. Moms and teens can make their posters however they like. IF there are moms and teens present who do not have other family members with them, they can make the collage on their own for their family. Dyads can share their posters with the group once activity has ended.

FACILITATOR directions: Facilitators can walk around and help dyads as needed, help people find images, comment on what people are doing.

Group Discussion: Allow people to share their posters and receive feedback from the group!

Wrap-Up and Goal Setting (10 min.)

Skills: Increased ability to set a goal that is realistic, clear, not too easy or too difficult and that has a clear end point; and increased ability to problem-solve in order to optimize success and to plan for potential obstacles.

Identify a short-term goal (for the week) that is related to the plan you just developed.

For example, if your family decided to get into better physical shape as your long-term goal, the short-term goal might be to take a walk together twice this week.

Appendix A: Check-In and How to Identify a Barrier to Accomplishing Goal

Discuss goal set at last session:
Life project goal AND goal related to last week's session topic.

Don't Forget: The life project goal should be posted on the wall and referenced to throughout the intervention. This can be done in a number of ways. For example:

During the check-in, conduct a quick general follow-up with the participants (i.e., is everyone keeping their life project goal in mind and working towards it?)

During the check-in, conduct a more specific follow-up asking members for their progress with their goals.

Some of the life project goals my not entail weekly small goals. If so, there is no need for a weekly check-in. You can do a quick reminder and then move on to the next participant.

Directions

For participants who accomplished their goals:
Praise efforts and success
Relate to FTD and Feeling Thermometer

Feeling thermometer: 10
Physical reaction: "deep breath, tension released in shoulders"
Thinking: "I can accomplish this goal"
Doing: "Bragged about how I accomplished my goal"

-OR-

For participants who did not accomplish their goals:
Praise efforts
Relate to FTD and Feeling Thermometer

Feeling thermometer: 100
Physical reaction: "shaky hands, tightened stomach"
Thinking: "I'm never going to be able to do this"
Doing: "Giving up"

Don't Forget: Positive reframe and yet maintain accountability (i.e., if they did not accomplish the goal, it is because they were trying to take care of themselves by not overstressing themselves.)

How to change above negative loop to a positive loop

What positive thing could you have said to yourself instead?
If you said this positive thing to yourself, what would you have done instead?
Where would you have been on the feeling thermometer?

Don't Forget: Help participant identify choices they have that impact their feelings, thoughts, and behaviors.

Emphasize the impact of cognitive errors on behavior.

Generate feedback from group members on how to alter the negative loop to a positive one, including altering unhelpful thoughts, positively reframing the situation, or correcting cognitive distortions.

Identify barrier to accomplishing goal

Don't Forget: Make sure that original goal was realistic. Use this as an opportunity to emphasize the importance of setting realistic goals in order to optimize success.

Problem-solve barrier to accomplishing goal

State the problem/potential obstacles

Make a goal (Realistic and Specific)

Actions—Make a list of all the possible actions you could take and evaluate the pros and cons of each option

Reach a decision about which action you want to try

Try it and review it

Chapter 8

Manualized Treatment for Anxiety-Based School Refusal Behavior in Youth

Christopher A. Kearney, PhD, Stephanie Stowman, MA, Courtney Haight, MA, and Adrianna Wechsler, MA

School refusal behavior refers to child-motivated refusal to attend school and/or difficulties remaining in classes for an entire day. The behavior includes school-aged youth who are completely absent from school for extended or limited periods of time, who skip classes or sections of a school day, who are chronically tardy to school, who display severe morning misbehaviors in an attempt to miss school, or who attend school with great dread and persistent pleas for future nonattendance. School refusal behavior affects about 5%–28% of youths at some point in their lives and can lead to severe short- and long-term problems if left unaddressed. School refusal behavior is represented fairly equally among boys and girls, and peak onset is 10–13 years of age. Entry into kindergarten, first grade, middle school, and high

The material in this chapter is adapted with permission from the therapist guide for *When Children Refuse School: A Cognitive-Behavioral Therapy Approach* (2nd ed.), published by Oxford University Press (2007). For the complete program, please visit the TreatmentsThatWork companion Web site at http://www.oup.com/us/ttw.

school may be particularly problematic for some children (Kearney, 2001; Kearney & Silverman, 1996).

School refusal behavior has been a vexing problem for parents, educators, and psychologists since the early twentieth century. This is due to the often urgent nature of the problem as well as its extensive symptom heterogeneity. Children with school refusal behavior commonly display a wide range of internalizing and externalizing symptoms such as general and social anxiety, depression, social withdrawal, fear, fatigue, worry, somatic complaints, running away from home or school, noncompliance and defiance, arguing, verbal and physical aggression, tantrums, and clinging. Many of these youths show a wide range of diagnoses as well. Clinicians and researchers have not reached consensus on how to conceptualize, organize, assess, and treat this population based on the many forms of school refusal behavior (Egger, Costello, & Angold, 2003; Kearney, 2003; Kearney & Albano, 2004).

An alternative model for conceptualizing this population is to consider the function of school refusal behavior. In this model, youths are presumed to refuse school for one of four main reasons, or functions:

- To avoid school-based stimuli that provoke negative affectivity.
- To escape from aversive social and/or evaluative situations at school.
- To pursue attention from significant others.
- To pursue tangible rewards outside of school.

The initial two functions refer to youths who refuse school for negative reinforcement, or to evade aversive stimuli at school. The latter two functions refer to youths who refuse school for positive reinforcement, or to pursue salient rewards outside of school. Youths may also refuse school for two or more functions.

The focus of this chapter is the first function: to avoid school-based stimuli that provoke negative affectivity. Negative affectivity refers to general feelings of sadness and anxiety or diffuse dread about school. Many younger children refuse school because a stimulus provokes this negative emotional state, which is often manifested by crying, reluctance to enter a school building, withdrawal, clinging, and somatic complaints such as stomachaches and headaches. Common examples of general school-based stimuli that provoke negative affectivity in children include riding the school bus, entry into the school building, and transitions between classes. However, many children cannot specifically identify which stimulus causes their negative affectivity. This functional condition is analogous to anxiety-based school refusal behavior, often referred to simply as *school refusal* in the research literature (Hanna, Fischer, & Fluent, 2006; Suveg, Aschenbrand, & Kendall, 2005).

BRIEF OVERVIEW OF CONSIDERATIONS REGARDING ANXIETY-BASED SCHOOL REFUSAL BEHAVIOR

The treatment of anxiety-based school refusal behavior involves considerations that may not exist when treating anxious children without school refusal behavior. First, a child absent from school will typically present with an urgent situation because of immediate risk of academic decline, social alienation, intense distress, family legal problems for educational neglect,

and parent financial stress from missing work. Second, clinicians who address this population must be prepared for time-consuming sessions and consultations with various people such as teachers, guidance counselors, principals, school-based social workers and psychologists, pediatricians, and child psychiatrists. Frequent contacts with families between sessions are often necessary as well.

Third, school refusal behavior must be monitored and addressed frequently. This may necessitate daily use of logbooks, attendance records, and behavior report cards from a teacher. Fourth, legitimate school-based threats or other problems that could justify a child's nonattendance should be fully assessed and resolved prior to clinical treatment. Examples include bullying or other threats, poor match between a student's academic needs and his curriculum, and student-teacher conflict.

Finally, successful treatment outcome must be determined by anxiety reduction and increased attendance. Anxiety should be reduced at least 75% (using self-ratings of distress) and full-time attendance should occur for at least two weeks prior to considering treatment termination. Clinicians are also encouraged to engage in frequent follow-up contact with families. Special attention should be paid to times that present high risk for slips or relapse, particularly following holiday breaks from school, extended weekends or family vacations, or summer.

BRIEF SUMMARY OF EVIDENCE REGARDING THIS TREATMENT APPROACH

Cognitive-behavioral strategies to treat child anxiety in general, and anxiety-based school refusal behavior in particular, have been well-developed and tested over the past two decades. Cognitive-behavioral strategies for these populations most commonly include three sets of techniques based on the main components of anxiety: physiological, cognitive, and behavioral. First, somatic control exercises help children manage aversive physiological anxiety symptoms such as muscle tension, hyperventilation, and accelerated heart rate. These exercises include relaxation strategies, such as tensing and easing various muscle groups, and breathing retraining to help children engage in regular and deep inhalation and exhalation. In extreme cases, these techniques may be supplemented with anxiolytic medication.

Second, cognitive therapy helps children think more realistically and flexibly in anxiety-provoking situations. Cognitive therapy for youths typically involves identifying underlying beliefs or thoughts that are automatic and maladaptive, engaging in strategies to restructure the beliefs or thoughts, and evaluating whether the strategies were effective. Cognitive strategies may include hypothesis-testing of specific thoughts, decentering, examining alternative causes, and reducing absolutist thinking. Readers are referred elsewhere for a detailed description of cognitive procedures with children (Friedberg & McClure, 2002; Reinecke, Dattilio, & Freeman, 2003).

Third, exposure-based practices help children gradually increase school attendance and manage anxiety-provoking situations such as conversations with others or tests. Exposure-based practice is thought to help children habituate to anxiety-provoking stimuli, fully process information regarding anxious events, and increase self-efficacy. Exposure-based practices are often used in conjunction with somatic control exercises, as in systematic desensitization, but may be accelerated in urgent cases involving school refusal behavior (Heyne & Rollings, 2002).

Other cognitive-behavioral strategies for these populations include psychoeducation about components of anxiety, social skills and assertiveness training, self-monitoring of key behaviors, and parent-based contingency management. Children with anxiety-based school refusal behavior may receive other, more family-based treatments if they refuse school for tangible reinforcement as well. The general goal of these cognitive-behavioral techniques is to help children master control over physiological, cognitive, and behavioral aspects of anxiety to engage more adaptively in various settings and receive social and other reinforcement from others.

Several large-scale studies support the use of cognitive-behavioral procedures for anxious children in general (Barrett, Dadds, & Rapee, 1996; Kendall, 1994; Silverman et al., 1999a, 1999b). These studies were based on decades of previous work indicating that cognitive-behavioral treatment procedures are effective for adults with anxiety disorders. Indeed, cognitive-behavioral strategies are now considered the treatment of choice for anxious children (Albano & Kendall, 2002). Large-scale treatment outcome studies also support the use of cognitive-behavioral strategies for youths with anxiety-based school refusal

behavior (Bernstein et al., 2000; King et al., 1998; Last, Hansen, & Franco, 1998). Evidence has accrued in support of cognitive-behavioral strategies for anxiety-based school refusal behavior within a functional model as well (Chorpita, Albano, Heimberg, & Barlow, 1996; Kearney, 2002; Kearney, Pursell, & Alvarez, 2001; Kearney & Silverman, 1999).

INTRODUCTION TO THE TREATMENT MANUAL

The treatment approach exemplified in this chapter comes from the second edition of *When Children Refuse School: A Cognitive-Behavioral Therapy Approach: Therapist Guide* (Kearney & Albano, 2007a). The manual comprises eight chapters: three chapters cover aspects of school refusal behavior, screening, assessment, and consultation, four chapters cover detailed treatment procedures for each of the four functions of school refusal behavior, and one chapter covers slips and relapse prevention. Each treatment chapter also includes special circumstances relevant to that particular function. Examples pertinent to anxiety-based school refusal behavior include methods for gradually reintroducing a child to school and criteria for keeping a child home from school.

Each treatment chapter is arranged into eight sessions. This structure represents a general guide and not a fixed timeline. Treatment chapters progress from Session 1, which typically involves setting the stage for treatment by providing a rationale for procedures used and educating clients about the nature of a child's school refusal behavior and, if pertinent, his or her anxiety. Session 2 includes an intensification of treatment procedures, Sessions 3–4 include maturing treatment strategies, Sessions 5–6 include advanced treatment strategies, and Sessions 7–8 include end-stage treatment strategies.

The *Therapist Guide* has a companion workbook for parents who use it in conjunction with a therapist (Kearney & Albano, 2007b). The procedures are generally tailored to reduce anxiety and gradually increase a child's school attendance. Following is a reprint of Chapter 4 of the *Therapist Guide*, which is designed specifically for youths who refuse school to avoid stimuli that provoke negative affectivity. Key procedures include psychoeducation, somatic control exercises, and exposure-based practices.

References

Albano, A. M., & Kendall, P. C. (2002). Cognitive behavioural therapy for children and adolescents with anxiety disorders: Clinical research advances. *International Review of Psychiatry, 14*, 129–134.

Barrett, P. M., Dadds, M. R., & Rapee, R. M. (1996). Family treatment of childhood anxiety: A controlled trial. *Journal of Consulting and Clinical Psychology, 64*, 333–342.

Bernstein, G. A., Borchardt, C. M., Perwein, A. R., Crosby, R. D., Kushner, M. G., Thuras, et al. (2000). Imipramine plus cognitive-behavioral therapy in the treatment of school refusal. *Journal of the American Academy of Child and Adolescent Psychiatry, 39*, 276–283.

Chorpita, B. F., Albano, A. M., Heimberg, R. G., & Barlow, D. H. (1996). A systematic replication of the prescriptive treatment of school refusal behavior in a single subject. *Journal of Behavior Therapy and Experimental Psychiatry, 27*, 281–290.

Egger, H. L., Costello, E. J., & Angold, A. (2003). School refusal and psychiatric disorders: A community study. *Journal of the American Academy of Child and Adolescent Psychiatry, 42*, 797–807.

Friedberg, R. D., & McClure, J. M. (2002). *Clinical practice of cognitive therapy with children and adolescents: The nuts and bolts.* New York: Guilford.

Hanna, G. L., Fischer, D. J., & Fluent, T. E. (2006). Separation anxiety disorder and school refusal in children and adolescents. *Pediatrics in Review, 27*, 56–63.

Heyne, D., & Rollings, S. (2002). *School refusal.* Malden, MA: BPS Blackwell.

Kearney, C. A. (2001). *School refusal behavior in youth: A functional approach to assessment and treatment.* Washington, DC: American Psychological Association.

Kearney, C. A. (2002). Case study of the assessment and treatment of a youth with multifunction school refusal behavior. *Clinical Case Studies, 1*, 67–80.

Kearney, C. A. (2003). Bridging the gap among professionals who address youth with school absenteeism: Overview and suggestions for consensus. *Professional Psychology: Research and Practice, 34*, 57–65.

Kearney, C. A., & Albano, A. M. (2004). The functional profiles of school refusal behavior: Diagnostic aspects. *Behavior Modification, 28*, 147–161.

Kearney, C. A., & Albano, A. M. (2007a). *When children refuse school: A cognitive-behavioral therapy approach: Therapist's guide* (2nd ed.). New York: Oxford University Press.

Kearney, C. A., & Albano, A. M. (2007b). *When children refuse school: A cognitive-behavioral therapy approach: Parent workbook* (2nd ed.). New York: Oxford University Press.

Kearney, C. A., & Silverman, W. K. (1996). The evolution and reconciliation of taxonomic strategies for school refusal behavior. *Clinical Psychology: Science and Practice, 3*, 339–354.

Kearney, C. A., & Silverman, W. K. (1999). Functionally-based prescriptive and nonprescriptive treatment for children and adolescents with school refusal behavior. *Behavior Therapy, 30*, 673–695.

Kearney, C. A., Pursell, C., & Alvarez, K. (2001). Treatment of school refusal behavior in children with mixed functional profiles. *Cognitive and Behavioral Practice, 8*, 3–11.

Kendall, P. C. (1994). Treating anxiety disorders in children: Results of a randomized clinical trial. *Journal of Consulting and Clinical Psychology, 62*, 100–110.

King, N. J., Tonge, B. J., Heyne, D., Pritchard, M., Rollings, S., Young, D., et al. (1998). Cognitive-behavioral treatment of school-refusing children: A controlled evaluation. *Journal of the American Academy of Child and Adolescent Psychiatry, 37*, 395–403.

Last, C. G., Hansen, C., & Franco, N. (1998). Cognitive-behavioral treatment of school phobia. *Journal of the American Academy of Child and Adolescent Psychiatry, 37*, 404–411.

Ollendick, T. H., & Cerny, J. A. (1981). *Child behavior therapy with children.* New York: Plenum.

Reinecke, M. A., Dattilio, F. M., & Freeman, A. (Eds.). (2003). *Cognitive therapy with children and adolescents: A casebook for clinical practice* (2nd ed.). New York: Guilford.

Silverman, W. K., Kurtines, W. M., Ginsburg, G. S., Weems, C. F., Lumpkin, P. W., & Carmichael, D. H. (1999a). Treating anxiety disorders in children with group cognitive-behavioral therapy: A randomized clinical trial. *Journal of Consulting and Clinical Psychology, 67*, 995–1003.

Silverman, W. K., Kurtines, W. M., Ginsburg, G. S., Weems, C. F., Rabian, B., & Serafini, L. T. (1999b). Contingency management, self-control, and education support in the treatment of childhood phobic disorders: A randomized clinical trial. *Journal of Consulting and Clinical Psychology, 67*, 675–687.

Suveg, C., Aschenbrand, S. G., & Kendall, P. C. (2005). Separation anxiety disorder, panic disorder, and school refusal. *Child and Adolescent Psychiatric Clinics of North America, 14*, 773–795.

Session 1: Starting Treatment

Materials Needed

- Model of Anxiety
- Anxiety and Avoidance Hierarchy
- Feelings Thermometer
- Relaxation and Deep-Breathing Scripts
- Relaxation Log
- Blank audiotape

Session Outline

- Teach a child about anxiety.
- Work with a child to create an Anxiety and Avoidance Hierarchy.
- Teach a child relaxation training and deep diaphragmatic breathing.

School refusal behavior is often motivated by a desire to avoid symptoms of dread, anxiety, panic, or depression associated with certain school-related stimuli. For children who avoid stimuli that provoke such negative affectivity, the main goal of treatment is to change avoidance behavior and build coping and active school attendance behaviors. Treatment for this condition will involve:

- Building an anxiety and avoidance hierarchy of stimuli
- Teaching somatic management skills to decrease negative emotional arousal
- Conducting systematic exposure to anxiety cues identified on a hierarchy in a step-by-step fashion
- Gradually reintegrating a child to school
- Having a child access self-reinforcement to cope with transient negative emotions

Treatment thus involves training a child to use self-control procedures. During this treatment program, you will teach a child to identify personally relevant objects and situations that provoke negative affectivity and to use specific somatic skills to prevent her from spiraling into a full-blown anxiety reaction. These somatic skills can also be used to prevent the start of an anxiety spiral. Gradually, the child will enter situations that are most anxiety-provoking while using these somatic management skills.

The majority of your time will be spent with the child, but you should invite parents into the last portion of each session to access their input and review the session. Each session will detail specific homework assignments that involve parental support and active participation and that should become a family activity. Parents are invaluable resources for distracting or involving other children and managing a situation to provide uninterrupted family time to focus on homework assignments.

Psychoeducation

Initial treatment involves helping a child understand the nature and process of anxiety. As a child's understanding of anxiety progresses, you can help her observe her own anxiety reactions, identify where anxiety reactions occur, and use specific skills or tools to cope with negative emotions. The following is an example of how to explain the process of anxiety to a child. Simplify this for younger children or those with special needs. Utilize a flip chart or paper to illustrate and present the model to the child (Figure 8.1).

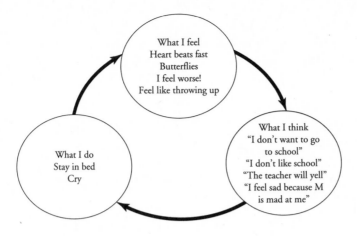

Figure 8.1 Model Of Anxiety

When you say that you're scared (anxious, upset), it feels like there's one big ball of bad stuff rolling over you, and there's nothing you can do to stop it. It's like a train is going to run you over! If we think of feeling anxious in that way, then we stay upset and feel like we can't handle the situation. But being upset (anxious) is really made up of three parts.

First is what you feel; all those feelings in your body that let you know you're scared. Things like your heart beating fast, shaking, your hands feeling sweaty, and butterflies in your stomach are all signals that you're scared. (Draw a circle and label it "What I feel.")

The second part to being scared is what you say to yourself. Usually, you say something like, Get me out of here, I'm afraid, I can't do this, I want to go home, or I need my Mom or someone to help me. (Draw a circle and label it "What I think.")

Finally, the third part to being scared is what you do when you're scared. This is usually something like leaving a place, or avoiding going to a place, or trying to be near someone who can help you feel better. (Draw a circle and label it "What I do.")

After presenting the model, ask the child for personally relevant responses to each of the three components of anxiety: What I feel, What I think, and What I do. With the child, begin to identify targets for change within each component. Cognitive-behavioral treatments rely heavily on the Socratic method, or questioning a client so she becomes an active participant in the therapy process. Questioning leads the client to uncover her own biases, beliefs, behavioral patterns, and coping resources. You will initially lead the questioning process, but as the questioning method becomes a learned response, the child will be able to engage independently in the process of deductive, rational thinking. The following is a sample dialogue of questioning a child. In the dialogue, C represents the child and T represents the therapist.

Case Vignette

T: *Let's look at the three circles here on the board. This one is called "What I feel," meaning those feelings in my body. This one is called "What I think," and this one is "What I do." Think for a moment about the last time you were nervous going to school. Do you remember when that was?*

C: *Yes. I had to go to school last week, and didn't want to go.*

T: *Okay, think about that time. Was it in the morning, before school?*

C: *Yes. Mommy woke me up and told me to get dressed for school.*

T: *And what were you thinking about when Mom said to get dressed?*

C: *I don't know. I didn't want to go.*

T: *Okay, there's one thing you were thinking, "I don't want to go." We'll put that right here in this circle. (Therapist writes "I don't want to go" in the thinking circle). What happened next?*

C: *I stayed in bed. And then Mommy came and yelled at me.*

T: *So, right here (begins to write in the "Things I do" circle) we'd put "Stayed in bed." That's something that you did when you thought about not wanting to go to school. What happened next, after Mommy yelled at you?*

C: *I started to cry.*

T: *(Writes "Cry" in the behavior circle) What were you thinking about that made you cry?*

C: *I don't like school. I get scared that I'll get yelled at by the teacher.*

T: *(Writes "I don't like school" and "The teacher will yell at me" in the thinking circle) When you think about having to go to school, and worry that the teacher will yell at you, do get any funny feelings in your body?*

C: *I feel sick. Like I'm going to throw up.*

T: *So, the feeling you get is an upset stomach, maybe like having butterflies?*

C: *Yeah. And my heart beats really fast.*

T: *(Writes "Heart beats fast" and "Butterflies" in the feelings circle) This is a good start. See, we're looking now at what goes on inside you when you get afraid.*

Next, describe for the child the way in which these three components interact to spiral into overwhelming feelings of anxiety:

T: *Let's look at these circles. When you were in bed (points to the "What I do" circle), you were thinking that you didn't want to go to school because you don't like it, and the teacher might yell at you. Right?*

C: *Yeah.*

T: *Did it make you feel better to think about what could go wrong at school?*

C: *No.*

T: *Did your butterflies feel better when you cried?*

C: *No. I felt worse.*

T: *And what did you tell yourself then?*

C: *That Mommy was mad at me. And I was sad that she yelled at me.*

T: *(Writes "I feel sad because Mommy is mad at me" in the thinking circle) Look at this now. Each time something happens in one circle, something else happens in another circle. (Draws arrows from each circle, linking to the next circle in the chain) So, when you tell yourself the teacher will yell at you, your butterflies get worse. And so you don't get out of bed. Then Mom comes in and yells, and you think about that, and you get sad. See, our feelings have three parts to them, and they each work on one another.*

Emphasize the role of the physical sensations of anxiety, how these sensations spiral to uncomfortable levels, and the resulting avoidance behavior that occurs. Introduce a child to the skills she will learn to address each component. Relaxation and deep breathing will be used to manage physical feelings of anxiety; step-by-step practices of entering anxious situations will be used to change avoidance and escape behaviors; self-reinforcement, thinking realistically, pride, and praise will be taught to change negative thoughts that accompany anxiety. Inform the child you will help her gradually return to school by taking bigger and bigger steps as time goes on. In addition, inform the child you will be nudging her to attend school more and more during treatment.

Building an Anxiety and Avoidance Hierarchy

The Anxiety and Avoidance Hierarchy (AAH) is a list of objects or situations most upsetting to a child that will be actively targeted during treatment. The information is organized into gradual steps so a child may begin with the easiest (or lowest) item and progress toward

Problem: School refusal due to anxiety about being away from parents

Situations or Places That Scare Me!	Anxiety Rating	Avoidance Rating
1. Staying in school all day without calling Mom and Dad	8	8
2. Staying in school all morning, and not calling Mom or Dad, or going to the nurse	8	8
3. Riding the school bus all by myself	7	8
4. Waiting for Mom, and she's late to pick me up	6	7
5. Staying with the babysitter, and Mom doesn't call home to check on us	5	5
6. Getting my school clothes ready the night before school	5	3
7. Having tutoring at the school, without Mom there	4	2
8. Going to school to get my homework, and visiting with my teacher	3	2
9. Going to lunch at school	3	2
10. Meeting with the tutor while Mom goes shopping	3	2

Figure 8.2 Sample AAH

the most difficult (highest) hierarchy item. Most children progress through several hierarchies during treatment until all upsetting situations or activities are challenged. Figure 8.2 represents a sample AAH for a 7-year-old girl who refused to attend school due to separation concerns. You may download multiple copies from the TreatmentsThatWork™ Web site at www.oupcom/us/ttw.

To create an AAH, review information gathered from the child and parents during sassessment and note additional objects or situations currently avoided. Organize the information by writing each object or situation on a separate index card. Keep several blank cards for additional information you uncover during treatment. Present the index cards to the child and ask her to sort the situations into categories based on the Feelings Thermometer (Figure 8.3). The Feelings Thermometer will help a child identify and rate the degree of anxiety/general distress experienced in each situation. Ratings range from 0 (none) to 8 (very, very much). Based on the child's ratings, construct the first 10-item AAH using the 10 lowest-ranked items. For the remainder of treatment, have the child rate her anxiety about

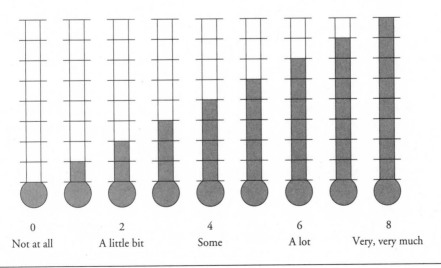

0	2	4	6	8
Not at all	A little bit	Some	A lot	Very, very much

Figure 8.3 Feelings Thermometer

these objects or situations at each session to provide you with feedback and an ongoing measure of behavior change. Ask parents to complete AAH ratings separately from the child, thereby providing valuable cross-informant information and a broader and more accurate view of a child's presentation and functioning. Begin all sessions with one AAH form for the child and one for each parent.

Relaxation Training and Breathing Retraining

The next treatment component is to teach a child relaxation training and deep diaphragmatic breathing using the scripts below. Ideally, this segment should be audiotaped for a child to use at home. If a tape recorder is not available, parents can use the Relaxation and Deep Breathing Scripts included in the parent workbook or they can download them from the Treatments ThatWork™ Web site at www.oup.com/us/ttw.

Relaxation training involves talking a child through a series of muscle tension and relaxation exercises, each designed to teach her to discriminate physical sensations of tension and calmness. Begin the relaxation process by asking a child to find a comfortable position in the chair or couch. Next, have her close her eyes or let her gaze settle and focus on one spot in the room. At each step of the process, focus the child on letting go of tension and feeling calm and relaxed. The child should isolate each muscle group one at a time, so give ongoing direction to her to tense only a particular muscle. Instruct a younger child to watch and emulate as you perform the step and use imagery to help her follow the exercises. Introduce deep breathing (into the stomach or diaphragm) to prolong relaxation and make it more complete.

The entire process of relaxation should last about 20 minutes. Parents may be called into the session for a discussion and summary at this point. To facilitate a child's learning of the treatment model and procedures have the child tell the parents about the session. Add comments or guide the child to give a more complete summary of the session as needed. At this point, you may wish to discuss with parents how they can assist their child with the homework. For example, a parent could be encouraged to keep distractions to a minimum while the child practices the relaxation procedures.

Relaxation Script (modified from Ollendick & Cerny, 1981)

Have the child recline in a comfortable position and either close her eyes or focus the eyes on one spot on the wall or ceiling. Legs and arms should not be crossed; have the child take off her shoes and loosen any tight clothing such as belts.

I would like you to sit as comfortably as possible in your chair. During the next few minutes, I am going to give you some instructions about tensing and releasing different muscle groups. I want you to listen carefully and do what I ask you to do. Be sure not to anticipate what I say; just relax and concentrate on my voice. Any questions? (Answer questions as they occur) Okay, put your feet on the floor, and put your arms on the arms of the chair. (Child focuses or closes eyes as desired.) Try to relax as much as possible.

Using this tension-release relaxation protocol, tensed muscles are held in place for approximately five seconds. The procedure is audiotaped.

Hands and Arms

Make a fist with your left hand. Squeeze it hard. Feel the tightness in your hand and arm as you squeeze. Now let your hand go and relax. See how much better your hand and arm feel when they are relaxed. Once again, make a fist with your left hand and squeeze hard. Good. Now relax and let your hand go. (Repeat the process for the right hand and arm.)

Arms and Shoulders

Stretch your arms out in front of you. Raise them up high over your head. Way back. Feel the pull in your shoulders. Stretch higher. Now just let your arms drop back to your side. Okay, let's stretch again. Stretch your arms out in front of you. Raise them over your head. Pull them back, way back. Pull hard. Now let them drop quickly. Good. Notice how your shoulders feel more relaxed. This time let's have a great big stretch. Try to touch the ceiling. Stretch your arms out in front of you. Raise them way up over your head. Push them way, way back. Notice the tension and pull in your arms and shoulders. Hold tight, now. Great. Let them drop very quickly and feel how good it is to be relaxed. It feels good and warm and lazy.

Shoulders and Neck

Try to pull your shoulders up to your ears and push your head down into your shoulders. Hold in tight. Okay, now relax and feel the warmth. Again, pull your shoulders up to your ears and push your head down into your shoulders. Do it tightly. Okay, you can relax now. Bring your head out and let your shoulders relax. Notice how much better it feels to be relaxed than to be all tight. One more time now. Push your head down and your shoulders way up to your ears. Hold it. Feel the tenseness in your neck and shoulders. Okay. You can relax now and feel comfortable. You feel good.

Jaw

Put your teeth together real hard. Let your neck muscles help you. Now relax. Just let your jaw hang loose. Notice how good it feels just to let your jaw drop. Okay, bite down hard. That's good. Now relax again. Just let your jaw drop. It feels so good just to let go. Okay, one more time. Bite down. Hard as you can. Harder. Oh, you really are working hard. Good. Now relax. Try to relax your whole body. Let yourself get as loose as you can.

Face and Nose

Wrinkle up your nose. Make as many wrinkles in your nose as you can. Scrunch up your nose real hard. Good. Now relax your nose. Now wrinkle up your nose again. Wrinkle it up hard. Hold it just as tight as you can. Okay. You can relax your face. Notice that when you scrunch up your nose, your cheeks and your mouth and your forehead all help you and they get tight, too. So when you relax your nose, your whole face relaxes too, and that feels good. Now make lots of wrinkles on your forehead. Hold it tight, now. Okay, you can let go. Now you can just relax. Let your face go smooth. No wrinkles anywhere. Your face feels nice and smooth and relaxed.

Stomach

Now tighten up your stomach muscles real tight. Make your stomach real hard. Don't move. Hold it. You can relax now. Let your stomach go soft. Let it be as relaxed as you can. That feels so much better. Okay, again. Tighten your stomach real hard. Good. You can relax now. Settle down, get comfortable and relax. Notice the difference between a tight stomach and a relaxed one. That's how we want to feel. Nice and loose and relaxed. Okay. Once more. Tighten up. Tighten hard. Good. Now you can relax completely. You feel nice and relaxed.

This time, try to pull your stomach in. Try to squeeze it against your backbone. Try to be as skinny as you can. Now relax. You do not have to be skinny now. Just relax and feel your stomach being warm and loose. Okay, squeeze in your stomach again. Make it touch your backbone. Get it real small and tight. Get as skinny as you can. Hold tight now. You can relax now. Settle back and let your stomach come back out where it belongs. You can feel really good now. You've done fine.

Legs and Feet

Push your toes down on the floor real hard. You'll probably need your legs to help you push. Push down, spread your toes apart. Now relax your feet. Let your toes go loose and feel how nice that is. It feels good to be relaxed. Okay. Now push your toes down. Let your leg muscles help you put your feet down. Push your feet. Hard. Okay. Relax your feet, relax your legs, relax your toes. It feels so good to be relaxed. No tenseness anywhere. You kind of feel warm and tingly.

Conclusion

Stay as relaxed as you can. Let your whole body go limp and feel all your muscles relaxed. In a few minutes it will be the end of the relaxation exercise. Today is a good day. You've worked hard in here and it feels good to work hard. Okay, shake your arms. Now shake your legs. Move your head around. Open your eyes slowly (if they were closed). Very good. You've done a good job. You're going to be a super relaxer.

Breathing Retraining Script

Ask the child to imagine going on a hot-air balloon ride. As long as the hot-air balloon has fuel supplied by the child's breathing, destinations are unlimited. Ask the child to breathe in through her nose and out through her mouth with a SSSSSSSSS sound. You may encourage this process through imagery, such as having a picture of a hot-air balloon nearby. If necessary, have the child count to herself slowly when breathing out. The following is an example: Imagine going on a ride in a hot-air balloon. Your breathing will give the balloon its power. As long as you breathe deeply, the balloon can go anywhere. Breathe in through your nose like this (demonstrate). Breathe slowly and deeply. Try to breathe in a lot of air. Now breathe out slowly through your mouth, making a hissing sound like this (demonstrate). If you want, you can count to yourself when you breathe in and out.

Homework

Practice the relaxation and breathing procedure at home every day, twice a day if possible, between sessions. A relaxation log is provided in the parent workbook and multiple copies may be downloaded at the Treatments That Work™ Web site at www.oup.com/us/ttw. Following each practice, the child should note any difficulties she encountered, such as inability to concentrate or falling asleep during the practice. If a child is too young to write or may not be able to comply with this instruction independently, then a parent should question the child and record any difficulties on the relaxation log.

- The child and parent should continue to complete the daily logbooks.
- Encourage the child and parent to record any specific situations or experiences that arise during the week.
- Encourage general adherence to a regular school-day schedule, even if only in the morning prior to school. This includes early wakening, dressing and preparing for school as if going, and completing school assignments.

Session 2: Intensifying Treatment

Session Outline

- Review homework from last session.
- Prepare the child for exposure.
- Conduct systematic desensitization using one of the easier items from the child's Anxiety and Avoidance Hierarchy from session 1.
- Conduct imaginal desensitization.

In session 2, begin to expose a child to school-related objects or situations that provoke her anxiety. Systematic desensitization is a therapeutic process of confronting anxieties in a step-by-step fashion through imagination (imaginal exposure) and real-life situations (in vivo exposure). The effectiveness of systematic desensitization has been well documented as a treatment for anxiety disorders in children and adults. Imaginal systematic desensitization will be followed by in vivo desensitization exercises. For the child and parent, these in vivo practices are called "Show That I Can" or STIC tasks. Parent support and participation in establishing and conducting these home-based STIC tasks is essential for treatment success.

Preparing a Child for Systematic Desensitization

Explain the term "systematic desensitization" to the child if she is an adolescent and can understand more complex concepts.

Case Vignette

T: *Let me ask you something. Do you know how to ride a bike? Or swim? Or do you ski or ride horses? (Probe until you find some activity the child can perform with some skill)*

C: *Yes, I can ride a bicycle. I learned that when I was 5 or 6.*

T: *Okay, tell me about what you do when you want to go (biking, skiing, horseback riding).*

C: *Well, I get my bike out of the garage, and I ride it up the street or to my friend's house.*

T: *Okay, you have to get the bike out of the garage. What do you think about when you're riding your bike?*

C: *Nothing. I mean, I think about what me and my friend are going to do. Like maybe we'll play video games.*

T: *Are you riding your bike in the street or on the sidewalk?*

C: *Well, I have to ride on the sidewalk. But sometimes I have to cross the street, so I look both ways.*

T: *And what are you doing with your hands, feet, and eyes when you ride?*

C: *Nothing. I just pedal and hold the handlebars. And I have to look where I'm going.*

T: *Okay. So, what you're telling me is that you get on the bike, ride along the sidewalks and street, pedal along, and watch where you're going, and you do not think about those things. Instead, you think about what you're going to do with your friend. Right?*

C: *Yeah, I guess.*

T: *Sure, it's automatic that you ride now, and watch out for where you're going. You've learned how to do these things, haven't you? (Child nods) And you do not even think about how you're doing these things anymore. But do you remember when you first went out on the bike? Do you remember that it used to be scary?*

Using Socratic questioning, question the child and prompt her to recall the first time riding a bike or doing some similar activity that requires skill. Then, ask her about physical feelings, thoughts, and behaviors that may occur in someone learning to ride for the first time. Ask the child as well about her personal reactions during her initial learning experiences. Focus the child on how initial steps to learning this skill were small, but with practice she developed skill and mastery. The main point to convey is that continued practice and over-learning has made the situation easy and automatic. Next, ask the child about what happened to her initial anxieties:

T: *Why aren't you scared of falling off the bike now?*

C: *Because I don't fall anymore. And if I do, I may get scraped, but it gets better.*

T: *So, even if you do fall, you know you're going to be okay. Right?*

C: *Yeah, I've fallen. I just have to get on the bike again. That way I don't get scared again.*

T: *Right! That's exactly right! You have practiced riding your bike, and you started out in steps. Someone helped you, and you used training wheels. Then you took them off when you started feeling more comfortable and less nervous. Right? So you did this step by step and, as you developed more skill, you became less nervous. Now you do not even think about how you were once nervous.*

Introduce the concept of taking steps, one at a time, and mastering each step until little or no anxiety is felt. The imaginal desensitization process can be presented to the child as "practicing thinking about troubling situations." Systematic desensitization involves training a child in progressive muscle relaxation procedures and then alternating the presentation of relaxing scenes with talking through a scene from the child's anxiety hierarchy. When the child indicates that her anxiety is at an uncomfortable level during an anxious scenario, you quickly switch back to the relaxing scene. The child is instructed to raise her hand when anxiety becomes uncomfortable.

Constructing the Anxiety Scenario

Begin with one of the easier steps from the child's AAH. This will be the first situation to confront imaginally. Ask the child about what she thinks will happen in the situation and develop a scenario about that situation based on what the child thinks and is anxious about. You may embellish the scenario to some degree. Often, parents are surprised at the graphic nature and intensity of their child's anxieties. However, note that these are the child's anxieties and, left to her imagination, can continue to develop unchecked. Hence, you must guide a child in thinking about these anxieties, mix in relaxing scenes so the thoughts themselves are no longer frightening, and discuss what is realistic for any given situation. The goal of desensitization is to gradually get a child to listen to an entire anxiety scenario "as if watching a movie" and realize that the scene is not that scary itself. Another goal is to have the child recognize that almost any scenario can be coped with in a positive, proactive way. A sample scenario, using situation 8 from Sandy's AAH (Figure 8.2), follows:

It's after 2 o'clock, and you and your mother are driving to school to see your teacher. You have to go in and get your own homework. You haven't been in school for 3 weeks and haven't really seen any of the other kids or the teacher. The last time you were there you felt real funny in your stomach, and you felt like throwing up. As you get closer to school, you start to feel a bit dizzy and start to sweat a bit. You look up at Mom and want her to turn the car around, but she says you have to get the work. Mom has to stay in the car, because there's no place to park, so you have to go in alone. Mom drives up to the front door of the school. Some kids are there, and some teachers, but not anyone you know. You open the car door and feel really dizzy now, and your stomach feels like you're on a roller coaster. You start to walk up to the door, and you feel really shaky and sweaty. These are the feelings that you get sometimes that scare you. What if you get sick?

You look back, and Mom is moving the car and is now pulling out of the school driveway. You walk in through the door and feel so dizzy that you have to hold on to the wall to stay standing. Some kids walk by and laugh. You're really feeling scared now, and it's getting harder to breathe. What if you faint, and no one comes to get you and help you? What if Mom just stays in the car? You start walking down the long hall to the classroom, and when you get there, several kids are in line to see the teacher, so you have to wait. It's really hot in the classroom, and you feel like you might throw up. You're so dizzy now and can taste real sour stuff coming up in your throat. You feel dizzy and faint and wish that the teacher would look at you and help you, but she's talking to someone else. You can feel it coming now: it's at the top of your throat. You yell out for help, and when you do, you get sick all over the place. The teacher and all the kids are looking at you now, with wide eyes. You feel really sick and really embarrassed. If only your mother had come in with you!

Tracking Anxiety during Desensitization

Throughout systematic desensitization, ask a child to rate her anxiety levels using the Feelings Thermometer or other measurement scale. Record the child's ratings. This way, you can illustrate, using charts or graphs, what happened to the child's anxiety during desensitization. These charts or graphs will show how a child gradually mastered her anxiety over the course of treatment.

Some children are able to track their own anxiety levels. Recording their own ratings gives children instant information about how they handled certain situations. The ratings can illustrate how they coped with panic symptoms, separation concerns, fears of specific objects or situations, or any other situation where anxiety ratings can be taken and recorded. You may suggest that parents keep their child's ratings in a log or notebook to remind her of progress made during therapy.

Conducting the Imaginal Desensitization

Audiotape the following desensitization procedure for later processing and for home use. Desensitization begins by instructing the child to raise her hand whenever anxiety becomes uncomfortable. Give the child a copy of the thermometer to keep on her lap. You will first conduct a relaxation procedure with the child. During initial sessions, you may wish to present a full relaxation procedure. With repeated practice, you may change the relaxation induction to (1) include breathing retraining, (2) focus on being relaxed in general, and/or (3) focus on releasing tension in specific parts of the body. Instruct the child to listen to you and follow your voice. Ask the child to listen and imagine the scene in her mind as if it is actually happening.

Explain that the child will relax first and you will then talk her through a challenging scene. When anxiety becomes uncomfortable, the child should raise a hand to signal this to you and point to the level of discomfort on the thermometer. Ask the child to switch to thinking about something pleasant, such as being on a beach, in the park, or some place relaxing and pleasing for her. Once anxiety declines to a level of 0 or 1, present the troubling scene again. This switching back and forth should continue until the child can tolerate listening to the scene completely without indicating uncomfortable levels of anxiety.

As the child progresses through each scene, ask her to wait to raise a hand until anxiety reaches a level of 4 or 5. This allows her to develop increased tolerance and eventually habituate to sensations and feelings of anxiety. As tolerance increases, these feelings will lose their ability to signal the child to escape or avoid and will allow her to try new situations while tolerating normal levels of arousal. If necessary, divide the anxiety scenario into smaller steps or less volatile scenes. The desensitization process should always end with a relaxation scene.

Processing the Imaginal Desensitization

Invite a parent into the session to discuss the child's progress. To facilitate understanding of desensitization, play a portion of the audiotape for the parent. Encourage the child to explain and demonstrate the process to the parent. Ask the child about what happened to her anxiety during the practice. The typical response is that anxiety dropped during the session and the child's tolerance increased with repeated presentations. Illustrate habituation of anxiety during desensitization by drawing an inverted-U curve of the child's anxiety ratings (Figure 8.4).

If the child did not habituate (i.e., anxiety did not drop), then praise her for any effort or degree of participation and process that may have been particularly diffcult. Divide the scenario into smaller steps or less volatile scenes. Be sure to praise and encourage a child for making any step, regardless of how small. By praising a child for her efforts, you will also be modeling this behavior for parents. Typically, desensitization begins slowly and the pace increases with time. This may occur in one session or across two or more sessions if necessary.

As noted, the child and parent should be presented with a graphic illustration of the habituation curve. This visual medium provides additional feedback to the child about her specific reaction to a feared stimulus. Note that ratings may be made on a more traditional 0-to-100 scale (SUDS) or may parallel the 0-to-8 scale on the Feelings Thermometer. As an example, compare in the diagram above Sandy's anxiety about riding the school bus in her first imaginal desensitization session with her anxiety in a later in vivo desensitization practice (Figure 8.5).

Illustrations allow a child to receive concrete information about her initial concerns about riding the bus. In this case, for example, initial anxiety ratings during imaginal practice began near 3 and quickly reached their worst level of 8. However, Sandy can clearly see from her later chart that her anxiety during in vivo situations now starts on a lower level, peaks at a lower level, and dissipates much faster than before. You can help children learn that what they imagine is often worse than what will actually occur, and that they can handle the situation despite anxiety.

Habituation Curves

Examples follow of various habituation curves and some cautionary notes for their interpretation. First, in the "inverted-U" curve shown in Figure 8.4, beware that some children will give lower anxiety ratings over time to please the therapist or escape the exposure. Check for this

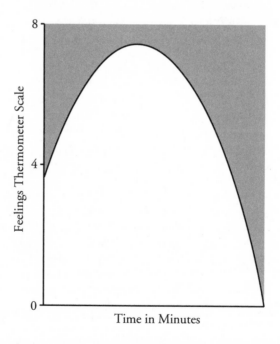

Figure 8.4 'Inverted-U' Habituation Curve

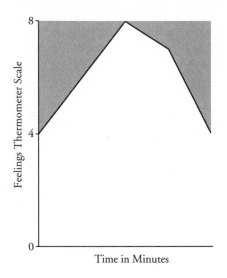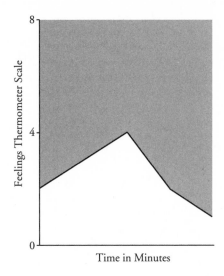

Figure 8.5 Sample First Imaginal vs. Later In Vivo desensitization

by examining a child's thoughts and behaviors in extended exposures. Second, the "peaks and valleys" curve indicates uneven but continued habituation (Figure 8.6). In this situation, therapists should check for automatic thoughts. This curve may represent a child focusing on negative outcomes at various times. A focus on the child's cognitive restructuring skills may be in order.

Third, the "steady climb" curve indicates that anxiety is increasing and habituation is not occurring (Figure 8.7). This may indicate that a hierarchy item is too challenging or complex for a child. Divide the item into smaller steps or consider that the child is not yet ready for exposure. If this is the case, then continue to work on somatic management and/or begin cognitive restructuring if applicable. Fourth, the "bottoms out" curve indicates a suspiciously fast

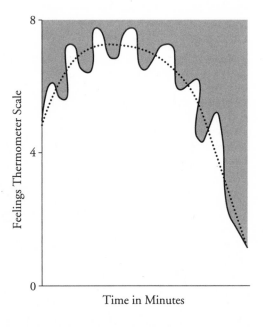

Figure 8.6 Peaks and Valleys Habituation Curve

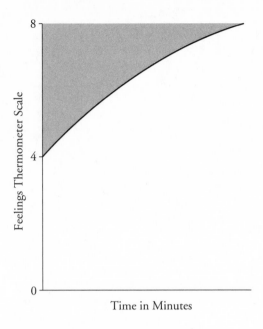

Figure 8.7 Steady Climb Habituation Curve

decline in anxiety (Figure 8.8). In this situation, a child may be trying to escape the exposure. In later sessions, this curve may indicate an appropriately faster habituation, but the level of anticipatory anxiety is still high. In this case, continue somatic management and/or begin cognitive restructuring if applicable. Finally, the "steady state" curve indicates that anxiety remains at a high level and a child is neither habituating nor getting worse (Figure 8.9). This may indicate that a hierarchy item is too complex or the child is focusing on anxiety instead of the situation. In the latter situation, check for automatic thoughts.

Homework

Homework assignments after session 2 may require more assistance from parents and may include the following:

- The child should continue to practice the relaxation procedure using the audiotape or relaxation scripts just before bedtime each night.
- At least once daily, the child should listen to the desensitization tape and go through an imaginal procedure (STIC task). The parent can assist by asking for anxiety ratings or by keeping other children from interrupting the procedure. Encourage a parent to talk with the child after each practice. You can model this process, which should involve focusing the child on how anxiety dissipated during desensitization. Also, instruct parents to praise and encourage a child for attempting and/or completing each practice.
- Provide the child and parent with structure for each day. Beginning with the next school day after this session, the parent should wake the child about 90 to 120 minutes before school is scheduled to start and implement the normal school-day routine. The child should only complete schoolwork and read school-related books when home during the day.
- Instruct the child and parent to continue to maintain the daily logbooks, noting any specific issues or situations that may arise during the week.

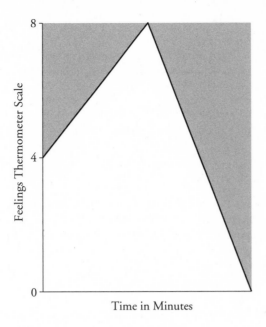

Figure 8.8 'Bottoms Out' Habituation Curve

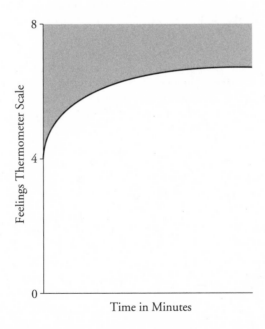

Figure 8.9 'Steady State' Habituation Curve

Sessions 3 and 4: Maturing of Treatment

Session Outline

- Review child's progress with systematic desensitization from previous session and address any problems encountered.
- Introduce the child to in vivo desensitization by working initially on her easiest item from the Anxiety and Avoidance Hierarchy.

Sessions 3 and 4 will continue to focus on systematic desensitization, with an introduction to in vivo desensitization. In vivo desensitization involves having a child gradually enter an anxiety-provoking situation and use relaxation techniques to manage anxiety. Parents are expected to arrange a time and place for in vivo desensitization and help a child engage the situation. Parental involvement is, of course, determined by your consideration of the child's age, developmental level, and severity of diagnosis or problem.

Continuing the Systematic Desensitization

Review the child's progress listening to the home-based desensitization tapes (STIC tasks) and process any problems encountered during the week. If the child reports noncompliance with the STIC task, ask her about difficulties completing the task. Some children avoid doing homework to avoid rising feelings of anxiety. If this is so, divide the scenario into smaller and more manageable steps. Plan strategies with the child to increase compliance. You may wish to incorporate coping scenes known as emotive imagery during the desensitization. If a child is having a particularly difficult time listening to a scene and is unable to habituate to anxiety, then present images of the child and a favorite athlete or superhero confronting and coping with the situation. An example of this type of desensitization follows:

You are waiting for your mother to pick you up after school, but she is late! As you stand out front, the other kids are all being picked up, and the teachers have gone back into the school or driven home. It is really getting late, and you are worried that something may have happened to Mom. What if something bad happens to you? You notice that the sky is getting dark, and big thunderclouds are coming. It starts to thunder, and flashes of lightning are happening. You try to go back into the school, but now the door is locked! Where is Mom? You are really scared now and feel like crying. You think something terrible must have happened to Mom, and now you could get caught in the lightning. But wait! You start to think, "What would (name of child's famous role model) do in this situation?" There must have been times when he had to wait for his parents, and probably he was alone and outside too. Would he cry if he were here? What would he tell you to do? Picture (name of child's famous role model) standing next to you. He says, "Okay, you're afraid that something bad happened to Mom, but why else could she be late?" You answer, "Well, maybe she's in traffic, and there are a lot of cars. Or, maybe she had to run an errand and it's taking a bit longer than she thought." (Name of famous role model) tells you, "Yeah! Good thought! She could just be running late. Now, what should you do about the weather here?" Now picture yourself telling (name of famous role model) "Well, I suppose I could stand under the awning, and wait by the door. That way I can see Mom when she comes, and I'll be out of the storm." "Great job," says (name of famous role model). "Take some deep breaths, and wait by the door for her. She'll be here soon." (Name of famous role model) gives you a high-five, and you feel so proud! Now, picture yourself going to the door, standing under the awning, and waiting calmly for Mom.

Some children avoid doing STIC tasks because they anticipate that getting better means getting back into school more quickly. If so, focus a child on goals of the program and examine whether additional factors (e.g., attention-seeking, tangible rewards for staying home) need to be addressed more directly in treatment.

Treatment progresses sequentially with the continued development of scenarios for each AAH item. A specific hierarchy item is considered complete when a child can listen to an entire scene completely and report minimal anxiety ratings without switching to a neutral, relaxing scene.

Introducing the Child to the In Vivo Desensitization

In vivo desensitization involves entering and confronting real-life situations or activities. Begin by prompting a child to think about the difference between imaginal confrontation of an anxiety-provoking situation and actually entering the situation. A sample dialogue for how you may present this to a child follows:

Case Vignette

T: *Let's think about something. Remember when we talked about how you learned to ride a bicycle?*

C: *Yes, from practice.*

T: *Right. And you've been doing a great job here, practicing here and at home imagining doing these things that make you upset.*

C: *Yes, I "Show That I Can" all the time. I do my practice every day!*

T: *Yep. That's great! Let's think about something. Suppose that you didn't know how to ride a bicycle. Suppose it was back to that time before you learned how to do that. Can you remember that?*

C: *Yes, I remember.*

T: *Okay. Now, suppose that I show you a movie about how to ride a bicycle. And you watch the movie again and again. But, you just watch the movie; you never really get to try a bicycle. Do you think it would be easy to just get on a bike and ride?*

C: *No, I have to practice on a bike. I'd be all wobbly and could fall down if I don't practice.*

T: *Right! So, watching the movie may help you to know what it looks like to ride, and it may show you some things to think about while you ride. But you really have to try a bicycle again and again to practice and learn how to ride.*

C: *Right. You have to get on the bicycle to learn how to ride it.*

T: *Well, the same thing goes here. We've been imagining going into these situations that scare you, and you've been doing a great job of learning that you do not have to be scared. But we need to help you really go into these situations and practice really being there. Do you understand what I mean?*

C: *So, I have to ride the school bus?*

T: *Well, eventually, yes. But first, we'll only practice for real the situations we've done in here and on tape. And we'll work up to the bus and those other things that are really scary for you. We'll do this step by step, just like we do in your imagination. We'll first do it in your imagination, and then we'll do it for real. Taking it easy, going one step at a time, and we'll get Mom and Dad to help out here and there.*

Conducting the First In Vivo Desensitization

Initiate in vivo desensitization by having the child role-play one of the easier items from the AAH. This role-play, made as close to reality as possible, will involve the child acting out and confronting an anxiety-provoking situation. For example, if a child is anxious about being alone either at school or home, construct a situation where she waits in a therapy room by herself for a period of time. Initially, set up the situation to be minimally anxiety-provoking and encourage the child to use relaxation and deep-breathing skills to manage anxiety. As the child develops tolerance of the situation, slowly make the situation more challenging and encourage her to refrain from safety behaviors to make herself feel better. Following are examples of trials in graduated in vivo desensitization for a child afraid to be left waiting alone:

1. Sitting alone in the therapy room for 3 and then 5 minutes, knowing that the therapist is in the hall.
2. Sitting alone in the therapy room for 5 and then 10 minutes, knowing that the therapist may not be in the hall.
3. Sitting alone in the therapy room for 10 minutes, with the lights dimmed, and knowing that the therapist is not in the hall.
4. Sitting alone in the therapy room, not knowing how long it will be, with lights dimmed, the therapist not in the hall, and Mom or Dad told not to be in the waiting room.

Desensitization trials begin with assistance from the therapist and with relatively easier situations, and demands increase with each successive trial. The child's expectations also are addressed, as she first knows what to expect in the situation (e.g., trial 1, knowing the therapist is in the hall) but is later exposed to unknowns (e.g., trial 4, not knowing how long it will be). This process is designed to build a child's ability to cope with ambiguous, challenging, and often uncontrollable situations. Anxiety often results from feeling unable to control a situation or predict what could happen in any situation, along with concern that something very negative will occur. These desensitization procedures are focused on teaching a child that even when a person does not have total control in a situation, she can still cope effectively and the worst scenario is not likely to occur. The child learns to tolerate normal levels of arousal while gathering information about her coping resources and skills.

Review each session's progress with the child and parent. Encourage the child to tell her parent about the in vivo desensitization. Offer corrective information or detail during the child's summary. Shape the child's ability to accurately communicate the process and progress of these treatment sessions. In addition, review with the child and parent progress in managing the daily routine. Provide instructions on what steps to take next in adjusting to the school routine. For example, you may suggest that the next STIC task involve a trip to the school library or meeting after school hours with a teacher to collect homework. These tasks combine the in vivo desensitization process with the STIC tasks. Discuss potential problems with adherence to the school schedule, and make recommendations as needed.

Setting the Pace of, and Assistance with, the In Vivo Exposures

There are several ways to conduct in vivo practices to manipulate the pace of the exposure. A slower pace is ideal for younger children, those with special needs, and those with exceptionally high levels of anxiety. Moving slower allows a child to fully habituate to anxiety and build trust that she will not be forced into anything overwhelming.

In assisted exposure, you or the parent performs the exposure with the child. This allows a child to receive support from a trusted individual and observe a model who manages the situation. These procedures are especially helpful in early sessions, when confronting an anxious situation for the first time, or when more challenging exposures are developed. Educate parents, however, about the difference between modeling, where one shows a child how to manage the situation, and rescuing, where one takes over and does the situation for the child. A child's anxiety may interact with parents' natural tendencies to comfort their children and lead to rescuing. Therefore, instruct parents to allow their child to experience normal rises in anxiety. Modeling and assisted exposure keep the focus on the child, with the goal of having her confront anxious situations alone.

Several steps make up this process. First, model for the child how to deal with the situation as the child observes. This gives the child a chance to observe how you process and manage a difficult situation. Second, help the child manage the situation together as a team (i.e., with the therapist and/or parents as coaches). Third, have the child manage the situation on her own as words of encouragement are given by a "coach." Prompt the child to use the somatic control exercises during this procedure. Fourth, have the child engage in the situation on her own while verbalizing self-reinforcement for performing the in vivo exposure.

Massed exposure or flooding involves having a child confront a stressor at a high intensity. Rather than gradually progressing up the AAH, the therapist chooses a higher item and begins there. Relaxation procedures are typically downplayed, so the advantage of flooding is less time. The child simply enters the anxiety-provoking situation and endures it until anxiety naturally dissipates. Flooding is not often used with young children, when anxiety is extreme, at the beginning of therapy, for children with chronic school refusal behavior, or for children with social and/or evaluative anxieties. Deciding to use more rapid exposure or flooding depends on a child's progress to this point and whether she understands the reason for this process.

Homework

Homework assignments after sessions 3 and 4 may include the following:

- Continue to practice relaxation at bedtime using audiotape or relaxation scripts from the parent workbook.
- At least once daily, the child should listen to and conduct a tape (imaginal) desensitization procedure.
- An additional STIC task will be assigned, which will involve a minimum of three different days practicing an in vivo desensitization. You, the child, and parent should agree on which task to assign. The in vivo desensitization may involve any of the following: practice at home, such as practicing staying alone in a room or the house for varying periods of time; allowing the parent to leave the house and staying with a sitter for varying periods of time; visiting the school bus stop in the morning; visiting the school or some room at the school; or similar situations. Be sure the parent agrees to find time to assist the child with these in vivo practices.
- Encourage adherence to a regular school-day schedule, including early wakening, dressing and preparing for school, and completing school assignments. Bear in mind that parents may inadvertently reinforce a child for not going to school. For example, a parent may find it easier to take a child to the store or on errands; however, these types of outings reinforce a child's avoidance of school, increase dependence on the parent, and convey that it is acceptable to be home. Arranging for a sitter or, in the case of responsible older children, leaving the child alone for specified periods is preferred to taking her on such excursions.

Sessions 5 and 6: Advanced Maturing of Treatment

Session Outline

- Review the week's progress and examine any difficulties encountered during in vivo desensitization.
- Conduct in vivo exposures involving increased school attendance.

Sessions 5 and 6 involve helping a child move more swiftly and aggressively through the AAH. You may want to schedule two or three sessions per week to facilitate progress or arrange therapy sessions at school or in places outside the office to conduct assisted in vivo practices. Begin to place greater responsibility on the child for identifying challenging situations. Over time, the child will learn to construct and conduct her own exposures and reframe anxiety-provoking situations as positive opportunities to address challenges. The main goal of this phase of treatment is to train a child to recognize when negative emotions occur and immediately set up an exposure and take coping action rather than avoid or escape. The therapist is the expert and the one who assumes responsibility during treatment to transfer his or her knowledge of coping with negative emotions to the parents and child by modeling for and training a parent to conduct in vivo desensitization at home, and helping the child practice anxiety management skills. Through systematic homework assignments, the parent likewise becomes an active and crucial part of the transfer process by fostering a child's sense of control and mastery of negative emotions.

Review of Assigned In Vivo Desensitization and STIC Tasks

Review the week's progress and examine difficulties encountered during in vivo desensitization practices. Examples of assigned tasks include visiting the school and/or teacher, staying alone for increasingly longer periods, and approaching and remaining in other situations. Emphasize the importance of using relaxation and deep-breathing techniques to remain calm during difficult situations and stay in a situation rather than avoiding or escaping. In addition, review the child's progress adhering to a school schedule and her initial attempts at attending classes or school functions.

Stepping Up the STIC Tasks: Eliminating Safety Signals

As treatment continues, increasingly more challenging situations are presented to the child for in vivo desensitization within and between sessions. One focus of the child's desensitization practices should be to enter difficult situations without help or use of "safety signals." A safety signal is any object or person one relies on to feel better or less anxious in a situation. Although a safety signal may lessen a child's anxiety in the short-term, the long-term use of safety signals maintains anxiety and prevents a child from learning she can manage the situation.

Those with anxiety disorders often rely on safety signals when confronting anxiety-provoking situations. These individuals, for example, carry water bottles, medication, or cellular telephones in the mistaken belief they "need" these things to prevent panic attacks or access help. Similarly, the presence of a safe person (e.g., friend) is often interpreted as someone who can "save" the individual from untoward consequences of a panic attack. Of course, a panic attack only produces discomfort that will pass even if a person does nothing.

Anxious children will likewise develop safety behaviors and safety signals. For example, an anxious child may become more "clingy" or in need of attention and reassurance. Although parents want to comfort their child, frequently doing so may prevent her from learning to manage normal levels

Table 8.1
Negative Emotions and Behaviors and Accompanying Safety Signals

Negative emotions or behaviors	Safety signals
Worry: "What if" thinking; reassurance-seeking; anxiety in new or changing situations; perfectionism.	Repeated questioning; needing to know every detail and plan; carrying everything in the book bag (anxiety about leaving something behind); rewriting and erasing to get a paper "perfect."
Panic: Fear of the sudden rush of certain body sensations, such as a racing heart, sweating, dizziness, shortness of breath, or shaking.	Having someone always close by "just in case" (e.g., friend, parent); carrying certain objects to feel better (e.g., water, medicine, cellular telephones or beepers); checking the heartbeat or pulse; dropping out of sports or gym activities.
Anxiety about specific objects or situations: Anxiety about fire drills, riding the bus, insects or animals, thunderstorms, a ringing bell, small places like classrooms, doctors, needles, or the dark.	Watching a weather report and anticipating a storm; sleeping with the lights on or needing someone to sleep with the child; earplugs.
Separation anxieties: Anxiety that something terrible will happen when separated from home or loved ones, and then two people will never see each other again.	"Shadowing" or clinging to Mom or Dad; always being in sight of Mom or Dad; never being alone; needing much reassurance if a separation is going to occur.
Sadness, the "blues," or depression: Being down more days than not; feeling hopeless or that things will never work out; feelings of worthlessness or guilt; loss of interest in usual activities; irritability; crying; thoughts of death or harming self.	Clinging; not wanting to be alone; having someone else (parent, friend) solve or handle one's problems due to beliefs that "I can't ever get things right" or "I don't deserve this."

of discomfort. Children with anxiety disorders who refuse to attend school due to these negative emotions can often be "bribed" into entering these situations with assistance. For example, some children will ride the school bus only if a certain sibling or friend accompanies them. If the "safety" child is absent, the anxious child resists riding the bus. Similarly, adolescents with panic attacks may require elaborate safety measures such as carrying a cellular telephone in case they need to call for help. Adolescents with panic attacks find it difficult to be away from home or their primary caretaker for fear that no one else will understand or be able to help them if an attack occurs.

Increasing the complexity and challenge of the STIC tasks is important to uncover, and then dispose of, as many of these unnecessary and unhelpful safety signals as possible. Table 8.1 lists some common safety signals for children who refuse school. Help a child construct in vivo practices to confront and challenge these negative emotions. As each practice progresses, accompanying safety signals will be systematically taken away to give the child the opportunity to learn for herself how to manage the situation alone.

In Vivo Practices

Increasing the challenge of the STIC tasks, along with decreasing the use of safety signals, will give a child much-needed experience with managing diffcult situations. Begin with an imaginal desensitization so the child is prepared for the in vivo practice situation. The imaginal desensitization will involve describing the child confronting a stressful or anxiety-provoking situation and not engaging in a safety behavior. If the child is progressing fairly rapidly, then move quickly to in vivo desensitization. Following are examples of in vivo desensitization plans for three of the most common forms of negative distress in a school refusal population.

Example 1: The Clinging Child—"Don't Leave Me Alone!"

Problem Focus

School refusal due to anxiety about something terrible happening to Mom or Dad, or being kidnapped or killed, or getting lost and not being able to find the way home.

Safety Behaviors and Signals

Needing to call home every hour during the school day; needing Mom and Dad to call home every hour when they go out without the children; having Mom or Dad always arrive early to pick up child from school; having Mom or Dad drive down the same streets to prevent getting lost.

In Vivo Desensitization Plans

Practice going for increasingly longer periods of time without talking to Mom or Dad, and gradually work up to not knowing their whereabouts. Telephone calls initially can be stretched to every 90 minutes, then to twice in the morning and once in the afternoon, then to once only in the morning, and then to no calls at all. A similar schedule would apply when the parents go out without the children: call home every 90 minutes, then every 2 hours, then once during any 4-hour period, and then not at all.

In vivo practice for anxiety about not being picked up on time would involve having the parent arrive 5 minutes late and giving a plausible excuse (e.g., stuck in traffic), then 10 minutes late with an excuse, then 10 minutes late without an excuse, and then 20 minutes late (working up to 45 minutes). To increase the challenge in this situation, employ "confederates," or assistants who are unknown to the child, who will walk by or ask for directions. Concurrently with this type of exposure, instruct the child about what to do to stay safe if a parent is running late: wait inside the school building and inform the office staff where you are; stay outside and inform a teacher or an adult who is well known that you are waiting for your parents; do not approach strangers; if a stranger approaches you, walk quickly toward a group of kids, an adult who you know, or someone in authority such as a police officer or crossing guard. The goal of this type of exposure is to enhance a child's tolerance for normal inconveniences and to develop the necessary skills to manage and remain safe in an ambiguous situation.

To desensitize anxiety about getting lost, blindfold a child (using a mask or scarf) and, without talking, take the child on a walk around the office building or outside area. Lead the child by the hand, but refrain from conversation. The child's inability to see the surroundings will arouse anxiety and worry. By increasing the practice time, the child will again learn to tolerate an ambiguous situation. Next, ask parents to simulate getting lost by driving on unfamiliar roads and occasionally mumbling, "Oh boy, where are we?" Instruct parents not to give any reassurance to the child and stay "lost" for increasing periods. Tell the parent to verbalize a plan for finding the correct street while remaining calm and in control: "Okay, let's see where we are. Breathe slowly, relax. This is Hylan Boulevard, and I know that it runs into New Dorp Lane at some point. Take it easy, stay calm and relaxed. I'll keep driving in this direction for another mile. Okay! There's New Dorp Lane! I knew I could find it if I just remained calm!"

Example 2: Pushing the Panic Button—"I Feel Sick and I Need Help!"

Problem Focus

Panic attacks occur in various situations or places, and may cause nausea, dizziness, shortness of breath, heart palpitations, sweating, shaking, numbing or tingling sensations, and feelings of unreality. These attacks seem to come "from out of the blue" and may have happened to the child in school, on the bus, in public places such as malls and movie theaters, and/or in crowds.

Safety Behaviors and Signals

Carrying a paper bag in case of hyperventilation, a bottle of water to keep the throat "open," and a cellular telephone to call for help; needing to have Mom available by telephone at all times; parents rearranging their work schedules to drive the child to and from school to avoid the bus that "triggers my panic attacks"; attending school only for half days because panic is more likely to occur in the afternoon; staying home to rest in bed each afternoon to stave off

Table 8.2
Interoceptive Exposure Exercises for Target Sensations

Spinning in a chair	Dizziness, lightheadedness
Running in place or up stairs	Shortness of breath, racing/pounding heart
Breathing through a straw	Shortness of breath, chest tightness
Staring at a light and then reading	Visual disturbances, unreality
Shaking head from side to side	Lightheadedness
Tensing all muscles, and holding them very tight	Muscle tension, tingling sensations
Hyperventilation	Shortness of breath, pounding heart, lightheadedness, tingling sensations
Putting your head down below the knees, and then "popping" up very quickly	Lightheadedness, dizziness, unreality

panic; being given an open pass by the teacher to go to the school nurse at any time during class if any panic symptoms are felt (on average, spending at least 1 hour each morning with the nurse), and then lying on a cot.

In Vivo Desensitization Plans

For those with panic attacks, interoceptive exposure exercises help desensitize a child to the physical sensations of panic. Interoceptive conditioning is the process of learning to be afraid of physical sensations. Individuals who experience panic begin to feel a change in their physical state and become vigilant about the change and scared of its implications. They thus typically avoid running up stairs, aerobic activity, drinking caffeinated beverages, or other situations or activities that may cause physical changes. One key to overcoming panic is to learn to tolerate normal physical arousal and changes without becoming frightened and distressed. Interoceptive exposure involves the systematic provocation of these sensations over repeated trials to reduce anxiety. Construct a hierarchy of sensations that scare a child and begin exposure with the least anxiety-provoking sensation, then gradually progress to exercises designed to elicit the sensation at higher and higher intensities. Typical exercises and their targets are listed in Table 8.2.

The goal of having a child engage in these exercises is to teach her that these sensations are temporary, predictable, and controllable. Most importantly, the child learns that changes in physical states are normal and harmless. Forewarn parents that a child will be somewhat uncomfortable, but only temporarily. The sensations of a panic attack are harmless and will eventually dissipate even if the child does nothing. Most importantly, the child will learn that normal functioning does not have to be altered because she experiences panic attacks.

Encourage the child to enter situations she avoids. Instruct the child to gradually leave safety signals (e.g., paper bags, cellular telephones, water bottles) at home. Slowly increase school attendance and limit visits to the nurse. These steps involve cooperation with the teacher and school nurse, so be prepared to communicate how they may coach the child to comply with the desensitization. Similarly, practice at home will involve spending less time in bed and an increasing amount of time engaging in physical activities (e.g., bike riding) that arouse physical sensations. Instruct the child to use deep breathing whenever anxiety is aroused and to remain in the situation despite experiencing panic-like sensations.

For further detail regarding this technique, read Mastery of Your Anxiety and Panic, Therapist Guide, 4th Edition, available from Oxford University Press.

Example 3: The Worrier—"What If, What If, What If?"

Problem Focus

Excessive worry about new situations, changes in routine, or doing things perfectly or to an unrealistic standard; difficulty with concentration and resting and sleeping well; complaints of muscle tension or aches; and repeatedly asking the same question, in the same manner.

Safety Behaviors and Signals

Constantly seeking reassurance from parents, teachers, and peers; teacher reporting that the child is "always at my desk"; child needing to know what the family's plan is for every day of the week and having difficulty if plans are changed or unexpected events occur.

In Vivo Desensitization Plans

Teach the child to experience less-than-perfect or less-than-desired circumstances and accept consequences without asking for reassurance. For example, ask a child who is an extreme perfectionist and puts undue pressure on herself to purposely make mistakes on homework papers or in sporting activities (e.g., strike out in baseball). Similarly, ask a child overly preoccupied with looking perfect to wear something wrinkled, have messy hair, and not use the mirror to check on her appearance. Do not provide reassurance to the child. Instruct parents to refrain from responding to her when she repeatedly asks, "Do you think this is okay?" Help parents set limits on reassurance-seeking. When the in vivo desensitization involves making mistakes on schoolwork, ask the teacher to expect a change in the child's work and to prepare some worksheets that will not enter into the child's official grade. Teach the child that even if mistakes occur, there are usually no long-term consequences, and most mistakes can be remedied.

For a child overly concerned with details of plans and activities, teach her to confront unknown and changing experiences. Have the parent schedule an outing that involves several planned stops (e.g., first to the mall, then to Grandma's house, then to the library). Typically, children who worry excessively will want to know all details of each stop, such as how long they will be there, what will happen, and who else may be involved. Instruct parents to change the order of the plans (e.g., go to Grandma's first) and the length of time the child expects to be in each place (e.g., leaving ahead of schedule or staying longer in one place). As the child begins to adjust, have parents advance desensitization by confronting established expectations (e.g., Grandma is not at home, the library is closed) and canceling an individual element of the plan. Lastly, tell parents to cancel an entire scheduled outing at the last minute without giving notice to the child.

Homework

Homework assignments after sessions 5 and 6 may include the following:

- Practice the relaxation tape at bedtime and complete daily logbooks.
- STIC tasks will involve various in vivo desensitization plans, in addition to imaginal desensitization as needed.
- Attendance in school will be increased over the course of these sessions, with the goal of having the child attend most of the day, every day.

Sessions 7 and 8: Completing Treatment and Preparing for Termination

The main focus of this latter part of treatment is to have a child spend increasingly longer periods of time in school, with the eventual goal of full-time attendance. Initially, you may wish to accompany the child to school or arrange your scheduled appointments in a private office of the school building during the day (e.g., a non-academic class period such as study hall). These assisted exposures may prompt a child to progress more rapidly to full-time attendance. Once the child has returned to school, however, therapy appointments should be avoided during school hours. Appointments may continue at school after school hours if appropriate. At this point, have the child take most of the responsibility for treatment and apply what was learned in real-life situations. Continue to implement techniques from previous sessions to help the child achieve this goal.

Chapter 9

The Children of Divorce Intervention Program: Fostering Children's Resilience through Group Support and Skill-Building

Procedures for Facilitating a Supportive Group Intervention with Second and Third Grade Children

JoAnne Pedro-Carroll, PhD

Each year in the United States, over one million children experience the dissolution of their parents' marriage, marking the beginning of a series of life changes and adjustments, ranging from emotional to economic. Divorce is an enormously stressful process for families, and especially for children. Although the form of children's responses varies by age and developmental level, most children react initially to their parents' separation with distress. Indeed, if

This chapter is reproduced with permission from the Children's Institute's Children of Divorce Intervention Program (CODIP), which publishes procedures manuals for conducting support groups. To see the other available manuals and program materials that are available, visit http://www.childrens institute.net/catalog/manuals/.
Acknowledgements: "The Children of Divorce Intervention Program" is the property of Children's Institute. It is reprinted here with permission of Children's Institute, Rochester, New York. Complete copies of this and other CODIP manuals and materials may be obtained from Children's Institute, 274 N. Goodman St. D 103, Rochester, NY 14607, or www.childrens institute.net.

given a choice, the vast majority of children would vote a resounding "NO!" to their parents' breakup. For young children especially, divorce can be a confusing, frightening time, during which they feel little control over the myriad changes they face. These reactions are to be expected, but a number of studies, including our own research on evidence-based preventive interventions, show that much can be done to prevent early reactions from becoming long-term problems.

The Children of Divorce Intervention Program (CODIP) model presented in this Handbook is based on an awareness of the well-documented risks that parental divorce poses for children, the protective factors that shape trajectories of outcomes over time, and a belief that divorce does not inevitably have to mean long-term trauma for children. A number of studies show that how children fare in the aftermath of divorce depends in part on the amount of support they receive from significant adults in their lives, especially their families, schools and other systems that affect their development. Children's coping resources also play an important role in their potential for risk or resilience in the aftermath of divorce. Those competencies and coping skills are an integral part of this intervention model for children of all ages. Four CODIP manuals have been developed for children of different ages: kindergarten and 1st grade, 2nd and 3rd grades, 4th through 6th grades, and 7th and 8th grades. While the goals and objectives embedded in these interventions remain relatively constant, the specific issues and techniques vary according to the developmental differences of the age groups.

Thus, CODIP is designed specifically to enhance children's capacity to cope effectively with the many challenges and changes that are synonymous with divorce.

The program's two main goals are to:

1. Reduce the stress of parental divorce by providing a supportive group environment.
2. Build competence by teaching specific skills that can help children cope with the many challenges posed by parental divorce.

This program is a selective preventive intervention program, built on the premise that early, timely intervention for children in stressful circumstances can provide important protective benefits. It is not intended for children with severe or chronic emotional difficulties that warrant more intensive treatment. This curriculum was designed to address psychological reactions and developmental characteristics of 7- and 8-year-olds. Children of divorce, at this age, often react to parental divorce with intense sadness. Fears and worries, feelings of loss and longing for the family unit, hopes and wishes for parental reconciliation, anger, guilt and misconceptions are quite common. These clinical themes and methods for effective coping are embedded in the activities in this manual.

Developmentally relevant aspects of Wallerstein's (1983) concept of psychological tasks facing children of divorce are also reflected in the curriculum. Specifically, the six hierarchical, divorce-related coping tasks identified are:

1. Acknowledging the reality of the divorce and achieving a realistic cognitive understanding.

2. Disengaging from parental conflict and resuming the child's agenda.
3. Resolving the many losses that divorce imposes.
4. Resolving problems of anger and self-blame.
5. Accepting the permanence of divorce.
6. Achieving realistic hope about one's future relationships.

Mastering these sequenced tasks, starting at the time of the parental separation and continuing through late adolescence, enables the child to integrate the experience of parental divorce and to develop the capacity to trust and love in the future. To that end, the program emphasizes the importance of developing a supportive group environment in which these tasks are addressed and incorporated into intervention goals.

The program has four primary units:

1. Feelings, families and family changes.
2. Coping skills: Learning how to handle feelings and problems.
3. Child-parent relationships.
4. Children's perceptions of themselves and their families.

Although CODIP uses a variety of techniques, it is important for practitioners to use their own sensitivity and creativity to engage children in the group process and make it relevant and supportive for each child. Any single technique or approach is but one aspect of a more comprehensive effort to realize the larger goals of helping children express and understand their feelings and resolve or cope effectively with personal problems. And beyond those objectives lies the program's ultimate and most important goal: to foster children's resilience and healthy adjustment.

This curriculum is intended as a guide for conducting a preventive intervention program, not group psychotherapy. Carefully controlled research has been conducted on this program, providing an evidence base of CODIP's effectiveness. Results of those evaluation studies have shown significant improvements in children's home and school adjustment from the perspectives of parents, teachers, group leaders and the children themselves (Pedro-Carroll, 2005; Pedro-Carroll & Jones, 2005; Pedro-Carroll, 2001; Alpert-Gillis, Pedro-Carroll & Cowen, 1989; Pedro-Carroll & Alpert-Gillis, 1987; Pedro-Carroll & Cowen, 1985,

1987; Pedro-Carroll, Cowen, Hightower & Guare, 1986; Sterling, 1986; Pedro-Carroll, Alpert-Gillis & Cowen, 1992; Pedro-Carroll & Alpert-Gillis, 1997). A follow-up study found that improvements in program children's social, emotional and school adjustment were still in evidence two years later on multiple measures of healthy development (Pedro-Carroll, Sutton & Wyman, 1999). In 1991, CODIP was the recipient of the National Mental Health Association's Lela Rowland Award for Exemplary Prevention Programs in the United States. In 2005, CODIP received the Program Excellence Award from the Department of Health and Human Services, Substance Abuse and Mental Health Services Administration, and is cited as an Exemplary Program by the Association of Family and Conciliation Courts (AFCC) and the New York State Department of Education. Based on converging evidence of the efficacy of this intervention, CODIP has been widely disseminated throughout the US and countries around the world.

CURRICULUM OVERVIEW

The CODIP model for 7- and 8-year-old children is a 15-session supportive group intervention. The program's overarching goal is to prevent or minimize the behavioral and emotional problems that children experience following parental divorce. To achieve this goal the program's structure and curriculum are based on five fundamental objectives.

1. Foster a supportive group environment. Support is emphasized throughout the program. The group format itself is designed to provide children with much needed social support. Contacts with peers who have gone through comparable experiences can help children realize that they are not alone in their situation and that they are not different from other children.
2. Facilitate the identification and expression of emotions and divorce-related feelings. Most people who are going through a major life transition find it difficult to understand and cope with a range of intense emotions. Young children are vulnerable to being overwhelmed by stressful emotional experiences, because they lack the coping skills of older children and adults. Accordingly, the program seeks to increase children's understanding of the universality of emotions, enhance

their ability to identify and label feelings in themselves and others and to learn to express feelings appropriately. Concepts such as "All feelings are okay" are developed as the group aims to provide a safe, supportive atmosphere in which all feelings are accepted.
3. Promote understanding of divorce-related concepts and encourage exploration and clarification of divorce-related misconceptions. Helping children achieve a realistic understanding of what divorce *does* and *does not* mean is another important program objective. Children are often confused about their family situation. To minimize such confusion, the program develops concepts such as "divorce means that a child's parents decide not to live together anymore" and "divorce is a grown-up problem that is not something that children cause or can fix."
4. Teach relevant coping skills including social problem solving skills. Another important program element is to provide children with skills that can help them cope better with the many challenges they face. Social problem solving teaches children how to think, not what to think. As children learn to generate alternative solutions and anticipate their consequences, they can cope more effectively with everyday problems. Such skills may be especially beneficial for children who must deal with the major stresses associated with parental divorce.
5. Enhance positive perceptions of self and families. The program also emphasizes positive regard for self and one's family. Many children of divorce feel "different" or "defective" (e.g., "If I were only a better kid, my parents would have stayed together."). Thus, helping children to focus on their unique and special qualities is important. Family esteem (e.g., awareness and acceptance of non-traditional family structures and the ability to see the positive family changes that have occurred since the parental separation) is stressed, as well as self-esteem.

These five objectives are addressed in a structured, sequential, detailed program curriculum. The curriculum has four primary units, with three to five 45-minute sessions each:

1. Feelings, families and family changes.
2. Coping skills: Learning how to handle problems and feelings.

3. Child-parent relationships.
4. Children's perceptions of themselves and their families.

Each session includes goals, activities (e.g., stories, puppet play, interactive games), required materials, procedures and review questions. Brief abstracts of the four major units and the 15 sessions of the curriculum follow.

PART I: FEELINGS, FAMILIES AND FAMILY CHANGES

Sessions 1–4 focus on:

* Introducing children to the support group.
* Establishing a safe, supportive, and consistent environment.
* Building children's emotional vocabulary.
* Clarifying basic feeling concepts.
* Defining and explore the concept of family.
* Introducing the topic of divorce.
* Exploring children's feelings about divorce in general.

Session 1 seeks to establish the group as a safe, supportive place and clarify the purpose of the group. The latter includes helping children better understand divorce and handle feelings and problems that sometimes happen with divorce. Selecting a group name and introducing a group puppet, whose parents are also divorced, also help build cohesiveness.

Session 2 focuses on identifying feelings, developing a vocabulary of "feeling" words, and introducing feeling concepts such as the "universality" of emotions, and that all feelings are ok, while all behaviors aren't always acceptable. Pictures of facial expressions and a feelings "grab bag game" are used to facilitate children's understanding and regulation of emotion and introduce ways to self-soothe when faced with distressing emotions.

Session 3 deals with families, "something everyone has feelings about." The idea that there are all kinds of families, each being unique and special, is emphasized through:

(a) a book that promotes awareness and acceptance of non-traditional families; and
(b) an exercise that helps children identify, reflect on, and share their own family situations, using wooden family figures.

Session 4 begins to apply feeling words and feeling concepts to children's divorce experiences. A book is used to describe children's common reactions to divorce. The goal is to facilitate children's awareness, expression, and acceptance of such divorce-related feelings. Common divorce concepts and misconceptions are also considered.

PART II: COPING SKILLS: LEARNING HOW TO HANDLE PROBLEMS AND FEELINGS

The general objectives of sessions 5–9 are:

* Clarifying the concepts of "problem" and "solution."
* Clarify the relationship between problems and feelings.
* Expand children's coping abilities by teaching them the strategy of social problem solving.

  a. Teach children the basic social problem solving steps:
  Identify the problem—"What is the problem?"
  Generate alternative solutions—"What are all the things I could do?"
  Anticipate the consequences—"What might happen next?"
  Choose an alternative—"Choose what looks best and try it!"
  b. Emphasize that there is more than one solution to any problem.

* Help children learn to distinguish between problems they can and cannot solve.
* Encourage children to apply social problem solving to personal, divorce-related problems.

Sessions 5–9 teach social problem solving skills that children can use to cope with "not so good" feelings, and problems. Rather than telling children what to think, they are taught how to think when experiencing a problem. As children learn to think of alternative solutions and anticipate consequences of their behavior, they are better able to cope with daily obstacles. Research has shown that effective social problem solving skills are closely related to children's self-confidence, good peer relationships, and overall positive adjustment.

Social problem solving skills may be especially beneficial for children who must cope with a highly stressful situation such as parental divorce. Children of divorce are often faced with difficult new problems that they are not prepared to handle. Teaching social problem solving skills is one way to prepare them to cope with such problems. Social problem solving skills can help children reduce the stress and confusion inherent in the divorce process, and help them gain control over aspects of a situation over which they originally had no control (i.e., the parents' decision to separate/divorce).

The goals of these sessions are to teach children the four basic social problem solving steps and to apply them to personal divorce-related problems.

Although children learn all four social problem solving steps, two aspects of the process are emphasized in these sessions. The first is the generation of alternative solutions (i.e., Step 2). The ability to generate alternatives has been shown to relate more closely to children's adjustment than any other step. Thus, one primary objective of the social problem solving sessions in this manual is to teach children to think of as many different solutions as possible for personal, divorce-related problems. Teaching children the difference between solvable and unsolvable problems is another important aspect of problem solving. Understanding locus of control helps to empower children to effectively solve what they can, and disengage from uncontrollable problems, and focus their efforts instead on age appropriate activities. Problems that have negative consequences regardless of the number or type of solutions children try are "unsolvable." Some divorce-related problems are "unsolvable" because children have no control or power over certain aspects of the divorce process (e.g., parents in protracted conflict or parents who decide to move). Teaching children to distinguish between divorce-related problems they can and cannot solve (i.e., control) minimizes feelings of frustration, self-blame, and confusion. Children are given opportunities to develop and practice problem solving methods through diverse exercises and games. Increasingly, the new skills are applied to divorce related problems and feelings.

Session 5 introduces all four problem solving steps with an emphasis on generating alternatives. Children are asked to generate solutions to problem situations depicted in pictures. A point highlighted in the discussion is that there are usually many solutions to a problem.

Session 6 focuses on generating alternative solutions, anticipating consequences, and evaluating solutions. Choosing the best solution involves first anticipating and then evaluating possible consequences of each. A Tic-Tac-Toe game is used as a vehicle for practicing the four social problem solving steps.

Session 7 applies the social problem solving steps to divorce-related problems.

Puppet plays by leaders and children are used to help group members apply these newly learned coping skills to typical divorce-related interpersonal problems of early latency children (e.g., fear of abandonment, loyalty conflicts, longing for the non-custodial parent). Leaders guide children in applying the problem solving steps to selected scenarios.

Session 8 teaches the distinction between problems that children can solve (e.g., wanting more friends) and cannot solve (e.g., getting parents back together). Children who understand and accept that some divorce-related problems are beyond their control feel less self-blame, frustration, and confusion. Children are encouraged to disengage from "unsolvable" problems and become more involved in age-appropriate activities. The Red-Light Green-Light game helps children learn to discriminate between their own solvable and unsolvable problems.

Session 9 reinforces children's efforts to apply problem solving skills to their own problems through a problem solving "show-and-tell," and an engaging board game called Daring Dinosaurs, designed to reinforce skills and concepts taught in the program thus far.

PART III: CHILD-PARENT RELATIONSHIPS

The general objectives of sessions 10–12 are:

- Further explore children's personal conceptions and feelings about divorce.
- Encourage children to express feelings about parents and parent child relationships and assist them in clarifying related issues.
- Assist children in applying social problem solving concepts to personal divorce-related problems.

Sessions 10–12 continue to explore children's feelings about divorce. These sessions focus on children's relationships with their parents. Relevant divorce-related concerns (e.g., loyalty conflicts, fears of abandonment, reconciliation fantasies, feelings of rejection and loss), are highlighted. Further application of social problem solving skills to divorce-related problems is encouraged when applicable.

Session 10 explores children's personal feelings about divorce through the use of a book and a question-and-answer activity. Feelings toward parents are emphasized. For example, leaders ask while reading the book: "When Niki got mad that her mother went out on a date, how did she show it? Is it okay to feel angry at your mother?"

Session 11 focuses on children's perceptions and feelings about parent child issues through puppet play. Children are helped to understand their parents' feelings, as well as their own. Problem solving skills are applied to the problem scenarios in the plays. The following is an example of a dilemma acted out and resolved by the children using problem solving skills: "Sam's parents are divorced. His father is moving to another city. Sam is worried that if his father could move away and leave him maybe someday his mother might go away too. Sam is talking about his problem with his friends Mike and Chris."

Session 12 uses a board game to review and consolidate important program concepts, and encourage further exploration of parent-related issues. With only three sessions remaining, group termination is also introduced. Although children are initially told how many meetings there will be, ending the group and discussing ways to ask for support and help when needed becomes an important theme from this point on.

PART IV: CHILDREN'S PERCEPTIONS OF THEMSELVES AND THEIR FAMILIES

The general objectives of sessions 13–15 are:

- Enhance children's self-esteem.
- Promote children's positive feelings about their families.
- Foster children's awareness of positive post-separation family changes.
- Explore termination issues and facilitate the working through of termination-related feelings.
- Encourage children to seek continued support from their environment.

Sessions 13–15 deal with children's perceptions of themselves and their families. Activities seek to enhance children's self-esteem and to develop awareness of positive family changes. The unit also emphasizes termination issues. The end of the group may reactivate feelings of loss related to those experienced around the family dissolution. The goal of the termination process is to facilitate working through this issue in a supportive group context.

Session 13 strives to enhance children's perceptions of themselves and others. Each child completes an 8-page booklet describing his/her characteristics, likes, feelings, wishes, and place in the group and family. Children complete sentences in ways that best describe how they think and feel. Termination is discussed in relation to items dealing with the group (e.g., "My favorite thing about the group has been _____."). Positive post-divorce experiences are discussed in relation to items dealing with the family (e.g., "Divorce can be hard on kids. Divorce can also make things better for kids and their families. One thing that is better now in my family is _____.").

Session 14 emphasizes children's special strengths as group members (e.g., being a good problem solver, being supportive). In the You're a Special Person game, members are first asked to list positive qualities of children. Next, papers with each person's name are circulated and group members write down the positive qualities that describe particular children. Children's and leaders' reactions to the ending of the group are explored further. Children are involved in planning a small party for the last group meeting.

Session 15, the final session, deals with children's experiences and feelings about the group. Children are encouraged to maintain relationships with fellow group members; others (e.g., parents, teachers, friends) to whom they can reach out for support are identified. The group ends with a celebration and children receive certificates of achievement in "Caring and Sharing."

Program Implementation

Although CODIP can be conducted in a variety of settings, schools are a natural locus for such groups because of the accessibility of large numbers of children sharing similar experiences who can continue in their supportive relationships after the groups end. School based mental health professionals are ideal candidates for group leaders because of the potential continuity of their contacts with program children and their families. Whether such groups are school or community based however, it is important that they have a consistent, private meeting place with regularly scheduled (approximately 45-minute) weekly sessions. Groups for primary aged youngsters tend to work best with 4–7 children. It is ideal for groups to be co-led by a male and a female leader, although that is not always possible. Although the manual refers to group leaders throughout, it is possible for sessions to be conducted by a single leader, perhaps with reductions in group size. Clearly, the success of a program such as CODIP depends heavily on the interest, care and sensitivity of those who conduct it, i.e., the leaders. Leaders are important role models for establishing trust, encouraging active involvement, sharing feelings, providing support and empathy, and setting appropriate limits. Their ability to discuss emotionally laden issues comfortably helps set the tone and climate of the group situation.

Group Leader Training

For best results, it is recommended that CODIP leaders receive training prior to and during the initial implementation of the program. This provides the opportunity for interaction and support from colleagues who are engaged in similar activities.

In addition, it affords the opportunity to learn from others what might be typical in the program. Typically, leader training and supervision in CODIP includes two components:

1. Preparatory training sessions before the program begins.
2. Consultation and supervision meetings throughout the intervention period, as needed.

Preparatory training addresses the following broad topics: the impact of divorce on families with a particular emphasis on early latency children; developmental issues of this age group; the rationale for preventive interventions with children of divorce; temporal stages in adjustment to divorce; risk and protective factors that mediate children's adjustment; psychological tasks facing children of divorce; group process and facilitation techniques; and a preview and discussion of curriculum materials. Readings of relevant research literature is used extensively throughout. Ongoing supervisory meetings with leaders have the following objectives:

- Review the events of the preceding sessions and their substantive or management problems.
- Review curriculum materials for the next meetings.

- When indicated, consider and act on curricular modifications to achieve program objectives.

Group Facilitation Techniques

Early school-aged children are not always able to verbalize their feelings clearly, especially in early meetings. Perhaps the most important challenge CODIP leaders face is facilitating a supportive group environment in which children can freely and trustingly express important feelings. Leaders are essential role models in this regard. The following are some of the approaches that CODIP leaders have found helpful in creating a supportive group environment:

Empathic Responding

Many children find it easier to recount experiences or events to the group, than to identify central feelings associated with them. An empathic response, i.e., one that helps the child identify such feelings, is very helpful.[1] Take the following as an example:

CHILD: *I think it was my fault that my parents broke up because they always fought about me; I could hear my name come up while I was trying to go to sleep and they were arguing.*

LEADER: *An empathic (feeling-oriented) response might be: It must have been pretty scary to hear them argue and maybe even more upsetting to think that they were fighting over you.*

Such a response brings the child's central feelings to the surface and paves the way to deal further and more constructively with them. Although an important ultimate goal is to help children clarify misconceptions such as assuming responsibility for the divorce, a constructive first step is responding empathetically to their feelings.

When going through difficult changes, children may be somewhat defensive, or guarded about sharing their feelings. Some may get silly or obstreperous to deflect emotional issues. It is important to deal with defensiveness empathetically, but directly, for example, "Sometimes it's hard to talk about how we feel if we're not sure what people will think . . ."

Sensitivity to "Hidden" Agendas or Nonverbal Cues

Children often communicate feelings nonverbally, through facial expressions or posture. It is important to be in tune with a child's expressions or tone of voice. For example, if children look or sound apprehensive about having friends at their house after parents have separated, the following comment may help them identify their fears: "It sounds like you have some worries about other kids finding out about your parents' divorce. What do you think might happen?"

Specifying a Statement

Children often make sweeping generalizations in their efforts to express the intensity of their feelings. Helping them sort out and identify specific situations and their associated feelings can help.

CHILD: *Everything's terrible since my parents split up.*

LEADER: *Divorce can be really hard sometimes—a lot of kids feel this way. Tell us about some of the things that are hard for you?*

Refocus on the Topic

Group discussion may sometimes digress to unrelated topics, especially as an attempt to avoid difficult, painful topics. A redirective prompt can help, "I know you enjoy baseball, Jeff, but can you think of some ways to help Jane solve her problem with her Dad?"

Group Process Issues

A striking observation in many CODIP groups is that children of divorce often start with the erroneous assumption that they are the only ones who have had certain types of divorce-related experiences. Learning that others have encountered similar experiences is comforting and supportive. Actively involving other members of the group is one way of achieving that goal.

Involving the Whole Group

Comments or questions which elicit the participation of other children helps foster a sense of commonality and mutual support. Examples of such responses include, "John, that sounds like the experience you described last week," or "Has anyone else here had a similar experience?"

Encouraging Participation

Some children are reticent about sharing feelings and experiences with the group. Encouraging such children to participate without pressuring them is an important leader skill. Children respond at their own individual pace; a withdrawn child may need a number of sessions before he/she comes to believe that the group really is a safe place in which to disclose intimate personal information. Comments that convey group interest, support, and acceptance reassure the wary participant, for example, "You don't have to talk about this today if you don't want to, but when you're ready, we'd really like to hear," or "I bet everyone here has had times when they felt like they were the only one who had such feelings and didn't want anyone else to know, but we're finding out that it can really help to talk about it."

Reinforcing Support among Group Members

One of CODIP's most basic underlying goals throughout the program, is to foster support among group members. Leaders can help achieve that goal both by modeling supportive behavior themselves and by reinforcing children's supportive comments, for example, "It was really helpful that so many of you let Mark know that you felt the same way as he does about what's happening in your family."

Clarifying and Summarizing

Near the end of each session, it is helpful to remind children when the session will end (e.g., "in 5 minutes") and to summarize the important aspects of the meeting, for example, "Today we worked on solving problems and learned that there are some problems that can't be solved—like trying to get our parents back together. You all helped Eve figure out a way to solve a tricky problem she was having with her stepmother. Eve, we'll look forward to hearing how it worked next Tuesday at 2:00, when we meet."

Setting Limits

At times in group meetings limits must be set on disruptive behavior. Children need and want limits; they feel safer knowing the parameters of acceptable behavior. Problems of under-controlled behavior are not infrequent among children of divorce. Setting limits in such instances can help strengthen children's self-control skills, reduce their guilt and anxiety, insure the physical and emotional well-being of group members and permit leaders to remain accepting and empathic. Although limits must be clear and consistent, they can best be put in a friendly but firm way that minimizes resentment. They should be phrased in a way that doesn't challenge the child's self-respect, i.e., succinctly and impersonally. For example, the phrasing, "Time is up for today," is more effective than "Your time is up and you have to go." Sometimes a subtle, nonverbal cue, for example, sitting next to a disruptive child, patting his/her arm, or making eye contact, is all that is needed to remind him/her of an appropriate limit. It is helpful to work on more chronic disruptive (limit-threatening) problems with the group, by involving members in a discussion of how the behavior affects the group and eliciting suggestions for solving the problem.

Confidentiality

An important aspect of the group is to foster a safe environment in which children can discuss personal feelings and problems. Leaders should make it very clear to participants that the group is a safe place to talk about any feelings they may have. It is essential that children also be assured that, with the exception of potential risk of danger to themselves or others, the things they say in the group are confidential and that members, as well as leaders, must respect that confidentiality. At the same time, members should be encouraged to talk with their parents about their own feelings and relevant matters that the group raises for them. (Session 1 provides more detailed information on the handling of confidentiality.)

Parent Involvement

Although this program is primarily for children, important benefits can accrue from involving parents in introductory meetings to explain its purpose and rationale, and responding to their questions and concerns at that time. Additionally, encouraging parents and children to talk throughout the program about divorce-related feelings and experiences can often help reduce within-family tensions and can open lines of parent-child communication.

Keep in mind that while these techniques are helpful tools for group facilitation, each leader has his/her own unique style when working with children. The techniques and exercises included are simply vehicles toward achieving the goals of enhancing children's adjustment. If a modification of a technique seems in order for a particular group of children, it is certainly appropriate to use creativity and clinical judgment and adapt the curriculum accordingly.

Children's groups tend to develop cohesiveness and support more slowly than adult groups, so do not be discouraged if children seem so preoccupied at first with their own issues that supportive responses are slow to emerge. The active involvement of leaders is a key ingredient in modeling and encouraging children's participation and mutual support among group members. Although the CODIP leadership experience is understandably challenging, it can also be an immensely rewarding experience.

Session 1: Getting to Know Each Other

Goals

- Begin to establish a safe, supportive environment among children.
- Provide a focus and structure for the upcoming meetings.

Procedure

1. Distribute name-tags.
2. Conduct the introductory, ice-breaking exercise, the Name Game.
3. Introduce the group purpose.
4. Clarify the group structure.
5. Name the group.
6. Introduce the group puppet.
7. Distribute stickers.

Materials

- Name-tags.
- Puppets.
- Stickers.

Overview

Session 1 seeks to establish the group as a safe, supportive place and clarify the purpose of the group. The latter includes helping children better understand divorce and handle feelings and problems that sometimes happen with divorce. Selecting a group name and introducing a group puppet, whose parents are also divorced, help build cohesiveness.

Procedure

1. Distribute name-tags. Have name-tags prepared for the children and distribute them at the start of the session. The name-tags should be kept in the group room until the last session.
2. Ice-breaking exercise. Begin with an introductory, ice-breaking exercise such as the Name Game to help children get acquainted and feel comfortable with each other. First seat the children in a circle. Leaders start the game by saying their own names. The first child then repeats the leader's name and adds his/her own name (e.g., "That's Miss Davis and I'm Billy."). This process continues until the last child has repeated everyone's name. The game can be repeated. During the second round each person can add something he/she likes to do in addition to his/her name (e.g., "That's Miss Davis, that's Billy, and I'm Sue and I like to draw."). (Note: Leaders can have the children turn over their name tags during this exercise.)
3. Introduce the group purpose. Leaders should note that although the Name Game tells us that kids are different in some ways (i.e., what they like), all kids in this group have one thing in common. Leaders ask if anyone knows what that thing is and why we are meeting. Allow ample time to explore children's fantasies about why they are in the group and what they expect to be doing. Leaders can summarize the discussion by stating the group commonality.

LEADER: *Even though each of you is different, you all have one thing that's the same. Each of you has parents who no longer live with each other. Does anyone know what this is called? (Children respond.) That's right, it's called a separation or divorce.*

> *Leaders should explain that divorce can be kind of tough for kids because it can cause not-so-good feelings and problems, and when we have such feelings it helps to talk about them. Clarify the purpose of the group, i.e., to help children better understand divorce; and learn how to handle some not-so-good feelings and problems that sometimes happen with divorce. Leaders can also begin to describe some of the activities that the group will be doing (e.g., drawing, reading books, watching films, playing with puppets).*

4. Clarify the group structure. Explain the specifics of the meeting: Leaders should clarify when, where, and how many times the group will meet. Emphasize that it is important that they attend each meeting as there will be many things to learn and fun things to do. Review confidentiality rule: Leaders should point out to the children that for groups to be fun they need to have rules (e.g., "One person talks at a time."). One rule that should be discussed in the first session is the confidentiality rule (e.g., "No repeating what anyone else says outside this room," or "Only our own thoughts and feelings can be shared outside our group."). Leaders should allow time to discuss the meaning and rationale behind the confidentiality rule. Leaders should also be sure that children understand that they will inform the child if they feel it is necessary to talk with his/her parents about issues that have arisen in the group. It is OK and desirable to talk about his/her own group experience with parents or friends. Parent-child communication should be encouraged throughout the program.
5. Name the group. In order to foster group identity and supportive peer relations it is very useful for the children to select a name for their group. Ask the children to suggest possible names for the group and then help them select a name acceptable to all.
6. Introduce the group puppet. Leaders can introduce the puppet as a "very special friend" who also has parents who don't live together, and wants to learn about divorce. Explain that in order for this friend to feel like he/she belongs in the group, it's important to give the puppet a name. Children can be asked to think of names for the puppet by next session.
7. Distribute stickers.
   End the session on a positive note by giving each member a sticker as a reminder of their special role in the group. Also, briefly review the session.
8. Review questions.
   • What is the same for all the children in the group?
     (All the children have parents who do not live together.)
   • Why is it important not to talk about what other children said in the group?
     (Be sure the confidentiality rule is clear.)
   • Is it OK to talk to your parents about what you learn here?
     (Emphasize that it is acceptable and helpful to talk with parents' about what they are learning.)
   • What are you going to think about for next week?
     (i.e. puppet's name.)
     See you next at (day and time)!

Session 2: Focus on Feelings

Goals

- Help children recognize and identify feelings in themselves and others.
- Introduce basic feelings and feeling concepts.

Procedure

1. Review the purpose and rules of the group.
2. Follow-up last week's session by naming the group puppet.
3. Introduce the topic of feelings.
4. Read the book, *I Feel: A Picture Book of Emotions*, by George Ancona or *The Boys' and Girls' Book of Dealing with Feelings*, by Eric Dlugokinski, PhD.
5. Play the Feelings Grab-Bag game.
6. Distribute Feeling Faces sheets.

Materials

- Name-tags.
- Puppets.
- The book, *I Feel: A Picture Book of Emotions,* by George Ancona (1977) or any other age appropriate book dealing with children's emotions such as *The Boys' and Girls' Book of Dealing with Feelings,* by Eric Dlugokinski, PhD (1993).
- Grab bag of 18 Feeling Faces.
- Poster of feeling words.
- Extra copies of the Feeling Faces sheet.

Overview

Session 2 focuses on identifying feelings, developing a vocabulary of feeling words, and introducing feeling concepts such as the universality of emotions. Pictures of facial expressions and a Feelings Grab-Bag game are used to facilitate children's understanding of feelings.

Procedure

1. Review of previous session. Review the group purpose with the children to clarify the group's focus and to be sure that children understand the concept of "divorce." Also review any group rules discussed in the last session (e.g., confidentiality, one person talks at a time).
2. Name the puppet. Follow-up on the last session by having children decide the puppet's name. If children have not thought of names, the group can have a brainstorming session. After a name is chosen, start to develop the puppet's unique "identity" by asking children specific questions about the puppet's background (e.g., Does the puppet live with his/her mother or father? Does he/she have any brothers and sisters?) and personal characteristics (e.g., friendly, shy, talkative, likes chocolate ice cream). The puppet's personality can continue to be developed in future sessions.

    This unfolding process has two purposes:
    a. develop group cohesion, and
    b. elicit children's perceptions of their own attributes and life experiences in a non-threatening manner.

3. Introduce the topic of feelings

The puppet can be used to introduce the topic of feelings:

This has been quite a day for (puppet's name) because he/she has been making lots of new friends and talking about his/her family. How do you think (puppet's name) feels right now? (Ask each child to name a feeling.) Yes, those are all feelings that (puppet's name) might be having.

There are three ways to find out how someone feels. First we can see how people feel with our eyes. I can tell (puppet's name) feels happy right now because I can see (puppet's name) is smiling.

Also we can hear how people feel with our ears. When I hear someone crying (puppet cries) I know he/she feels sad, and when I hear someone laughing (puppet laughs) I know he/she feels happy.

The third way to tell how someone is feeling is to ask him/her. If I want to know how (puppet's name) is feeling, I can ask 'How do you feel right now?' (puppet responds) or if I want to know how (puppet's name) felt last night, I can ask that too—'How did you feel last night?' (Puppet responds.)

Everybody has feelings—all different kinds of feelings. That's what we'll be talking about today.

4. Read the book, *I Feel: A Picture Book of Emotions,* by George Ancona or *The Boys' and Girls' Book of Dealing with Feelings,* by Eric Dlugokinski, PhD.

LEADER: *Now we are going to look at a special book all about feelings. Let's use our eyes to see how the children in the book are feeling.*

Leaders can encourage participation by covering the feeling word and having children guess what feeling the picture conveys. It is helpful for leaders to ask children about specific situational or behavioral clues they used to guess the feeling. Children can be asked to suggest why the child feels the way he/she does (e.g., the girl may feel proud because she just painted a special picture). The following feeling concepts should be emphasized in the process of reading the book:

- Everyone has feelings.
- Some feelings are good and some are not-so-good.
- All feelings are okay—they are all special and important.
- People can feel differently about the same thing.
- Feelings can change.
- Everything we do and everything that happens to us causes feelings.

5. Play the Feelings Grab-Bag game. Tell the group that it can now have a chance to act out the different feelings that it just read about by playing the Feelings Grab-Bag game.

The grab-bag can be a box or paper bag containing the 18 feelings on the Feeling Faces sheet. The paper should be cut into squares with each square containing one feeling and the corresponding face. The slips of paper can then be put into a bag or box. These feeling names are the ones discussed in the previous exercise. Thus, children can learn about each feeling both from vicarious (i.e., pictures) and experiential (i.e., role-playing) perspectives.

One feeling that is not illustrated in the book, but is included on the sheet and in the exercise, is "guilty." This feeling is included since feeling responsible for the divorce is a relevant age-specific reaction to parental divorce. A poster of the 18 feelings can be displayed during the game to help the children recall the feeling words: *happy, sad, angry, shy, good, lonely, excited, proud, jealous, silly, scared, hurt, sorry, loving, guilty, confused, embarrassed, frustrated.*

To play the game, leaders should first role-play the exercise to demonstrate the technique. The feelings can either be acted out non-verbally (e.g., "I'll show you with my face what the feeling is."), or verbally (e.g., I'll tell you about a time when I felt this way.). After the feeling is acted-out, have children attempt to guess the feeling word. Each child can then choose and act out a feeling from the grab-bag while other children try to guess the feeling. After children have guessed the feeling, have them describe situations when they have felt that way. This discussion time is a valuable opportunity for using children's responses to illustrate the basic feeling concepts discussed earlier. If desired and time permits, leaders can have all children act out the feeling. The same procedure (i.e., role-playing and discussion) can be used for all feelings in the grab-bag.

6. Distribute Feeling Faces sheets. Distribute copies of the Feeling Faces sheets to the children to take home. Leaders can suggest that the children color the faces, play the Feelings Grab-Bag game with others, and especially share the paper with their parent(s).

7. Review questions.
   - Are all feelings okay?
   - How can you tell how someone is feeling?
   - Can people feel differently about the same thing?
   - Do feelings change?

Session 3: All Kinds of Families

Goals

- Explore the concept of family—promote awareness and acceptance of non-traditional family structures.
- Help children understand that each family is unique and special.
- Help children identify and reflect on their own family composition.
- Allow children to get accustomed to talking about their families (and feelings) in a relatively non-threatening context.

Procedure

1. Review basic feelings and feeling concepts.
2. Introduce the concept of families.
3. Read the book, *All Kinds of Families,* by Norma Simon, or a similar book dealing with families.
4. Conduct the My Family exercise.

Materials

- Name-tags.
- Poster of feeling words.
- The book, *All Kinds of Families,* by Norma Simon (1976).
- Family figures.

Overview

Session 3 deals with families, "something everyone has feelings about." The idea that there are all kinds of families, each unique and special, is emphasized through:

  a. a book that promotes awareness and acceptance of non-traditional families; and
  b. an exercise that helps children identify, reflect on, and share their own family situations, using wooden family figures.

Procedure

1. Review basic feelings and feeling concepts. Leaders should review the main points of the last session (e.g., all feelings are okay). Going over the poster of feeling words is useful.
   Last week we learned that everyone has feelings. We learned that there are a lot of different ways that people can feel when things happen to them; some feel good, some not-so-good, but all feelings are okay to have. Another thing we learned is that our feelings can change: something that at one time made us sad or angry, may not bother us so much at another time.
2. Introduce the concept of families. Today, we are going to talk about something that everyone has feelings about: families. Everyone here is part of a family. Families are made up of people like brothers and sisters. Can someone tell us who else may be in a family (e.g., mother, cousin, grandfather)?
3. Read and discuss the book, *All Kinds of Families.* The main purpose of this activity is to promote children's awareness and acceptance of non-traditional families in general, and their own families in particular. Many children of divorce feel different

or defective because they do not live in a two-parent home. The book's message is that there are all kinds of families and all families are special.

As you go through the book, encourage the children to relate the material to their own families (e.g., "Is your family little, middle-sized, or big?"). Also highlight the many references to families affected by separation and divorce, as well as the feelings discussed.

Now, we are going to read a special book about all kinds of families. As we read it, think about how the families in the book are like or unlike your own.

After reading the book, leaders can highlight the following:

Sometimes children whose parents are divorced or separated feel embarrassed or different from other kids, but we know all families are special.

4. Conduct the My Family exercise. "My Family" helps the children identify, reflect upon, and share their family composition with the group through the use of wooden family figures. Whereas the previous activity emphasizes that there are many kinds of families, this exercise stresses that each family is unique and special. Explore the family compositions of the children by having each child take a turn setting up family dolls or figures to represent his/her family members and telling the group something about them. If desired, the children can also similarly discuss the puppet's family.

We have just talked about many kinds of families and a little about your families too. Now each of you will have a chance to show us who is in your family.

5. Review questions.
    *   What is a family?
    *   Are there many kinds of families?
    *   How are families different from one another?
    *   Are all families special?

Session 4: Divorce Is a Grown-Up Problem

Goals

- Help children to understand the concept of divorce and clarify common misconceptions.
- Provide a supportive atmosphere for group members to share divorce-related feelings.
- Help children identify common feelings and reactions to divorce (e.g., denial, fear of abandonment, guilt, sadness).

Procedure

1. Introduce the concept of divorce.
2. Show pictures from Sinberg's or Brown's book.
3. Read the book, *Divorce Is a Grown Up Problem: A Book about Divorce for Young Children and their Parents,* by Janet Sinberg or *Dinosaurs Divorce,* by L. K. Brown and M. Brown.

Materials

- Name-tags.
- The book, *Divorce Is a Grown Up Problem: A Book about Divorce for Young Children and their Parents,* by Janet Sinberg (1978) or *Dinosaurs Divorce,* by L. K. Brown and M. Brown (1986).

Overview

Session 4 begins to apply feeling words and feeling concepts to children's divorce experiences. A book is used to describe children's common reactions to divorce. The goal is to facilitate children's awareness, expression, and acceptance of such divorce-related feelings. Common divorce concepts and misconceptions are also considered.

Procedure

1. Introduce the concept of divorce. Leaders can introduce the concept of divorce by focusing on the group commonality and children's feelings and reactions.

Last week, we talked about our families and feelings about our families. Changes in our families cause us to have a lot of different feelings—feelings that can be pretty tough to understand. Everyone here has had a change in their family—their parents are separated or divorced. When I say *divorce* what is the first word that pops into your head?

Leaders should write responses on a blackboard or poster board, and highlight both the common themes and the diverse reactions to divorce.

2. Show pictures from *Divorce Is a Grown Up Problem* or *Dinosaurs Divorce.* Once the concept of divorce is introduced, leaders can facilitate a discussion of divorce by showing pictures from the book. The pictures can be used as a projective technique where children make up stories about what has happened in the picture and describe each character's feelings. The pictures should show specific situations or feelings common to young children's divorce experience (e.g., loyalty conflicts, parental conflicts, fear of abandonment).

3. Read *Divorce is a Grown Up Problem* or *Dinosaurs Divorce*. Introduce the book by saying that many children have parents who are divorced or separated, and that many children have a lot of feelings that are sometimes hard to talk about. Ask group members to be listening for all the different feelings the child in the book is experiencing.

After reading the book, discuss relevant issues. One way to facilitate discussion is to return to specific pictures, and ask children to talk about the feelings and reactions portrayed: confused, scared, angry, lonely, sad, guilty, different, reconciliation fantasies, and eventual adaptation.

4. Review questions.
   • What are some reasons parents decide to separate? Does it mean that they don't love their children anymore?
   • What are some of the feelings that children have about their parents' separation?

Session 5: Introducing Social Problem Solving

Goals

- Introduce social problem solving concepts.
- Emphasize that there are many ways to solve problems.

Procedure

1. Introduce the concepts of *problem* and *solution*.
2. Clarify the relationships among problems, solutions and feelings.
3. Review the four steps in the Social Problem Solving cartoon.
4. Illustrate alternative solutions thinking with the aid of pictures (and puppets if desired).
5. Distribute the Social Problem Solving cartoon.

Materials

- Name-tags.
- Copies of the Social Problem Solving cartoon.
- Puppets.

Overview

Session 5 introduces all four problem solving steps with an emphasis on generating alternatives. Children are asked to generate solutions to problem situations depicted in pictures. A point highlighted in the discussion is that there is usually more than one solution to a problem.

Procedure

1. Introduce the concept of a problem and a solution. Leaders should introduce the concept of a problem and give examples of nondivorce-related problems:

We've been talking a lot about divorce and some unhappy feelings and problems that children may have when that happens. For the next few meetings we're going to talk about what kids can do about those problems. But first, we need to think about what a problem is. Everybody has problems: some have to do with divorce but many don't.

Give an example, for instance, you lose a toy that belongs to a friend.

"Can anyone think of another problem?"

2. Clarify the relationships among problems, solutions and feelings. Leaders can sharpen the definition of what a problem is by clarifying the relationship between problems and feelings:

There are all different kinds of problems—math problems, reading problems, and problems between people. The kinds of problems we'll be talking about give someone an unhappy or upset feeling. We have just thought of several examples of problems. How might you feel if _____ (repeat example)?

Leaders should then define a solution and its relationship to feelings.

Most problems can be solved or fixed. We have to do or say something to make the problem stop or go away. The way we solve a problem is called a solution.

Give an example of a problem and a solution to illustrate.

How do you think someone feels when they think of a good solution to a problem? (Children respond.)

That's right—solving a problem helps us stop feeling upset and start feeling good. For the next few sessions, we'll be learning about ways to solve all kinds of problems that give us unhappy feelings.

3. Review the Social Problem Solving cartoon. Leaders should review the steps of social problem solving using the problem solving cartoon. Children will be able to understand the abstract concepts better if leaders use a concrete example when reviewing each step in the cartoon.

Today we're going to learn about all the steps you go through to solve a problem. I'm going to show you a cartoon of a little boy who has a problem. Jimmy just lost his brand new lunch box at school. Let's look at the first picture. What is the problem? (Children respond.)

How do you think Jimmy feels? (Children respond.)

So the first step in solving a problem is to decide what is the problem. The next step is to think of all the things you can do to solve the problem. Can you think of something Jimmy could do? (Children respond.)

That's one thing he could do. Can anyone think of something else Jimmy could do?

Leaders then repeat the two alternative solutions while drawing children's attention to Step 2 of the cartoon. It is important for leaders to convey non-judgmental acceptance of all alternatives generated. In other words, avoid the suggestion that solutions given might be wrong.

The next step is to think about what might happen next if you were to try to solve the problem. If Jimmy was to do _____, what might happen next? (Children respond.)

Leaders should then repeat Step 3 with the other alternative solutions.

The last step in solving a problem is to choose the best way and to try it! What do you think is the best solution? (Children respond.)

Leaders should then repeat the four sequential steps in the cartoon.

4. Illustrate alternative solutions thinking. For the rest of the session, leaders should focus on the first two steps of social problem solving: stating the problem and thinking of alternative solutions. Other than giving children a brief overview of social problem solving steps, the goal of this session is to highlight the fact there are many ways to solve problems (not just divorce-related problems). Leaders should use pictures of problem situations (about three) to illustrate alternative solution thinking. If desired, leaders can have a puppet present the problem situations or model responses for the children. Children should be encouraged to think of as many solutions as possible to each problem scenario. Non-judgmental acceptance of all solutions offered is important. Getting a few bad solutions is fine and such responses can become part of a useful stockpile of solutions when discussing consequences during later sessions. Furthermore, leaders should build on the previous five sessions by clarifying the feelings associated with each problem situation.

5. Distribute copies of the Social Problem Solving cartoon. Give a copy of the Social Problem Solving cartoon to each child. To foster parent-child communication, children should be encouraged to take the cartoon home and share what they have learned with their parents. An extra copy of the cartoon should be kept in the room for future reference.

6. Review questions.
   - What is a problem? (e.g., Something that gives a person an unhappy or upset feeling.)
   - What is a solution?
   - Is there only one way to solve a problem?
   - What are the first two steps in the cartoon?

Session 6: Developing Problem Solving Skills

Goals

- Continue encouraging children to generate alternative solutions to problems.
- Help children evaluate the quality (i.e., consequences) of generated solutions.

Procedure

1. Play the Tic-Tac-Toe game to facilitate discussion of alternative solutions and consequences to general problems.

Materials

- Name-tags.
- Blackboard and chalk or poster paper and marker.
- Ten cards: five of which have an X drawn on them and five of which have an O drawn on them.
- Social Problem Solving cartoon.

Overview

Session 6 focuses on generating alternative solutions, anticipating consequences, and evaluating solutions. Choosing the best solution involves first anticipating and then evaluating possible consequences of each. A Tic-Tac-Toe game is used as a vehicle for practicing the four social problem solving steps.

Procedure

1. Play the Tic-Tac-Toe game. The Tic-Tac-Toe game is divided into four parts. Each part corresponds to a social problem solving step in the cartoon.

Review problem solving steps: Leaders should begin the session by reviewing what a problem is and the four social problem solving steps in the cartoon. The Tic-Tac-Toe game can be introduced as a way to practice the steps in the cartoon.

Last session we talked about what a problem is and ways to solve problems. We have just gone over all the steps to solve a problem in this problem solving cartoon.

Leader holds up cartoon.

Today we are going to play a game to help us better learn those steps.

Select a problem scenario (Step One)

In order to play the game leaders should choose a general problem not related to divorce. (NOTE: The problem should have as many alternative solutions as possible.) Examples of problem scenarios are:

- Carl is teasing Joey and calling him names.
- Ann just got a new bicycle and Tom would like to try riding it.
- Ann forgot to take her lunch to school.
- Peter borrowed Tim's plane and then broke it by accident.
- Bob grabbed a truck that Jim was playing with.

- Sue wants new mittens in the store but she doesn't have any money.
- Jane was drying the supper dishes and broke one.
- Sam wanted his father to buy him a special toy for his birthday but his father said "No, it costs too much money."

Example:

Before we play the game, we need to have a problem. For example, what if _____.
Why is that a problem? What is _____ feeling?
Leader holds up a picture, provides points to Step One in the cartoon.
Right. Those are all not-so-good feelings. Now that we understand the problem, let's play a game to help _____ solve his/her problem.

Generate Alternatives (Step Two)

This part of the game, which is based on traditional Tic-Tac-Toe, can be a useful and fun way for children to practice generating alternative solutions. On the right side of a blackboard or large poster paper, leaders should draw a Tic-Tac-Toe field (i.e., #), leaving room on the left side to write down the alternative solutions generated by children. Place ten cards (five of which have an "X" drawn on them and five of which have an "O" drawn on them) face down in a stack. Children can then take turns generating solutions to the problem. Each time a solution is given by a child, he or she can draw a card and place it (using tape) on the Tic-Tac-Toe field; at the same time a leader can write the solution on the board or poster. During this part of the game, leaders should accept all solutions regardless of how inappropriate, outlandish, or similar they are. Children will have an opportunity to evaluate their solutions later in the game. This portion of the game is "over" when children can no longer think of alternative solutions, the "X"s or "O"s have won, or the game has ended in a tie.

NOTE: The Tic-Tac-Toe game is merely a vehicle for children to practice thinking of alternative solutions. Leaders may wish to create other games for children to practice the social problem-solving steps.

Anticipate Possible Consequences (Step Three)

After all solutions are written down, leaders should facilitate a discussion of each solution and its possible consequences. Consequential thinking can be introduced by encouraging children to think ahead to "what might happen next" if they were to try a solution.

As we can see from this game, there are lots of ways to solve a problem. From this written list we can see that some ways may be better than others. In order to choose the best way, it's important that we think ahead to what might happen next if we were to try out a solution.

Leaders point to Step Three in the cartoon. Leaders can help children anticipate consequences by focusing on the possible short- or long-term consequences for the person trying the solution.

Example:

If Joey hit Carl for calling him names what might happen next? (Children respond.) That's one thing that could happen. What else might happen next? (Children respond.) What might happen later on? (Children respond.)

If the problem scenario involves two people, leaders can help children anticipate short- or long-term consequences by focusing on the behavioral or emotional reactions of the person being "acted upon."

Example:

If Joey hit Carl for calling him names, what might Carl do (say/feel) next? (Children respond.) What might Carl do (say/feel) later on? (Children respond.)

Choose an Alternative Solution (Step Four)

Once children have discussed the possible consequences of each solution, leaders can help them evaluate and choose the best solution. The evaluation process encourages children to think beyond immediate, positive effects of solutions. For example, a socially inappropriate solution may solve the child's immediate problem (i.e., he/she reaches his/her goal and feels good) but can have later, negative consequences. The following questions can be used to facilitate a discussion of solutions and their consequences.

Is that the best way to solve the problem? Would _____ really solve his/her problem?
Is that solution a good idea? Why or why not?
Would anyone be upset with the solution?
Will that solution make things better?

After each solution has been evaluated, leaders can draw a face next to the solution to describe a good, a not-so-good, or a mixed outcome. The pictures provide a visual evaluation of each solution and its consequences. Children can then choose the best solution, based on the discussion of consequences.

2. Review questions.
   • What can we do if we have a problem? (Think of lots of ways to solve it.)
   • How do you choose the best solution? (Think of what might happen next.)

Session 7: Divorce-Related Issues . . .
Problem Solving with Puppets

Goals

- Begin applying social problem solving skills to personal, divorce-related problems.

Procedure

1. Review problem solving steps.
2. Introduce the application of the social problem solving steps to personal, divorce-related problems.
3. A leader performs a puppet play to review the social problem solving steps and to practice applying these steps to divorce related problems.
4. Children and leaders perform puppet plays of divorce-related problems.
5. Assignment: Think of a problem to work on during the next session.

Materials

- Name-tags.
- Social Problem Solving cartoon.
- Puppets.
- Grab bag of common, divorce-related problem situations.

Overview

Session 7 applies the social problem solving steps to divorce-related problems. Puppet plays by leaders and children are used to help group members apply these newly learned coping skills to typical divorce-related interpersonal problems of early latency children (e.g., fear of abandonment, loyalty conflicts, longing for the non-custodial parent). Leaders guide children in applying the problem solving steps to selected scenarios.

Procedure

1. Review the problem solving steps. Begin the session by reviewing the four steps in the Social Problem Solving cartoon.
2. Introduce the application of the social problem solving steps to personal, divorce related problems.

We have been talking about different ways to solve problems. Children whose parents don't live together often have lots of problems that they want to solve. All of you can probably think of what some of those problems might be. (Have children generate several such problems.)

3. Perform a puppet play. A puppet show is a useful vehicle for helping children apply their problem solving skills to divorce-related problems. Choose an interpersonal divorce-related problem that early-latency aged children often experience (e.g., fear of abandonment, loyalty conflicts, longing for the noncustodial parent, anger at the custodial parent). Select a topic that is particularly relevant to group members. The play should illustrate each step in the problem solving cartoon and encourage child participation.

An example of a puppet play illustrating loyalty conflicts follows.

We have been talking about ways to make a problem better. We found that there are lots of different ways to solve a problem and feel better. Today (one group leader) is going to put on a puppet show for you. We're going to see all the ways that Billy Bear and Lela Lion thought of to make a problem better. Listen carefully so we can help them solve the problem too.

A leader role-plays the following script using two puppets, while the other group leader sits with the children and facilitates group participation:

Billy Bear (BB) is on stage looking sad when his friend, Lela Lion (LL) arrives.

LL: *What's the matter, Billy Bear? You look really sad!*

BB: *Well, I feel really sad. You know my parents got a divorce and I live with my mom. The problem is that dad wants to take me to a ball game Saturday afternoon but I already promised to help my mom with the grocery shopping then.*

LL: *So—what is the problem?*

BB: *The problem is my dad wants to take me to a ball game at the same time am supposed to go shopping with my mom and I'm really upset! I want to go to the ball game with dad but I don't want to hurt mom's feelings. Sometimes it seems like I have to choose between my mom and dad and that's really tough on me! What should I do?*

LL: *Gee, it must be a problem because you look sad and upset. (Turns to children.) Can you think of some way to solve Billy Bear's problem? (Children respond.)*

NOTE: *If children generate a solution, leaders can incorporate the idea into the puppet play. If not, leaders can use the following script.*

   There are lots of things you can do to solve your problem. One solution is to sneak out of the house to meet your dad. That way you won't have to go grocery shopping with your mom.

BB: *(Looking pensive) Hmmm . . . that's one idea. But if I sneak out of the house, what might happen next? (Turns to children.) What do you think? (Children respond.)*

LL: *Your mom could find out and would be hurt and angry.*

BB: *But I don't want my mom to be hurt and angry. I don't think sneaking out would really solve my problem because I'd still feel upset. You know, that's just one solution. You said there were lots of ways to solve my problem. What else can I do? (Turns to Children.) (Children respond.)*

LL: *I have another way to solve your problem. You could ask your mom if the two of you can go grocery shopping on Sunday instead of Saturday.*

BB: *If I ask my mom to go on Sunday, what might happen next? (Turns to children.) (Children respond.)*

LL: *Your mom could say "yes" because she can spend time with you on Sunday. Also, you get to spend time with both of them and you don't have to choose between them! Wouldn't that solution help you feel happier?*

BB: *(Turns to children.) Well, now I have two ways to solve my problem. I could sneak out of the house or I could ask my mom to go grocery shopping on Sunday. What do you think is the best way for me to solve my problem? (Children respond.) Yes, I think asking my mom to go shopping on Sunday would be the best solution to try. The leader can now role-play Billy Bear trying out the solution.*

4.   Children and group leaders conduct puppet plays.
   Children can now be involved in puppet plays in a semi-structured format. The puppet plays can focus on divorce-related problem situations drawn out of a problem grab bag or generated by the children. The grab bag should contain common, divorce-related problems, such as the following "Problem Scenarios:"
   a.   Bill's problem: Bill really misses his dad a lot. Today he feels very lonely. Bill is talking to his Uncle Joe and Aunt Barbara.
   b.   Kim's problem: Kim is in a special school play. She wants both of her parents to come, but they don't get along with each other. What could she do? Kim is talking to her friends Chris and Beth.

Procedure: A grab bag containing cards with one of three roles (i.e., puppeteer, Announcer, audience) can be used to determine each child's part in the production (i.e., each child draws a card which determines his/her role). Depending on the size of the group, there can be one adult puppeteer, one or two child puppeteers, and one child announcer with the rest of the group serving as the audience.

Role of the Announcer: The announcer can state the name of the play, introduce the characters, and lead the audience in applause after the play is over.

Role of the Puppeteers: Puppeteers decide on who shall play which character in the play. The leader-puppeteer can steer the play in appropriate directions, facilitating each puppeteer's participation. Leaders will probably need to guide the puppeteers through the problem solving steps.

Role of the Audience: The audience should be encouraged to participate as much as possible in the play, without being disruptive. Their primary role can be to suggest solutions to problem situations when appropriate. Each member of the audience can be given a banner (e.g., a paper flag taped to a pencil) with one of the problem solving steps on it (e.g., "What is the problem?"). As the play proceeds, members of the audience can indicate which problem solving step is being dealt with in the play.

5. Assignment. To prepare for the next session, leaders should ask children to think of one problem—divorce-related or not—that they would like to solve. Inform the children that each child will get a chance to work on solving his/her problem with the group.

6. Review question.
   • Do you know what problem you want to work on during our next meeting?

Session 8: Solvable Problems vs. Unsolvable Problems

Goals

- Teach children to differentiate between problems they can solve and those they cannot solve.
- Encourage children to use their energy for age-appropriate, adaptive activities.
- Help children distinguish between wishes and beliefs.
- Continue to apply social problem solving skills to divorce-related problems.

Procedure

1. Introduce the concept that some problems cannot be solved.
2. A leader performs a puppet play of an unsolvable problem (i.e., parental reconciliation).
3. Play the Red-Light Green-Light game with divorce-related problems.

Materials

- Name-tags.
- Puppets.
- Red and green "lights" for each child (e.g., red and green circles cut out of construction paper).
- Grab bag of several common divorce-related problems.

Overview

The main purpose of this session is for children to learn the difference between problems they can solve and those they cannot solve. Children who understand and accept that some divorce-related problems are beyond their control (i.e., are "unsolvable") will feel less self-blame, frustration, and confusion. Children can be helped to see the difference between "wishing" and "believing" that they can solve a certain problem (e.g., leaders can emphasize that many children wish that their parents will get back together and that is okay; however, when children really believe that they are able to make it happen, they end up feeling angry, disappointed, guilty and frustrated). Leaders should encourage children to disengage from "unsolvable" divorce-related problems and find more age-appropriate, adaptive activities (e.g., becoming more actively involved with school and friends, rather than expending energy devising ways to reunite parents).

A second purpose of this session is for children to apply social problem solving skills to personal, real-life situations.

Procedure

1. Introduce the concept that some problems cannot be solved. Introduce the notion that some problems are beyond children's control and cannot be solved.

In the last couple of meetings we've learned ways to solve problems that give us a sad or upset feeling. We've solved a lot of problems using the four steps in the problem solving cartoon (hold up cartoon). But some problems just can't be solved even if you try really hard and follow all those steps, even if you are a great problem solver.

Leaders should illustrate the concept through several examples of general, unsolvable problems. Emphasize that everybody has unsolvable problems (e.g., physical characteristics he/she wants to change; events or situations he/she does not like) and that a person's inability to solve or control a problem is not a reflection of the person's self-worth or abilities.

2. Puppet play of an unsolvable problem. To illustrate further the concept of an unsolvable problem, a leader should do a puppet-play about children's responses to a common "unsolvable" divorce-related problem. One such problem is children's wish to reunite their parents. Rather than saying immediately that a problem is beyond their control, leaders can help children reach that conclusion themselves by encouraging them to generate alternative solutions and think of possible consequences to those solutions.

We want to act out a problem for you that may or may not be solvable. You can help us decide if the problem can or cannot be solved by using the four steps in the cartoon.

A leader can then speak through the puppet to introduce the problem selected.

Hi, friends. I'm feeling kind of sad today. You know my mom and dad got a divorce and dad doesn't live with us anymore. Mom says that sometimes sad things make people happier in the long run. She says that someday I'll understand but some day seems so far away. I want my mom and dad back together again right now! There must be something I can do to solve my problem. Please help me think of all the things I could do to get my parents back together. (Children respond.)

A leader can then use the puppets to act out all the possible solutions and consequences given by children. Writing down children's solutions on a blackboard or poster can be helpful. Leaders can then summarize by reviewing the list of solutions and helping the children decide the problem cannot be solved. For example, leaders can point out that the parents' decision to separate is a "grown-up problem" (Sinberg, 1978) and not one that children can solve, no matter how hard they try.

After reaching that sobering conclusion, leaders should explore how children feel about not being able to change or control aspects of their family lives. The exercise can be ended on a positive note by helping children think of activities that are under their control and would help them adapt to the situation by asking, "What could help you feel better?" (e.g., writing to their mother or father, seeing friends, talking with their parents about how they feel.)

3. Play the Red-Light Green-Light game.

Purpose
   a. help children learn the difference between problems they can solve and those they cannot solve;
   b. apply social problem solving concepts to "real-life" problems; and
   c. promote the pairing of solutions and consequences. The game also encourages group members to help each other with social problem solving concepts.

Leaders can introduce the game in the following way:

Last time we met, we asked each of you to think of a problem you would like to solve. Well, today we're all going to help you solve your problem and work on some other problems children have when their parents don't live together, by playing the red-light green-light game.

Use the analogy of a stoplight to describe how children decide on the solvability of presented problems.

Who knows what the colors of a stoplight mean? (Children respond.)

Right. Green means "go" and red means "stop." We're going to use these green and red lights to decide if a problem can or cannot be solved. (Hold up a green circle and a red circle cut from construction paper.)

What color would you hold up if you think a problem can be solved? (Children respond.)

That's right, you hold up a green light. What color would you hold up if you think that the problem cannot be solved? (Children respond.) That's right. You would hold up the red light. If we decide a problem is a green light—that it can be solved—let's go ahead and think of some solutions and decide which one is best to try. If we decide a problem is a red light—that it cannot be solved—let's think of some things to do that might help us change our not-so-good feelings.

Give each child a green paper circle and a red paper circle.

Overview of how to play the game: Call on each child to tell the group what problem he/she would like to solve. If a child has not thought of a problem he/she can draw a problem out of the Problem Grab bag. After the problem is stated, the children can decide whether the problem can or cannot be solved (green light or red light). If the problem is solvable, the child can generate one or two solutions (with the help of the group if necessary) and be assisted by the group in deciding which solution would be best to try. If the problem is not solvable, the child can generate one or two ways he/she (or someone with this problem) might deal with their not-so-good feelings about it.

Step One: Can the Problem Be Solved?

Example:

Mary, can you tell the group what problem you would like to work on (or have drawn from the grab bag)? (Child responds.)

Now, everyone hold up the green light if you think this problem can be solved or hold up the red light if you think it cannot be solved.

Leaders should then explore the group's responses.

Jim, you held up a red light. Can you tell the group, why? Ann, you held up a green light. Why? (Child responds.)

Step Two: For Solvable Problems

If it is decided that the problem is solvable, the child can be asked to generate a solution to the problem. (The group can also help generate a solution if necessary.) After a solution is offered, the child offering it should immediately be asked to evaluate the consequences of the solution. The group can then help the child decide whether or not that would be the best solution.

Tell us how you would solve that problem. So, you would do _____ to solve the problem. (Child responds.)

What might happen next if you _____? (Child responds.)

Let's help Mary with the problem. Does that sound like the best solution or do you think Mary should stop and think of another solution? (Children respond.)

Do you think Mary should try that solution?

Leaders can again explore the group's responses.

Mary, your friends have told you what they think. How do you feel about (thinking of another solution/trying your idea)?

If a child can think of two solutions, the group can help him/her decide on the better one.

Step Two: For Unsolvable Problems

If it is decided that the problem is not solvable, ask the child, and then the group, what the child could do to change his/her not-so-good feelings.

We have decided that Mary's problem is not solvable. When we decide that we cannot solve a problem sometimes it makes us have some not-so-good feelings. How do you feel about not being able to solve your problem, Mary? (Child responds.)

Now, we have a different problem: How could Mary help herself feel better? Mary, can you think of something that you could do to feel happier? (Child responds.)

Everybody, can you think of things that Mary could do to feel happier? (Children respond and can be asked whether the solutions offered by others would make her happier.)

Step Three: Encourage Child to Try the Chosen Solution

After the "best solution" for a child's problem is selected, encourage the child to try out the solution. Inform the children that each child will get a chance to discuss his/her problem solving efforts with the group in a "Problem Solving Show and Tell" next week. If a child has not presented a problem help him/her think of one to work on. Once again the problems can be either divorce- or nondivorce-related.

Hints for Leaders: Leaders should be prepared for children who do not have problem scenarios by providing a grab bag of common, divorce-related problems (e.g., Steve's problem: Sometimes when Steve's father is supposed to visit him, he does not come). The problems in the grab bag should be relevant to the children in the group.

The ideal situation is when children are interested and responsive to a discussion of problems and solutions. However, children may require considerable prompting and encouragement by the leaders. Also, leaders should be prepared to spend only a few minutes at a time with any given child to maximize participation and maintain group interest. Leaders may wish to modify the discussion or game rules to save time or maintain group interest. However, at the end of the exercise each child should have one real-life problem to work on before the next meeting.

3. Review questions.
   • Can every problem be solved? Why not?
   • What problem are you going to work on?
   • What is the solution you're going to try?

Session 9: Consolidating Skills . . . CODIP Daring Dinosaurs Game

Goals

- Further consolidation of social problem solving skills.
- Review basic feelings, feeling concepts, family concepts and divorce-related issues.

Procedure

1. Problem Solving Show and Tell: Review and discuss outcomes of children's solutions.
2. Play the CODIP Daring Dinosaurs game.

Materials

- Name-tags.
- Cards depicting good, not-so-good and mixed outcomes.
- The CODIP Daring Dinosaurs game, consisting of one board, two dice, cards and six playing pieces.

Overview

Session 9 reinforces children's efforts to apply problem solving skills to their own problems through a Problem Solving Show and Tell and promotes consolidation of problem solving skills and concepts learned thus far, through an engaging board game.

Procedure

1. Problem Solving Show and Tell. This exercise allows children to report their real life problem solving experiences within a supportive, encouraging environment. Follow-up on last session's assignment (i.e., actually trying an alternative solution) by asking children, "what happened" (i.e., the consequences). One way to facilitate discussion and evaluation of children's alternative solutions is to have children engage in a "Problem Solving Show and Tell." Leaders can have each child tell the group how his/her solution worked out. Each child can then summarize his/her experience by holding up an appropriate sign depicting a good, a not-so-good, or mixed outcome.

During our last meeting we asked each of you to try to solve a problem you're having. Today we want to find out how the solution you tried worked out. Each of you will get a chance to tell the group the steps you went through to solve your problem. Then, each of you can hold up one of these three pictures to describe what happened.

Leader can hold up the three cards and describe outcomes associated with each face.

If the solution resulted in a positive outcome, leaders can praise the child on his/her social problem solving skills. If the solution outcome was not-so-good or mixed, leaders can help the child determine if the problem was unsolvable or if another alternative solution could be tried. All children should be praised for their efforts, and their feelings should be acknowledged and supported. Emphasize that even though children may have tried hard, some problems can't be solved or may be very difficult to solve and that fact has little to do with the child's efforts or personal qualities. Leaders should either encourage children to continue to use their problem solving skills (i.e., with difficult but solvable problems) or to disengage from the problem situation (i.e., with unsolvable problems).

Some children may have forgotten, or may not have had a chance to try their solution. Leaders can encourage those children to continue trying because they will get another chance to share their experience in the next session.

2. Play the CODIP Daring Dinosaurs game. This game is meant to be a review of skills and concepts learned so far.

The CODIP Daring Dinosaurs game is a board game in which children roll the dice to determine how many squares to move on the board. There are two categories of cards, Thoughts and Feelings: "How do children feel when their parents fight?" and "John's dad is late picking him up for a visit. What can John do to feel better?"

The game is played by having children take turns rolling the dice, moving their playing pieces, and selecting and responding to a card. If a child cannot answer a question, other children can be invited to help. The leaders may want to increase children's interest in the game by providing a "surprise" (e.g., a ribbon) for whomever reaches the finish mark first. However, at the end of the session all children can be given some sort of surprise (e.g., a sticker).

The questions on the cards are meant as a review. Leaders can facilitate and clarify discussion of children's responses throughout the game. This game gives leaders a chance to see how far children have progressed in understanding divorce-related issues and social problem solving skills.

Leaders should review all printed cards to be sure that they reflect the basic concepts from previous sessions with particular emphasis on social problem solving. Leaders should also feel free to "stack the deck" so that the most relevant cards are placed on top.

The content of the cards should cover most of the topics explored in previous sessions. However, to reflect individual groups' unique experiences, blank cards are included with the game. Leaders can write individualized cards to reflect problems and situations discussed in their groups.

Reminder—Encourage children to use their social problem solving skills during the upcoming week.

Session 10: Between Child and Parent

Goals

- Increase children's ability to identify and express feelings about their parents.
- Further explore children's personal perceptions and feelings about divorce.
- Help children recognize the difference between their thoughts and actions.
- Assist children in applying social problem solving concepts to divorce-related problems.

Procedure

1. Introduce the book, *Two Homes to Live In,* by Barbara Shook Hazen, or a similar book dealing with children's reactions to a break up.
2. Read and review the book, *Two Homes to Live In,* by Barbara Shook Hazen.

Materials

- Name-tags.
- Puppets.
- The book, *Two Homes to Live In,* by Barbara Shook Hazen (1978).

Overview

Session 10 explores children's personal feelings about divorce through the use of a book and a question-and-answer activity. Feelings towards parents are emphasized.

For example, leaders ask while reading the book:

When Niki got mad that her mother went out on a date, how did she show it? Is it okay to feel angry at your mother?

Procedure

1. Introduce the book, *Two Homes to Live In,* by Barbara Shook Hazen. Leaders can introduce the book's main character, Niki, with the aid of a puppet:

Hi, my name is Niki. I'm 8 years old, just like some of you. I like bicycles and kittens, just like some of you, too. There's another way we're alike. My mom and dad are divorced. That means they aren't married anymore and you know, that can be pretty hard on me sometimes. Right now I'd like to tell you about how I feel about divorce. Later on I'd like to hear about how you feel, and what you do to help yourself feel better. You know, we can learn from each other and help each other out. After all, we kids have to stick together.

2. Read and review the book. Leaders should review the important points in the book by asking children specific questions such as those listed below. These issues should be discussed with regard to children in the group as well as to Niki. It is important to point out that while things worked out well between Niki and her mother and father this is not always possible. Help the group to explore how children feel when things do not work out this way (when they do not have "two homes to live in"). To make this review more action-oriented, the questions can be put on cards and drawn out of a grab bag.

- Why did Niki's parents decide not to live together anymore?
- Was it because of something Niki did?
- If Niki's parents don't love each other anymore, does that mean they will stop loving Niki, too?
- What are some of the things Niki missed about not having her dad live with her?
- When Niki's dad said that he and her mom were getting a divorce, what did Niki do? How did Niki feel?
- Niki's mom said, "Divorce is sad, but sometimes sad things make people happier in the long run." What does she mean by this?
- Niki's mom said that it was good to cry. Why? How did Niki feel after she cried? What else could Niki do to feel better (e.g., generate alternative solutions)?
- What scary thoughts do you think Niki had when her dad was late?
- Does thinking or wishing something make it happen? (Highlight the distinction between thoughts and actions.)
- When Niki got mad that her mom went out on a date, how did she show it? Is it OK to feel angry? Help children understand that it's OK to feel or say they're angry but it's not OK to hurt others when they are angry (e.g., hitting parents, breaking windows). Leaders can then discuss appropriate ways of handling angry feelings by having children use their social problem solving skills.
- Niki wished that her parents would get back together. Is it OK for kids to wish that their parents will get back together? Is getting parents back together a problem children can solve? What did Niki wish for that could happen?
- How did Niki's feelings about divorce change?

Session 11: Child-Parent Relationships ... Puppet Performances

Goals

- Explore children's perceptions and feelings about parent-child issues.
- Help children perceive what the family change has meant for their parents as well as for themselves.
- Apply social problem solving skills to divorce-related problems.

Procedure

1. Puppet play by a group leader.
2. Puppet play by leader(s) and children.

Materials

- Name-tags.
- Puppets.

Overview

Session 11 focuses on children's perceptions and feelings about parent-child issues through puppet play. Children are helped to understand their parents' feelings, as well as their own. Problem solving skills are applied to the problem scenarios in the plays. The following is an example of a dilemma acted out and resolved by the children using problem solving skills: "Sam's parents are divorced. His father is moving to another city. Sam is worried that if his father could move away and leave him maybe someday his mother might go away, too. Sam is talking about his problem with his friends Mike and Chris."

Procedure

1. Puppet play by a group leader. A leader can do a puppet play about a parent-child issue relevant to early latency-aged children. Examples of such issues include the day one parent moved out of the family home, concern about the well-being of one or both parents, intense longing for the non-custodial parent, feelings of rejection, loyalty conflicts, fears of abandonment, anger toward one or both parents for their decision to separate, feeling lonely and neglected by one or both parents, feeling jealous and angry about a parent dating or remarrying, and feeling responsible for the divorce. Children can be actively involved in the puppet play by using the procedure described in Session 8. In the puppet play it is important to explore not only the perceptions and feelings of the children, but also of the parents as well.

   Examples of puppet play scenarios for this exercise (as well as the next exercise) follow:

   - Sam's parents are divorced. Sam's father moved to another city. Sam is worried that if his father could move away and leave him maybe someday his mother might go away too. Sam does not want to be all alone. Sam is talking about his feelings with his friends Mike and Jim.

- Sara is very angry. She does not like her mother going out on dates. Sara is talking to her mother about her feelings.
- Beth is 9 years old. She lives with her mother and her little brother. Beth is worried about her mother. Beth thinks her mother is sad and lonely; sometimes at night Beth can hear her crying. She also is worried about her mother because she is working so hard at her job and at home. Beth is talking to her friend Mona.
- Michael is angry at his mom. He thinks it was her fault that his dad moved away. Michael doesn't know what to do about his feelings. He also doesn't understand how he could be so mad at someone he loves. He is talking with his two best friends.
- Denise is going to her mother's apartment for a visit. She really wants to see her mom but she is not sure whether or not she wants to meet her mother's new boyfriend who will also be there.

2. Puppet play by leader(s) and children. One or two children at a time can perform a puppet play with a group leader (see Session 8). The play ideas can be drawn from a grab bag of appropriate plots (see previously), or generated by the children depending on the degree of structure group leaders feel is needed. The group leader and children in the audience should play an active role in discussing with the characters what is happening in the play and suggesting alternative solutions to problem situations. Both leaders (one as puppeteer and one as audience member) should facilitate the children's exploration of issues and feelings raised in the plays.

Session 12: Consolidating Skills . . . CODIP Daring Dinosaurs Game

Goals

- Review and consolidate important divorce concepts.
- Explore further parent-related issues.
- Introduce group termination.

Procedure

1. Play the CODIP Daring Dinosaurs game with an emphasis on parent-related issues.
2. Discuss group termination.

Materials

- Name-tags.
- The CODIP Daring Dinosaurs game.
- Calendar.

Overview

Session 12 uses a board game to review and consolidate important program concepts, and encourage further exploration of parent-related issues. Group termination is also introduced. Although children are initially told how many meetings there will be, termination becomes an important theme from this point on.

Procedure

1. Play the CODIP Daring Dinosaurs game. The game is played to review and consolidate important divorce concepts and to explore further parent-related issues. (See Session 9 for a description of the game and how to play it.) Parent and parent-child issues should be highlighted in the cards selected for play (e.g., "You've just been to your dad's apartment and had a great time. Is it OK to tell your mom?"; "Do kids ever worry about who is going to take care of them?"). Leaders can draw from previous group discussions related to parent-child issues when selecting and writing their own cards. Some of the cards should focus on having children apply their social problem solving skills to problem scenarios involving these issues (e.g., "Pretend that you are visiting your dad but you really miss your mom. Show two things you could do.").
2. Discuss group termination. Discuss group termination during the last 5–10 minutes of the session.

Over the past several weeks we have shared special times together. We've read books, performed puppet plays, played games and talked about our thoughts and feelings. Soon our group will be ending. Can anyone guess how many more meetings we have left? (Children respond.)

After today, we only have three more meetings. Let's look at this calendar and circle the dates we will be meeting.

Leaders can then facilitate a group discussion of reactions to the group ending.

Usually, children will initially appear to be unaffected by the fact that the group is ending. However, children often have strong feelings as the loss of the support group is symbolic of the loss of their family as they once knew it. Even though some children's feelings may not be as strong as others, all children will have some reaction to the group ending. Some children may talk directly about the group ending while others may refer to it indirectly through their feelings about other events or situations. Therefore, throughout the remaining sessions leaders will need to take a very active role in listening for themes of loss (e.g., sadness, loneliness, anger or disappointment), relating those themes to group termination, and inviting all children to share their feelings. It is very helpful for leaders to share their own feelings about the group ending so that children have an accepting role model for expressing feelings.

Leaders should be sure that the group's ending is discussed in each of the three remaining sessions. If leaders wait for children to mention the group ending, there is the risk of sessions slipping by without having members "work through" the ending of a group that has been a part of their lives for four months. Many leaders have found it helpful for children to have the opportunity to meet again to discuss new changes and reinforce the supportive connections made in CODIP. Keep in mind the possibility of "booster sessions" or alumni meetings in the future.

3. Review question.
   • How many more sessions are left?

Session 13: I Am Special

Goals

- Promote children's self-esteem.
- Increase children's awareness of themselves as unique individuals and their relationships with others.
- Highlight positive post-divorce family changes.

Procedure

1. Each child completes an *I Am Special* book.
2. Discuss termination issues.

Materials

- Name-tags.
- *I Am Special* book for each child (included at end of this session).
- Crayons and markers.
- Instant or digital camera for group pictures (if available).

Overview

Session 13 strives to enhance children's perceptions of themselves and others. Each child completes an eight-page booklet describing his/her characteristics, likes, feelings, wishes, and place in the group and family. Children complete sentences in ways that best describe how they think and feel. Termination is discussed in relation to items dealing with the group (e.g., "My favorite thing about the group has been _____."). Positive post-divorce experiences are discussed in relation to items dealing with the family (e.g., "Divorce can be hard on kids. Divorce can also make things better for kids and their families. One thing that is better now in my family is _____.").

Procedure

1. Each child completes an *I Am Special* book. "I am Special" is a self-esteem exercise that personalizes important program concepts. The seven-page booklet first deals with the individual child's own characteristics, likes, feelings, and wishes. The book then facilitates the child's examination of his/her place in the group and in his/her family. Specifically, the child is asked to focus on positive post-divorce family experiences.

Thus, the goal of this exercise is not only to enhance children's self-esteem, but to focus on the positive family changes that have occurred since the parental separation or divorce (e.g., parents who fight less, children spending special times with each parent). One way to illustrate this concept is by referring to the book, *Two Homes to Live In,* where Niki's mom says, "Divorce is sad, but sometimes sad things have to happen to make people happier in the long run." Leaders should ask the children for examples of how family situations may improve, or get better after a divorce. It is important to emphasize the sense of hope for a brighter future that their parents may have had in making the decision to divorce.

A leader can introduce the exercise in the following way.

Now, we are all going to do a special activity. Each of you will get your own *I Am Special* book to fill out just like this one. When everyone is finished, people can share their books with the group if they would like.

Leaders should sit with the children as they are working on their books to discuss the questions and answers and to help those that may need assistance. If enough time is available, children can be encouraged to share their books with one another. (*Note:* If an instant camera is available, leaders can take pictures of the children to be placed in the book. If a camera is not available, children can simply draw a picture of themselves.)

2. Discuss termination issues. Leaders can also raise the topic of group termination while children are working on their books. For example, leaders can discuss with the children what activity they have enjoyed most during the group. By helping the children to reflect back on group experiences, leaders can deal with the children's feelings associated with being in the group and with having the group end. Leaders can then ask children how they feel about having only two more meetings left.

3. Review questions.
    *   Is each person special?
    *   In what ways are people different from one another?
    *   In what ways are people the same as one another?
    *   What do you like about belonging to this group?
    *   What do you like about belonging to your family?
    *   What things might get better in a family after a divorce?
    *   How many more meetings do we have left?

Session 14: You're a Special Person

Goals

- Enhance self-esteem by focusing on each child's unique strengths, particularly strengths as a group member.
- Foster a smooth termination of the group.

Procedure

1. Consolidate the group experience.
2. Play the You're a Special Person game.
3. Discuss group termination.

Materials

- Name-tags.
- Construction paper.
- White writing paper.
- Markers.

Overview

Session 14 emphasizes children's special strengths as group members (e.g., being a good problem solver, being supportive). In the You're a Special Person Game, members are first asked to list positive qualities of children. Next, papers with each person's name are circulated and group members write down the positive qualities that describe particular children. Children's and leaders' reactions to the ending of the group are explored further. Children are involved in planning a small party for the last group meeting.

Procedure

1. Consolidate the group experience. With only one session remaining, it is important for leaders to tie up any loose ends. This may mean exploring divorce-related topics that need further discussion, allowing children to work on specific personal problems, or completing a group activity.

    Leaders can also use this time to review the new skills that children have learned in the group (e.g., social problem solving skills) and some common ways to handle problems (e.g., talking to a parent or friend about how they feel). It is important that leaders emphasize and encourage children to practice their new skills outside of the group with family members and friends.

2. Play the You're a Special Person game. Leaders can promote children's self-esteem by helping them recognize their special strengths. One way to do this is to have the children play the You're a Special Person game. The format for this game may vary based on leaders' creativity and preference, but the goal is to provide each child in the group with realistic positive feedback from the other members. It is important to emphasize that each child has contributed to the group in some significant way (e.g., being supportive, caring, sharing, helpful, a good listener, identifying feelings, suggesting solutions to problems, good puppeteer), and that each child has special personal qualities (e.g., friendly, strong).

How to play: Ask members to name as many positive qualities or characteristics (preferably related to the group process) as they can. List those characteristics on the board. Then, distribute writing paper (mounted on heavier construction paper for long term durability) with a different child's name written on each of the sheets of paper. Group members should be asked to write down on each child's paper some of the characteristics listed on the board which describes that particular child. The papers are then rotated around the group, so that each child has the opportunity to contribute written comments for the other group members. Each group member then reads the comments for another child, while co-leaders facilitate a discussion of each person's unique contributions and strengths.

Note: While children may appear self-conscious and "giggly" about this exercise, they frequently keep their "warm fuzzy" list long after the group ends!

3. Discuss group termination. Leaders should remind the children that the next meeting is the last meeting and then ask them to share their thoughts and feelings about the group ending. It is important for leaders to point out common reactions among group members to the group ending. It is also helpful for leaders to share their own feelings about the group ending. One way to facilitate a discussion is for leaders to ask children to recall how they felt the first time the group met and to compare those feelings with their present feelings.

Leaders should inform children that there will be a party at the end of the last meeting (i.e., after the group discussion and activity). Invite the children to think of special activities to do during the party and suggest that each child may bring "goodies" to share if he/she chooses.

Session 15: Saying Goodbye

Goals

- Review children's group experience.
- Emphasize and encourage both the continued support among group members and the increased communication between children and parents.
- End the group on a positive note.

Procedure

1. Review children's experiences of being in the group.
2. Explore children's feelings about the group ending.
3. Hand out certificates of achievement.
4. Have a party.

Materials

- Name-tags.
- Poster paper and markers.
- Certificates of Achievement (included at end of this session).
- Materials for a party.

Overview

Session 15, the final session, deals with children's experiences and feelings about the group. Children are encouraged to maintain relationships with fellow group members; others (e.g., parents, teachers, friends) to whom they can reach out for support are identified. The group ends with a celebration and children receive certificates of achievement in "Caring and Sharing."

Procedure

1. Review children's experiences of being in the group. Leaders can begin by stating that this is the last session and asking children what it was like to participate in the group. As children give comments, leaders can write them on a piece of poster paper. Examples of questions that can be used to facilitate this review process are:
   - What were some of the good things about being in the group?
   - What were some of the hard things about being in the group?
   - What was the most important thing you learned?
   - How did it feel to talk about yourself in front of other kids?
   - Is there anything about the group that you would want to change?
   - What would you tell other kids whose parents are separated or divorced about the group?
2. Explore children's feelings about the group ending. After children have reviewed the 4-month group experience, leaders can encourage an exploration of children's feelings about the group ending. It is important that leaders model this discussion by sharing their own feelings about the group ending and what the group has meant for them. Children should be reassured that school-based group leaders can be contacted after the sessions end, should a child wish to talk. Leaders should also help children identify other people in their lives to whom they can turn for ongoing support after the group ends (e.g., other group members, friends, relatives, counselors, teachers).

Leaders should mention that many parents are interested in both understanding how their children feel about divorce, and knowing what happens in the divorce groups. They can encourage children to continue talking with each parent about their problems or feelings. Leaders can also ask children to think of ways to share some aspect of the group with their parents (e.g., talking about an enjoyable activity; drawing a picture of an important divorce concept, or sharing what they have learned). To further encourage and model parent-child communication, leaders can invite children to share "what happened" when they talked with parents about the group.

3. Hand out certificates of achievement. Leaders can give each child a certificate of achievement (e.g., for Caring and Sharing) and praise him/her for special contributions to the group. Leaders can review comments made during the "You're a Special Person" exercise in Session 15, by emphasizing children's unique contributions to the group (e.g., being a good listener, making a useful suggestion to a problem, helping another group member).

4. Have a party. Aside from having fun, the purpose of the party is to end the group on a positive note, with a message that children can always contact leaders in the future if they wish.

Selected Bibliography

Ancona, G. (1977). *I Feel: A picture book of emotions.* New York: E. P. Dutton. (Out of print—obtain book from public library.)

Brown, L., & Brown, M. (1986). *Dinosaurs divorce.* New York: Little, Brown & Company.

Curtis, J. L. (1998). *Today I feel silly: And other moods that make my day.* New York: Harper Collins.

Dlugokinski, E. (1988). *The boys' and girls' book of dealing with feelings.* Raleigh, NC: Feeling Factory, Inc.

Hazen, B. S. (1977). *Two homes to live in: A child's eye view of divorce.* New York: Human Services Press.

Simon, N. (1976). *All kinds of families.* Chicago: Albert Whitman & Company.

Sinberg, J. (1978). *Divorce is a grown up problem: A book about divorce for young children and their parents.* New York: Avon Books. (Out of print, obtain book from public library.)

Note

1. For more information about training or program consultation contact the author at Children's Institute, 274 N. Goodman St. Rochester, New York 14607.

References

Alpert-Gillis, L. J., Pedro-Carroll, J. L., & Cowen, E. L. (1989). Children of Divorce Intervention Program: Development, implementation and evaluation of a program for young urban children. *Journal of Clinical and Consulting Psychology, 57,* 583–587.

Pedro-Carroll, J. L. (1996). The Children of Divorce Intervention Program: Fostering resilient outcomes for school-aged children. In G. W. Albee & T. P. Gullotta (Eds.), *Primary prevention works* (pp. 213–238). Thousand Oaks, CA: Sage Publications.

Pedro-Carroll, J. L. (2001). The promotion of wellness in children and families: Challenges and opportunities. *American Psychologist, 56,* 993–1004.

Pedro-Carroll, J. L. (2005) Fostering resilience in the aftermath of divorce: The role of evidence-based programs for children. *Family Court Review, 43,* 52–64.

Pedro-Carroll, J. L., & Alpert-Gillis, L. J. (1987). Helping children cope: Preventive interventions for children of divorce. *The Community Psychologist, 20,* 11–13.

Pedro-Carroll, J. L., & Alpert-Gillis, L. J. (1997). Preventive interventions for children of divorce: A developmental model for 5 and 6 year old children. *Journal of Primary Prevention, 18,* 5–23.

Pedro-Carroll, J. L., & Cowen, E. L. (1985). The Children of Divorce Intervention Project: An investigation of the efficacy of a school-based prevention program. *Journal of Consulting and Clinical Psychology, 53,* 603–611.

Pedro-Carroll, J. L., & Cowen, E. L. (1987). The Children of Divorce Intervention Program: Implementation and evaluation of a time limited group approach. In *Advances in family intervention, assessment, and theory* (Vol. 1, pp. 281–307). Greenwich, CT: JAI Press.

Pedro-Carroll, J. L., & Jones, S. (2005). A play based intervention to foster children's resilience after divorce. In L. A. Reddy, T. M. Files-Hall, & C. E. Shaefer (Eds.), *Empirically based play interventions for children* (pp. 51–75). Washington, DC: American Psychological Association.

Pedro-Carroll, J. L., Alpert-Gillis, L. J., & Cowen, E. L. (1992). An evaluation of the efficacy of a preventive intervention for 4th–6th grade urban children of divorce. *Journal of Primary Prevention, 13,* 115–130.

Pedro-Carroll, J. L., Sutton, S. E., & Wyman, P. A. (1999). A two-year follow-up of a preventive intervention for young children of divorce. *School Psychology Review, 28,* 467–476.

Pedro-Carroll, J. L., Cowen, E. L., Hightower, A. D., & Guare, J. C. (1986). Preventive intervention with latency-aged children of divorce: A replication study. *American Journal of Community Psychology, 14,* 277–290.

Sterling, S. E. (1986). *School-based intervention program for early latency-aged children of divorce.* Unpublished Ph.D. dissertation, University of Rochester, Rochester, New York.

Wallerstein, J. S. (1983). Children of divorce: The psychological tasks of childhood. *American Journal of Orthopsychiatry, 53,* 230–243.

Chapter 10

Discovering Forgiveness: A Guided Curriculum for Children Ages 6–8

Robert D. Enright and Jeanette Knutson Enright

Both counseling and teaching are about giving life to our students in the form of relevant and exciting tools that they will use for a lifetime. Forgiving someone who was unjust, casting aside the bitterness that can become an unwanted companion, and recapturing emotional health are life-giving. Through this curriculum, you will be helping establish a foundation of forgiveness in young children. Many years from now, because we are in a world that is not always fair, some of the children, now grown, may find themselves in unhappy marriages, or stifling jobs, or in other situations that cause them deep distress and unhappiness. We wish it were not so, but we also know the realities of this world. Your guiding the students in forgiveness now may help them adjust to that marriage or to deal with that tyrannical boss in ways that are life-giving

and positive precisely because you took the time when they were quite young to lay the foundation of forgiveness for them. What you do now may make a major difference for some of these children in the distant future. You have the opportunity to give them the gift of forgiveness.

We cannot think of a more worthwhile activity for them. We know one child who was so angry with his father, who abandoned the family years before, that he could not sit still long enough to learn. He was angry, the teacher was frustrated, and the other students sensed the unhappiness that pervaded the classroom. The child had the courage to forgive and everyone benefited. The child's grades improved and he became quieter in a healthy, reasonable sense.

The practice of forgiveness can cut through our angers, disappointments, and resentments to give all involved a fresh start. As you forgive, you can be set free from the prison of resentment. As you offer forgiveness to another, he or she has the chance to begin anew with you, trying to be more civil, more respectful, more kind. Those around you may benefit because you are less likely to carry your anger into other situations. You are less likely to displace your anger onto those who don't deserve such treatment.

As we practice forgiveness, we learn that it is full of surprises. As educators and scientists who have studied forgiveness for decades, we have seen remarkable improvements in the emotional health and well-being of children, adolescents, young and middle-aged adults, and the elderly as they learned to forgive. We have seen lives transformed.

Forgiveness, of course, has a long history, dating back thousands of years to the writing in Genesis where Joseph forgives his brother and half-brothers for selling him into slavery in Egypt. The New Testament tells the story of the Prodigal Son, who is unconditionally forgiven by his father, who runs to him, hugs him, and has a party in his honor. Why? The father forgives because he loves his son. Forgiveness is like that. It has a way of lavishing love on those who were unfair. Other ancient traditions, such as Buddhism, Hinduism, and Islam, all have positive stories of people forgiving others who acted unfairly. In fact, we have yet to encounter an ancient text that talks unfavorably of forgiveness. The wisdom of the ages suggests that forgiveness is worth exploring.

Forgiveness can be defined this way: When you are unjustly hurt by another person, you forgive when you struggle to give up the resentment (to which you are actually entitled because you were unfairly treated) and you strive to offer the offending one compassion, benevolence, and love (knowing that yours is an act of mercy and therefore not necessarily deserved by the person).

Forgiveness has three paradoxes embedded in it.

1. A forgiver gives up resentment even though the world might tell him or her to cling to the resentment. Why cast off the resentment? Be strong . . . show your anger . . . don't let the person get away with this! A forgiver gives up resentment nonetheless.
2. A forgiver seems to be doing all of the giving and the offender all of the taking. After all, that person hurt you, so why should you give the gift of compassion, benevolence, and love? Is it not their turn to give to you, not the other way around? A forgiver gives these gifts nonetheless.

3. A forgiver, who reaches out to the other person with concern and care, often finds that he or she (the forgiver), is the one who is emotionally healed.

As you learn more about forgiveness, you will see that it is not always what it seems to be. Forgiveness is not something weak, but strong. Giving a gift to one who was unfair is a lavish act of love and mercy. Forgiveness does not make us a door mat, to be walked on by others. When we forgive, we can and should stand up for our rights.

Forgiveness is not the same as condoning or excusing. When we forgive, we label the other person's actions as wrong; we do not find an excuse for that person's actions. Forgiveness is not equated with forgetting. Having scientifically studied forgiveness now for years, we can say that we have never—not once—seen anyone who forgets the wrong done against them when they forgive. Yes, people may remember in new ways, but they do not develop a curious moral amnesia upon forgiving.

Forgiveness and reconciliation are not the exact same. When a person forgives, he or she unilaterally offers an end to resentment and institutes compassion and love. The other person might spurn this gift, but the gift-giver is the one who decides whether or not to give it. When two or more people reconcile, they come together again in mutual trust. To reconcile is to trust the other person again. To forgive is to offer love, but not necessarily to trust the other person unless he or she resolves not to offend in the same way again (within reason), repents, and offers recompense. One can forgive and then not reconcile if the other remains in his or her hurtful ways.

As you work with children on forgiveness, please keep in mind some basic issues to guard the children's rights and safety. Consider the following four ideas.

1. Forgiveness is a choice of the forgiver. Counselors, teachers, parents, or anyone else should not demand that a child forgive someone. If a child does not want to forgive, we must respect that.
2. Forgiveness does not mean that a child automatically enters into a relationship with a bully or anyone who is a danger to the child. Please remember that forgiveness and reconciliation are not the same thing.
3. Please avoid putting pressure on the group as children learn to forgive. This is not like math class or any other class where children

get good grades for performing better and more than others. We should avoid making forgiveness into a competition. Try to get the children to enjoy this, again keeping in mind that it is their choice.

4. Even if a child does not want to forgive someone, you should decide whether or not it is appropriate for the child to at least learn about forgiveness. Understanding forgiveness is not the same as practicing it. A skeptic might say that this is just a subtle way of getting a child to practice it. We disagree. When handled sensitively, you can have the child listen and learn without the pressure to perform acts of forgiveness.

RESEARCH SUPPORTING FORGIVENESS AS AN INTERVENTION

Forgiveness intervention shows much promise as a means of reducing anger and related emotional health variables (Lin, Mack, Enright, Krahn, & Baskin, 2004; Reed & Enright, 2006). Forgiveness intervention is relatively new, having first emerged in the early 1990s as a model of helping adult clients recover emotionally from deep injustices (Hebl & Enright, 1993). A person who forgives reduces resentment and offers goodness to an offender, without condoning, excusing, forgetting, or necessarily reconciling (see Enright & Fitzgibbons, 2000; Worthington, 2005). The one who forgives tries to think about the one who acted unfairly with a broader perspective than just the offense itself (the cognitive process of reframing) and to cultivate kindness, respect, generosity, and even love toward the offender (while, at the same time, protecting oneself as necessary if the other is not trustworthy).

Forgiveness therapy programs have helped the following kinds of samples to statistically significantly reduce anger, anxiety, and/or depression in randomized, experimental and control group designs with pre-tests, post-tests, and follow-up testing: elderly women hurt by family and others (effect size across mental health variables was 0.72; Hebl & Enright, 1993), parentally love deprived adolescents (Al-Mabuk, Enright, & Cardis, 1995), incest survivors (overall effect size for all participants of 1.44; Freedman & Enright, 1996), men hurt by the abortion decision of a partner (Coyle & Enright, 1997), college students (overall 0.75 effect size; McCullough, Worthington, & Rachal, 1997), in-patient drug rehabilitation patients (overall effect

size of 1.58; Lin et al., 2004), divorced adults (effect size of 0.3; Rye, Pargament, Pan, Yingling, Shogren, et al., 2005), emotionally-abused women (within-experimental group effect size of 1.79; Reed & Enright, 2006), and middle school students in Seoul, Korea (Park, 2003).

A manual similar to the one in this volume (using Dr. Seuss books primarily rather than Disney stories primarily) showed that children in first and third grades (Primary 3 and 5) in Belfast, Northern Ireland, when taught by their classroom teachers, reduced anger in statistically significant measures more than their control group counterparts. The third-grade children also decreased more in psychological depression and increased more in forgiveness than the control group children (Enright, Knutson Enright, Holter, Baskin, & Knutson, 2007).

Given the findings across the above studies, it is not surprising that Baskin and Enright (2004) found in a meta-analysis of forgiveness interventions that those implemented with a *group* format, across all mental health variables, showed a 0.59 effect size, and similarly, that those implemented with an *individual* format showed a 1.42 effect size. According to Lipsey (1990), both of these effect sizes can be considered large. Thus forgiveness interventions have been shown to be effective in a variety of applications with children, adolescents, and adults.

The Curriculum

The main point of this curriculum is to introduce the children to the basics of forgiveness. When we use that term—*the basics of forgiveness*—we are talking about the central foundation that will allow the children to build forgiveness skills as they develop through their lives. The basics of forgiveness include five issues: inherent worth, moral love, kindness, respect, and generosity.

The students who engage in this curriculum will meet characters who are not all bad or all good, but who have very human mixtures of the two. The children will learn that the world is not divided into the good people who forgive and the bad people who do not. Instead, they will see that we all are capable of anger at times and we all are capable of struggling to forgive. The children will learn that forgiveness does not come easily because we do not always feel like being good. Yet, it is that struggle to be good that makes us moral beings who make a difference in other people's lives.

The Structure of the Discovering Forgiveness Curriculum. At first, instead of concentrating on forgiveness per se, the children will be focusing on five of the basics of forgiveness, *those major ingredients involved in forgiving another person:* the idea of inherent worth, and the virtues of moral love, kindness, respect, and generosity. The children are introduced to these concepts in the first seven lessons. These concepts are explained below.

Inherent Worth. This is the important idea that a person is a person no matter what he or she does. It is akin to the idea that we are to love the sinner, but hate the sin. As children begin to see beyond what people do to what they are like inside themselves, they will be laying an important foundation for forgiving.

Moral Love. When we morally love someone, we love him or her unconditionally, despite his or her flaws. Certainly, someone who morally loves another can ask fairness of him or her. Yet, the one who morally loves has the other person's best interest at heart. Moral love is not a selfish or self-centered love. It has that lavish notion of love that Joseph showed to his brothers. Moral love underlies true forgiveness.

Kindness. When people are kind, they tend to be warm-hearted, concerned about the other person, humane. People who practice being kind are laying the foundation for forgiving. Some people talk about the "change of heart" that occurs when someone forgives. The heart-of-stone becomes the softened heart.

Respect. When someone shows respect, he or she is highly regarding the other person. Some people think that respect must be earned. People possess intrinsic value to such a degree that we should respect all persons. We respect, not because of what people *do*, but because of whom they *are*. As children practice respecting all people, they make forgiveness easier in the future.

Generosity. To be generous is to give abundantly. It is a gift-giving that surprises and delights the recipient. If children can learn to be generous, they will be in a better position to understand what it means to give a gift of forgiveness to someone who hurts them.

To repeat, our intention in the first seven lessons is not to have the children understand or to practice forgiveness, but to understand five of the important aspects of forgiveness.

The next part of this curriculum is intended to once again introduce the above five "basics of forgiveness" in the specific context of forgiveness. We are not asking children at this point to forgive anyone. Instead, we are asking them to *understand* how inherent worth looks in the context of forgiveness as described in stories. We ask children to understand kindness and moral love, respect and generosity all within the context of forgiveness. We do this through stories that illustrate these points.

Finally, we ask the children to think about someone who has hurt them unfairly. We then have them try to forgive that person by exercising the idea of inherent worth, and the virtues of moral love, kindness, respect, and generosity toward that person. This final part is the practical aspect of the curriculum. Prior to this, we are setting the stage for actual forgiving.

Forgiveness encompasses more than the practice of inherent worth and the exercise of the virtues of moral love, kindness, respect, and generosity. This is a curriculum based on the principles of developmental psychology. We want to start small, start with some of the basics, and keep it somewhat simple. We save the complexity and greater subtlety for later grades.

A word on our choice of curricular materials is in order. Our intent here is to make the exploration of forgiveness interesting and fun. One does not learn to play football by being thrust into highly competitive, serious situations too early. At first, it is sufficient for the children to run out onto the field on a warm afternoon, kick the ball around, and not worry yet about all the rules and regulations. It is the same with forgiveness. Its introduction should be somewhat light, free of lots of rules, and fun.

For the reason above, many (but not all) of books and DVDs that we chose are by the Disney Company because of their fun and their ability to teach the serious moral message. If the children can begin to understand the five basics (inherent worth, moral love, kindness, respect, and generosity), if the children can begin to understand how those five basics are part of forgiveness, and if the children can practice forgiveness using these five basics, you as the counselor, teacher, or parent will have laid the foundation for a lifetime of forgiving. You will have done something life-giving for your children.

Lesson 1: All People Have Deep Worth, Part I

Main Ideas of the Lesson

In lessons 1 and 2, the children will learn about the concept of inherent worth. The term "inherent worth" refers to the goodness that is a natural part of all people. It is not earned nor can it be taken away.

In today's lesson, the children will learn that people differ in a number of ways. These differences in personal appearance, possessions, abilities, achievement, places of residence, personalities, or cultural groups are certainly important, but they do not determine worth. A focus on individual differences based on such external features may interfere with us seeing the worth of all as members of the human family.

A person has worth simply because he or she is a person. No person is to be used, manipulated, or disrespected. We are to treat each person as persons of great worth. Each person has a heart and has the capacity for goodwill. We do acknowledge that not all people seem interested in offering beneficence, kindness, and so forth, nevertheless, all are capable of goodwill.

Introduction to the Lesson

Explain to the children, "Today we will begin a discovery of forgiveness. Over the next few months, we will learn about forgiveness, personal worth, love, kindness, respect, and generosity. In the first six lessons, we will not be learning about forgiveness, but about the importance of seeing the deep worth of all people and practicing love, kindness, respect, and generosity. In the final lessons, we will learn about forgiveness. What do you think it means to forgive?"

Please clarify this for the children: "When we've been unfairly hurt, we may need to forgive the person who was unfair. Forgiveness can occur as we choose to see the deep worth of the person who was unfair. As we look at the deep worth of the person and see that he or she is capable of being kind and that he or she may be hurting, our hearts may begin to soften and our anger may begin to fade. Forgiveness never says that unfairness is good, but that even when a person is unfair, he or she is good."

You may continue telling the children "In this first lesson, you will learn that all people have deep worth. You will also learn what gives people deep worth."

What do you think it means to say that all people have deep worth? All people are valuable in and of themselves. All people are worthy of love, kindness, respect, and generosity. No person is to be mistreated, used, or disrespected.

What gives people worth? A person has worth simply because he or she is a person. Personal appearance, possessions, abilities, achievement, places of residence, personalities, or cultural groups do not determine worth. It is not earned nor can it be taken away.

"We are now going to read the Walt Disney story entitled, *The Fox and the Hound*. In this story, you will meet a dog named Copper and a fox named Tod. Please watch for signs that Copper and Tod saw the deep worth of one another."

Read Aloud the Story, *The Fox and the Hound*

Discussion Questions

1. What is today's story about?
2. After a brief discussion about the "The Fox and the Hound," hold up the picture found on Page 8 of the book (a big tree, Copper the dog playfully laying with his

feet on a root of the tree, and Tod the fox happily looking back at Copper). Ask the children if they remember when Big Mama told Dinky and Boomer, "It's very unusual for a fox and a hound to be so friendly. It just isn't done! But they do like each other."

3. Why do you think that "Big Mama" thought it was unusual for a fox and a hound to be so friendly?

4. Why do you think Copper the hound and Tod the fox liked each other? *They both liked to run and play. They lived close to each other. They were about the same age. They were nice to each other. They were similar in many ways.*

5. If hounds and foxes don't usually like each other, why might Copper and Tod have been able to be friends? *They must have realized that people are important just because they are people. It doesn't matter what group they belong to, their possessions, where they live, what they look like, or their culture.*

6. There came a point when Copper and Tod were no longer friends. What happened that changed their friendship?

7. When Copper was very angry with Tod, do you think that Copper saw Tod as having deep worth? Why or why not?

8. Did Tod have deep worth even though Copper was angry with him? Why or why not?

9. How was Copper able to stop being angry with Tod?

10. Copper became able to see the deep worth of Tod. Tod saw the deep worth of Copper. They realized their worth didn't come from being either a fox or a hound. What else does not matter when deciding whether a person has deep worth?

Activity

Through this activity, the children will learn that all people have deep worth regardless of possessions (wealth), place of residence, appearance, personality, physical health, or group membership. A person has value because he or she is a person. Each person has a heart and is capable of goodwill. Deep worth cannot be earned or taken away.

The children will first draw, color, and cut-out a large picture of a dog (Copper) or a fox (Tod). Their picture of a dog or fox should come close to filling a standard 9 x 12 sheet of paper.

Next, the children will make costumes and props for their cut-out friend, Copper or Tod. Ask the children to draw, color and cut-out the following pictures: paper money representing great wealth, a small house or shack (obviously poor), a moustache, a pair of glasses, a pair of crutches, a frowning face, hats and head pieces representing different countries (France, Asia, Middle-East, and so forth), and a red heart. Please feel free to vary the items provided the children learn the message that a person's deep worth does not come from possessions, place of residence, appearance, personality, physical health, or group membership.

Once the children have drawn, colored, and cut-out all of the pictures, ask them to select the costumes or props they would first like to hold up to their Copper or Tod friend. Now, ask the children to hold the selected item up to Copper or Tod. Ask, "Is Copper (Tod) now different than before you put the . . . on him? Is he still Copper (Tod)? How do you know?" *He has the same heart. The hat, money, or house didn't change who he is.* Continue this process for all of the items.

Please keep in mind that the students may require more discussion regarding some of the concepts. For example, the idea that a person has deep worth even if he or she lives in another part of the world or has lots of money is quite abstract when compared with the idea that a person is of value even if he or she has a moustache. It is not necessary that every item be held up to Copper (Tod). It is important that the children understand that while Copper (Tod) might be different on the outside, he is still the same on the inside.

We have found great benefits in giving each child the gift of a stuffed animal to use instead of a paper cut-out as it can be a constant reminder of the important message that all people have deep worth.

Conclusion

The term *inherent worth* refers to the goodness that is a natural part of all people. It is not earned nor can it be taken away. People differ in a number of ways. These differences in personal appearance, possessions, abilities, achievement, places of residence, personalities, or cultural groups are certainly important, but they do not determine worth. A person has worth simply because he or she is a person. No person is to be used, manipulated, or disrespected. We are to treat each person as persons of great worth. Each person has a heart and has the capacity for goodwill. We do acknowledge that not all people seem interested in offering beneficence, kindness, and so forth. For those who are uninterested in offering beneficence, for example, you still may wish to ask them the all-important question: Do all people have worth even if you do not feel kindly toward such a person?

Lesson 2: All People Have Worth, Part II

Main Ideas of the Lesson

In this lesson, the children will again learn that all people have deep inherent worth. The term inherent worth, as discussed in lesson 1, refers to the goodness that is a natural part of all people. It is not earned nor can it be taken away. This deep worth does not rest on personal differences (appearance, possessions, abilities, achievements, personality, group membership or other things that set people apart from one another). A person has worth simply because he or she is a person. We will learn about inherent worth outside of the context of forgiveness.

Today, we will be extending our views of what gives each person deep worth to include a discussion of those qualities that unite all people as members of the human family: all people experience various hardships, good times, and feelings; all have similar basic needs; have similar physical make-up (eyes, nose, legs, arms, etc.), bodily functions (blood circulation, respiration, digestion), emotions (love, anger, sadness), and all can think and reason. The ways people are the same do not give people deep worth.

All people have worth because they are members of the human family. No person is to be used, manipulated, or disrespected. We are to treat each person as persons of great worth.

Introduction to the Lesson

Please review the main ideas of lesson 1 with the following questions.

1. What is deep personal (inherent) worth?
2. What gives people deep worth? A person has worth simply because he or she is a person.
3. What does not give people worth? *Personal differences like possessions, homes, work, appearance, and group membership.*
4. How are we to show that all people have deep worth? We show that others have deep worth through love and kindness.

Today, we are again going to learn about personal worth. However, today we will be focusing on the ways that people are the same. We will ask the question whether a person's deep worth comes solely from experiences, feelings, or body make-up.

Show Part I (Chapters 1–15) of Walt Disney's, *Snow White and the Seven Dwarfs*

Introduce the characters and summarize the main ideas of the story before showing part I of the DVD. We will leave it up to you to decide whether it is appropriate for the children to view chapter 7, "Flight through the Woods" as it may be somewhat frightening.

Discussion Questions

1. What happened in today's story?
2. Do you remember when Snow White and the animals fell asleep in the Dwarfs' little home in the forest? The Dwarfs returned home from a day of work to find their home cleaned, the dishes washed, and soup cooking in the fireplace. They

were confused. They were angry. They were frightened. Up the stairs they climbed. They were ready to protect themselves from what must be a horrible monster. They approached one of the beds. They pulled back the covers and there it was. A beautiful girl. Snow White awakened! The Seven Dwarfs looked at her in surprise. She looked at them in surprise.

3. What did Snow White first do when she saw the dwarfs?
4. What do you think Snow White saw when she looked at each of the dwarfs? *She saw their differences (she guessed each of their names), but she also saw their worth. She was kind to them.*
5. What do you think the Dwarfs saw when they looked at Snow White? *They saw her deep worth. They protected her.*
6. What are some of the ways that Snow White and the Seven Dwarfs were the same? Do they have worth simply because they're the same? *No. They have worth because they are people. They have worth as members of the human family.*
7. In what ways are you and I the same? In what ways are you the same as your friends? In what ways are you the same as people in your family?
8. Do you think all people have deep worth? Why or why not?
9. Do you have deep worth? Why or why not?
10. What gives you deep worth?
11. Was this deep worth earned? Can it ever be taken away?

Activity

The children will sing the song "Snow White Lost in the Woods" to the tune of "The Farmer in the Dell." Please notice that the words to the song follow the actions, written in italics and put in parentheses.

(Join hands and circle right while singing. Place one or more persons in the center. They will pretend to be Snow White. Those forming the circle will pretend to be the Dwarfs.)

Snow White lost in the woods.
Snow White lost in the woods.
Abandoned by hate, but saved by love.
Snow White lost in the woods.

(While still holding hands and singing, walk to the center to closely surround Snow White(s) in a supportive way.)

Along came the critters.
Along came the critters.
Abandoned by hate, but saved by love.
Along came the critters.

(Return to a full size circle. Drop hands. Stand still. Continue singing.)

Snow White found a home.

(Wave to the persons in the center of the circle while singing. Those in the center should wave back to the persons forming the circle while singing.)

Snow White met the Dwarfs.

(Those in the center should hold their hands up to their eyes as they look at the people pretending to be the Dwarfs.)

She saw their worth.

(Everybody in the center of the circle should wrap their arms around their body as if they were hugging themselves.)

> She acted in love.
> Snow White saw their worth.

(The students forming the circle should hold their hands up to their eyes as they look at those in the center of the circle.)

> The Dwarfs saw her worth.

(Wrap your arms around your body to give yourself a hug.)

> The Dwarfs acted in love.

(Repeat hands to eyes.)

> They saw her worth.

(Repeat arms around selves.)

> They acted in love.
> A happy home was formed.

(The people in the center join the big circle. Shake hands with one another. Join hands and continue circling while singing.)

> She valued Doc and Bashful.
> She valued Happy and Sleepy.
> She valued Sneezy.
> She valued Dopey.
> She valued Grumpy, too.

Conclusion

Review the main ideas of the lesson. All people experience various hardships, good times, and feelings; all have similar basic needs; have similar physical make-up (eyes, nose, legs, arms, etc.), bodily functions (blood circulation, respiration, digestion), emotions (love, anger, sadness), and all can think and reason. The ways people are the same do not give them worth.

All people have worth as members of the human family. No person is to be used, manipulated, or disrespected. We are to treat each person as persons of great worth.

Lesson 3: Love, a Foundation for Forgiveness

Main Ideas of the Lesson

In today's lesson, we will begin to learn about the virtue of love.

Webster's dictionary defines love as "feelings of strong attachment, liking, or fondness for another person." Love is more than a feeling. It is a decision to treat others with kindness, respect, and generosity through our thoughts, words, and actions. Love asks us to give of ourselves for the benefit of others.

Love helps us to see the deep worth of all people and it is an expression of all peoples' deep worth. Communities can experience positive change through love.

Introduction to the Lesson

Briefly review lesson 2. All people experience various hardships, good times, and feelings; all have similar basic needs; have similar physical make-up (eyes, nose, legs, arms, etc.), bodily functions (blood circulation, respiration, digestion), emotions (love, anger, sadness), and all can think and reason. The ways people are the same do not give people deep worth.

All people have worth because they are members of the human family. No person is to be used, manipulated, or disrespected. We are to treat each person as persons of great worth.

In this lesson, we will discuss the virtue of moral love. Love is a feeling of warmth or fondness toward a person. It is more than a feeling though. It is deciding to treat others with kindness, respect, and generosity through thoughts, words, and actions.

Please review part I of, *Snow White and the Seven Dwarfs* (chapters 1–15). Show part II of the *Snow White and the Seven Dwarfs* DVD (chapters 16–27). We will leave it up to you to decide whether chapter 21, "The Poison Apple," is appropriate to show to the children. It may be slightly disturbing.

Discussion Questions

1. What happened in today's portion of *Snow White and the Seven Dwarfs*?
2. Were there any signs of love in the movie? What were they?
3. In what ways did Snow White show love toward the Dwarfs? She cooked and cleaned for them. She didn't judge them. She didn't care if they were "grumpy."
4. How do you think her love made the Dwarfs feel?
5. Snow White cooked, cleaned and helped seven busy people. She did this day after day. Do you think it was sometimes hard for Snow White to be loving? Why or why not?
6. Why do you think she could be loving day after day even though it may have been difficult? *She was willing to give of herself to help them. She chose to be kind, respectful, and generous in love even if she didn't feel like it.*
7. In what ways did the Dwarfs show love toward Snow White? How do you think that made Snow White feel?
8. How do people you know show love toward you? How does it make you feel when you are given love from family and friends?
9. How do you show love toward others? How do you feel when you give love?
10. Is it possible for you to *safely* show love toward people you don't know very (children at your school, clerks in a store, neighbors, and so forth)?

11. What are some ways you could *safely* show love toward people in stores, restaurants, at school, in your neighborhoods, and so forth?
12. Is there something we can do to be worthy of love? Why or why not? Are you worthy of love? Why?
13. How might loving hearts help communities?

Activity

The following activity will help the children to understand the virtue of love. Begin by having the children make one large "fruit of love tree" together as a group. Next, ask them to draw, color, and cut-out pictures of fruit. The children will draw pictures of loving acts, cut from magazines pictures of loving acts, bring photographs from home, or write about loving acts and attach them to the cut-outs of fruit. Finally, these pieces of "love fruit" will be hung on the "fruit of love tree." You may decide to have each child make their own "fruit of love tree" and hang them together in a display to create a "Forest of Love" symbolizing the effects that love can have on an entire community.

Conclusion

Love has been described as "feelings of strong attachment, liking, or fondness for another person." Love is more than a feeling. It is a decision to treat others with kindness, respect, and generosity through our thoughts, words, and actions. Love asks us to give of ourselves for the benefit of others. Love helps us to see the deep worth of all people and it is an expression of all peoples' deep worth. Communities can experience positive change through love.

Lesson 4: Kindness, a Foundation for Forgiveness

Main Ideas of the Lesson

In this lesson, the children will learn about kindness. An understanding of kindness will help people forgive. We will not yet be discussing kindness as it relates to forgiveness.

Kindness is an expression of love. Webster's dictionary defines kindness as a "demonstration of goodness, benevolence, sympathy, and grace." We show kindness through thoughts, words, and actions. Kindness, as with love, can have a positive effect on entire communities.

Introduction to the Lesson

Review the main ideas of lesson 3. Love has been described as "feelings of strong attachment, liking, or fondness for another person." Love is more than a feeling. It is a decision to treat others with kindness, respect, and generosity through our thoughts, words, and actions. Love asks us to give of ourselves for the benefit of others. Love helps us to see the deep worth of all people and it is an expression of all peoples' deep worth. Communities can experience positive change through love.

Today we are going to learn about kindness. What is kindness? How can we show kindness?

Show part I ("The Honey Tree") of *The Many Adventures of Winnie the Pooh* DVD. Ask the children to watch for acts of kindness.

Discussion Questions

1. What was today's story about?
2. Were there any acts of kindness in the story? What were they?
3. How did Christopher Robin treat Winnie the Pooh?
4. How did he behave toward all of the animals in the Hundred Acre Forest?
5. Why do you think Christopher Robin was able to be kind over and over again to Pooh and all of the animals?
6. Was it careless or wrong for Christopher Robin to be kind over and over again? Why or why not?
7. What are some ways that others have been kind to you? How did this kindness make you feel?
8. What are some of the ways that you have been kind to others?
9. Is it possible to show *safely* show kindness to people other than your family and friends? How? *We can say please and thank-you. We can smile or be helpful.*
10. How do you think your kindness make others feel?
11. Have you ever had a chance to keep being kind to someone day after day after day?
12. What do you think our families, schools, and communities would be like if people were kind to one another over and over again?

Activity

The children will continue learning about kindness through journaling. They will write and draw pictures about kindness, personal worth, love, respect, generosity, and forgiveness given and received. The children may listen to music (classical, favorite children's tunes, or songs with a kindness theme) while journaling once or more a week.

Conclusion

Review the main ideas of the lesson. Kindness is an expression of love. It is a "demonstration of goodness, benevolence, sympathy, and grace." We show kindness through thoughts, words, and actions. Kindness, as with love, can have a positive effect on entire communities.

Lesson 5: Respect, a Foundation for Forgiveness

Main Ideas of the Lesson

In today's lesson, the children will learn about respect. We will discuss respect apart from forgiveness.

Respect is treating others as we would like to be treated. We can show respect through thoughts, words, and behaviors. Those who understand that all people have deep worth through love are able to show respect. All people are worthy of respect. Consistent respectful thoughts, feelings, and behaviors can change communities for the good.

Introduction to the Lesson

Review the main ideas of lesson 4. Kindness is an expression of love. It is a "demonstration of goodness, benevolence, sympathy, and grace." We show kindness through thoughts, words, and actions. Kindness, as with love, can have a positive effect on entire communities.

Tell the children that in today's lesson they will learn about *respect*. They will learn about respect by discussing its opposite, *disrespect*. What is respect? *We treat others as we would like to be treated*. What is disrespect? *We do not treat others as we want to be treated. We do not see the person's worth*.

Read the book, *Dumbo*. We are going to learn about respect by discussing its opposite, disrespect. Ask the children to watch for signs of disrespect and respect.

Discussion Questions

1. What is the story, *Dumbo* about?
2. Were there any signs of respect in the story? What were they? Why were these behaviors respectful?
3. Were there signs of disrespect? What were they? Why were these behaviors disrespectful?
4. Do you think Dumbo felt that he had deep worth? Why or why not?
5. Have you ever been treated with respect? How?
6. How did you feel when you were treated with respect?
7. Have you ever shown respect to a person? What did you do? Why did you show respect?
8. How did the person act when you were respectful? What did he or she say?
9. Are all people worthy of respect? Why or why not?
10. Are you worthy of respect? Why or why not?
11. What might our school, families, and communities be like if all people were respectful over and over again?

Activity

Today's activity will help the children learn about respect. The children will make a list of the ways they *have* shown respect toward people in their families, schools, neighborhoods, and communities and the ways they *could* show respect toward people in their families, schools, neighborhoods, and communities.

Some examples of respectful behaviors are: saying please and thank you, being careful with others' property, sharing toys or food, helping others with work, or complimenting others.

Conclusion

Review the main ideas of the lesson. Respect is treating others as we would like to be treated. We can show respect through thoughts, words, and behaviors. Those who understand that all people have deep worth through love are able to show respect. All people are worthy of respect. Consistent respectful thoughts, feelings, and behaviors can change communities for the good.

Lesson 6: Generosity, a Foundation for Forgiveness

Main Ideas of the Lesson

In today's lesson, we will discuss generosity apart from forgiveness. As is the case with kindness and respect, generosity grows out of a loving heart. Generosity can involve giving our time, possessions, feelings (love, kindness, respect, forgiveness, and so forth) to others. Our thoughts, words, and actions can be generous. All people are worthy of receiving generosity.

Introduction to the Lesson

Review the main ideas of the previous lesson. Respect is treating others as we would like to be treated. We can show respect through thoughts, words, and behaviors. Those who understand that all people have deep worth through love are able to show respect. All people are worthy of respect. Consistent respectful thoughts, feelings, and behaviors can change communities for the good.

Tell the children that today they will learn about generosity. Ask the children, "What is generosity? It is the giving of our time, possessions, feelings (love, kindness, respect, forgiveness, and so forth). How can we be generous?" We can be generous in the giving of our time, possessions, love, and kindness.

Show part II ("The Blustery Day") of *The Many Adventures of Winnie the Pooh* DVD. Ask the children to watch for signs of generosity in the story.

Discussion Questions

1. What happened in our story, *The Blustery Day?*
2. What are some of the ways that Pooh, Piglet, and others were generous toward one another?
3. When Piglet offered his house to Eeyore, what did Eeyore do and say? How do you think Eeyore felt?
4. Generosity can sometimes be difficult. Think of Piglet when he first offered his home. Did Piglet seem happy and joyous to offer his home or quiet and a little bit sad?
5. Piglet's generosity was mixed with some sadness. How did Piglet change *after* he was generous to Eeyore?
6. How did Piglet's generosity spread? *Winnie the Pooh showed generosity to Piglet by offering to let him live with him.*
7. What are some of the ways that people have been generous to you?
8. How did their generosity make you feel? Did it make you feel more generous? Why or why not?
9. What are some of the ways that you have been generous to others?
10. How do you think your generosity made them feel?
11. Are all people *worthy* of generosity? Why or why not?
12. Are you *worthy* of generosity? Why or why not?
13. How might our schools, families, and communities change if every person was generous over and over again?

Activity

This activity will help the children continue to learn about generosity. The teacher (person in authority) and children will have an opportunity to recognize others' loving, kind, respectful, generous, and, in future lessons, forgiving behaviors and to be recognized for their own loving, kind, respectful, generous, and, in future lessons, forgiving behaviors. The children may be recognized through certificates, special opportunities (time at the computer or playtime), and words of praise. We realize that it is important for the children to be loving, kind, respectful, generous, and forgiving because they value these behaviors, but encouraging these virtues on a regular basis (with tangible rewards)may help the children to develop an appreciation for them.

Conclusion

Review the main ideas of the lesson. Generosity grows out of a loving heart. Generosity can involve giving our time, possessions, feelings (love, kindness, respect, forgiveness, and so forth) to others. Our thoughts, words, and actions can be generous. All people are worthy of receiving generosity.

Lesson 7: The Meaning of Forgiveness

Main Ideas of the Lesson

In this lesson, the children will learn *what forgiveness is* and *is not*. Forgiveness is, "When unjustly hurt by another, we forgive when we overcome the resentment toward the offender, not by denying our right to the resentment, but instead by trying to offer the wrongdoer compassion, benevolence, and love; as we give these, we as forgivers realize that the offender does not necessarily have a right to such gifts."[1]

Forgiveness is not excusing, condoning, or putting up with injustice. Forgiveness is not blaming the self, forgetting the hurt (we remember the hurt in a different way), or pretending it didn't happen.

Forgiveness is not reconciliation. Forgiveness is an internal change of the heart. Reconciliation involves two people coming together in friendship. Forgiveness is possible without reconciliation. True reconciliation is not possible without forgiveness.

Forgiveness may result in less anger and sadness and more hopefulness. It may improve relationships. If people forgive one another over and over again, families, schools, and communities may benefit. Please remember that forgiveness is a choice. People should never be forced to forgive.

Introduction to the Lesson

Review the main ideas of the previous lesson. Generosity grows out of a loving heart. Generosity can involve giving our time, possessions, feelings (love, kindness, respect, forgiveness, and so forth) to others. Our thoughts, words, and actions can be generous. All people are worthy of receiving generosity.

Tell the children that in today's lesson, they will learn that when we forgive, we let go of our anger toward a person who was unfair. We are not required by any law to let go of our anger. We are not required to offer love, kindness, respect, and generosity to the person who was unfair. When we forgive, we do not excuse, condone, or put up with injustice. We do not blame the self, forget the hurt (we remember the hurt in a different way), or pretend it didn't happen. We *might* get along better with the person who was unfair, but if he or she keeps on hurting us, it may not be possible for us to continue a relationship. Forgiveness is a choice! We should never force or pressure anyone to forgive. You will always be allowed to choose to forgive, if and when you are ready."

Read the Story, *You're Not My Best Friend Anymore* by Charlotte Pomerantz

Please note that this book is no longer in print, but can be purchased through secondary sources on Amazon.com. Ask the children to watch for signs of forgiveness in the story.

Discussion Questions

1. Describe Molly and Ben's friendship.
2. How were Molly and Ben unfair to one another?
3. Was Molly angry with Ben? How do you know? Was Ben angry with Molly? How do you know?

4. Did Molly and Ben have a right to their anger? Why or why not?
5. When we forgive, our anger often gets less. Did Molly and Ben's anger get less? How can you tell?
6. When we forgive, we see that the person who was unfair has deep worth. Did Ben see Molly's deep worth? Did Molly see Ben's deep worth? How do you know?
7. When we forgive, our hearts often soften toward the person who was unfair. Did Molly and Ben's hearts soften toward one another? How can you tell?
8. Did Molly or Ben excuse or put up with injustice?
9. Did Molly or Ben blame themselves for the unfairness or pretend that it didn't happen?
10. If Molly had continued to be unfair with Ben, could Ben have forgiven her? Why or why not? *Ben could forgive Molly, but not enter into a friendship with her. Forgiveness is a change in the heart of a person. We can forgive and keep ourselves safe.*
11. If Ben had continued to be unfair toward Molly, could Molly have forgiven him? Why or why not? *Molly could forgive, but not enter into friendship. Forgiveness is a change in the heart of a person. We can forgive and keep ourselves safe.*
12. Did Molly or Ben forget the unfairness? Why do you think this?
13. What are some of the signs that Molly and Ben forgave one another?
14. If Molly and Ben had not been ready to forgive, should they have been forced to do so before they were ready? Why or why not?
15. What happened as a result of the forgiveness? Their friendship returned. They were less angry. They felt happier.

Activity

The children will continue to learn about forgiveness through this activity. They will write and illustrate a story about forgiveness. Ask the children to include the following: an injustice, a description of the anger or sadness that followed the unfairness, the lessening of anger as the deep worth of the person who was unfair is seen, and a willingness to offer love, kindness, respect, and generosity to the person who behaved unfairly.

Conclusion

Forgiveness is, "When unjustly hurt by another, we forgive when we overcome the resentment toward the offender, not by denying our right to the resentment, but instead by trying to offer the wrongdoer compassion, benevolence, and love; as we give these, we as forgivers realize that the offender does not necessarily have a right to such gifts."[2]

Forgiveness is not excusing, condoning, or putting up with injustice. Forgiveness is not blaming the self, forgetting the hurt (we remember the hurt in a different way), or pretending it didn't happen.

Forgiveness is not reconciliation. Forgiveness is an internal change of the heart. Reconciliation involves two people coming together in friendship. Forgiveness is possible without reconciliation. True reconciliation is not possible without forgiveness.

Forgiveness may result in less anger and sadness and more hopefulness. It may improve relationships. If people forgive one another over and over again, families, schools, and communities may benefit. Please remember that forgiveness is a choice. People should never be forced to forgive.

Lesson 8: Deep Worth Within Forgiveness

Main Ideas of the Lesson

In the previous lesson, the children learned the meaning of forgiveness. In lessons 8 (today's lesson), 9, and 10, they will begin applying what they've learned about forgiveness and what they learned in earlier lessons about inherent worth, love, kindness, respect, and generosity to the characters in the stories.

Today, we will discuss the concept of inherent worth as it relates to forgiveness. In lessons 1 and 2, we learned that the term "inherent worth" refers to the goodness that is a natural part of all people.

It is not usually difficult to see a person's deep worth when he or she is acting toward us in a loving and kind way, but if that person treats us with unfairness or unkindness, it may become very difficult for us to see his or her deep worth. Our hearts, once soft and loving, may become hardened with anger and hurt. Yet, if we persevere and work (often a struggle) to see the offender's deep worth, our hearts will once again become soft and loving once again. We may even become ready to reach out in love, kindness, respect, generosity, and forgiveness.

Forgiveness is a gift that can benefit individual people and society.

In this lesson, we will watch *The Fox and the Hound* DVD. This will extend the message that all people have deep worth as learned in Lesson 2 through the book, *The Fox and the Hound*. The children will now learn that even when we've been treated unfairly, it is possible for us to see the deep worth of our offenders and forgive.

Introduction to the Lesson

Review the main ideas of the previous lesson. Forgiveness means that we choose to become less angry with a person who was unfairly hurt us and willing to give love to that person. When we forgive, we do not excuse the person's hurtful behavior. We do not pretend and tell ourselves that we weren't hurt. We do not say that the unfairness was all right. Forgiveness does not always mean that the two people (the forgiver and forgiven) come back together in peace or friendship. There must be a sincere desire by both people to come back together. Forgiveness can help us to become less sad, less angry, more hopeful, and can improve our relationship with the person who hurt us.

Tell the children, "In this lesson we are going to continue learning about *forgiveness*. We are going to think about how unfair hurt can make our hearts hard with anger or sadness, but if we see the deep worth of the person who was unfair, our hearts may soften through forgiveness. We can choose to see the deep worth of one who was unfair and we can soften our hearts through forgiveness without being put in danger to be hurt again by the same person. Forgiveness can help entire communities."

Show the DVD, *The Fox and the Hound*.

Ask the children to watch for the ways that the different characters in the story (Tod, Copper, Widow Tweed, and Amos) show forgiveness. Describe what happens in chapter 18, "The Hunter Seeks Revenge" and in chapter 20, "Copper Saves Tod." The content of these chapters may contain scenes that could be frightening or upsetting to the children. We will leave this decision up to the teacher.

Discussion Questions

1. What happened in today's story?
2. Did any unfairness happen? What happened that was unfair? Who was unfair?
3. Do you remember when Chief was chasing Tod on the railroad tracks? A train was approaching on a high bridge. Tod was able to hide himself between the boards so that he wasn't injured, but Chief was forced off of the bridge. When Copper saw Tod looking over the railroad bridge from which Chief had fallen, he thought that Tod had been unfair and was to blame for Chief's injuries.
4. Did Copper at that time see Tod's deep worth? Why or why not? Did Amos and Chief see Tod's deep worth? Why do you think this?
5. Did Tod have deep worth even though Copper, Amos, and Chief were not able to see it at that time? Why or why not?
6. Did Copper, Amos, and Chief have deep worth even though they were now being unfair toward Tod? Why or why not?
7. What did Tod do at the end of the story? *He forgave them.*
8. How do you think Tod managed to forgive? *He thought kind thoughts. He saw their deep worth.*
9. If you were Tod, would you have been able to see the deep worth of Copper, Amos, and Chief even though they were unfair to you? Why or why not?
10. If you were Tod, would you have believed that you had deep worth even though you were being treated unfairly? Why or why not?
11. If you were Tod, would you have been able to forgive? Why or why not?
12. If people learned to forgive one another over and over again, could communities change? In what ways might they change?

Please let the children know that it is possible to see the deep worth of a person who's been unfair and yet remain safe. We can forgive a person who continues to be unfair without being a friend to him or her.

Activity

Teach the students the words and actions to the song *When You're the Best of Friends.*

Play the song from the DVD *The Fox and the Hound.*

You may either teach the words from the song on the DVD or have the children just listen to the song while doing the actions. If you have the students learn the words, they may either learn all of the words to the song or just "key" words. The lyrics and actions are below.

When You're the Best of Friends

Suggested Key Words or Verses: We have added a final verse to the song. We suggest the children learn and sing these words.

Tell the students, "If you so choose, you can think loving thoughts and feel loving feelings toward someone who has hurt you. If you so choose, you can even try to behave lovingly to that person, but be sure to keep yourself safe if that person is so angry as to endanger your safety." *(To the teacher: An example of loving and keeping one's distance is this: The student might think about the strengths of the bully [friendly, has helped him or her in the past] and might feel compassion toward the person, but then avoid interacting with him or her, especially when they are alone.)*

The italicized words in parentheses are the actions for the lyrics that directly follow. The words for the song follow the italicized words in parentheses.

(Join hands in a circle. Circle right) When you're the best of friends
Having so much fun together.
(Circle left) You're not even aware you're such a funny pair;
You're the best of friends.
(Drop hands. Stop circling.)
(Draw the corners of your mouth up in a smile.) Life's a happy game,
(While remaining in place, act silly—like a clown.) You can clown around forever
(Cover your eyes and turn your head from side to side as if to say no.) Neither one of
you sees your natural boundaries
(Draw the corners of your mouth up in a smile.) Life's one happy game.
(Join hands in a circle. Circle right.) If only the world wouldn't get in the way.
(Circle left.) If only people would just let you play.
(Drop hands. Stop circling.)
(Lift hands at your side and shrug your shoulders.) They say you're both being fools.
(Shake your finger at others as if you're scolding.) You're breaking all the rules.
(Join hands in a circle. Circle right.) They can't understand the magic of your wonder-
land.
When you're the best of friends
Sharing all that you discover.
When these moments are past
(Circle left) Will their friendship last.
Who can say
There's a way
Oh, I hope it never ends cuz you're the best of friends.
(Wrap arms around self and give yourself a hug.)
If hurt occurs, as it so often does.
Keep seeing the worth in the other.
Think loving thoughts, feel loving feelings, and a softened heart can return.
This will pave the way for forgiveness.

Conclusion

Conclude by summarizing the main ideas of the lesson. It is not usually difficult to see a person's deep worth when he or she is acting toward us in a loving and kind way, but if that person treats us with unfairness or unkindness, it may become very difficult for us to see his or her deep worth. Our hearts, once soft and loving, may become hardened with anger and hurt. Yet, if we persevere and work (often a struggle) to see the offender's deep worth, our hearts will once again become soft and loving once again. We may even become ready to reach out in love, kindness, respect, generosity, and forgiveness.

Forgiveness is a gift that can benefit individual people and society.

Lesson 9: Love within Forgiveness

Main Ideas of the Lesson

In lesson 3, the children learned that love is a feeling of strong attachment or liking for another person. We also learned that it is more than just a *feeling*. It is a *decision* to *behave toward others* with respect, kindness, and generosity. In today's lesson, through a study of conflict between our storybook characters, we will learn about love as it relates to forgiveness.

As previously discussed in lessons 7 and 8, anger and sadness are often a natural result of unfairness. Anger and sadness, if permitted to remain, may harden our hearts. The consistent practice of love can help us to once again soften our hearts, to see the deep worth of a person who was unfair, and to forgive.

We can offer love within forgiveness to a person who was unfair and yet remain safe. We do not necessarily enter into a friendship with a person who continues to be unfair. We can *safely* offer love to a person who was unfair by refusing to seek revenge, speak badly about him or her, or harm him or her in any way. We can *safely* offer love to a person who was unfair by interacting with him or her only in safe situations (when others are present), offering a smile, or a gift.

People with loving hearts, who forgive, can improve entire communities because they persist in seeing the deep worth in all people, even those who are unfair, and treating them with kindness, respect, and generosity.

Introduction to the Lesson

Review the main ideas of the previous lesson. It is not usually difficult to see a person's deep worth when he or she is acting toward us in a loving and kind way, but if that person treats us with unfairness or unkindness, it may become very difficult for us to see his or her deep worth. Our hearts, once soft and loving, may become hardened with anger and hurt. Yet, if we persevere and work (often a struggle) to see the offender's deep worth, our hearts will once again become soft and loving once again. We may even become ready to reach out in love, kindness, respect, generosity, and forgiveness. Forgiveness is a gift that can benefit individual people and society.

Tell the children, "When you have been unfairly hurt by another person, there are ways that you can *safely* show love toward him or her. This means that you can think loving thoughts, act in loving ways, and feel loving feelings without putting yourself in danger to be hurt again by the same person. We do not have to enter into a friendship with a person who continues to be unfair."

How can we *safely* offer love to a person who has behaved unfairly? We can refuse to seek revenge, speak badly about him or her, or harm him or her in anyway. We can *safely* offer love to a person who was unfair by interacting with him or her only in safe situations (when others are present), offering a smile, or a gift.

Play for the Children the *Cinderella* DVD or Video

Please ask the children to pay special attention to the ways Cinderella showed love. Although her stepmother and stepsisters caused her unfair hurt, Cinderella was able to continue walking in love. This helped her to forgive.

You may want to show only portions of the story if you feel it is too long. If you decide to show only portions of the story, we suggest you show Cinderella's unkind treatment at the beginning of the story up through her attendance to the ball.

Discussion Questions

1. What happened in the story of Cinderella?
2. In what ways did the stepmother and stepsisters unfairly hurt Cinderella?
3. How did Cinderella show love toward her stepmother and stepsisters?
4. If you were treated as Cinderella was treated, as a person of little worth, do you think it would be easy for you to show love? Why or why not?
5. How is it possible that Cinderella was able to show love toward her stepmother and stepsisters when she was treated so unfairly? *She recognized the deep worth of those who were unfair. She had practiced seeing peoples' worth and walking in love.*
6. Did Cinderella's stepmother and stepsisters deserve Cinderella's love? Why or why not? *Cinderella was not under any law to love them especially when they were unfair. But, the stepmother and stepsisters were still people of deep worth even though they had behaved unfairly.*
7. Love can change the hearts of others. Did Cinderella's love seem to change the hearts of her stepmother and stepsisters? How do you know?
8. Was Cinderella able to *safely* forgive her stepmother and stepsisters even though they remained unfair? What did she do and say that makes you think this?
9. How did a loving and forgiving heart help Cinderella?
10. Did Cinderella's love and forgiveness help her community? *The community received a loving Princess because of her soft and loving heart.*
11. What are some ways you to *safely* show love and forgiveness to a person who's been unfair?
12. How could your school, family, and community be helped through forgiveness?
13. Please help the children to understand that it is all right to be loving and forgiving toward a person who was unfair, but that they must be careful if the person continues to behave unfairly. They can forgive without entering into a friendship with a person who continues to be unfair.

Activity

The children will draw a picture showing some of the ways that we can *safely* offer love within forgiveness.

Conclusion

Love is a feeling of strong attachment or liking for another person. We also learned that it is more than just a *feeling*. It is a *decision* to *behave toward others* with respect, kindness, and generosity. In today's lesson, through a study of conflict between our storybook characters, we will learn about love as it relates to forgiveness.

As previously discussed in lessons 7 and 8, anger and sadness are often a natural result of unfairness. Anger and sadness, if permitted to remain, may harden our hearts. The consistent practice of love can help us to once again soften our hearts, to see the deep worth of a person who was unfair, and to forgive.

We can offer love within forgiveness to a person who was unfair and yet remain safe. We do not necessarily enter into a friendship with a person who continues to be unfair. We can *safely* offer love to a person who was unfair by refusing to seek revenge, speak badly about him or her, or harm him or her in anyway. We can *safely* offer love to a person who was unfair by interacting with him or her only in safe situations (when others are present), offering a smile, or a gift.

People with loving hearts, who forgive, can improve entire communities because they persist in seeing the deep worth in all people, even those who are unfair, and treating them with kindness, respect, and generosity.

Lesson 10: Kindness, Respect, and Generosity within Forgiveness

Main Ideas of the Lesson

In lessons 8 and 9 we discussed the difficulties and importance of seeing the deep worth of a person who was unfair and of offering love to him or her because of the anger and sadness that so often follows unfairness. In today's lesson, we will discuss the difficulties and importance of offering kindness (a demonstration of goodness, benevolence, sympathy, respect and grace), respect (treating others as we wish to be treated), and generosity (lavish giving of time, possession, and feelings like love and kindness) to a person who has been unfair. This is not an easy thing to do yet if we persevere, forgiveness may occur.

We can *safely* offer kindness, respect, and generosity. We can refuse to cause harm to the person or to his or her loved ones and property. We can give gifts of time, possessions, and kindness and love when it is safe to do so. We must take special precautions in offering kindness, respect, and generosity to a person who continues to be unfair. Kindness, respect, and generosity, given in the face of unfairness, can improve the quality of life in communities (schools, families, and neighborhoods).

Introduction to the Lesson

Review the main ideas of the previous lesson. Love is a feeling of strong attachment or liking for another person. We also learned that it is more than just a *feeling*. It is a *decision* to *behave toward others* with kindness, respect, and generosity. Anger and sadness are often a natural result of unfairness. Anger and sadness, if permitted to remain, may harden our hearts. The consistent practice of love can help us to once again soften our hearts, to see the deep worth of a person who was unfair, and to forgive. We can *safely* offer love within forgiveness to a person who was unfair.

Introduce today's lesson. Kindness, respect, and generosity toward a person who caused an unfair hurt can help us to forgive.

Show Part Three of the DVD, *The Many Adventures of Winnie the Pooh: "Winnie the Pooh and Tigger Too"*

Ask the students to look for signs of kindness, respect, generosity given to a person who was unfair. Please review the meanings of kindness, respect, and generosity before showing the film.

Discussion Questions

Let's think about the events of this story. Rabbit was happily working in his beautiful garden when all of a sudden along came Tigger!

1. What happened next in the story?
2. Why did Rabbit want to lose Tigger in the woods? *Rabbit was angry.*
3. When Rabbit had the idea to lose Tigger in the woods, was he showing kindness toward Tigger? Why or why not? Was Rabbit showing respect to Tigger? Why or why not? Was Rabbit being generous toward Tigger when he wanted him lost in the woods? Why or why not?
4. In what ways could Rabbit have solved the problem he was having with Tigger *and* treated him with kindness, respect, and generosity?

5. How might Rabbit's kind, respectful, and generous behavior have helped Tigger?
6. When people continue to be unkind, disrespectful and ungenerous, it has a way of spreading anger and sadness. Let's return to our story (see the DVD) where Rabbit insisted that Tigger should not bounce. Please pay careful attention to something very important: Rabbit is the only one smiling. Everyone else is frowning. Unkindness, disrespect, a lack of generosity, and an unforgiving attitude seem to spread anger and sadness. Now, let's take a look at the part where Rabbit seems to forgive—he offers kindness, respect, and generosity by letting Tigger bounce.
7. What happened to the sadness of all those in the Hundred Acre Wood once Rabbit becomes kind, respectful, generous, and forgiving? *Everyone starts smiling and dancing. Happiness spreads throughout the woods.*
8. What happened to Rabbit, in particular, when he became kind, respectful, generous, and forgiving of Tigger? *He smiled for the first time in the story. He was happy for the first time.*
9. Do you sometimes find it difficult to show kindness, respect, or generosity toward a person who has unfairly hurt you? Why or why not?
10. How might you *safely* show kindness, respect, and generosity toward a person who was unfair?
11. Could kindness, respectfulness, and generosity toward a person who was unfair help us forgive? Why or why not?
12. Could those who begin to be kind, respectful, generous, and forgiving make a difference for a whole community? Why? Why not?
13. Please help the children understand that we can *safely* be kind, respectful, and generous toward a person who was unfair, but that it may be necessary to be kind, respectful, and generous from a distance if the person continues in unfairness

Activity

Ask the children to write a letter from Rabbit to Tigger (the children will pretend to be Rabbit as they write the letter). Ask the children to include the following in their letters: (1) Write about your angry feelings (as Rabbit) toward Tigger (please remember you do have a right to the feelings of anger); (2) Explain that these angry feelings became too deep and revenge-filled; (3) Tell Tigger that you see him as a person of deep worth; and, (4) Offer love, kindness, respect, and generosity to Tigger.

Conclusion

Review the main ideas of the lesson. It is difficult, yet important, to offer kindness (a demonstration of goodness, benevolence, sympathy, respect and grace), respect (treating others as we wish to be treated), and generosity (lavish giving of time, possession, and feelings like love and kindness) to a person who has been unfair. This is not an easy thing to do yet, if we persevere, forgiveness may occur. We can *safely* offer kindness, respect, and generosity. We can refuse to cause harm to the person or to his or her loved ones and property. We can give gifts of time, possessions, and kindness and love when it is safe to do so. We must take special precautions in offering kindness, respect, and generosity to a person who continues to be unfair. Kindness, respect, and generosity, given in the face of unfairness, can improve the quality of life in communities (schools, families, and neighborhoods).

Lesson 11: Understanding Our Feelings

Main Ideas of the Lesson

In today's lesson, the children will learn about feelings (emotions) such as happiness, sadness, love, hate, anger, fear, peace, and so forth. We are especially interested in exploring those feelings connected with unfairness (anger and sadness). Forgiveness can help reduce theses emotions.

Webster's dictionary defines a feeling (emotion) as: "An affective state of consciousness in which joy, sorrow, fear, hate or the like is experienced; any agitated or intense state of mind, usually with concurrent physiological changes." Feelings can be pleasant or unpleasant and can bring forth positive or negative outcomes.

Anger is defined as a violent or revenge-seeking feeling often caused by unfairness. It can vary in depth from light to very deep and in length from short-lived to long-lasting. Anger is a healthy response to unfairness. Anger that is short-lived may actually protect us from further hurt and unfairness. Anger that does not leave or that deepens, on the other hand, can cause damage to our overall health, damage our relationships, and may even cause hurt to other people and property.

Sadness is marked by sorrow or unhappiness. Webster defines sorrow as, "anguish, mental suffering, or an expression of grief."

The children will begin learning in this lesson to forgive *for themselves* a person who was unfair. They will *privately* identify a person who treated them unfairly. *It is very important that each child's self-identified hurt remains absolutely private if this is in a classroom context.* Counselors should use their discretion if this is a counseling group activity. If the child was hurt numerous times by the same person, he or she should focus on *one* specific hurt. The children will continue to focus on this self-identified hurt in lessons 12, 13, 14, and 15.

Please remember that forgiveness is a choice. It is important that the children are given the freedom to decide when and if they are actually ready to forgive the person who was unfair.

Introduction to the Lesson

Review the main ideas of lesson 10. It is difficult, yet important, to offer kindness (a demonstration of goodness, benevolence, sympathy, respect and grace), respect (treating others as we wish to be treated), and generosity (lavish giving of time, possession, and feelings like love and kindness) to a person who has been unfair. This is not an easy thing to do yet, if we persevere, forgiveness may occur. We can *safely* offer kindness, respect, and generosity. We can refuse to cause harm to the person or to his or her loved ones and property. We can give gifts of time, possessions, and kindness and love when it is safe to do so. We must take special precautions in offering kindness, respect, and generosity to a person who continues to be unfair. Kindness, respect, and generosity, given in the face of unfairness, can improve the quality of life in communities (schools, families, and neighborhoods).

Tell the children that today they will learn about feelings. Feelings are a natural part of being human. Some feelings are pleasant (happiness, love, and peace). Some feelings are unpleasant (anger, sadness, or hate). Feelings themselves are not good or bad, but they may move us to act in good or bad ways. For example, when we are happy we often treat others with kindness and respect. When we are angry, we often hurt ourselves, others, or property. Sometimes we are just a little bit angry and sometimes we are very, very angry. Sometimes we are angry for a short time (a few minutes) or sometimes we are angry for a long, long time (days, weeks, months, or even years).

We will spend extra time in this lesson and the next talking about those feelings that follow unfairness (anger and sadness) because forgiveness can help both anger and sadness fade. Today is the first time they will begin learning *how* to forgive a person who treated them unfairly.

Ask the following questions.

1. What are feelings? What are some examples of feelings?
2. What is anger? Anger is a violent or revenge-seeking feeling often caused by unfairness. It can vary in depth from light to very deep and in length from short-lived to long-lasting.
3. What is sadness? *Sorrow or unhappiness.*
4. How do you feel when a person treats you unfairly (with unkindness or disrespect)? *Angry. Sad.*

Please note that today's lesson deviates from our usual pattern where we read a story, have a discussion, and then do an activity. We will instead read one section (there are four sections) at a time from the book written by Michaelene Mundy titled, *Mad Isn't Bad* and have a discussion following each section. We will then do the activity, "My Garden of Feelings."

Read the Section, "Mad Isn't Bad"

Discussion Questions

1. In today's story, we are learning about feelings, especially the feeling of anger. What are some of the feelings you've felt today? *Happiness, sadness, anger, love, or disappointment (or many others).*
2. Which feelings are pleasant (good)? Why are these feelings pleasant to you?
3. Which feelings are unpleasant (not so good)? Why are these feelings unpleasant to you?
4. Describe how it feels to be *angry. Cold inside. Anger can make us feel energized (temporarily).*
5. Describe how it feels to be *sad. Sadness can make us feel tired.*
6. Describe how *love* feels? *Happy. Warm inside.*
7. Might there ever be a time when anger is a good thing? When we've been treated unfairly. Why? It may protect us from further hurt.

Read the Section Titled, "What Makes You Mad?"

Discussion Questions

1. What are some things that might make you angry (mad)? Why might these things make you angry?
2. Angry feelings can be big or little. What are some things that might make you a little bit angry? What are some things that might make you very angry?
3. Angry feelings can last for a short time or for a long time. What are some things that might cause you to have anger that lasts for a short time? What are some things that might cause you to have anger that lasts for a long time?
4. Why might it help to know the cause of your anger?

Read the Section Titled, "What Does 'Mad' Feel Like?"

Discussion Questions

1. What does it feel like to be angry? When angry, you might feel like yelling, hitting, or running. You might feel stronger. You might feel more awake.

2. Sometimes people feel stronger when angry. Does anger really make you stronger? *No. Our strength can actually become less when angry for a long, long time.*

3. Sometimes people feel like they have more energy when angry. Does anger really make you have more energy? *No. We may feel more tired and lose energy if angry for a long time.*

4. Is it wrong or bad to feel angry or sad? Why? Why not? *No. Anger and sadness are just feelings. Feeling sad or angry for a short period of time is not harmful. It is our actions that are good or bad.*

Read the Section Titled, "Not-So-Good Ways to Let Out Anger"

Discussion Questions

1. Feelings can affect how we choose to behave. How do you behave when you are angry? How do you treat yourself and others? Why do you treat yourself and others in this way when angry?

2. How do you behave when you are sad? How do you treat yourself and others? Why do you treat yourself and others in this way when sad?

3. How do you treat yourself and others when you are happy? Why?

4. Do you think that you can choose to treat yourself and others with kindness and respect even if you are angry or sad?

5. What are some ways that could be harmful to let our anger out? *Hitting others. Destroying property. Yelling unkind things at people.*

6. What are some safe ways to get rid of anger? Talk with another person. Draw a picture. Play a game of football. Sing a song. Talk to a friend. Forgive.

Activity

The following activity *should not be skipped.* The children will identify a person who treated them unfairly. *Please tell the children that this activity is absolutely* private *and will not be discussed with others.* Again, counselors should use their discretion if this is a counseling group activity.

Begin the activity by saying, "We are now going to each think about a time when we were treated very unfairly. What does it mean to be 'treated very unfairly'? Now, please think of a time when a person was very unfair to you, a time when someone hurt you so deeply that you thought it was one of the most unfair things that ever happened to you. This should be an unfairness that hurt you—making you angry or sad on the inside (not a physical hurt). Do you have a person and an unfair situation in mind? Are you still angry with this person? If you are no longer angry with this person, please select a different unfairness."

Ask the children to think about this unfairness and to answer the following questions *privately.* The children's responses to the questions will not be discussed with one another.

1. When did this unfairness happen? Was it morning, afternoon, or evening?

2. What kind of a day was it?

3. Where were you when you were treated unfairly?

4. Who treated you unfairly? What did he or she do that was unfair?

5. Can you picture the person at the time of the unfairness? What was he or she wearing? Was he or she angry? Did he or she say unkind words?

6. How did you react at that time to the person who was unfair? Were you angry? Were you sad? What did you say? What did you do?

Please tell the children that they will continue to focus on this person and this unfairness in the remaining forgiveness lessons.

Conclusion

Conclude by summarizing the main points of the lesson. There are many different kinds of feelings (happiness, sadness, love, hate, anger, fear, peace, and many others). Feelings can be pleasant or unpleasant and can cause us to behave in either good or bad ways.

Feelings that can be helped by forgiveness are anger and sadness. Anger is a violent or revenge-seeking feeling often caused by unfairness. It can vary in depth from light to very deep and in length from short-lived to long-lasting. Anger is a healthy response to unfairness. At those times when we are feeling angry it is important that we choose to continue treating ourselves, others, and property with respect. Short-lived anger often serves to protect us from further hurt and unfairness. Long-lasting anger, on the other hand, can cause damage to our overall health, our relationships, and even to other people and property.

Sadness is marked by sorrow (anguish, mental suffering, or grief) or unhappiness.

Lesson 12: Forgiveness Can Set You Free from Anger

Main Ideas of the Lesson

In this lesson, we will discuss anger within the context of each student's unfair hurt that was privately identified in the activity section of lesson 11. In the day-to-day course of interacting with others, unfair and personal hurts often occur. Anger is a natural and healthy response to unfair hurts, but if that anger begins to live in the person's heart, an even deeper hurt may occur. Long-term and deep anger can damage a person's overall health and hurt relationships. Forgiveness can help to reduce anger.

In this lesson, the children will begin to explore their personal level of anger toward the person who caused them an unfair hurt. This is the hurt identified in the previous lesson.

Please remember that forgiveness is a choice. It is important that the children are given the freedom to decide when and if they are actually ready to forgive the person who was unfair.

Introduction to the Lesson

Review the main ideas of lesson 11. There are many different kinds of feelings (happiness, sadness, love, hate, anger, fear, peace, and many others). Feelings can be pleasant or unpleasant and can cause us to behave in either good or bad ways.

Feelings that can be helped by forgiveness are anger and sadness. Anger is a violent or revenge-seeking feeling often caused by unfairness. It can vary in depth from light to very deep and in length from short-lived to long-lasting. Anger is a healthy response to unfairness. Short-lived anger often serves to protect us from further hurt and unfairness. Long-lasting anger, on the other hand, can cause damage to our overall health, our relationships, and even to other people and property.

Sadness is marked by sorrow (anguish, mental suffering, or grief) or unhappiness.

Please tell the children that in today's lesson, we are going to continue our discussion of anger. As was the case in Lesson Eleven, today's lesson deviates from our usual pattern where we read a story, have a discussion, and then do an activity. We will instead read one section at a time from the book written by Michaelene Mundy entitled, *Mad Isn't Bad* and have a discussion following each section. We will then do the activity, "My Garden of Feelings."

Read the "Why You Need to Let Out Your Anger" Section

As with lesson 11, there are four sets of discussion questions. Please read each assigned reading and follow immediately with a discussion.

Discussion Questions

Please think about the same unfair hurt that you thought about in lesson 11 as you answer *privately* the following questions (you will not talk about this unfair hurt with others).

1. How angry are you with the person who treated you unfairly? Do you have a big anger or a little anger? Have you been angry for a short time or a long time?
2. Do you have a right to be angry with the person? Why or why not?
3. Could your anger keep you safe from being unfairly hurt again? How?
4. What might happen to you if you stay deeply angry for a long time? *Ruined relationships. Less healthy.* Why?

Read, "You Can Choose What to Do"

Discussion Questions

It is true that we can all choose how to behave when we've been treated unfairly. Think about the way you behaved when the person was unfair to you.

1. What did you say or do when the person treated you unfairly?
2. Did your words or actions make you feel *better* inside or *worse* inside? Why?
3. If your words or actions made you feel worse inside, what might you have said or done instead?
4. Deep and long-lasting anger can cause more hurt. How? Who could be hurt by deep and long-lasting anger? *Family members, friends, teachers, or ourselves.*

Read, "Get Help from Caring Adults"

Discussion Questions

It is often helpful to talk with caring adults when we have been unfairly hurt.

1. Is there an adult that you can talk to about your angry (or sad) feelings?
2. Have you talked to an adult about this hurt that we've been thinking about? How did it make you feel? Was he or she able to help you feel a little less angry?

Discussion Questions

We will not be reading the final section titled, "Forgiving Others—and Yourself" because it covers too many ideas that are not directly relevant to this particular lesson (forgiveness from God, forgiving oneself). We believe it will be more beneficial for the children if we remain focused on the topic of person-to-person forgiveness.

1. Have you considered forgiving the person who unfairly hurt you?
2. What might happen to your anger if you consider forgiving the person who was unfair? Why or why not?

Activity

The following activity should not be skipped.

The children will draw a picture called, "My Garden of Feelings."[3]

They can draw a flower, vegetable, or fruit garden. Tell the children, "Today you are going to draw a picture of a garden. This garden will be a way for you to 'show with a picture' how you feel inside. For example, if the plants in your garden are all mixed together, scattered with weeds, and colored in browns, blacks, and other dark colors—perhaps, you are feeling sad, confused, or angry. On the other hand, if the flowers, vegetables, or fruit in your garden are neatly arranged with bright colors (blues, purples, or yellows), perhaps you are feeling happy, peaceful, or energetic. If you are feeling somewhere in between the pleasant feelings and the unpleasant feelings, your garden may be a mixture of brown, black, yellow, green, blue, and other colors."

After the children have finished their pictures say, "Please look at your picture. Look at the colors you used. Look at how the plants, flowers, or vegetables are placed in your garden. How were you feeling as you drew the picture of your garden? How are you feeling now?" Please tell the children that if they are feeling sad or angry, they should talk to an adult about these feelings. The children will not discuss their feelings with the class. They will look at their pictures and think privately about their feelings.

Conclusion

Conclude by summarizing the main points of the lesson. It is common to feel angry after unfairness. We can feel angry and yet choose not to harm ourselves, others, or property. We have a right to feel angry when someone has unfairly hurt us. Yet, if we keep that anger inside of us, it may cause deeper hurt (it can make us feel sick, hurt other people, or hurt our relationships). Forgiveness can help us to feel less angry toward a person who causes us hurt.

Lesson 13: Exploring Forgiveness

Main Ideas of the Lesson

In today's lesson, we will once again discuss what forgiveness is and is not. A clear understanding of forgiveness is important in learning to forgive.

Following is the definition of forgiveness, "When unjustly hurt by another, we forgive when we overcome the resentment toward the offender, not by denying our right to the resentment, but instead by trying to offer the wrongdoer compassion, benevolence, and love; as we give these, we as forgivers realize that the offender does not necessarily have a right to such gifts."[4] As discussed in lesson 7, the person who forgives works to see that the person who behaved unfairly has deep worth, softens the heart in love, and becomes ready to give gifts of kindness, respect, and generosity.

When we forgive, we do not excuse, condone, deny, pretend, or forget (we see the person who was unfair in a different way) the unfairness. We acknowledge that the person's behavior was, is, and will always be unfair.

Forgiveness is not the same as reconciliation. When we reconcile with a person, two people once again come together in friendship. Forgiveness involves an internal change of heart. Forgiveness can occur without reconciliation. It is unlikely that true reconciliation can occur without forgiveness.

Forgiveness often restores relationships, reduces anger and sadness, and increases hopefulness and self-esteem. Please remember that forgiveness is a choice. It is important that the children are given the freedom to decide when and if they are actually ready to forgive the person who was unfair. We can forgive without putting ourselves at risk to be hurt again.

Introduction to the Lesson

Review the main ideas of lesson 12. We often feel angry when we've been treated unfairly. At those times when we are feeling angry it is important that we choose to continue treating ourselves, others, and property with respect. We have a right to feel angry when someone has unfairly hurt us. Yet, if we keep that anger inside of us, it may cause deeper hurt (it can make us feel sick, hurt other people, or hurt our relationships). Forgiveness can help us to feel less angry toward a person who causes us hurt.

Tell the children, "Today we are going to once again think about what forgiveness is and is not. Think back to lesson 7 where we learned what forgiveness is and is not? What did you learn forgiveness is? *Forgiveness is letting go of anger toward a person who was unfair, seeing that he or she has deep worth, softening our hearts in love, and becoming ready to offer gifts of kindness, respect, and generosity.*"

Read or Watch the Selected Story

In today's lesson, you may choose one of the children's favorite stories that were used in lessons 1 through 10 to teach what forgiveness is and is not.

Discussion Questions

1. What happened in today's story?
2. Was any person treated unfairly? If so, what happened that was unfair?
3. Are there any signs that the person who was treated unfairly began to forgive the person who behaved unfairly? What are these signs?

4. How did the person who was treated unfairly seem to think, act, and feel toward the one who was unfair?
5. Forgiveness is not excusing a person's unfair behavior or saying that their unfairness was all right. Did the person who was treated unfairly make excuses for the unfair behavior or say that the unfairness was all right?
6. Forgiveness is not pretending or denying that the unfairness happened. Did the person who was treated unfairly pretend or deny that the hurt happened?
7. Forgiveness is not forgetting the hurt. Did the person who was treated unfairly forget the hurt?
8. Forgiveness does not always mean that we come back together with a person who was unfair. Did the person who was unfairly hurt come back together in friendship with the person who behaved unfairly?
9. Should a person ever be forced to forgive? Why or why not?
10. Why might forgiveness be a good choice?

Activity

Ask the children to think about the same unfair hurt that they identified in lesson 11 as they reflect *privately* on the following questions.

1. Do you still think that the person's behavior was unfair? Why or why not?
2. Do you have a little bit of anger or a lot of anger toward the person?
3. Have you excused, pretended, denied, or forgot the unfairness? Why might it be dangerous to excuse, pretend, deny, or forget unfairness?
4. Would you consider forgiving the person who was unfair? Why or why not?
5. Can you forgive a person without being put at risk to be hurt again? Why or why not? *We can forgive without entering into a friendship with the person who was unfair.*

Conclusion

Review the main ideas of the lesson. The person who forgives works to see that the person who behaved unfairly has deep worth, softens the heart in love, and becomes ready to give gifts of kindness, respect, and generosity.

When we forgive, we do not excuse, condone, deny, pretend, or forget (we see the person who was unfair in a different way) the unfairness. We acknowledge that the person's behavior was, is, and will always be unfair.

Forgiveness is not reconciliation. Forgiveness involves an internal change of heart. Reconciliation involves two people coming together in friendship.

Forgiveness often restores relationships, reduces anger and sadness, and increases hopefulness and self-esteem. Forgiveness is a choice.

Lesson 14: A Fresh Look at a Person Who Was Unfair

Main Ideas of the Lesson

In today's lesson, the children will learn that if they can begin to see that the person who unfairly hurt them has deep worth, they may become ready to forgive. We will refer to this process of seeing the deep worth of our offenders as "seeing with new eyes." Lewis Smedes first used this phrase in his book, *Forgive and Forget*. We can work to see the deep worth of those who have been unfair even when angry.

We can "see with new eyes" a person who was unfair and acknowledge their deep worth without being put at risk to be hurt again by the same person.

Introduction to the Lesson

Review the main ideas of the previous lesson. The person who forgives works to see that the person who behaved unfairly has deep worth, softens the heart in love, and becomes ready to give gifts of kindness, respect, and generosity. Forgiveness is not excusing, condoning, denying, pretending, or forgetting (we see the person who was unfair in a different way) the unfairness. We acknowledge that the person's behavior was, is, and will always be unfair. When we forgive, we do not automatically come back together with the person in friendship. Forgiveness involves an internal change of heart. Forgiveness often restores relationships, reduces anger and sadness, and increases hopefulness and self-esteem. Forgiveness is a choice. We can forgive without putting ourselves at risk to be hurt again.

Review the Story (Lesson 7), *You're Not My Best Friend Anymore*

Discussion Questions

Ben and Molly had a big fight over which tent to buy with their saved money. Molly wanted a pup tent. Ben wanted an umbrella tent. They said unkind things to one another. Ben was angry. Molly was angry. They didn't talk for four days.

1. Did Ben see Molly "with new eyes" at first after she behaved unfairly? Why do you think this?
2. What does it mean to "see with new eyes"? *It means to see a person's deep worth. We see that the person has at times been kind and good.*
3. Did Molly see Ben "with new eyes" at first after he behaved unfairly? Why do you think this?
4. How was Ben seeing Molly by the time the party was over? How do you know?
5. How was Molly seeing Ben by the time the party was over? How do you know?
6. Why do you think Molly and Ben were able to move from deep anger with one another to softened hearts? *They realized that the fighting was not a wise thing to do. They thought about one another apart from their unfairness.*
7. What was Ben showing toward Molly when he offered to buy a pup tent? *Love and forgiveness.* What was Molly showing toward Ben when she offered to buy an umbrella tent? *Love and forgiveness.*
8. Do you think it was easy for Molly *at first* to see Ben's deep worth?

9. Do you think that it was easy for Ben *at first* to see Molly's worth?
10. How is it possible to show love and forgiveness toward a person who was unfair?
11. Are you ready to begin working so that you can "see with new eyes" those people who unfairly hurt you? Why or why not?
12. Can you begin to "see with new eyes" those who are unfair without being put at risk to be hurt again? Why or why not? *We can see a person's worth without entering into a friendship with the person.*

Activity

The children will learn to "see with new eyes" the person who treated them unfairly. This is the same unfair hurt previously identified by the children in lesson 11.

Together with the children, select a window in the classroom that will be referred to as a "Forgiveness Window." We will pretend that this window can help us to "see with new eyes" our great big world. We will pretend that this window can help us to "see with new eyes" the person who treated us unfairly. If there is no window, the children can make a pretend "Forgiveness Window" out of paper.

Tell the children, "Think about the person who hurt you. This is the same hurt you've been thinking about in lessons 11, 12, and 13. Please answer the following questions *silently and privately.*

1. How did you feel following the unfairness?
2. How are you feeling now about the unfairness?
3. Were you able to see the person's deep worth right after the unfairness? Why or why not?
4. Are you able to see that the person has deep worth now? Why or why not?
5. Did you feel love in your heart toward the person *right after he or she hurt you?* Why or why not?"

Please help the children understand that it is perfectly fine if they are not yet able to see the person's has deep worth. Forgiveness is a process. Each person must be allowed to go through forgiveness in his or her own time and at his or her own pace.

Following the silent and private reflection on the questions listed above, ask the children to go to the "Forgiveness Window." Remind the children that we are pretending that this window can help us to "see with new eyes" the great big world in which we live. Remind the children that we are pretending that this "Forgiveness Window" can help us to "see with new eyes" the person who treated us unfairly. It can help us to see clearly the deep worth of him or her. Tell the children that this window can help us to widen our view of the world. It can help us to widen our view of the person who was unfair. Sometimes when we are unfairly hurt, we begin think the world is unkind. Sometimes when we are hurt, we begin to think that all people are unkind. We may think that the person who behaved unfairly does not have any worth. We may live in a smaller world of anger and sadness. The "Forgiveness Window" can help us to see the world in a different way. As we look through the window, we can see the beauty of the world and the goodness of people. The "Forgiveness Window" can help us to see the person who unfairly hurt us in a different way. Let us now look through the window and begin to "see with new eyes." Let us see the person who unfairly hurt us in new ways. How are you now seeing the person who hurt you? Has this person ever shown kindness, respect, or generosity to you? What did he or she do that was kind? Was this person tired or upset at the time of the unfairness? If you can now see that the person has, at times, been kind, respectful, or generous, that does not now mean that the unfairness did not happen. The behavior was unfair even if you are now able to see his or her deep worth.

Conclude by asking the children the following question, "If you are now able to see that the person has deep worth even though he or she behaved unfairly, are your feelings changing toward the person? Are you beginning to feel more love and forgiveness toward the person?"

Conclusion

Forgiveness allows us to "see with new eyes" a person who was unfair. It helps us to offer love to him or her. We can safely see the deep worth of a person as we forgive.

Lesson 15: Forgiveness Gifts

Main Ideas of the Lesson

Thus far the children have learned that as we "see with new eyes" the worth of those who have behaved unfairly, forgiveness can occur. They've learned that through this process people's hearts, once hardened with anger, often become soft and loving. In today's lesson, the children will learn that forgiveness can be deepened as people become ready to give gifts of kindness, respect, and generosity to those who have been unfair.

Kindness, respect (treating others as we would like to be treated), and generosity (a lavish outpouring) to a person who has behaved unfairly can be very difficult. The process of seeing the offender's deep worth and maintaining a softened heart toward him or her can help one become ready to give the gifts of kindness, respect, and generosity.

Please continue to be patient with the children's readiness to forgive. It is likely that each child will be at a different point in their willingness to offer gifts to the person who was unfair. Kindness, respect, and generosity to a person who was unfair is not an easy thing to do and the ability to give them may depend on the depth of the hurt and the time that has passed since the unfairness. We have learned through many years of experience that people do eventually become ready to offer kindness, respect, and generosity through forgiveness. It may take a month, six months, or even a year for this to happen. Forgiveness is a choice. Every person must be allowed to forgive (and to give gifts within forgiveness) in his or her own time and his or her own way. The children can safely offer gifts of kindness, respect, and generosity to a person who was unfair.

As with the previous lessons where the children were learning to forgive for themselves, they will continue to focus on the one specific person who caused them an unfair hurt. The children will be encouraged to deepen their forgiveness by giving gifts of kindness, respect, and generosity.

Introduction

Please review the main ideas of lesson 14. If people can begin to see that the person who unfairly hurt them has deep worth, they may become ready to forgive. We will refer to this process of seeing the deep worth of our offenders as, "seeing with new eyes." We can "see with new eyes" a person who was unfair and acknowledge their deep worth without being put at risk to be hurt again by the same person.

Discussion Questions

1. In the story, *You're Not My Best Friend Anymore,* Ben and Molly were angry with one another. Why were they angry?
2. We know that eventually Ben and Molly began to see the other's worth. Eventually their hearts began to soften toward one another. Did Ben become ready to give a gift to Molly? What was his gift to her? Did Molly become ready to give a gift to Ben? What was her gift to Ben?
3. Did Molly or Ben become ready to give a gift of kindness, respect, or generosity? In what ways?
4. Were Ben and Molly able to give a gift of kindness, respect, and generosity without putting themselves in danger of being hurt again? Why or why not?
5. Do you think you would be able to give such gifts to a person who had treated you unfairly? Why or why not?

6. What are some ways that you could *safely* show kindness?
7. How might you *safely* show respect?
8. What are some ways to *safely* be generous to him or her?

Activity

The children will once again think about the person who treated him or her unfairly. Please tell the children that they are going to learn how to deepen forgiveness. They are going to learn about the kinds of gifts that can *safely* be given to a person who was unfair. Ask the children to *silently and privately* answer the following questions.

1. How are you now thinking about the person who was unfair? Do you see that the person has deep worth? Why or why not? It is all right if you are not yet ready to see his or her deep worth. You may see it in time.
2. How are you now feeling about the person? Do you have a softened and loving heart toward the person? Why or why not? It is all right if you are not yet ready to have a softened heart. You may feel loving toward him or her in time.
3. If you see the person's deep worth and have softened hearts toward him or her, are you ready to offer kindness? Why or why not?
4. What are some ways you could safely show kindness to the person?
5. What are some ways you could safely show respect to the person?
6. How could you safely show generosity toward the one who hurt you?

Conclusion

Thus far the children have learned that as we "see with new eyes" the worth of those who have behaved unfairly, forgiveness can occur. They've learned that through this process people's hearts, once hardened with anger, often become soft and loving. In today's lesson, the children will learn that forgiveness can be deepened as people become ready to give gifts of kindness, respect, and generosity to those who have been unfair.

Kindness, respect (treating others as we would like to be treated), and generosity (a lavish outpouring) to a person who has behaved unfairly can be very difficult. The process of seeing the offender's deep worth and maintaining a softened heart toward him or her can help one become ready to give the gifts of kindness, respect, and generosity.

Please continue to be patient with the children's readiness to forgive. It is likely that each child will be at a different point in their willingness to offer gifts to the person who was unfair. Kindness, respect, and generosity to a person who was unfair is not an easy thing to do and the ability to give them may depend on the depth of the hurt and the time that has passed since the unfairness. We have learned through many years of experience that people do eventually become ready to offer kindness, respect, and generosity through forgiveness. It may take a month, six months, or even a year for this to happen. Forgiveness is a choice. Every person must be allowed to forgive (and to give gifts within forgiveness) in his or her own time and his or her own way. The children can safely offer gifts of kindness, respect, and generosity to a person who was unfair.

As with the previous lessons where the children were learning to forgive for themselves, they will continue to focus on the one specific person who caused them an unfair hurt. The children will be encouraged to deepen their forgiveness by giving gifts of kindness, respect, and generosity.

This is the final lesson in our *Discovering Forgiveness* curriculum. We ask that you continue to keep the idea of forgiveness in front of the children even though their formal training through regularly scheduled stories, discussions, and activities is now over. *Congratulations! We expect the children (and you as their guide) will reap unexpected fruit from your efforts to forgive.*

Notes

1. Robert D. Enright, *Forgiveness Is a Choice* (2001), p. 25.
2. Robert D. Enright, *Forgiveness Is a Choice* (2001), p. 25.
3. The "My Garden of Feelings" activity was inspired by Anthony Holter, a former teacher in the United States and a graduate student at the University of Wisconsin–Madison.
4. Robert D. Enright, *Forgiveness Is a Choice* (2001), p. 25.

References

Al-Mabuk, R. H., Enright, R. D., & Cardis, P. (1995). Forgiveness education with parentally love-deprived late adolescents. *Journal of Moral Education, 24,* 427–443.

Baskin, T. W., & Enright, R. D. (2004). Intervention studies of forgiveness: A meta-analysis. *Journal of Counseling and Development, 82,* 79–90.

Coyle, C. T., & Enright, R. D. (1997). Forgiveness intervention with postabortion men. *Journal of Counseling and Clinical Psychology, 65,* 1042–1046.

Enright, R. D., & Fitzgibbons, R. P. (2000). *Helping clients forgive: An empirical guide for resolving anger and restoring hope.* Washington, DC: American Psychological Association.

Enright, R. D., Knutson Enright, J. A., Holter, A. C., Baskin, T., & Knutson, C. (2007). Waging peace through forgiveness in Belfast, Northern Ireland: Educational programs for mental health improvement of children. Manuscript submitted for publication.

Freedman, S. R., & Enright, R. D. (1996). Forgiveness as an intervention goal with incest survivors. *Journal of Counseling and Clinical Psychology, 64,* 983–992.

Hebl, J. H., & Enright, R. D. (1993). Forgiveness as a psychotherapeutic goal with elderly females. *Psychotherapy, 30,* 658–667.

Lin, W. F., Mack, D., Enright, R. D., Krahn, D., & Baskin, T. (2004). Effects of forgiveness therapy on anger, mood, and vulnerability to substance use among inpatient substance-dependent clients. *Journal of Consulting and Clinical Psychology, 72*(6), 1114–1121.

Lipsey, M. W. (1990). *Design sensitivity: Statistical power for experimental research.* Vewbury Park, CA: Sage.

McCullough, M. E., Worthington, E. L., Jr., & Rachal, K. C. (1997). Interpersonal forgiving in close relationships. *Journal of Personality and Social Psychology, 73,* 321–336.

Park, J. H. (2003). Validating a forgiveness education program for adolescent female aggressive victims in Korea. Unpublished doctoral dissertation. University of Wisconsin–Madison.

Reed, G. & Enright, R. D. (2006). The effects of forgiveness therapy on depression, anxiety, and posttraumatic stress for women after spousal emotional abuse. *Journal of Consulting and Clinical Psychology, 74,* 920–929.

Rye, M. S., Pargament, K. I., Pan, W., Yingling, D. W., Shogren, K. A., & Ito, M. (2005). Can group interventions facilitate forgiveness of an ex-spouse? A randomized clinical trial. *Journal of Consulting and Clinical Psychology, 73,* 880–892.

Worthington, E. L., Jr. (Ed.). (2005). *Handbook of forgiveness.* New York: Brunner/Routledge.

Part III

Treatment Manuals for
Clinical Problems

Chapter 11

Cognitive-Behavioral Treatment for Child and Adolescent Anxiety: The *Coping Cat Program*

Rinad S. Beidas, MA, Jennifer L. Podell, MA, and Philip C. Kendall, PhD, ABPP

Rinad S. Beidas, MA, Jennifer L. Podell, MA, and Philip C. Kendall, PhD, ABPP

RATIONALE AND DEVELOPMENT OF TREATMENT

Anxiety disorders are common psychological disorders experienced by youth (Warren & Messer, 1999), with reported rates of 10–20% in the general population and primary care settings (Chavira, Stein, Bailey, & Stein, 2004; Costello, Mustillo, Keeler, & Angold, 2004). Anxiety disorders in youth include generalized anxiety disorder (GAD), social phobia (SP), separation anxiety disorder (SAD), specific phobias, obsessive-compulsive disorder (OCD), and post-traumatic stress disorder (PTSD) (APA, 1994). In this chapter, we focus on treatment for the three main youth anxiety disorders: GAD, SP, and SAD.

Most anxiety disorders do not abate with time and if left untreated are linked to impairments into adulthood. Research indicates that anxious children experience related difficulties both socially (Strauss, Forehand, Smith, & Frame, 1986; Greco & Morris, 2005) and academically (King & Ollendick, 1989; Van

Amerigen, Manicini, & Farvolden, 2003). Additionally, anxiety disorders in youth are associated with psychopathology in adulthood such as subsequent anxiety disorders, depression, and substance abuse (Kendall, Safford, Flannery-Schroeder, & Webb, 2004). The consequences of untreated anxiety disorders in youth highlight the need for early intervention.

Cognitive-behavioral treatment (CBT) combines behavioral strategies (e.g., modeling, relaxation, in vivo exposures, and contingency maintenance) with cognitive strategies (e.g., problem-solving, appraisal of personal abilities and perceived threat). One structured version of CBT for youth anxiety which we have developed and researched is the *Coping Cat Program* which follows a therapist treatment manual (Kendall & Hedtke, 2006a) and uses a client workbook (Kendall & Hedtke, 2006b). This chapter summarizes the main components and strategies of the treatment manual. For added details (e.g., step by step administration procedures, "tips from the trenches") we recommend consulting the full manual and workbook

(Kendall & Hedtke, 2006a, 2006b; www.Workbook Publishing.com).

EVIDENCE FOR TREATMENT

CBT for youth anxiety disorders (i.e., the *Coping Cat Program* and variants of it) have been found to be effective in several randomized clinical trials conducted in the United States (Kendall, 1994; Kendall et al., 1997). Additional evidence for the efficacy of CBT has been provided by researchers in Australia (Barrett, Dadds, & Rapee, 1996), Canada (Manassis et al., 2002) and the Netherlands (Nauta, Scholing, & Emmelkamp, 2003). The results of these trials suggest that approximately 50–72% of children with anxiety disorders (i.e., GAD, SP, and/or SAD) who receive CBT no longer meet criteria for their presenting anxiety disorder following treatment.

Therapeutic gains have also been found to be maintained up to seven years posttreatment. In two follow-up studies of different samples of anxious youth (3.35 and 7.4 years after treatment), 80–90% of successfully treated children still did not meet criteria for their presenting anxiety disorder (Kendall & Southam-Gerow, 1996; Kendall et al., 2004). Reviews of this literature, applying Chambless and Hollon's (1998) criteria for evidence-based treatments, conclude that CBT for youth with anxiety disorders is efficacious (Albano & Kendall, 2002; Kazdin & Weisz, 1998; Ollendick & King, 1998).

INTRODUCTION TO THE TREATMENT PROTOCOL

The *Coping Cat* (Kendall & Hedtke, 2006a, 2006b) is a 16 session program of CBT for youth (aged 8–13), with GAD, SAD, and/or SP. The therapist manual (Kendall & Hedtke, 2006a) and client workbook (Kendall & Hedtke, 2006b) are used together: the manual guides the treatment, whereas the workbook contains client tasks which correspond sequentially with the treatment.

The *Coping Cat*, as in CBT, represents a synthesis of behavioral and cognitive strategies. Understanding social influences (e.g., family, peer) and the teaching of emotional management skills are also addressed.

The *Coping Cat* has two sections: the first focuses on psychoeducation, whereas the second emphasizes exposure to anxiety provoking situations. The first eight sessions focus on helping the child learn to identify when she is feeling anxious as well as an introduction of strategies to manage or ameliorate anxiety. These strategies are presented to the child as a tool set that she may carry with her and draw from when she is feeling anxious. The strategies include: identifying bodily arousal, engaging in relaxation, recognizing anxious thoughts, and problem-solving. These skills are taught in a sequence that allows the child to build skill upon skill. The last eight sessions focus on exposing the child to anxiety provoking situations (using a fear hierarchy) while using the skills the child has learned in the first eight sessions. Throughout, the therapist is a "coach," teaching the child the necessary skills and guiding the child to practice the skills.

It is important that the therapist be a 'coping model' for the child throughout treatment. A mastery model demonstrates success, whereas a coping model demonstrates the initial problem, a strategy to overcome the problem and then success. The therapist is a coping model by demonstrating anxiety, strategies that help one cope with the anxiety, and then success. The child participates with the therapist in role playing and the child is encouraged to role play scenes alone, practicing newly acquired skills.

Four important concepts are presented to the child in sequence. First, the child is taught to recognize how her body responds to anxiety. Second, the child learns to recognize anxious thoughts and expectations that she might have. Third, the child is taught ways to combat anxious thoughts and expectations through strategies such as problem-solving and coping thoughts. Fourth, the child is introduced to rewarding herself for partial or full success when facing anxiety provoking situations. These four concepts are presented in the education phase of treatment using a mnemonic FEAR, where F = Feeling Frightened? E = Expecting bad things to happen? A = Attitudes and Actions that can help and R = Results and Rewards.

After learning the FEAR plan during the psychoeducation portion of treatment, the child embarks upon the exposure tasks to practice the plan during anxiety provoking situations. The situations are individual to each child based on the child's specific anxieties. For example, exposure tasks for a male with social phobia (e.g., meeting a new peer) would be very different than exposure tasks for a female with separation anxiety (e.g., dealing with autonomy from parents). The exposure tasks are sequential: earlier exposure tasks (e.g., Session 10) are less anxiety provoking than later exposure tasks (e.g., Session 15). The last session includes the presentation of a child-created 'commercial' which gives the child a chance to show off the skills she has learned in treatment.

ISSUES TO CONSIDER WHEN CONDUCTING THE INTERVENTION

Clinicians and researchers have asked and researchers have investigated whether demographic variables (e.g., age, gender, socioeconomic status, comorbidity) affect treatment outcome. Let us consider each.

Age

The *Coping Cat Program* (Kendall & Hedtke, 2006a) is designed/recommended for children ages 7–13. For treatment of anxiety disorders in younger children (ages 4–7), please see the *Kiddie Cat* (Hughes, Hedtke, Flannery-Schroeder, & Kendall, 2005). For treatment of anxiety disorders in adolescents (ages 13–18), see the *C.A.T. Project Manual* (Kendall, Choudhury, Hudson & Webb, 2002). Data reported to date do not indicate that age influences the degree of positive benefit gained from treatment.

Format

The *Coping Cat Program* is an individualized therapy program for the child, with two parent sessions interspersed. Parents serve as consultants and collaborators in the treatment. For those who wish to work within a family therapy framework, with the parents as co-clients in the sessions, please see the family therapy manual (Howard, Chu, Krain, Marrs-Gracia, & Kendall, 2000). For those who wish to treat youth anxiety disorders within a group context, please see the group treatment manual (Flannery-Schroeder & Kendall, 1996).

IQ

The *Coping Cat Program* contains cognitive components that require the child to have at least average cognitive abilities. In our own work, a child is appropriate with an IQ of 80 and above. Please see Suveg and colleagues (in press) for an adaptation of the *Coping Cat* treatment with a cognitively delayed child.

Comorbidity

Most children come to our clinic with multiple anxiety disorders, as well as other forms of psychopathology such as attention deficit hyperactivity disorder (ADHD), and oppositional defiant disorder (ODD). Although comorbidity runs high, comorbid disorders present before treatment do not affect outcomes. In other words, both children with comorbid disorders as well as children without comorbid disorders improved when treated with CBT for their anxiety (Kendall, Brady, & Verduin, 2001; Kendall & Brady, 1995).

Gender and Ethnicity

Two factors that have not been found to affect treatment outcome are gender and ethnicity. CBT for anxious youth produces similar results regardless of gender or race. For example, although there are differences in attrition (Sood & Kendall, 2006), there are no differences in outcomes associated with child gender or ethnicity (Treadwell, Flannery-Schroeder, & Kendall, 1995).

Intake and Screening

The assessment of anxiety disorders in children and adolescents can be a challenging endeavor. Although there is no single universally accepted approach, a multi-method, multi-informant approach is preferred and practiced (Jensen, et al., 1999). Such an assessment involves the collection of information from parents, children, and their teachers, and from a variety of settings, including school, home, and peer interactions. This approach permits a thorough evaluation of presenting symptoms and resulting impairment (Achenbach, 1991; Achenbach, McConaughy, & Howell, 1987).

Clinical Interviews

Interviews are the most common method for assessing anxiety disorders in youth. Numerous interview schedules have been developed and tested. Semi-structured interviews for the assessment of anxiety disorders in children and adolescents provide a structured interviewing format, while also allowing for elaboration from informants as judged appropriate by a diagnostician.

We use the Anxiety Disorders Interview Schedule for Children—Parent and Child Versions for DSM-IV

(ADIS-C/P; Silverman & Albano, 1997). This semi-structured diagnostic interview is administered separately to parents and children. Although targeting anxiety disorders; the ADIS-C/P also assesses mood disorders externalizing disorders, and pervasive developmental disorders, providing information on possible comorbid conditions. Based on the symptoms, distress, and interference reported during independently administered child and parent interviews, the diagnostician assigns a composite Clinician Severity Rating (CSR) ranging from 0–8. CSRs of 0 indicate that no symptoms are present; CSRs between 1 and 3 indicate subclinical levels of impairment; whereas CSRs between 4 and 8 indicate a diagnosable (clinically significant) level of distress and impairment.

The ADIS-C/P has demonstrated favorable psychometric properties, including excellent retest reliability (Silverman, Saavedra, & Pina, 2001), convergent validity (March, Parker, Sullivan, Stallings, & Conners, 1997; Wood, Piacentini, Bergman, McCracken, & Barrios, 2002), and good inter-rater reliability (Rapee, Barrett, Dadds, & Evans, 1994). The ADIS-C/P has also been demonstrated to be sensitive to treatment-related changes (Kendall et al., 1997; Silverman, Kurtines, Ginsburg, Weems, Lumpkin, et al., 1999).

Although the use of semi-structured interviews is beneficial in diagnosing anxiety disorders in children and adolescents, the lack of concordance between children and parents as informants is a concern (Choudhury, Pimentel, & Kendall, 2003; DiBartolo, Albano, Barlow, & Heimberg, 1998). Specifically, research finds that parent-child agreement on observable, nonschool based symptoms is higher than that for unobservable, school-based symptoms (Comer & Kendall, 2004; Herjanic & Reich, 1982), most likely due to parents having increased access to the former. Parent-child agreement may also be affected by age, as the reliability of child report tends to increase with age, whereas the reliability of parent reports tends to decrease as the child ages (Edelbrock, Costello, Duncan, Kalas, & Conover, 1985). Again, the use of semi-structured interviews with parents and children as part of a multi-method assessment, in conjunction with self-report and other-report measures, is recommended.

Child Self-Report Measures

One of the most widely used methods for assessing youth anxiety is a self-report inventory. Numerous self-report inventories exist including the Multidimen-sional Anxiety Scale for Children (MASC; March et al., 1997), the Screen for Child Anxiety and Related Emotional Disorders (SCARED; Birmaher et al., 1999), the State-Trait Anxiety Inventory for Children (STAIC; Spielberger, 1973), the Negative Affectivity Self-Statement Questionnaire (NASSQ; Ronan, Kendall, & Rowe, 1994), and the Coping Questionnaire (CQ; Kendall, 1994). A selection of these measures is described below.

The MASC (March et al., 1997) addresses a multidimensional conceptualization of anxiety. This scale is a 39-item self-report inventory that assesses youth anxiety by examining four factors: physical symptoms (e.g., tension), social anxiety (e.g., rejection), harm avoidance (e.g. perfectionism), and separation anxiety. The factor structure has been shown to hold for boys and girls as well as for younger and older youth. In addition retest reliability for the MASC has been shown in past studies to be .79 in clinical samples (March et al., 1997) and .88 in school-based samples (March & Sullivan, 1999). Good three-month retest reliability has also been demonstrated (March & Albano, 1998).

The STAIC (Spielberger, 1973) consists of two separate 20-item inventories: the state scale, designed to assess present state and situation-specific anxiety, and the trait scale, designed to assess stability in anxiety across situations. Findings suggest that this measure is useful as a general screening instrument for anxiety (Barrios & Hartmann, 1988).

In addition to the self-report measures used to assess many of the general symptoms of anxiety, other self-report measures have been developed to specifically evaluate cognitive content, schemas and processes that have been implicated in the maintenance of anxiety (e.g., Ingram & Kendall, 1986, 1987). These measures include the NASSQ (Ronan et al., 1994) and the Coping Questionnaire (CQ: Kendall, 1994). The NASSQ examines the cognitive content of anxious children by measuring their self-talk. It measures the frequency of occurrence of negative self-statements on a 5-point scale and consists of separate items for younger and older children. The measure has been found to have good retest and internal reliability and to be sensitive to changes due to treatment (Kendall et al., 1997). The CQ assesses the child's perception of her ability to cope in stressful, anxiety-provoking situations, using three child-generated stressful situations. The CQ-C is sensitive to treatment gains (Kendall, 1994; Kendall et al., 1997).

Self-reports allow for a cost-effective examination of anxiety symptomatology. However, results from self-reports with children must be interpreted with caution for several reasons. Such measures may not adequately capture fears specific to the individual child (Kendall & Ronan, 1990), preventing the individualization of treatment. In addition, self-report instruments do not often account for developmental variability in comprehension—i.e., younger children may not be able to understand the questions posed or their corresponding response scales. Anxious children may respond in a socially desirable manner due to fear of negative evaluation, calling into question the validity of their self-report responses. The measures described herein may be less troublesome because each has a corresponding parent report form, which can be used in conjunction with child self-report.

Parent and Other-Report Measures

In addition to parent reports on the parent versions of child self-report measures just described (e.g., MASC-Parent, CQ-Parent), the impact of the child's anxiety on daily functioning can be assessed using the Child Anxiety Impact Scale-Parent Version (CAIS-P; Langley, Bergman, McCracken, & Piacentini, 2004). The CAIS-P measures functioning in a variety of domains and is comprised of three subscales: school, social, and home/family. The CAIS-P has demonstrated good internal consistency and construct validity, and results indicate that it is a useful measure of the impact of anxiety on child functioning (Langley et al., 2004).

The Child Behavior Checklist (CBCL; Achenbach & Edelbrock, 1983; Achenbach & Rescorla, 2001) is a parent rating scale (118-items) that assesses behavioral problems and social and academic competence. Although the CBCL does not differentiate between specific anxiety disorders, it discriminates between externalizing and internalizing disorders and provides information on the child's participation in social activities and peer interaction. The CBCL has been shown to effectively discriminate between youth with internalizing and externalizing disorders (Seligman, Ollendick, Langley, & Baldacci, 2004; see also Aschenbrand, Angelosante, & Kendall, 2005).

The Teacher Report Form (TRF; Achenbach & Rescorla, 2001) is a version of the CBCL designed for completion by teachers. The TRF allows for assessment of the child's classroom functioning and is use-ful in contrasting the child's behavior at home and at school. The TRF is particularly useful when assessing children whose primary concerns revolve around social interaction, classroom performance, or evaluation by peers. As with the CBCL, the TRF does not provide diagnostic clarity in regard to different subtypes of anxiety disorders.

The use of parent-report or other-report measures in the assessment of anxious children has some limitations. As described in Comer and Kendall (2004), parents or teachers may not be fully aware of the extent of the child's anxiety symptoms. Many of the child's observable anxiety symptoms may occur outside of parents' visibility, such as at school or when interacting with peers. Parents who are prone to anxiety themselves may also be more likely to over-report their child's anxiety symptoms (see Frick, Silverthorn, & Evans, 1994). Conversely, some parents may be likely to under-report symptoms either because they are unaware of the extent of the child's anxiety symptoms or they are concerned with providing socially desirable responses. Again, we recommend a multi-method assessment procedure that compiles information collected from various sources.

THE TREATMENT MANUAL

The *Coping Cat Program* (Kendall & Hedke, 2006a, 2006b) is an integrated cognitive behavioral treatment for youth with anxiety disorders, specifically GAD, SP, and SAD. The program incorporates exposure tasks, relaxation training, and role plays with an added emphasis on the child's cognitive information processing associated with her anxieties. The overall goal of the program is to teach youth to recognize signs of anxiety and use these signs as cues for the use of anxiety management strategies.

The treatment manual (Kendall & Hedtke, 2006a) describes CBT components such as psychoeducation, relaxation training, building a coping model, problem solving, contingent reinforcements, modeling, exposure tasks, and weekly homework. All are integrated within sessions of the 16 session treatment.

Psychoeducation

The psychoeducation component helps youth identify and discriminate their own (and others') emotional states. Many youth with anxiety experience physical symptoms, such as stomachaches or headaches, which they may attribute to an illness (as opposed to anxiety). Through psychoeducation youth are taught to discriminate when their somatic symptoms (i.e. headache) may be due to anxiety or illness by looking at the context in which these symptoms occur (i.e. only before reading aloud in front of the class). Other emotions are identified, named, and skills in their recognition are taught.

Relaxation

Practice in relaxation teaches youth to develop awareness and control over their own physiological and muscular reactions to anxiety. This procedure involves tensing and relaxing various muscle groups in order to allow the child to perceive sensations of bodily tension and to use these sensations as cues to begin relaxation. This increased awareness of somatic reactions to tension enables the child to use the aroused physical state as a warning signal to start the relaxation procedure.

Building a Coping Template

Throughout the program, youth are coached on how to think about anxious arousal. This involves the identification and modification of maladaptive self-talk, along with building a new way to view situations. The goal of building a new template for thinking is not that perceptions of stress will disappear, but that the formerly distressing perceptions and arousal, when seen through a coping template, will serve to prompt the use of coping strategies.

Problem Solving

The overall goal of problem solving is to teach children to develop confidence in their own ability to help themselves meet daily challenges. Children are shown that problems are part of everyday life and they are encouraged to inhibit their initial impulses (e.g., avoidance behavior). Problem solving involves helping the child define and formulate the problem into a workable situation with goals and alternatives. The therapist models brainstorming by generating both pragmatic and even improbable solutions. The child then evaluates the advantages and disadvantages of each solution—and is soon better equipped to select alternative solutions to problems.

Contingent Reinforcement

Reinforcement focuses on facilitating responses through reward. Many anxious children have unjustly critical beliefs and through contingent reinforcement the therapist emphasizes the importance of rewarding oneself for effort and partial success. Reinforcement provided contingent upon effort and nonavoidance help to modify and reduce anxious behavior.

Modeling

Modeling appropriate nonanxious behavior in anxiety-provoking situations is a main task for the *Coping Cat* therapist (see Nelson & Kendall, 2007). Through various role-plays the therapist models behavior appropriate to anxiety-provoking situations.

Exposure-Based Procedures

Exposure tasks involve placing the child in a fear-provoking situation, either imaginary or in vivo, helping her to acclimate, and providing opportunities for the child to use coping skills. The therapist works with the child to design a hierarchy of exposure tasks and the child gradually makes his or her way through the exposure tasks going from low anxiety provoking situations to high anxiety provoking situations. It is important that the child is able to have some degree of success in each exposure in order to build a sense of self-confidence and mastery.

A Feelings Thermometer (aka the Subjective Units of Distress [SUDS] rating) is a tool that the child uses to rate her anxiety on a scale from 0–8 during an exposure task. Please see the *Coping Cat* manual (Kendall & Hedtke, 2006a) for more details.

Show That I Can (STIC) Task

STIC tasks are weekly homework assignments to be completed outside the therapy setting. They provide the child with an opportunity to practice the skills learned in session. The child is rewarded for STIC task completion.

THE TREATMENT MANUAL WITH CASE ILLUSTRATIONS

To help bring the *Coping Cat Program* (Kendall & Hetdke, 2006a) to life,[1] we introduce two fictitious youngsters, Katie and Matt. As we describe each of the 16 sessions, we illustrate the treatment using Katie and Matt.

Katie, a 7-year-old female diagnosed with separation anxiety disorder, is afraid that bad things will happen to her mother and these worries are so distressing that she has difficulty being away from her mother for even brief periods of time. Katie attends first grade and makes multiple trips to the nurse's office with complaints of stomach and headaches. She calls her mother almost daily from school to check on her and Katie's mother reports that she picks Katie up from school early because of these physical complaints about once a week. Katie also has difficulty sleeping by herself and her mother sleeps with her most nights. Recently Katie has been invited to go on playdates at friends' houses but she refuses to go without her mother. During intake, Katie had difficulty being in the interview room without her mother.

Matt, a 12-year-old boy, was diagnosed with social phobia. He is easily embarrassed, and afraid that others will laugh at him when he interacts with them. He fears reading aloud in class, joining in a conversations, talking on the phone, asking questions, or speaking to strangers. Matt's distress impairs his social function; it gets in the way of his making/keeping friends. His distress is highly impairing to Matt, and gets in the way of his making/keeping friends. When Matt is faced with a social situation, he perspires and has difficulty maintaining eye contact. His heart beats very quickly and he finds it difficult to breathe. Matt expects that those around him will laugh at him if/when he speaks.

Session 1: Building Rapport

A main goal of the first session is to build rapport and get to know each other. The child-therapist relationship is important. We recommend that the first part of the session not focus on the child's anxiety—the time is best used by getting to know one another. Once that has been accomplished, the therapist can spend time introducing the child to an overview of the program. For example, the therapist can share logistics with the child (e.g., how often the two will meet) and discuss goals for the program. Time can be spent explaining to the child that the first eight sessions focus on recognizing anxiety, and the later sessions focus on knowing what to do about feeling anxious. Once the therapist has introduced the program, it is important for the child to feel free to ask any questions. This encourages the child's participation in the treatment, and puts an emphasis on the therapist and child being a collaborative 'team' working together.

At the end of the session the child is assigned an easy STIC task (homework) from the *Coping Cat Workbook* (Kendall & Hedtke, 2006b) and a reward is planned for completing the task. To illustrate, let's take a look at Matt's first session.

Matt enters the therapy room with his eyes cast downward. He sits hesitantly in a chair, and waits—what is going to happen? The therapist invites Matt to make himself comfortable and to look around and see if there are any interesting games that he would like to play. Matt searches the room and finds some video games. The therapist lets Matt know that they will save time (e.g., the last ten minutes) to play Super Mario Kart together. The therapist thanks Matt for coming and they engage in a "getting to know one another game" (asking each other questions). During this period, the therapist sees Matt start to relax.

After spending the first half hour getting to know one another, the therapist introduces Matt to some of the logistics of the *Coping Cat Program*. She lets him know that he will be coming in weekly, and that they are going to be doing some team work. Matt has told her that he worries about reading out loud in class, and the therapist tells Matt that they will be working on some skills that can help kids when they are feeling worried or scared. She tells him that in the beginning, they will simply focus on figuring out *when* he is worried—later on they will work on what to do about feeling worried. The therapist makes it a point to laugh and be comfortable with Matt, and to be encouraging when he talks or asks questions.

Matt is assigned a STIC task (Remember my name), and the therapist and Matt spend the last ten minutes playing Super Mario Kart (as promised).

Session 2: Identifying Anxious Feelings

The aim of this session is to help the child identify different feelings—to distinguish anxious or worried feelings from other feelings. To do this there is discussion about how different feelings have different physical expressions. The therapist and child collaborate to list various feelings and their corresponding physical expressions (in the *Coping Cat Workbook* pp. 6 and 8). Relatedly, they work to identify the child's own somatic responses to anxiety. Once the child understands that different feelings correspond to different expressions, the therapist works with the child to normalize the child's own experience of fears and anxiety. The therapist serves as a coping model by disclosing a time when the therapist felt anxious and how she handled it. The child and therapist discuss the child's own anxiety, including the types of situations that provoke anxiety, and the child's responses in the anxiety-provoking situation.

The therapist introduces the Feelings Thermometer—used to determine which situations are more anxiety provoking for the child (see the therapist manual for details). The therapist and child construct a fear hierarchy or fear ladder using the ratings from the Feeling Thermometer. Katie's Session 2 is an illustration. Just to refresh our memory, Katie is our seven year old female with SAD.

Katie is hesitant to be in the therapy room without her mother. After a review of what is going to happen and a firm and confident reminder that her mother will be in the next room, Katie is able to stay alone with the therapist. The session begins with a review of the STIC task and Katie and the therapist discuss the "feeling-great" situation that Katie recorded in her Coping Cat workbook. The therapist talks with Katie about how different feelings have different physical expressions. Katie and the therapist play a game, using pictures from magazines, to label pictures of people showing different emotions. Katie and the therapist identify certain facial or physical expressions (e.g., a smile, a clenched fist) that match to certain emotions (e.g., feeling happy, feeling angry). They discuss the idea that **all** people feel anxious at times and the purpose of the program is to help Katie learn to recognize when she is feeling anxious and how to make herself feel better.

Katie and her therapist start to construct a hierarchy of anxiety-provoking situations by categorizing the things Katie is afraid of into easy, medium, and challenging categories. Katie identifies being in the therapy room without her mother as a medium fear and going to a birthday party where her mom drops her off and leaves as the most challenging fear.

Before the session ends Katie is assigned a STIC task to complete at home—she is to record one anxious experience and one nonanxious experience in her Coping Cat workbook.

Session 3: What's That Your Body Is Saying?

This session emphasizes teaching the child to identify how her body responds to anxiety. A variety of techniques are used, culminating in the "F" step of the FEAR plan.

To begin, the child and therapist review the STIC task and an appropriate reward is given. If the child didn't do the STIC task, they do it then, together. Next, the therapist spends some time talking about somatic feelings that might occur when someone is feeling anxious, such as heart racing or an uneasy stomach. The child and therapist talk about different bodily sensations that may occur when an individual is faced with an anxiety provoking situation. Once the child is able to name some somatic responses that might occur, the child and therapist practice identifying these responses (via coping modeling and role-playing). The pair practice identifying somatic responses in various anxiety provoking situations, starting with the least anxiety provoking situation. When the child displays comfort identifying somatic feelings, it's time to introduce the "F" step. The "F" step stands for: Feeling Frightened?

At the end, the child is reminded that the next meeting will be with her parent(s). A STIC task is assigned based on tasks covered in the *Coping Cat Workbook* and a game is played to end session on a fun note.

> When Matt comes in today, he is feeling slightly less anxious than last time—he is beginning to learn the ropes. The therapist and Matt start the session by reviewing Matt's STIC task.
>
> They then focus on today's session: Identifying somatic expressions of anxiety. The therapist talks about possible bodily expressions of anxiety such as sweating, or getting red in the face. Funny, exaggerated examples make both laugh. The therapist asks Matt to think about possible ways someone might respond when anxious. Matt mentions having his heart beat quickly when he has to read in front of his class. Together, they discuss what kinds of somatic feelings they have during low anxiety provoking situations, medium anxiety provoking situations, and high anxiety provoking situations. This helps Matt zero in on what his body is telling him when he is feeling nervous. The therapist acts as a coping model for part of the session by letting Matt know what happens to her when she feels anxious. She introduces this process of learning to listen to your body as the "F" step.
>
> At the end of session, Matt is reminded that next session will be with his parent(s). The therapist checks with Matt about any information he shared with her that is off limits (not to be discussed with parents). A STIC task is assigned for Matt's next session and they play Super Mario Kart together for five minutes.

Session 4: First Parent Meeting

The goal of the first parent session is to facilitate parental cooperation and collaboration with the program, and to gather parent input. The therapist and parent(s) meet without the child to provide the parent(s) the opportunity to discuss any concerns they may have and to consider specific ways that the parent(s) can be involved in the program. The parents serve as consultants (i.e., provide the therapist with information about the child) and as collaborators (i.e., help with implementation of the program). During this parent session the therapist provides additional information about the program and gathers information about the parents' own understanding of anxiety. Let's turn back to Katie for an example.

> The therapist meets with Katie's mom because Katie's dad is unable to attend. The therapist briefly outlines the treatment program and explains Katie's involvement so far and what will happen in the remainder of treatment.
>
> Katie's mom has lots of questions about the things that Katie is going to be required to do and asks the therapist if she can sit in during the sessions so that she can help her daughter. The therapist recognizes that Katie's mother has been supporting/maintaining Katie's anxious avoidance (e.g., picking her up from school early). Katie's mom may not understand that although she is trying to help, her involvement in this way hinders Katie's progress. The therapist uses this opportunity to discuss with Katie's mom her own anxiety as well as the ways that she can be involved in treatment to help Katie. The therapist talks with Katie's mom to learn more about situations where Katie becomes anxious.

Session 5: Learning How to Relax

Prior to embarking upon the main goal of Session 5 (learning to relax), it is useful to briefly discuss the parent session with the child. Let the child know that her parents are very proud of her, and allow the child to ask any questions that may come up about the parent session. After discussing the parent session with the child, review the STIC task from Session 3 and reward the child.

Review the "F" step as you introduce the main topic of today's session: relaxation. The therapist may suggest to the child that when she is feeling anxious, her body gives her signals or cues. These signals may be associated with tension, which can be reduced by relaxation. The therapist explains relaxation, as well as useful ways to bring about this feeling. For example, deep breathing, progressive muscle relaxation, and relaxation aids such as relaxation CDs. It is useful to practice relaxing with the child (with the therapist as a coping model).

Once the child understands how to help herself become more relaxed, the therapist and child collaborate to identify when relaxation may be useful. For example, it is unlikely that the child can engage in full progressive muscle relaxation each time she is feeling anxious. However, the child may recognize that taking a few breaths and relaxing certain muscle groups might be useful. To end the session, the STIC task is assigned, and the therapist and child take a few moments to play a fun game or activity. Let's turn to Matt and see how he learns to relax.

When Matt arrives his therapist talks to him about last week's parent session. She tells him that his parents are very proud of him and support him every step along the way. Time is left for Matt to ask questions. After this, they go over Matt's STIC task and Matt trades in his points for a small soccer ball.

Today, the therapist is introducing relaxation as a technique for Matt to use when he feels anxious. She talks to him about how sometimes, when he has to speak in public or read aloud, his body gets tense. He agrees. She links this to the "F" step (Feeling frightened?) of the FEAR plan. The therapist explains that Matt's body provides cues when he is feeling nervous and they are signals for him to relax. The therapist asks Matt to imagine a situation where he is feeling relaxed and then to imagine a situation where he is feeling tense, and to compare the feelings.

Next, they practice deep breathing. The therapist asks Matt if he wants to turn down the lights—he does, and sits comfortably on a bean bag chair. She asks him to take a deep breath and then let it out slowly, focusing on how his body feels. They do this together a few times. She highlights to Matt how her body feels and how his might feel after taking deep breaths. She gives Matt a copy of his own relaxation tape, with the therapist's voice to help him practice these skills at home. They practice these skills together and then Matt's parents join. Matt is asked to teach relaxation to his parents.

At the end of the session, the therapist assigns Matt his STIC task from the Coping Cat Workbook, and they play a game of Super Mario Land together.

Session 6: Identifying and Challenging Anxious Self-talk

Session 6 introduces the role of personal thoughts and their impact on anxiety. The therapist uses pictures with blank thought bubbles to generate thoughts that might occur with different feelings. Through exercises in the *Coping Cat Workbook* (pp. 22–24) the child provides thoughts that could accompany various events. The therapist and child discuss self-talk, and the therapist facilitates the connection between thoughts and anxious feelings. Importantly, they work together to discriminate anxious self-talk from coping self-talk. The therapist models coping self-talk. During this session the "E" step of the FEAR plan is introduced. **E**xpecting bad things to happen? The child and therapist practice coping self-talk using the first two steps in the FEAR plan.

Katie and the therapist begin their session by reviewing the STIC task from last week. Katie reports that it was hard for her to relax when she was thinking about being away from her mom but after she listened to her relaxation tape at home two times she was able to relax.

Katie and the therapist discussed the anxious and nonanxious situations that Katie wrote about in her *Coping Cat Workbook* and the therapist called Katie's attention to the expectations and thoughts she reported in these situations. The therapist talks with Katie about the idea that thoughts are connected to feelings. Katie and the therapist work on a thought bubble exercise in Katie's workbook and during this exercise the therapist helps Katie differentiate between anxious self-talk and coping self-talk.

The therapist introduces the "E" step (Expecting bad things to happen) of the FEAR plan and helps Katie start to pay attention to what she is expecting might happen when she is anxious. Katie and the therapist practice coping self-talk and review the "F" and "E" steps of the FEAR plan. Katie is assigned a STIC task and the session ends with a game of Connect Four, one of Katie's favorites.

Session 7: Attitudes and Actions I Can Take to Help Myself Feel Better!

At the beginning, the therapist and child review the STIC task assigned in the *Coping Cat Workbook* and the child is rewarded appropriately. At this point it is also helpful to discuss the child's use of relaxation over the past few weeks. The therapist and child engage in a brief relaxation exercise and review the "F" and "E" steps. The therapist reminds the child that F and E allow the child to recognize how her body responds to anxiety and to recognize expectations that she may have about the situation.

The next step introduces the child to how she may change her reactions so that she may proceed even when feeling anxiety. The "A" step stands for **A**ttitudes and Actions that can help. Now that the child recognizes anxious arousal and thoughts, she can begin to deal with them. This session focuses on problem solving as a tool to deal with anxiety. Problem solving is a process. First, the child identifies what is making her feel anxious. Second, the child speculates what she might do to make the situation less anxiety-provoking. Third, the child identifies possible solutions that make sense. Last, the child selects the solution which makes the most sense, and proceeds.

The first use of problem solving should be easy and least anxiety-provoking. The therapist can begin with a problem that is concrete and relevant to the child, and show the child how to apply the problem solving process. The therapist slowly builds to practicing problem solving in more and more anxiety provoking situations.

Towards the end, homework is assigned and the therapist and child engage in a fun activity. Let's take a look at Matt in Session 7.

Matt and the therapist began by going over the STIC task and discussing Matt's use of relaxation over the past week. Matt let the therapist know that deep breathing helped him before he had to ask a friend about a homework assignment. It didn't help him as much when he had to read out loud in class. The therapist and Matt discuss possible reasons why this might be the case.

Next, the therapist reviews the "F" and "E" step with Matt by asking him to describe what they stand for. She introduces the idea that now that he knows how to make sense of his body and mind, he can learn how to cope with anxiety. She explains about the "A" step, which stands for "Attitudes and actions that can help." To illustrate the "A" step, the therapist discusses the process of problem solving. The therapist models problem solving by discussing a nonthreatening situation. She gives the following example: "You've misplaced your jacket somewhere at school. How would you try and find it?" She then thinks through this situation with Matt. Then, Matt tries to problem-solve a few different situations, including some that are anxiety-provoking situations.

To end the session, Matt is assigned his STIC task, and the therapist and Matt play a game of Jenga.

Session 8: Results and Rewards!

Session 8 introduces the last step of the FEAR plan: "R" **R**esults and rewards. The child is introduced to the concept of rating performance and rewarding oneself for effort. The therapist talks about self-reward and the pair discuss the concept of self-rating and being satisfied with one's effort.

The child and therapist collaborate on a list of rewards (e.g., going to the movies with friends, getting a new book or game) and specify what is required to earn the rewards. The therapist serves as a coping model by describing a situation where she experiences some distress but was able to cope with the anxiety, rate herself, and then give herself a reward. Before the end of session the child and therapist identify a stressful situation and apply the FEAR plan to get them through it.

The therapist informs the child that the next part of the treatment program involves practicing the skills that have been learned so far. The child and therapist will practice using the FEAR steps in situations where the child might be anxious or worried. The child is assured that the practice will happen gradually, starting with a situation that makes the child a little nervous. It is important to let the child know that the goal of treatment is not to remove all of the child's anxiety but to help the child identify it and cope with the anxiety. The therapist informs the child that she will experience some anxiety during these practice sessions but by going through the FEAR steps the child will be able to manage the anxiety. Let's now turn back to Katie.

Katie and the therapist begin by reviewing the STIC task from session 7. They discuss the plan of action that Katie has been working on when she is faced with an anxiety (e.g., being in school without her mom or sleeping in her bed alone). The therapist introduces the final step in the FEAR plan "R"—Results and rewards. The therapist talks with Katie about how people reward themselves when they are pleased with something they have done. Katie and the therapist create a list of rewards (e.g., stickers, time reading with mom) and identify scenarios in which Katie can earn rewards (e.g., making it through the school day without going to the nurse's office).

Katie and her therapist practice making self-ratings through role-plays. They review the steps of the FEAR plan and together create a FEAR card for Katie to keep with her when she is anxious. Katie and her therapist review Katie's fear hierarchy which includes walking into session without mom, having one day at school where she doesn't call her mom from the nurse's office, sleeping in her bed alone for one night, and finally attending a party without her mom.

The pair discuss that the next part of treatment involves practicing the things that Katie has learned. The therapist explains to Katie that she may feel anxious during the practice tasks but she can use the FEAR plan to help her get through them. The therapist tells Katie that she is going to meet with her mother again next time and asks Katie if there is anything that she doesn't want the therapist to talk about with her mother. The therapist assigns Katie a STIC task and at the end of session they read a few pages in a book that Katie brought from home.

Session 9: Second Parent Session

The second parent session provides an opportunity for the parent to learn more about the exposure tasks part of treatment. The therapist explains that these tasks provide opportunities to make sure the child practices the skills that have been learned.

Specifically, the therapist explains the rationale behind exposure tasks. The parents are reminded that the goal of treatment is not to "cure" anxiety, but to reduce the amount of distress experienced in previously anxiety provoking situations. This is accomplished through the repeated practicing of the FEAR plan in anxiety provoking situations. Parents are introduced to the idea that the child will likely feel some initial anxiety during the exposure tasks, and that this is beneficial because when the child applies her new skill set and experiences success, the anxiety is reduced and this improves her confidence and reduces anxiety in general.

Once the therapist has covered the key points regarding the exposure tasks, the parents are given an opportunity to ask questions. It is useful to encourage the parents to suggest situations in which they have noticed their child becoming anxious. Finally, the therapist may want to solicit the parent's assistance in the planning of exposure tasks at home. Let's see how Matt's parents fare in Session 9.

Today's session is dedicated to introducing Matt's parents to the exposure tasks portion of his treatment. Both parents are able to attend, and they arrive on time. The therapist begins by spending some time catching up, and then outlining the remainder of treatment. She highlights that Matt now has a way to cope with anxiety in social situations and that he will get to practice. By facing his anxiety he will gain mastery over his fears and lessen his anxiety in the future.

The therapist introduces the idea that exposure tasks are the best way for Matt to practice his new skills, and that it is normal for him to feel initial anxiety in these situations. At this point, Matt's mother interjects and asks if he is going to feel very upset. The therapist lets his mother know that the exposure tasks move at a very gradual pace, and that they will start with the least provocative one. Matt's father asks if Matt will be cured and the therapist tells Matt's father that the aim of the treatment is not to cure anxiety, because we all experience anxiety at one time or another, and in fact it can have an adaptive function. However, treatment is going to bring Matt's anxiety down to a normative level so that he can participate in social situations without feeling excessive distress.

Finally, the therapist asks if there are any particular situations that the parents can think of in which Matt needs practice. They volunteer reading aloud, calling friends on the phone, and joining in on conversations. The therapist tells Matt's parents that she may be involving them in some of the planning of exposure tasks and encourages them to call if they have questions or concerns.

Session 10: Facing Your FEAR: Low Anxiety-Provoking Situations

Session 10 involves "practice" (an exposure task) using the FEAR plan in a low anxiety situation. It is important for the child to have at least partial success.

The therapist and child talk about how the focus will shift from learning about thoughts and feelings to practicing coping in different situations. The therapist and child pick a low anxiety-provoking situation and practice using the FEAR plan through an imaginal exposure. Together they write out the child's FEAR plan for the specific situation in the *Coping Cat Workbook* (p. 44) and walk through all the steps during the imaginal exposure task. The child is asked for ratings on the Feelings Thermometer at different times during the imaginal exposure.

Once the child has walked through her FEAR plan in an imaginal exposure task, the child and therapist move to an in vivo exposure task (going into the real situation). They review relaxation exercises to remind the child that relaxation (i.e., taking a few deep breaths) can be a first response to feeling anxious.

Katie and the therapist begin by talking about how much Katie has improved in terms of coping and managing her anxiety as well as rewarding herself for her progress. Katie reported that she went to the nurse's office today because she had a stomachache but when she got there she was able to use her FEAR card. After doing some deep breathing and having a glass of water she returned to the classroom without calling her mom. The therapist praises Katie for her success at school and rewards her with a sticker of one her favorite characters, Ariel, from the Little Mermaid.

The therapist explains to Katie that today they are going to work on practicing the FEAR plan by imagining a situation that might make her a little anxious, such as having Katie imagine staying alone in the therapy room with the lights out for two minutes.

Katie and the therapist develop a FEAR plan for coping with the task and decide on a reward to be given for completing it. Katie and the therapist first practice the FEAR plan while imaging the situation. The therapist has Katie close her eyes and pretend that she is in the room alone. Katie explains the FEAR plan to the therapist saying that first she is going to ask herself if she's feeling frightened, what she is expecting might happen, what actions she can take, and how she will reward herself. Katie is able to successfully describe all the steps of the plan and completes the imaginal exposure task.

Katie and her therapist prepare for the in vivo exposure task. Throughout both the imaginal and in vivo exposure tasks Katie rates her own anxiety using the Feelings Thermometer. Katie is able to stay in the therapy room for two minutes with the lights out and as a reward Katie and the therapist find a comfortable spot to sit and read a chapter from the Little Mermaid. Before Katie leaves she completes a brief relaxation exercise and she and the therapist plan an exposure task for the next session. Katie is assigned a STIC task to review and to practice the FEAR plan in at least one anxious situation over the coming week.

Session 11: Facing Your FEAR: Low Anxiety-Provoking Situations

This session continues exposing the child to low anxiety-provoking situations. Session begins by reviewing the STIC task and the child is rewarded appropriately.

In this session the child practices coping with distress in several low anxiety-provoking situations. To prepare for each, the therapist and child develop a FEAR plan and record it in the *Coping Cat Workbook*. Once a FEAR plan is designed, the child role-plays its use in session. Finally, the child actually participates in the exposure task while using the FEAR plan. The child and therapist provide a rating of the child's anxiety and, after the exposure task, the child receives the planned reward.

The last part of session is to plan the exposure task for the next session (there will be an increase in difficulty) and the STIC task is assigned.

Matt comes in today feeling nervous about continuing the program. Last session, Matt and the therapist planned that the exposure for this week will be calling his grandmother on the phone. Using the phone is anxiety provoking for him because he worries about being unintelligible, not knowing what to say, or saying something stupid. He feels more comfortable calling his grandmother than phoning a friend.

Session begins with reviewing last weeks STIC assignment. Then the therapist and Matt begin preparing for calling his grandmother on the phone. They come up with a FEAR plan for this exposure, thinking through all the steps. Matt identifies that his body may be sweaty, and that he is worried that his grandmother may not be able to understand him. He comes up with the coping thought that his *grandmother will still care about him even if she is unable to understand him,* and problem-solves that he can repeat himself if he needs to. His reward will be spending time showing the therapist his latest book report (for which he received an A).

After designing the FEAR plan Matt practices calling his grandmother on a pretend phone. After this, it is time to actually give her a call. He picks up the phone and calls her, and gives the therapist SUDS rating before he makes the phone call, during each minute of the phone call, and after the call. Before beginning, his SUDS rating is very high (5), and it spikes even higher after the first minute. As he speaks to his grandmother about his day and gradually begins to immerse himself in the conversation, his SUDS ratings diminish. At the end he reports a SUDS rating of 1.

Matt and the therapist discuss what went well and what he might try in the future. Matt receives his reward—they share time reviewing his excellent book report. The pair plan the exposure task for session 12, and the STIC task is assigned.

Session 12: Facing Your FEAR: Moderate Anxiety-Provoking Situations

In session 12 the FEAR plan is applied in both imaginal and in vivo situations that produce moderate levels of anxiety for the child. The therapist prepares for the imaginal exposure task by describing the chosen situation and collaborating with the child to develop a FEAR plan for it: Make the imaginal situation as real as possible. As a coping model the therapist (acting as the child) models thinking through the situation out loud using the FEAR plan. The child then creates a FEAR plan for a slightly different situation with the therapist prompting the use of the FEAR plan. Following the imaginal exposure task, its time to prepare for and engage in in vivo exposure tasks. The child and therapist prepare for these by developing a FEAR plan (please see p. 53 in the *Coping Cat Workbook*), thinking through what might and might not happen and preparing for several likely aspects of the task. The therapist and child negotiate a reward for completion/effort. Let's check in on Katie and see how session 12 unfolds.

Katie and the therapist start session 12 by reviewing the STIC tasks that Katie was assigned. Together, they discuss two anxious experiences that Katie exposed herself to during the week and Katie describes how she coped with them and how she rewarded herself. Katie tells the therapist that this week she had four days where she didn't go to the nurse's office. Katie explained to the therapist that there were some days where she wanted to go to the nurse's office to call her mom but she was able to use her FEAR plan. Katie told the therapist that she had a stomachache because she was feeling frightened not because she was really sick. She told herself that bad things wouldn't happen if she didn't go to the nurse and as a reward she was able to stay in class where the students were working on their art projects, one of Katie's favorite activities. The therapist praised Katie for her effort using the FEAR plan and rewarded her with stickers.

Katie and her therapist discussed the practice situation that they were going to do today. The therapist spoke with Katie's mom during the week to arrange for her collaboration. For this task, Katie will go out to the waiting room and her mom will not be there (Katie's mom will actually be in another room down the hall). First Katie and the therapist practice, where Katie imagines what it would be like to walk into the waiting room and not know where her mom is. She takes the therapist through the steps of the FEAR plan, and they then undertake the real exposure task. Katie provides SUDS ratings throughout. Her SUDS rating is initially very high but as she goes through the steps of the FEAR plan her ratings decrease. Following this, Katie is rewarded and she and her therapist discuss the experience of the exposure task. Katie reports some new confidence, but also expresses concern that because of this confidence her mom may feel unwanted. Katie and the therapist discuss this, make sense of it (mom wants you to be confident) and comfort each other.

Session 13: Facing Your FEAR: Moderate Anxiety-Provoking Situations

This session begins by reviewing the STIC task and rewarding the child appropriately, and the session continues with practicing the FEAR plan in moderate anxiety-provoking situations. Together, the therapist and child come up with a FEAR plan that addresses the exposure task that was generated in Session 12. Prior to participating in the exposure task, the child practices with the therapist using imaginal exposure. Subsequently the child engages in the task and provides SUDS ratings. The child is rewarded for participation. The session ends by planning the next exposure task (a high anxiety-provoking situation) and the assigning of a STIC task. It is useful to mention to the child that there are only three sessions left, to mention the idea of the commercial, and to prepare her for the idea that she will be doing things on her own. Let's go to Matt's Session 13.

Matt comes to session ready to engage in the planned exposure task. He has been having good success and is eager to move forward.

To begin, the therapist and Matt review the STIC task from session 12, and Matt is rewarded appropriately. Next, Matt and the therapist develop the FEAR plan for the agreed upon exposure task for today—Matt will be reading a passage from a book in front of two members of the clinic staff. He anticipates that he will turn red, and expects that they might laugh at him if he mispronounces a word. However, his coping thought is that it is not likely that he will mispronounce a word since he has read the passage several times. And, even if he mispronounces something, it's no big deal. His reward will be getting ice cream with his therapist.

Matt practices reading the passage to his therapist and they discuss the FEAR plan. Matt is asked to describe how he is feeling while he practices.

Matt and the therapist go to a room where there are two clinic staff members whom Matt has never met before. He stands in front of them and reads a three minute passage. Afterwards, Matt and the therapist discuss how it went. Even though Matt turned a little red at first, and had a few anxious thoughts while reading, he was able to get through it (thinking coping thoughts). Although Matt felt anxious initially during the exposure, he soon felt calmer and was very proud of himself for going through with it.

To end, Matt and the therapist congratulate each other, and then plan the exposure task for session 14 which will be among the highest on his fear hierarchy. He is also assigned a STIC task.

Session 14: Facing Your FEAR: High Anxiety-Provoking Situations

Session 14 applies the skills for coping with anxiety in imaginal and in vivo situations that produce high levels of anxiety in the child. Just as in previous exposure tasks, the child and therapist prepare by developing a FEAR plan. During the imaginal exposure the therapist uses props to help create a situation of high anxiety and encourages the child to describe a situation that she can role play with minimal help from the therapist. Before the real exposure task, the therapist is careful to ensure that the child includes a plan to ensure success. The therapist remarks on specific aspects of the situation that might generate anxiety and the child, who is the new expert, walks the therapist through the FEAR plan. The child provides SUDS ratings and is rewarded for both effort and completion. Let's see how Katie does in a high anxiety-provoking situation.

Katie and the therapist begin session by reviewing the STIC task and Katie is rewarded for practicing the FEAR plan during anxious experiences that occurred during the week: (1) Katie's mom was late to pick her up from school one day (this had been arranged as an exposure task) and (2) Katie was able to stay in the house while her mom went to the store. Katie and the therapist prepare for today's exposure task which entails going for a walk around the office building with only the therapist, seeing mom and waving to her, but going back to the clinic without running up to mom.

Katie and the therapist practice the FEAR plan and the therapist helps Katie to identify aspects of the situation that may generate anxiety. Katie describes her feelings, somatic sensations, and self-talk regarding the upcoming task. Katie provides SUDS ratings before, during and after the exposure task and is rewarded for her effort. Katie and the therapist plan exposures for the remaining sessions with the help of Katie's mother. The therapist reminds Katie about the "commercial" that she can produce in the final session. The therapist explains that the commercial is something to show others what she has learned and to teach them about managing anxiety.

Session 15: Facing Your FEAR:
High Anxiety-Provoking Situations

Session 15 continues to engage the child in exposure to situations that cause anxious distress. The session begins with a review of the STIC task. Additionally, the therapist and child discuss ideas for the commercial.

Most of session is spent preparing and engaging in the exposure task. The therapist and child prepare for it by designing a FEAR plan. Finally, the child engages in the planned exposure task. The therapist and child discuss the child's performance afterwards and the child is rewarded. A last exposure task is planned for session 16.

It is important to discuss the end of treatment. The therapist lets the child know that the next session is the last one, and remarks on the child's progress to date. To introduce this idea, it is useful to briefly summarize what the child has learned over the past 15 weeks, and to communicate confidence in the child's new abilities. Finally, the therapist assigns the last STIC task. In between this session and the last, the therapist gathers materials needed for the commercial. Let's check in on Matt.

To begin, Matt and the therapist review the STIC task. Unfortunately, Matt had a death in his family, was busy almost every night, and wasn't able to complete his STIC task. The therapist and Matt complete the STIC task together. Next, Matt and the therapist brainstorm ideas for the commercial. Matt says that he would like to do something involving basketball, so the therapist agrees to have a basketball hoop and a basketball on hand for the last session.

Most of the session today is spent on the exposure to a high anxiety-provoking situation. Matt and the therapist prepare for one of the situations highest on Matt's fear hierarchy: calling a classmate on the telephone. Matt and the therapist begin by talking about the FEAR plan for this particular exposure. They discuss how Matt's body might be feeling, what he might be expecting, and actions he can take to make himself feel better. They agree that his reward is staying up late this weekend (this was agreed upon by his parents prior to session).

After practicing with his therapist, Matt reports being ready to call a friend, Timothy. Although his SUDS rating is high, he picks up the phone and makes the call. The call goes through and he spends about five minutes on the phone with his friend. When he gets off the phone, he has a triumphant grin on his face, and is very excited that he was able to do it. The therapist and Matt discuss what was easier for him and what was more difficult. Together, they plan the last exposure, which will be reading aloud to a group of six people, including some who will be disinterested and some who will not understand what he is saying.

The therapist reminds Matt that the program will be completed soon. She tells him how proud she is of him and lets him know that she thinks he is ready to be on his own at school and at home. They talk a bit about Matt's feelings toward ending treatment: He is excited to be able to do activities that he wasn't able to do before, but he is sad about ending. She tells him that in a few months, she'd love him to call her on the phone and let her know how he is doing, and he agrees.

Session 16: Primetime!

Congratulations! You made it. The goal of the last session is to have a final practice using the FEAR plan and to allow the child the pleasures of "producing" a commercial. The commercial is where the child client celebrates and teaches others about the program and her successes. Prior to this session the therapist prepares the room for taping the commercial. The commercial should be fun and should be a celebration of how far the child has come since the beginning of treatment.

After the commercial is filmed, the parents are invited to watch the commercial and the child, who is the now the expert, reviews and explains the FEAR plan/acronym. It is important for the therapist to note that the child has made great gains, but there may be areas in need of improvement and that there will be times that are difficult in terms of coping with anxiety. In commemoration of the child's completion of the program she receives an official certificate of completion. Let's check in on Katie.

Katie enters the clinic by herself and explains to the therapist that her mom dropped her off and is parking the car. The therapist is exuberant, and praises Katie for coming into the clinic by herself. Katie explains that even though she was nervous about walking in without her mom she used her FEAR plan and was able to do it.

Katie and the therapist run through one final imaginal and in vivo exposure task and then Katie starts her commercial. Katie, with the help of her mother, has written a song about the FEAR plan—and the song is to the tune of The Little Mermaid's "Under the Sea." Katie practices parts of the song for the therapist and then she sings it though. Katie and the therapist show the recording to her mother. Katie, the therapist, and her mother review Katie's progress and discuss treatment termination. The session ends with a shared pizza to celebrate the gains.

Notes

1. We recommend that anyone interested in treating an 7–13 year old anxious child consult the therapist manual (Kendall & Hedtke, 2006a) and accompanying client workbook (Kendall & Hedtke, 2006b). For teens, see the related *C.A.T. Project* treatment materials. For more information about the printed materials and the training videos and DVDs, visit the website at www.Workbook Publishing.com. For more information about the Child and Adolescent Anxiety Disorders Clinic (CAADC), visit our website at www.childanxiety.org.

References

Achenbach, T. M. (1991). *Integrative guide for the 1991 CBCL/4–18, YSR, and TRF.* Burlington: University of Vermont.

Achenbach, T. M., & Edelbrock, C. (1983). *Manual for the child behavior checklist and revised child behavior profile.* Burlington: University of Vermont, Associates in Psychiatry.

Achenbach, T. M., & Rescorla, L. A. (2001). *Manual for school-age forms & profiles.* Burlington: University of Vermont, Research Center for Children, Youth, Families.

Achenbach, T. M., McConaughy, S. H., & Howell, C. T. (1987). Child/adolescent behavioral and emotional problems: Implications of cross-informant correlations for situational specificity. *Psychological Bulletin, 101,* 213–232.

Albano, A. M., & Kendall, P. C. (2002). Cognitive behavioral therapy for children and adolescents with anxiety disorders: Clinical research advances. *International Review of Psychiatry, 14,* 129–134.

American Psychiatric Association (APA). (1994). *Diagnostic and statistical manual of mental disorders* (4th ed.). Washington, DC: Author.

Aschenbrand, S. G., Angelosante, A. G., & Kendall, P. C. (2005). Discriminant validity and clinical utility of the CBCL with anxiety disordered youth. *Journal of Clinical Child and Adolescent Psychology, 34,* 735–746.

Barrett, P., Dadds, M., & Rapee, R. (1996). Family treatment of child anxiety: A controlled trial. *Journal of Consulting and Clinical Psychology, 64,* 333–342.

Barrios, B. A., & Hartmann, D. B. (1988). Fears and anxieties. In E. J. Mash & L. G. Terdal (Eds.), *Behavioral assessment of childhood disorders* (2nd ed., pp. 196–264). New York: Guilford Press.

Birmaher, B., Brent, D. A., Chiappetta, L., Bridge, J., Monga, S., & Baugher, M. (1999). Psychometric properties of the Screen for Child Anxiety Related Emotional Disorders Scale (SCARED): A replication study. *Journal of the American Academy of Child and Adolescent Psychiatry, 38,* 1230–1236.

Chambless, D. & Hollon, S. (1998). Defining empirically supported treatments. *Journal of Consulting and Clinical Psychology, 66,* 5–17.

Chavira, D., Stein, M., Bailey, K., & Stein, M. (2004). Child anxiety in primary care: Prevalent but untreated. *Depression and Anxiety, 20,* 155–164.

Choudhury, M. S., Pimentel, S. S., & Kendall, P. C. (2003). Childhood anxiety disorders: Parent-child (dis)agreement using a structured interview for the DSM-IV. *Journal of the American Academy of Child and Adolescent Psychiatry, 42,* 957–964.

Comer, J. S., & Kendall, P. C. (2004). A symptom-level examination of parent-child agreement in the diagnosis of anxious youths. *Journal of the American Academy of Child and Adolescent Psychiatry, 43,* 878–886.

Costello, E., Mustillo, S., Keeler, G., & Angold, A. (2004). Prevalence of psychiatric disorders in children and adolescents. In B. Levine, J. Petrila, & K. Hennessey (Eds), *Mental health services: A public health perspective* (pp. 111–128). New York: Oxford University Press.

DiBartolo, P. M., Albano, A. M., Barlow, D. H., & Heimberg, R. G. (1998). Cross-informant agreement in the assessment of social phobia in youth. *Journal of Abnormal Child Psychology, 26,* 213–220.

Edelbrock, C., Costello, A. J., Duncan, M. K., Kalas, R., & Conover, N. C. (1985). Age differences in the reliability of the psychiatric interview of the child. *Child Development, 56,* 265–275.

Flannery-Schroeder, E., & Kendall, P. (1996). *Cognitive behavioral therapy for anxious children: Therapist manual for group treatment.* Ardmore, PA: Workbook Publishing.

Frick, P. J., Silverthorn, P., & Evans, C. (1994). Assessment of childhood anxiety using structured interviews: Patterns of agreement among informants and association with maternal anxiety. *Psychological Assessment, 6,* 372–379.

Greco, L., & Morris, T. (2005). Factors influencing the link between social anxiety and peer acceptance: Contributions of social skills and close friendships during middle childhood. *Behavior Therapy, 36,* 197–205.

Herjanic, B., & Reich, W. (1982). Development of a structured psychiatric interview for children: Agreement between child and parent on individual symptoms. *Journal of Abnormal Child Psychology, 10,* 307–324.

Howard, B., Chu, B., Krain, A., Marrs-Garcia, A., & Kendall, P. (2000). *Cognitive-behavioral family therapy for anxious children: Therapist manual.* Ardmore, PA: Workbook Publishing.

Hughes, A. A., Hedtke, K. A., Flannery-Schroeder, E., & Kendall, P. C. (2005). *Kiddie cat therapist manual: Cognitive-behavioral family therapy for anxious children (ages 3–7 years).* Unpublished manual.

Ingram, R. E., & Kendall, P. C. (1986). Cognitive clinical psychology: Implications of an information processing perspective. In R. E. Ingram (Ed.), *Information processing approaches to clinical psychology* (pp. 3–21). New York: Academic Press.

Ingram, R. E., & Kendall, P. C. (1987). The cognitive side of anxiety. *Cognitive Therapy and Research, 11,* 523–537.

Jensen, P. S., Rubio-Stipec, M., Canino, G., Bird, H. R., Dulcan, M. K., Schwab-Stone, M. E., et al. (1999). Parent and child contributions to diagnosis of mental disorder: Are both informants always necessary? *Journal of the American Academy of Child and Adolescent Psychiatry, 38,* 1569–1579.

Kazdin, A. E. & Weisz, J. (1998). Identifying and developing empirically supported child and adolescent treatments. *Journal of Consulting and Clinical Psychology, 66,* 18–35.

Kendall, P. C. (1994). Treating anxiety disorders in children: Results of a randomized clinical trial. *Journal of Consulting and Clinical Psychology, 62,* 100–110.

Kendall, P. C. & Brady, E. U. (1995). Comorbidity in the anxiety disorders of childhood: Implications for validity and clinical significance. In K. D. Craig & K. S. Dobson (Eds.), *Anxiety and depression in adults and children Banff international behavioral science series* (pp. 3–36). Thousand Oaks, CA: Sage Publications, Inc.

Kendall, P. C., & Hedtke, K. (2006a). *Cognitive-behavioral therapy for anxious children: Therapist manual* (3rd ed.). Ardmore, PA: Workbook Publishing. Retrieved January 18, 2007, from www.workbookpublishing.com

Kendall, P. C., & Hedtke, K. (2006b). *The Coping Cat Workbook* (2nd ed.). Ardmore, PA: Workbook Publishing. Retrieved January 18, 2007, from www.workbookpublishing.com

Kendall, P. C., & Ronan, K. R. (1990). Assessment of childhood anxieties, fears, and phobias: Cognitive-behavioral models and methods. In C. R. Reynolds & R. W. Kamphaus (Eds.), *Handbook of psychological and educational assessment of children: Personality, behavior, and context* (pp. 223–244). New York: Guilford Press.

Kendall, P. C. & Southam-Gerow, M. (1996). Long-term follow-up of treatment for anxiety disordered youth. *Journal of Consulting and Clinical Psychology, 64,* 724–730.

Kendall, P., Brady, E., & Verduin, T. (2001). Comorbidity in childhood anxiety disorders and treatment outcome. *Journal of the American Academy of Child and Adolescent Psychiatry, 40,* 787–794.

Kendall, P., Choudhury, M., Hudson, J., & Webb, A. (2002). *The C.A.T. project manual.* Ardmore, PA: Workbook Publishing. Retrieved January 18, 2007, from www.workbookpublishing.com

Kendall, P. C., Flannery-Schroeder, E. C., Panichelli-Mindel, S., Southam-Gerow, M., Henin, A., Warman, M., et al. (1997). Therapy for youths with anxiety disorders: A second randomized clinical trial. *Journal of Consulting and Clinical Psychology, 65,* 366–380.

Kendall, P. C., Safford, S., Flannery-Schroeder, E., & Webb, A. (2004). Child anxiety treatment: Outcomes in adolescence and impact on substance use and depression at 7.4-year follow-up. *Journal of Consulting and Clinical Psychology, 72,* 276–287.

King, N. J., & Ollendick, T. H. (1989). Children's anxiety and phobic disorders in school settings: Classification, assessment, and intervention issues. *Review of Educational Research, 59,* 431–470.

Langley, A. K., Bergman, R. L., McCracken, J., & Piacentini, J. C. (2004). Impairment in childhood anxiety disorders: Preliminary examination of the Child Anxiety Impact Scale-Parent Version. *Journal of Child and Adolescent Psychopharmacology, 14,* 105–114.

Manassis, K., Mendlowitz, S., Scapillato, D., Avery, D., Fiksenbaum, L., Freire, M. et al. (2002). Group and individual cognitive-behavior therapy for childhood anxiety disorders: A randomized trial. *Journal of the American Academy of Child and Adolescent Psychiatry, 41,* 1423–1430.

March, J. S., & Albano, A. M. (1998). Advances in the assessment of pediatric anxiety disorders. *Advances in Clinical Child Psychology, 20,* 213–241.

March, J. S. & Sullivan, K. (1999). Test-retest reliability of the Multidimensional Anxiety Scale for Children. *Journal of Anxiety Disorders, 13,* 349–358.

March, J. S., Parker, J., Sullivan, K., Stallings, P., & Conners, C. (1997). The multidimensional anxiety scale for children (MASC): Factor structure, reliability, and validity. *Journal of the American Academy of Child and Adolescent Psychiatry, 36,* 554–565.

Nauta, M., Scholing, A., & Emmelkamp, P. (2003). Cognitive-behavioral therapy for children with anxiety disorders in a clinical setting: No additional effect of cognitive parent training. *Journal of the American Academy of Child and Adolescent Psychiatry, 42,* 1270–1278.

Nelson, W. M. & Kendall, P. C. (2007). *The coping cat therapist: Session-by-session guide.* [DVD]. Ardmore, PA: Workbook Publishing.

Ollendick, T. H., & King, N. J. (1998). Empirically supported treatments for children with phobic and anxiety disorders: Current status. *Journal of Clinical Child Psychology, 27,* 156–167.

Rapee, R. M., Barrett, P. M., Dadds, M. R., & Evans, L. (1994). Reliability of the *DSM-III-R* childhood anxiety disorders using structured interview: Interrater and parent-child agreement. *Journal of the American Academy of Child and Adolescent Psychiatry, 33,* 984–992.

Ronan, K., Kendall, P., & Rowe, M. (1994). Negative affectivity in children: Development and validation of a questionnaire. *Cognitive Therapy and Research, 18,* 509–528.

Seligman, L. D., Ollendick, T. H., Langley, A. K., & Baldacci, H. B. (2004). The utility of measures of child and adolescent anxiety: A meta-analytic review of the Revised Children's Anxiety Scale, the State-Trait

Anxiety Inventory for Children, and the Child Behavior Checklist. *Journal of Clinical Child and Adolescent Psychology, 33,* 557–565.

Silverman, W. K., & Albano, A. M. (1997). *Anxiety Disorders Interview Schedule for DSM-IV: Child and Parent Versions.* Boulder, CO: Graywind Publications Incorporated.

Silverman, W. K., Saavedra, L. M., & Pina, A. A., (2001). Test-retest reliability of anxiety symptoms and diagnoses with anxiety disorders interview schedule for *DSM-IV*: Child and parent versions. *Journal of the American Academy of Child and Adolescent Psychiatry, 40,* 937–944.

Silverman, W., Kurtines, W., Ginsburg, G., Weems, C., Lumpkin, P., & Carmichael, D. (1999). Treating anxiety disorders in children with group cognitive-behavioral therapy: A randomized clinical trial. *Journal of Consulting and Clinical Psychology, 67,* 995–1003.

Sood, E. D., & Kendall P. C. (2006). Ethnicity in relation to treatment utilization, referral source, diagnostic status and outcomes at a child anxiety clinic. Presented at the annual meeting of the Association for Behavioral and Cognitive Therapies, Chicago, IL.

Spielberger, C. (1973). *STAI manual for the State-Trait Anxiety Inventory.* Lutz, FL: Psychological Assessment Resources, Inc.

Strauss, C. C., Forehand, R., Smith, K., & Frame, C. L. (1986). The association between social withdrawal and internalizing problems of children. *Journal of Abnormal Child Psychology, 14,* 525–535.

Suveg, C., Comer, J., Furr, J., & Kendall, P. C. (in press). Adapting manualized CBT for a cognitively-delayed child with multiple anxiety disorders. *Clinical Case Studies.*

Treadwell, K., Flannery-Schroeder, E., & Kendall, P. (1995). Ethnicity and gender in relation to adaptive functioning, diagnostic status, and treatment outcome in children from an anxiety clinic. *Journal of Anxiety Disorders, 9,* 373–384.

Van Amerigen, M., Manicini, C., & Farvolden, P. (2003). The impact of anxiety disorders on educational achievement. *Journal of Anxiety Disorders, 17,* 561–571.

Warren, S. C., & Messer, S. B. (1999). Brief psychodynamic therapy with anxious children. In S. W. Russ & T. H. Ollendick (Eds.), *Handbook of psychotherapies with children and families* (pp. 219–239). New York: Kluwer Academic/Plenum.

Wood, J. J., Piacentini, J. C., Bergman, R. L., McCracken, J., & Barrios, V. (2002). Concurrent validity of the anxiety disorders section of the Anxiety Disorders Interview Schedule for *DSM-IV*: Child and parent versions. *Journal of Clinical Child and Adolescent Psychology, 31,* 335–342.

Chapter 12

A Cognitive Therapy Intervention for Adolescent Suicide Attempters: An Empirically-Informed Treatment

Michele S. Berk, PhD, Gregory K. Brown, PhD, Amy Wenzel, PhD, and Gregg R. Henriques, PhD

Adolescent suicidal behavior is a significant public health problem in the United States. Suicide is the third leading cause of death in the United States for youth aged 10–19 (Hamilton, Miniño, Martin, Kochanek, Strobino, et al., 2007), and approximately one-third of youth who die by suicide have made previous suicide attempts (United States Public Health Service, 1999). A history of previous suicide attempts is one of the strongest predictors of future suicide attempts and suicide deaths among teens (Lewinsohn, Rohde, & Seely, 1993; Shaffer, Garland, Gould, Fisher, & Trautman, 1988). Identifying and targeting groups at high risk for suicide is a key suicide prevention strategy, as outlined in the *National Strategy for Suicide Prevention* (United States Department of Health and Human Services, 2001). Adolescent suicide attempters constitute a high risk population in need of intensive suicide prevention efforts. Indeed, the death or

serious injury of a teen due to a potentially preventable cause, such as suicidal behavior, is a particularly tragic outcome.

The present chapter focuses on suicide prevention in adolescents by describing an empirically-based, cognitive-behavioral intervention for recent suicide attempters, developed by Aaron T. Beck and colleagues at the University of Pennsylvania (see Brown, Tenhave, Henriques, Xie, Hollander, et al., 2005). Although this treatment was originally developed and tested with adult suicide attempters, the present chapter will describe an adaptation of the intervention for use with adolescents. At present, there are few psychosocial treatments that have been demonstrated to be effective in reducing suicide attempts in teens. Moreover, recent data suggesting that anti-depressant medications may increase suicidality in children and teens (United States Food and Drug Administration, 2004) highlights the importance of developing effective psychotherapy interventions for suicidal adolescents. Psychosocial interventions that incorporate cognitive

We would like to thank Stephanie R. Alley, MA, for her assistance with preparation of this chapter.

and behavioral approaches have demonstrated some initial promising results in decreasing suicide attempts and/or suicide ideation, suggesting the potential value of adapting Beck's cognitive therapy intervention for use with adolescents. This literature is summarized briefly below.

There have only been a few randomized controlled trials supporting a beneficial effect of treatment on suicidal behavior and/or self-injury behavior in adolescents. In one randomized trial, multi-systemic therapy (MST), an intensive, home-based intervention that uses behavioral principles to intervene across multiple systems relevant to the adolescent (e.g., family, community), decreased rates of youth self-reports of suicide attempts at one year follow-up (Huey et al., 2004) to a greater degree than hospitalization. In another study, adolescents who had engaged in at least two episodes of deliberate self-harm (DSH; self-injurious behavior both with and without the intent to die) in the past year were randomized either to a group therapy approach that included cognitive-behavioral strategies, such as problem-solving, anger management, and decreasing hopelessness and depression, or to routine care. Results showed that youth assigned to the group therapy condition were significantly less likely to engage in DSH and had a longer time to the first repeat DSH episode than those receiving routine care (Wood, Trainor, Rothwell, Moore, & Harrington, 2001). Empirically-supported interventions that reduce suicidal ideation include those that increase social support (King, Kramer, Preuss, Kerr, Weisse, et al., 2006) as well as those that incorporate a family-based approach focusing on problem solving (Harrington et al., 1993).

Quasi-experimental trials have also yielded encouraging results for cognitive-behavioral interventions. Rathus and Miller (2002) conducted an open trial of a downward extension of Dialectical Behavior Therapy (DBT) for adolescents (DBT-A). DBT was originally developed by Marsha Linehan to treat chronically suicidal adult women with Borderline Personality Disorder (see Linehan, 1993) and incorporates a range of cognitive-behavioral strategies, as well as practices derived from Eastern philosophy and religion, such as mindfulness and radical acceptance. Adaptations made specifically for adolescents include shortening the length of treatment (from one year to sixteen weeks), including parents in the treatment, simplifying the language and materials, and including a new skills module addressing developmental issues central

to adolescence (see Miller, Rathus, & Linehan, 2007). Adolescents who received DBT-A showed a significant pre/post treatment decrease in suicidal ideation, as well as significantly fewer hospitalizations than those youth receiving treatment as usual. However, the overall number of suicide attempts in this study, across conditions, was too small to permit meaningful between-group comparisons. Rotheram-Borus and colleagues (2000) examined the impact of a one-time, family-based, cognitive-behavioral crisis intervention session conducted in the Emergency Department (ED). All participants, regardless of whether or not they received the ED-intervention, also received a brief, outpatient follow-up treatment. At 18 month follow-up, those receiving the ED intervention showed greater adherence to the outpatient treatment and reduced depression than those who did not receive the ED intervention.

Cognitive-behavioral approaches have also shown efficacy in the adult literature on the treatment of suicidal behavior. For example, DBT is superior to treatment as usual as well as treatment by experts in the community in decreasing parasuicidal behaviors, including suicide attempts (e.g., Linehan, Armstrong, Suarez, Allmon, & Heard, 1991; Linehan et al., 2006). A recent randomized clinical trial conducted by Gregory K. Brown and colleagues at the University of Pennsylvania comparing a brief cognitive therapy intervention plus enriched care (i.e., usual care plus case management) to enriched care alone demonstrated that cognitive therapy reduced the re-attempt rate in half, relative to the enriched care group (Brown et al., 2005). The cognitive therapy intervention, which consists of approximately ten outpatient, individual sessions, targets the cognitions that were activated just prior to the individual's suicide attempt and focuses on suicidal behavior as the primary target of treatment (Berk, Henriques, Warman, Brown, & Beck, 2004; for a comprehensive description of this treatment, see Wenzel, Brown, & Beck, in press).

The present chapter describes a cognitive therapy intervention for adolescent suicide attempters. As detailed above, cognitive behavioral treatment approaches have shown promise in decreasing suicidal behavior and ideation in adolescents. The results obtained by Miller and colleagues using DBT-A support the notion that treatments originally created for suicidal adults can be of benefit to adolescents, with appropriate developmental modifications. Empirical research demonstrates that cognitive-behavioral treatment approaches are effective with children and adolescents, across a variety of psychiatric disorders (see Friedberg & McClure, 2002). Because of its robust demonstration of a reduction in subsequent suicide attempts among adult suicide attempters, the application of the cognitive therapy approach with teens may potentially be of great benefit. Elements of this intervention are currently being studied in the Treatment of Adolescent Suicide Attempters study (TASA), (TASA, n.d.), a large, multisite trial funded by the NIMH for adolescent suicide attempters.

COGNITIVE THEORY AND THERAPY FOR SUICIDE ATTEMPTERS

Previous work on the cognitive model of the emotional disorders and, in particular, depression (Beck, 1976; Beck, Rush, Shaw & Emery, 1979) provides the framework for the intervention for suicidal behavior described in this chapter. According to cognitive theory, the manner in which people think about and interpret life events determines their emotional and behavioral responses to those events (Beck, 1976; Beck et al., 1979). Hence, a cognitive model considers maladaptive cognitions to be the central pathway to suicidal behavior (e.g., Rudd, Joiner & Rajab, 2001; Weishaar & Beck, 1990; Wenzel et al., in press). According to cognitive theory, suicidal behavior is conceptualized in terms of the cognitions that occurred just prior to the patient's suicide attempt.

Research has shown that various types of cognitions are associated with suicidal thoughts and behavior in adolescents. In a study of hospitalized adolescents, results indicated that adolescents' expectations that they would attempt suicide in the future prospectively predicted suicide attempts in the years following hospital discharge (Goldston, Daniel, Reboussin, Reboussin, Frazier, et al., 2001). In this same study, among past suicide attempters only, hopelessness predicted future suicide attempts (although this relationship disappeared after controlling for depression), and survival and coping beliefs decreased this risk. Kienhorst and colleagues (1995) conducted semi-structured interviews with a sample of 14–21 year olds in the Netherlands who had attempted suicide within the previous year. The most common precipitant to the suicide attempt was the desire to escape or get relief from painful emotions or situations, as expressed in thoughts such as, "I wanted

to get relief from a terrible state of mind." Using a sample of inpatients with suicidal ideation, ages 7–17 years old, Wagner and colleagues (2000) found that attributional style became more positive (e.g., less internal, stable, and global) and hopelessness decreased when suicidal ideation had resolved. In a sample of 8–13 year old inpatients, Asarnow and colleagues (1987) found that suicidal behavior was associated with children's perceptions of their families as low in control and cohesiveness and high in conflict, and that suicidal children spontaneously generated fewer cognitive coping strategies (e.g., self-soothing statements) during a problem-solving task. Similarly, using a predominately Latina sample of female suicide attempters ages 12–17, Rotheram-Borus and colleagues (1990) found that suicide attempters were characterized by poor interpersonal problem solving and a wishful thinking style of coping. Finally, in an inpatient sample of 175 children ages 6–13, Nock and Kazdin (2002) showed that, after controlling for depressed mood, negative automatic thoughts (as assessed by the *Automatic Thoughts Questionnaire*) were associated with a current suicide attempt, as well as with suicidal ideation. In addition, among current suicide attempters, hopelessness was correlated positively with suicide intent. Taken together, these findings suggest that a cognitive therapy approach is appropriate for use with adolescent suicide attempters and that suicide-related cognitions are an important target of treatment because maladaptive cognition is a central feature of adolescent suicidal behavior.

OVERVIEW OF THE COGNITIVE THERAPY INTERVENTION

The treatment follows general principles of cognitive therapy and includes a specific set of cognitive and behavioral strategies designed to decrease suicidal thoughts and behavior. The overall goal of the treatment is the prevention of future suicide attempts. One unique aspect of the intervention is that the suicidal behavior itself is the primary target of treatment, rather than it being approached as secondary to an underlying psychiatric disorder. Hence, all issues brought forth by the adolescent and his or her family in therapy are discussed and conceptualized in terms of their relation to his or her suicidal behavior.

The therapy was developed as a brief and flexible intervention that can be used in a variety of settings and as an adjunct to other treatments. The therapist is highly active and directive in using a range of cognitive and behavioral techniques to help the adolescent develop alternative ways of thinking and behaving during periods of acute emotional distress rather than engaging in suicidal behavior. Therapy sessions are highly structured and follow standard cognitive therapy practices such as a mood check, a review of the previous session's content, setting an agenda, and regular homework assignments (for a review see Beck, 1995; see also Friedberg & McClure, 2002). Each session follows the basic structure shown in Table 12.1. Each therapy session also includes assessment and monitoring assess suicide ideation, intent, and plans, access to lethal means, acute psychiatric symptoms, hopelessness, drug and alcohol use (because this may lead to impulsive, dangerous behavior), and current environmental stressors, as these factors are crucial in determining current suicide risk (for a comprehensive discussion of risk factors for adolescent suicidality see Gould, Greenberg, Velting, & Shaffer, 2003; Wenzel et al., in press).

The intervention is designed as a 10-session protocol and is divided into early, middle, and late phases. The treatment includes four main targets: (a) behavioral strategies, (b) affective coping strategies, (c) cognitive strategies, and (d) the family relationship. The therapy is focused on decreasing both

Table 12.1
General Session Structure

1. Set Agenda
2. Mood Check and Suicide Risk Assessment (assess suicide ideation, intent, and plans, access to lethal means, acute/worsening psychiatric symptoms, hopelessness, drug and alcohol use and current environmental stressors)
3. Review Session Number (Discuss Anticipated Termination)
4. Bridge from Previous Session
5. Review Homework
6. Set Agenda (includes session-specific interventions, e.g., constructing safety plan, making a list of items for the hope box, etc.)
7. Review of Agenda Items/Session Body
8. Assign Homework (homework should be related to session content, e.g., practice coping skills on the safety plan, create a hope box)
9. Final Summary and Session Feedback
10. Review Safety Plan and Emergency Numbers
11. Make Appointment for Next Session
12. Check-in with parents (as needed)

immediate and long term risk of subsequent suicide attempts, and it is recommended that the clinician begin treatment as soon as possible after the suicide attempt. Early intervention is crucial with this patient population, as 10% of adolescent suicide attempters reattempt within 3 months, 12%–20% within one year and 20%–50% in 2–3 years (Spirito, Lewander, Levy, Kurkjian, & Fritz, 1994; see also Boergers & Spirito, 2003).

The treatment is specifically designed for adolescents who have recently attempted suicide rather than adolescents who engage in non-suicidal self-injury behavior (NSSIB) or who have suicidal ideation only. A suicide attempt is defined as self injurious behavior with a non-fatal outcome, in which there is some evidence, either implicit or explicit, of intent to kill oneself (O'Carroll, Berman, Maris, Moscicki, Tanney, et al., 1996). Determining whether an adolescent has made a suicide attempt can be a challenge for the clinician. Adolescents are often unwilling or unable to accurately report their intent for engaging in self-injurious behavior. Moreover, adolescents may not accurately understand the lethality of various methods and often over-estimate the potential lethality of suicide attempt methods (Harris & Myers, 1997). Hence, the potential lethality of a suicide attempt may not necessarily correlate with the degree of suicide intent. It is recommended that the clinician consider a number of factors in determining whether an adolescent's self-injurious behavior should be classified as a suicide attempt. These factors should include the teen's report of suicidal intent and the perception of the expectation for death as a result of the act, the parent's report of the teen's suicidal intent, the reports of other relevant informants, and the lethality of the attempt (e.g., if the youth took 50 pills, but denies this was a suicide attempt, the clinician may decide to classify this as a suicide attempt based on the potential lethality).

girl interrupted: Winona Ryder

PARENTAL INVOLVEMENT

One of the primary modifications needed in using the treatment with adolescents is the inclusion of the family. Family members play a crucial role in the adolescent's treatment in a variety of ways. First, parents are typically responsible for taking adolescents to their therapy appointments. Hence, their engagement in treatment is necessary for treatment compliance.

Second, parents are a critical part of the ongoing assessment process, as they can provide important information about the suicide attempt, symptoms of psychopathology, warning signs of suicidal escalation, treatment progress, and the success/failure of therapy interventions. Third, parents are needed to monitor youth safety in the home, to assist the youth in using his or her safety plan, and to contact mental health professionals during a suicidal crisis. Fourth, parents are responsible for insuring that the home is safe and free of lethal means and means for self-harm. Fifth, parents can facilitate the treatment by serving as "collaborators" (Kendall, 2000), in coaching the youth to use what he or she learned in treatment outside of the session. Sixth, parent/child conflict is often the trigger for teen suicidality (for a review, see Miller & Glinski, 2000), so resolution of these issues is a key target of treatment. Because the focus of the treatment is on the adolescent, family members should be referred to other providers to deal with their own mental health or substance abuse problems. These problems are addressed in the treatment only in terms of their direct impact on youth suicidality.

The amount of session to session participation of parents should be based on clinical judgment and should take into account the adolescent's age and degree of independence from the family (see Asarnow, Tompson, & Berk, 2005). It is recommended that parents be involved in removing lethal means from the home, developing the safety plan, and monitoring youth safety in the home. In addition, family members may be involved in learning the basic treatment approach and interventions that their son or daughter is learning so that they can facilitate (and not interfere with) the application of these strategies. The therapist should conduct a brief check-in with parents at the end of every session to review safety, treatment progress, and the interventions learned in treatment. Because family conflict is typical during the adolescent phase of development, as well as a frequent trigger of teen suicidality, in most cases, it will be of benefit to teach family communication and problem-solving skills. The decision of whether or not to conduct family versus collateral sessions with parents depends on the youth's degree of autonomy from the family and the degree of current family conflict, and again, is best determined by clinical judgment. Family sessions are not recommended until the parent can be in the room with the youth without a high level of conflict and criticism.

EARLY PHASE OF TREATMENT
(SESSIONS 1–3)

The initial therapy sessions set the stage for the remainder of the treatment by focusing on engaging the adolescent and family in treatment, orienting them to the cognitive model, and developing a list of problems and goals for therapy. In addition to establishing the framework that will guide the therapy, three key interventions are introduced in the early phase of treatment: (a) developing a safety plan for suicidal emergencies, (b) obtaining a narrative description of the events leading to the suicide attempt, (c) conducting a suicide risk assessment and removal of lethal means, (d) developing the cognitive conceptualization, and (e) establishing goals for treatment.

Adolescent suicide attempters have been shown to have poor compliance with outpatient treatment (Trautman, Stewart, & Morishima, 1993; Spirito et al., 1992). Hence, we recommend that the therapist take an active role in keeping the teen and family in therapy. This is in contrast to the more typical approach in which the patient and family are considered responsible for staying engaged in treatment. Interventions that can be used to increase treatment compliance include: calling parents/teens to remind them of scheduled appointments, problem-solving impediments to regular attendance, increasing therapist availability to reschedule appointments and to see patients on a walk-in basis, and providing practical assistance with transportation (e.g., providing tokens for public transportation). As noted above, it is necessary to work with parents to insure treatment compliance. Adolescents are typically reliant on their parents for transportation to and from therapy appointments. Parents often have multiple practical barriers to treatment compliance such as work schedules, household responsibilities, and care of other children in the home. Moreover, parents may experience shame or guilt about their son/daughter's suicide attempt and have a lack of understanding of the importance of treatment and/or how treatment works. It is of critical importance that these obstacles are addressed with parents, in order to facilitate the teen and family's participation in treatment.

Session 1

Table 12.2 shows an outline of interventions that should be conducted in Session 1. The first therapy session has several important goals, including a review of the limits of confidentiality, risk assessment, removal of lethal means from the home, overview of the treatment approach, education about the cognitive-behavioral model, and the establishment of the initial safety plan. Each of these elements is described below.

Review of the Limits of Confidentiality

A review of the limits of confidentiality should be conducted at the beginning of the first session. In establishing rapport with the teen and gaining his or her trust, it is important that confidentiality be discussed openly. Privacy from parents is likely to be an issue of importance to most teens, who are in the process of establishing independence. Moreover, due to the high risk nature of this population and the need to have an open dialogue with parents regarding safety, therapists should be clear with teens from the outset what the limits of confidentiality are. A sample script for speaking with suicidal teens about confidentiality is shown in Table 12.3.

Although the details may vary by state, parents typically have access to their son/daughter's treatment records, and there is no legal protection that keeps information shared by teens in psychotherapy confidential from their parents. However, most therapists working with teens try to offer some degree of privacy regarding details of non-urgent issues (e.g., peer and romantic relationships) in order to facilitate trust and collaboration. In particular, because safety is of paramount importance in working with this population, it is recommended that the therapist inform the teen that *any* information pertaining to his or her safety will need to be shared with parents and that they are entitled to know information needed to keep their son/daughter safe. Sharing this in advance is important in avoiding later feelings of betrayal that can damage the therapeutic relationship if a disclosure is made. In our experience, when the need to share information with parents is framed as part of the therapist's care and concern for the patient's well-being, it is received well by most youth. The therapist can reassure the patient that if a disclosure needs to be made, he or she will work together with the youth to determine the best way of conveying the information their parents. Therapists should also communicate to youth and parents that limits of confidentiality include child abuse (and elder abuse in some states) and danger to others, according to state laws.

Risk assessment and removal of lethal means. Because teens who have made past suicide attempts are at high risk for future suicide attempts, a comprehensive assessment of suicide risk should be conducted during the initial phase of treatment (for a comprehensive review of risk assessment, see the *Practice Guideline for the Assessment and Treatment of Patients with*

Table 12.2
Outline of Session 1*

1. Review of Limits of Confidentiality
2. Discuss and Plan Removal of Lethal Means
3. Overview of the Treatment (e.g., short-term, focus on suicidal behavior)
4. Description of the Cognitive-Behavioral Model
5. Construction of the Safety Plan (including both youth and family versions)
6. Assign Session Specific Homework (e.g., practice elements of the safety plan)

---

*Note that Items 1–5 should be also be conducted with the parents.

Table 12.3
Script for Reviewing Confidentiality with Youth and Parents

Youth

"Before we begin talking today, I want to tell you how confidentiality between you and me will work. A lot of what you tell me is private, but there are certain things that are not private. My number one goal is your health and safety. That takes priority over anything else that we do together. So, if you tell me anything that makes me concerned that you might be in danger of harming yourself or somebody else, or that you are unsafe in anyway, I will need to share this information with people who will help me keep you safe, like your parents, other doctors, or the police. Second, if I hear anything about child abuse or abuse of an elderly person, I am obligated to report that to the authorities (follow appropriate guidelines according to individual state law). Your parents are entitled to receive information from your therapist about how you are doing. I will do my best to give this information in general terms and to not share specific details, except in the situations I have already mentioned. It is your choice what you decide to tell me today. You do not have to tell me anything that you don't want to, but I hope that you will be honest with me as you can, so I can be as helpful to you as possible. I know you have been coping with some tough situations and that is why you are here today."

Parent

"Before we begin, let me review with you how confidentiality works. Everything you and your child tell me will remain private, except under certain circumstances. First, if you or your son/daughter tells me information that makes me concerned that he or she might be in danger of harming him/herself or somebody else, I will need to share this information with people needed to keep him/her safe, such as other doctors and/or the police. The primary goal of this treatment is to keep your son/daughter safe and I will let you know immediately any information that pertains to his or her safety and or risk of harming him/herself. Second, if I hear anything about child abuse/neglect or abuse/neglect of an elderly person, I am obligated to report that to the authorities. During the course of treatment, I will let you know how your son/daughter is doing and discuss how you can help him/her. In order to give your son/daughter some privacy so that he or she feels comfortable talking with me, I will try to give you information about his or her discussions with me in general terms and not share specific details of situations your son/daughter has described, except in the situations I have already mentioned."

Suicidal Behaviors; APA, 2003). In addition to this initial assessment, an ongoing assessment of suicidal thoughts and behavior should be conducted during each therapy session. Monitoring of suicidal ideation, intent, and plan, as well as hopelessness and depression can be conducted both by clinical interview and using standardized self-report measures such as the *Beck Depression Inventory II* (BDI-II; Beck, Steer, & Brown, 1996) and the *Beck Hopelessness Scale* (BHS; Beck & Steer, 1993). Items 2 (Pessimism) and 9 (Suicidal Thoughts and Dying) of the BDI-II are of particular relevance. Measures designed especially for children and adolescents, such as the *Children's Depression Inventory* (CDI; Kovacs & Beck, 1977) and the *Hopelessness Scale for Children* (HSC; Kazdin, Rodgers, & Colbus, 1986) can also be used. In addition, parents should also be questioned regarding their observations of suicidal thoughts or behavior in the youth, as youth may not always be reliable reporters. Other risk factors for suicidal behavior such as substance use, compliance with psychiatric medications, exacerbation of psychopathology, and environmental stressors (e.g., family or peer conflict), should also be assessed.

It is of critical importance that the therapist works with the teen and family to insure that potentially lethal means are removed from the home and/or secured safely. Access to lethal means is associated with suicide deaths (Brent, Perper, Moritz, Baugher, Schweers, et al., 1993; Kellermann et al., 1992). In particular, every effort must be made to remove guns from the home, as research shows that adolescents may use guns in suicide attempts if they are available (Marzuk, Leon, Tardiff, Morgan, Stajic, et al., 1992). The family may also wish to remove or secure any knives and pills (i.e., prescription and over the counter medication). Other methods may also be removed if they youth has used them in the past or expressed ideation about them, such as ropes/belts that can be used for hanging. Locks can be placed on windows if the youth has tried or threatened to jump. Parents should be told about the increased risk of suicide when lethal means are available, and the rationale should be given that not having ready access to lethal means decreases the teen's ability to act on suicidal impulses (e.g., "like a person on a diet not keeping cake and cookies in the house").

Of importance, when a patient is in a suicidal crisis, we use a collaborative team approach in which crucial clinical decisions, such as whether or not to hospitalize him or her, are made in consultation with the treatment team. In addition to consulting about crisis situations, we also hold a weekly group supervision meeting during which therapists discuss ongoing cases and provide each other with feedback and support. We recommend that therapists working with this population have access to other mental health professionals for case consultation and support. In addition, therapists should be aware of the procedures for emergency hospitalization in their work setting.

Overview of the Treatment Approach and Education about the Cognitive Model

In the first session, the adolescent and parents should be informed about the structure of the treatment. For example, they should be told that the treatment is short-term, that it involves approximately ten sessions, and that the primary focus will be on preventing suicidal behavior. Next, the therapist should review the cognitive-behavioral model on which the treatment is based (e.g., the connection between thoughts, feelings, and behaviors, as well as physiological cues of emotional arousal). A diagram explaining the relationships among thoughts, feelings and behavior is often useful for illustrating cognitive model, as well as more creative approaches for younger adolescents, such as conceptualizing thoughts, feelings and behaviors as a "baseball diamond" (for a description, see Friedberg & McClure, 2002).

Developing a Safety Plan

It is often difficult for suicidal adolescents to plan and implement adaptive coping strategies during a suicidal crisis, because they may be overwhelmed by strong negative emotions and have difficulty thinking logically (see Wenzel et al., in press). For this reason, the therapist and patient work together from the very beginning of treatment to develop a detailed safety plan that can be easily accessed for use in future crisis situations. The initial safety plan is expanded throughout the therapy as new skills are learned and consists of a list of coping strategies that range from those the adolescent can perform on his or her own to a plan for contacting emergency services.

The safety plan should include the following components, (a) warning signs of the potential for suicidal behavior, (b) coping strategies, (c) how to contact responsible adults for assistance in a crisis. Warning signs may include thoughts (e.g., "I can't take it anymore"), feelings (e.g., acute depressed mood), or behaviors (e.g., isolating oneself) that the youth or parent has identified as preceding a suicide attempt in the past. Coping strategies typically include simple behavioral tasks (e.g., going for a walk, calling a friend, or watching a funny movie). These activities function as a way for patients to distract themselves and prevent suicide ideation from escalating (Wenzel et al., in press). Coping strategies that are learned during the middle phase of therapy, such as using coping cards or a hope box may also be incorporated into the safety plan later in the treatment. The safety plan always includes the telephone numbers of (a) family members and other responsible adults, (b) the therapist, (c) the psychiatric emergency department, and (d) other crisis hotlines that handle emergency calls (such as 1-800-273-TALK). Adolescents are instructed to contact their parents or another responsible adult (e.g., a relative or a teacher or school counselor if they are at school), the therapist or the emergency room if they are in danger of engaging in self-harm behavior and other coping strategies have failed to help.

At the end of the first session, the adolescent and therapist should have agreed upon an initial safety plan that he or she can use prior to the next session if a crisis occurs. The safety plan should be reviewed with the parent, so he or she can assist the patient with its use. The parent's role in assisting the youth with carrying out the safety plan should be reviewed in detail. In addition, the feasibility of the safety plan should always be checked with the parent. For example, the adolescent may suggest a coping strategy, such as "staying overnight at a friend's house" or "buying new clothes," which is either not possible or not allowable by the parent. The safety plan should be written down and copies given to the youth and parents. The youth may be encouraged to carry a copy of the safety plan with him/her at all times.

Parents should also be given a copy of the safety plan or a modified version that describes the responsibilities of the family. The family safety plan should include warning signs that the teen is at increased risk and what the family should do at varying levels of danger (e.g., coach youth to use coping strategies, call the therapist, take youth immediately to the emergency room). Family members should be told to take any communication seriously from the teen regarding suicide ideation or suicide intent. The family safety plan should include (a) strategies for talking adolescents about their suicide ideation and (b) a plan for monitoring adolescents to ensure that they are not left unattended. The family should also be instructed to negotiate a "truce" around conflicts related to the adolescent's suicidal behavior until family members have learned more effective communication skills. Figures 12.1 and 12.2 show examples of adolescent and parent safety plans.

TEEN SAFETY PLAN

Warning Signs (When I am to use the Safety Plan):

☐ Wanting to go to sleep and not wake up
☐ Wanting to hurt myself
☐ Thinking "I can't take it anymore."

Coping Strategies (Things I can try to do on my own):

☐ Listening to music
☐ Drawing or painting
☐ Playing videogames
☐ Sending email/using the computer
☐ Going for a walk
☐ Watching a comedy on television
☐ Eating ice cream
☐ Exercising
☐ Other: _____

Contacting Other People:

☐ Calling my parents: _____ Phone: _____
☐ Calling other adults: _____ Phone: _____

Contacting a Health Care Professional during business hours:

☐ Calling my therapist: _____ Phone: _____
☐ Calling my psychiatrist: _____ Phone: _____

The following agencies or services may be called 24 hours a day/7 days a week:

☐ Calling the psychiatric ED: _____ Phone: _____
☐ Calling National Suicide Prevention Lifeline   Phone: 1-800-273-TALK

Figure 12.1 Adolescent Safety Plan (adapted from Wenzel et al., in press).

FAMILY SAFETY PLAN

Warning Signs That My Child is At High Risk for Suicidal Behavior:

☐ He or she says "I want to go to sleep and not wake up"
☐ He or she says "I want to hurt myself"
☐ He or she says "I can't take it anymore."
☐ He or she appears agitated and irritable.
☐ He or she gets a bad grade at school.

Plan for Monitoring Safety (check all that apply):

☐ Removal of lethal means from our home
☐ Regularly checking in with my son/daughter to assess if he or she is feeling suicidal
☐ Locks on doors and windows leading out of the house
☐ Locks on doors and windows on second story of home
☐ Removal of car keys/driving privileges
☐ Removal of lock on bedroom door or removal of bedroom door
☐ Not allowing my son/daughter to leave home alone
☐ Not allowing my son/daughter to be alone at any time, even at home
☐ Decreasing family conflict/arguments
☐ Other: _____

Parent Plan of Action:

If my son/daughter is has any of the warning signs listed above I will:

1. Ask calmly and directly about suicidal thoughts, plans, and intent.

2. If he or she reports suicidal thoughts only and believes he or she can stay safe, I will coach him/her to use the coping strategies listed above.

3. If he or she reports starting to implement a specific plan for suicide, the intent to carry the plan out, and/or inability to keep him/herself safe, I will take him/her to the nearest emergency room.

Figure 12.2 Family Safety Plan (adapted from Wenzel et al., in press).

Sessions 2 and 3

As shown in Table 12.4, Sessions 2 and 3 focus on obtaining a timeline of the most recent suicide attempt, developing a cognitive case conceptualization, creating a list of the key problems that will need to be addressed during treatment in order to decrease suicidality, and selecting the interventions that will be used to target these problems.

Obtaining a Timeline of the Suicide Attempt

The cognitive case conceptualization that guides treatment is created from the adolescent's description of his or her suicide attempt. Hence, in sessions 2 and 3, the adolescent is asked to tell the story of the suicide attempt in detail. This description includes the events leading up to the suicide attempt, the teen's cognitive, emotional and behavioral reactions to these events and the details of the suicide attempt itself. It is also helpful to ask the teen to describe what happened immediately after the suicide attempt in order to identify potential reinforcers of suicidal behavior (Linehan, 1993). The teen is instructed to tell the story of the attempt in "real time," as if "you are watching a movie of that day." It is assumed that suicide attempts are multi-determined and thus are likely to involve multiple triggers (e.g., situational, cognitive, emotional, physiological, and behavioral). Attempting to gather information from each of these domains also serves as an assessment tool to identify the areas that are most salient to teen and, thus, the types of interventions that are most likely to be successful. For example, if the teen is unable to report cognitions that occurred prior to the attempt but is able to describe behaviors occurring prior to the attempt, then the therapist may have more success focusing on behavioral coping strategies. This exercise also yields important information about proximal triggers of suicidality, which can then be highlighted as "warning signs" that the teen may be at increased risk for engaging in suicidal behavior.

In our experience, some teens may have trouble with this exercise, such as tolerating the distress associated with the discussion of the suicide attempt, finding the exercise tedious, having difficulty accessing their memories of the attempt, or feeling ashamed. The therapist can assist the teen by making the task as concrete as possible and by presenting a clear rationale for asking them to re-tell the story, such as "So that I can be of the most help possible to you, it is important that I really understand what happened from your point of view. There is no right or wrong answer. I need to understand what happened so we can work together to prevent it from happening again." The therapist should guide the teen with a series of prompts, such as: "What happened next?" "When that happened, how did you feel?" "What was running through your mind at that point?" Some may find it helpful to imagine that they are describing a sequence of events in a movie and they can be asked to replay the events in "slow motion." Another helpful approach is for the adolescent and therapist to create a written timeline together. Youth often need visual aids to facilitate their memory. The timeline can be referenced throughout the

Table 12.4
Outline of Sessions 2 and 3

1. Obtain a Timeline of the Most Recent Suicide Attempt*

2. Obtain Relevant Psychiatric History

3. Develop a Cognitive Case Conceptualization

4. Develop a Problem List

5. Select Intervention Strategies

*Note: Item 1 should also be conducted with parents.

Received "D" on math test. Felt angry, ashamed, hot, and shaky. Had thought: "Nothing I do turns out right." Sat through the rest of class feeling terrible.

Walked in the house and Mom immediately asked about my math test. Told her about the "D." She got angry and said, "Why can't you try harder? You will never make it in life with such bad grades."

Went into bathroom and took out bottle of Tylenol. Had thought: "Things will be easier for everyone if I just end it now." Cried. Felt very sad and like my body was very heavy.

Mom came into my room yelling at me about starting my homework. I was awake. I didn't feel sick yet or anything. When mom saw the pills she started screaming, "Did you take these?!" When I said yes, she started crying and called 911.

The ambulance came and took me to the hospital. Mom rode in the ambulance with me. I kept thinking, "I can't believe I did something so stupid."

| 2 pm | 3 pm | 3:15 pm | 3:20 pm | 3:25 pm | 3:30 pm | 3:35 pm | 3:40 - 4 pm | 4 pm |

Got a ride home from school with a friend. Talked with my friend about the bad grade. Felt a little bit better.

Felt angry, sad, and hopeless. Had thought: "She's right. I am a failure. Nothing will ever work out for me. I might as well die."

Went into my room and took a handful of Tylenol. Laid down on my bed. Felt sad and also relieved that I wouldn't feel bad anymore soon.

In my room with Mom waiting for the ambulance to arrive. Mom was crying and asking me how I could do this to myself. She told me she loved me and apologized for yelling at me about my grades. I felt a little bit better and regretted taking the pills. I started to worry about the pills hurting me.

Figure 12.3 Timeline

course of therapy. For example, as various strategies for managing suicidal crises are introduced, the clinician can go back to the timeline and ask teens where in the sequence of events that a particular intervention or coping strategy would have been most useful in preventing a suicide attempt. See Figure 12.3 for an example of a timeline.

Parents should also be given the opportunity to tell the story of the suicide attempt from their perspective. Hearing the parent's story serves multiple purposes, including (a) verifying the accuracy of the teen's account and obtaining details the teen was not able to recall, (b) helping parents identify "warning signs" of future suicidal crises, (c) identifying of family-based triggers, and (d) identifying of family responses that may be reinforcing of suicidal behavior. As noted above, the clinician should use his or her clinical judgment as to whether the parent should tell his or her story with the youth present. A separate meeting is recommended if the parent is likely to be angry or critical toward the adolescent.

In addition to obtaining detailed information about the most recent suicide attempt, the therapist should also conduct a standard intake assessment, focusing on psychiatric diagnoses, history of the present episode and past psychiatry history, past history of suicidal behavior, previous psychiatric treatment, family history of psychiatric disturbance and suicidal acts, medical history, psychosocial history, developmental history, drug and alcohol use, and mental status examination. This information is important in identifying distal risk factors for suicide attempts (e.g., a diagnosis of Major Depressive Disorder and past suicide attempts).

Developing a Cognitive Case Conceptualization

Based on the information obtained from the timeline of the suicide attempt, as well as the standard psychiatric interview, the therapist formulates a cognitively-based case conceptualization that guides the treatment and selection of intervention strategies. In addition to the key cognitions associated with the suicide attempt, as well as the proximal triggers, the conceptualization should include distal risk factors for suicide attempts (e.g., impulsivity, poor problem solving ability, psychiatric diagnosis, past suicide attempts), as well as protective factors (e.g., reasons for living, no access to lethal means). Because adolescents' lives are intertwined with their families, family risk and protective factors should also be included in the conceptualization. For example, family conflict is a common precipitant to adolescents' suicide attempts (for a review, see Miller & Glinski, 2000; Wenzel et al., in press).

The conceptualization should also include the cognitions associated with the suicide attempt. These cognitions may take the form of core beliefs, intermediate beliefs, or automatic thoughts. Core beliefs are global statements about the self, world, or others, that are deeply held, usually developed in childhood, and apply across situations (e.g., "I'm worthless"). Intermediate beliefs consist of attitudes, rules, and assumptions about the world that are derived from the core belief and often occur in conditional or "if-then" form (e.g., "If I get a bad grade, then I am worthless"). Finally, automatic thoughts are the most superficial level of cognitions, occur rapidly, briefly, and without intention, are often triggered by a given situation (e.g., "I can't do anything right, I might as well be dead"), and are also derived from core beliefs. The therapist should attempt to elicit as many of these types of cognitions as possible from the adolescent. This can be done during the timeline exercise described above or by asking questions such as, "What was going through your mind before you attempted suicide?" Adolescents may have difficulty identifying the various types of cognitions listed above. If this is the case, the therapist can hypothesize the types of cognitions that may have been present. For example, if the teen describes attempting suicide to escape negative emotions, the therapist may speculate that the corresponding automatic thought was "I can't tolerate these feelings."

Although cognitive variables are important in *understanding* the teen's suicidal behavior, he or she may or may not *respond* to intervention strategies that focus on identifying and restructuring negative cognitions. In these cases, the therapist can apply behavioral interventions designed to achieve cognitive change (e.g., the use of distraction skills to help patients see that they can tolerate the pain). In general, although the suicide attempt is conceptualized in cognitive terms, interventions used with adolescents may more often focus on behavioral and affective coping strategies and family issues. The specific interventions that are chosen may be based on those interventions that are most likely to prevent another attempt as well as those interventions that the teen is most likely to use during a suicide crisis. The therapist should continue to update the conceptualization as new data are gathered throughout the course of treatment. Thus, the cognitive case conceptualization not only facilitates an understanding of the patient in light of cognitive theory, it also guides the specific intervention strategies that the therapist can implement.

Developing a Problem List and Selecting Intervention Strategies

After the therapist has developed a cognitive case conceptualization, a problem list should be developed to guide the selection of interventions. The therapist should identify the most important skills deficits that contributed to the suicide attempt that will need to be modified in order to prevent a future suicide attempt. For example, the problem list may include: (a) coping with rejection by a group of popular kids at school, (b) the cognition "I can't tolerate the emotional pain," (c) coping with depressed mood, and (d) poor emotion regulation abilities. Hence, interventions that may be used include: (a) social skills training and working with the youth on developing a supportive circle of other friendships and strengthening family support, (b) restructuring of the cognition "I can't tolerate the pain" either by Socratic questioning or behavioral experiments (see Friedberg & McClure, 2002, for a detailed discussion of how to use these procedures with adolescents), (c) assisting the youth in obtaining treatment for depression, such as medications and/or psychotherapy specifically targeting depression, and (d) teaching affect regulation skills, such as relaxation or other self-soothing strategies.

The Middle Phase of Treatment (Sessions 4–8)

The middle phase of treatment targets suicidal behavior in depth by focusing on both cognitive and behavioral change. The interventions conducted in this phase include cognitive restructuring, the creation of coping cards and a hope box, teaching behavioral and affect regulation skills, and family-based interventions. Table 12.5 presents a therapist outline for Sessions 4–8. The order in which to use these interventions is left up to the therapist's judgment. In addition, the choice of which interventions to use should be determined by the conceptualization created in the initial sessions, the level of cognitive development, and the nature and degree of family difficulties.

Cognitive Strategies

In the middle phase of treatment, therapist and patient work together to identify and modify the key thoughts that became activated when he or she was suicidal, a process called *cognitive restructuring*. Standard cognitive therapy strategies such as Socratic (guided, open-ended) questioning, the recognition of cognitive distortions, dysfunctional thought records, behavioral experiments, and role-plays should be used to create a set of adaptive alternatives to each belief (for a discussion of the use of the techniques with adolescents, see Friedberg & McClure, 2002). It may be necessary for the therapist to assist the adolescent in creating alternative responses, such as by giving them a list of positive thoughts from which to choose. The therapist should ask the youth to rate how much they believe each alternative response on a scale of 1 to 10. Only thoughts that the youth believes at an 8 or higher should be selected for use in a future suicidal crisis, and it make take several sessions to identify such thoughts. However, this level of belief in the thoughts is crucial in ensuring that they will be helpful to the teen in a suicidal crisis.

Coping cards. Each suicide-promoting thought and set of alternative responses is placed on a coping card. Coping cards are small wallet-sized cards that the teen can easily carry around with him/her. The primary purpose of the coping cards is to provide the patient with an easily accessible way of "jump-starting" adaptive thinking during a suicidal crisis. In a crisis, the patient is often highly distressed and may have difficulty accessing positive thoughts on his or her own. In this case, he or she can simply pull out and read a coping card. We also recommend to patients that they read the cards regularly when not in crisis to practice the more adaptive ways of thinking they have learned in treatment so that such thoughts eventually become accessible on their own. A rationale can be given to patients, "just like training for a tennis match by practicing your serve over and over, you need to train your mind to think positively by reading these cards over and over." An example of a coping card is presented in Figure 12.4. Coping cards should be reviewed with parents, so that parents can remind the

Table 12.5
Outline of Sessions 4–8

1. Develop Cognitive Coping Strategies (e.g., cognitive restructuring, problem-solving skills, coping cards, hope box)
2. Develop Behavioral Coping Strategies (e.g., distraction, relaxation, self-soothing)
3. Develop Affective Coping Strategies (e.g., feeling thermometer technique)
4. Develop Family Coping Strategies (e.g., family positives, family commitment and engagement, family communication, family contingency management, family high expectations and positive reinforcement)

```
┌─────────────────────────────────────┐
│                                     │
│  **Negative Thought:**              │
│  I can't tolerate the pain.         │
│                                     │
│                                     │
│  **Alternative Response:**          │
│  1) I can handle it.  I have always │
│       handled it in the past.       │
│                                     │
│  2) I am capable of feeling good.   │
│                                     │
│  3) I have things to look forward to. │
│                                     │
│  4) I have gotten through it before. │
│                                     │
└─────────────────────────────────────┘
```

Figure 12.4 Example of a Coping Card (adapted from Berk et al., 2004).

teen of his or her alternative responses during a crisis. It may also be helpful to give school personnel copies of the coping card, so they can be assistance to the youth if a crisis occurs at school. If the adolescent's suicide-promoting thoughts are directly related to their relationship with their parents, such as "my parents won't love me anymore if I fail a class in school and therefore I might as well die," it may be helpful for the parent to create a coping card for the youth. For example, the parent can write down (in his or her own handwriting) the alternative response, "I will always love you, no matter what happens," which the youth can carry around with him/her as a reminder. Copies of coping cards should be placed in the hope box, as described below.

Problem Solving Strategies

Adolescents may attempt suicide as a way to address situations that they perceive to be unsolvable (Esposito, Johnson, Wolfsdorf, & Spirito, 2003). It is important conceptualize the suicide attempt with the teen as a maladaptive problem-solving strategy and to teach him/her problem solving skills that lead to safe choices. There are many cognitive-behavioral strategies for teaching teens how to solve problems. In general, these approaches teach a series of steps, including (a) identifying the problem, (b) brainstorming all possible solutions, (c) evaluating the pros and cons of each possible solution, and (d) choosing a solution to implement. These same strategies can be taught to parents to be used for solving family problems effectively. Problem solving strategies are best taught to adolescents and families by using neutral or generic problems (e.g., negotiating household chores) first, before moving on to more "hot" topics.

Construction of a hope box. In a suicidal crisis, it is often difficult for youth to identify and remember positives, coping skills, and reasons to live. To combat this problem, the youth should be asked to create a "hope box" for use during suicidal crises. The hope box is a box or other type of container in which the youth places items and mementos that elicit positive feelings, cue him or her to use coping skills, and serve as reminders of reasons to live. For example, items that may be placed in the hope box include photographs of favorite people and places, postcards, letters, gifts, coping cards, or a scented candle. The youth is instructed to put the hope box in a safe place where he or she can easily access it (e.g., in the bedroom closet) when feeling suicidal. If appropriate, assigning parents a role in creating the hope box gives them an active part to play in helping their child and can help to decrease their feelings of helplessness.

Table 12.6
Sample Items That Can Be Included in the Hope Box

- Photographs of family, friends, favorite places, pets, etc.
- CDs, tapes, MP3s of favorite songs
- Videos or DVDs of favorite television shows or movies
- Favorite books, magazines, comic books
- Favorite foods (e.g, chocolate, tea bags—should be non-perishable)
- Favorite scents (e.g., perfume, scented candles, incense)
- Videogames
- Crossword puzzles, word search puzzles
- Coping Cards
- Letters
- Favorite gifts (e.g., a bracelet from a friend)
- Paper, pencils, paints, etc. (if the teen likes to draw or paint)

For example, parents may find this task useful as an activity they can work together on with their child, such as by accompanying their child to the bookstore to buy his or her favorite book of poetry to put in the hope box.

The hope box intervention is best conducted after the youth has learned cognitive and behavioral coping skills. Cues to use the coping skills that have been identified should be placed in the hope box. For example, adolescents can put in a CD with their favorite song, a videotape with their favorite funny television show, and their coping cards. Distraction methods (e.g., listening to a favorite song, word search puzzles) and self-soothing techniques (e.g., techniques that improve mood via hearing, smell, sound, taste and touch) are particularly amenable to the hope box. The hope box should be assigned for homework and the youth should be instructed to bring it to show the therapist in the following session. Reviewing the items in the hope box with the youth helps strengthen the therapeutic alliance by allowing them to "show and tell" the therapist about their life and their likes and dislikes. Sample items that can be included in a hope box are shown in Table 12.6. This intervention should be conducted with most teens due to its importance in crisis management.

Behavioral Coping Skills

A range of behavioral strategies can be taught to teens in order to safely manage suicidal thoughts and behavior. Distraction techniques can be extremely useful in helping patients to tolerate short-term distress without resorting to self-injury. Almost any activity can serve as a distracter (e.g., reading, watching television or movies, talking to friends, counting backwards from 100, physical exercise) as long as it is compelling enough to the patient to demand a shift in his or her attention. Creating intense physical sensations (e.g., holding ice cubes, taking a hot or cold shower, drinking hot tea) can be particularly helpful as a substitute for self harm (Linehan, 1993). Relaxation techniques can be taught to decrease the physiological arousal associated with painful emotions and to prevent impulsive responses. Emphasizing the short-term nature of most suicidal crises can also be of use as a motivator to tolerate distress rather than escape from it via self-injurious behavior. The therapist can help the teen focus on the short term nature of negative feelings by using the "time projection" technique (Friedberg & McClure, 2002), which involves asking teens "How will you feel in 1 week, 3, weeks, 3 months, 1 year, etc.?" Finally, self-soothing activities (e.g., taking a hot bath, eating a favorite food, petting a kitten) can also function to decrease negative mood states and offset suicidal behavior. It can be helpful to have the teen select self-soothing strategies from each of his or her five senses (Linehan, 1993). Each behavioral skill that the patient finds useful should be added to his or her safety plan.

Affective Strategies

Adolescents who make suicide attempts or hurt themselves often describe wanting to rid themselves of overwhelming or painful emotions as the reason for their suicide attempt (see Kienhorst et al., 1995; Linehan, 1993; Miller et al., 2007). The capacity to understand and identify emotions, their physiological, cognitive, and behavioral aspects, and the situations that trigger various emotions, gives an adolescent the capability of developing a more thoughtful response to those situations. One way to target this is by using the "Feeling Thermometer" intervention (Miller, Rotheram-Borus, Piacentini, Graae, & Castro-Blanco, 1992). Adolescents are taught the metaphor that escalating emotions are like a rise in temperature until they are at the "boiling point" where they are at risk for engaging in dangerous behaviors. The goal is to learn to "cool down" and "lower the temperature" before reaching the boiling point. Once the youth and therapist understand the process by which emotional escalation occurs, they can identify the appropriate cognitive and behavioral skills needed to decrease it. These skills should be added to the safety plan.

The adolescent should be given a diagram to look at during the exercise that represents a thermometer, such as a vertical line with the number one at the bottom, going up to ten at the top. The therapist can label the number one "feeling the best" and the number ten "feeling the worst." For younger adolescents, happy and sad faces may also be used at the appropriate ends of the scale. A brief script for conducting this intervention is provided here (Miller et al., 1992; for an adaptation see also Berk & Asarnow, 2005).

At times, when we are experiencing really bad feelings, all we want to do is get rid of them. Sometimes, the only way we can think of to do this is by hurting ourselves. Does this sound like what happened with you?

I want to teach you ways to handle painful emotions without having to hurt yourself.

The first step is to learn how to identify your emotions and when they are starting to head up to a danger point.

Take a look at this picture (show adolescent the feeling thermometer diagram). We call this a "feeling thermometer." It is similar to the kind of thermometer that measures when you have a temperature when you are sick, in that the higher you get, the worse you feel. Zero is the best you ever feel, totally at ease, calm, content, like everything is ok with the world. Ten (10) is the worst you ever feel, when your feelings are so painful you can't stand them and all you want to do is make them stop. This is the point when you are in danger of hurting yourself.

I want to use this picture to help you (1) identify what your danger point is and (2) at what point on the thermometer you know that you are heading up to your danger point, so you can catch it and turn it around before it is too late.

Family Strategies

Whereas cognitive therapy for adult suicidal patients focuses on family problems in the broader context of helping patients improve their social support networks, cognitive therapy with suicidal adolescent patients focuses directly on improving family functioning. Several interventions can be conducted with the family as needed, including (a) increasing positive affect and support within the family, (b) improving family communication, (c) improving the family's problem solving ability (described above in the section on teen problem solving), (d) contingency management of problematic behaviors, and (e) decreasing parents' high expectations and improve the positive reinforcement of the teen (see Wenzel et al., in press, for further discussion of these interventions). These goals serve to decrease vulnerability factors for future suicidal acts (e.g., family conflict) and increase protective factors such as family support and cohesion. Family interventions are highly recommended when family dysfunction was identified by the patient as a proximal factor leading to the suicide attempt.

Increasing Positive Affect and Support within the Family

Prior to engaging the teen and family in change-based interventions, it is important to enhance positive affect and support, as a means of mobilizing the family to do the work that will be needed. The family may be experiencing a great deal of negative affect toward one another, due to conflicts existing prior to the suicide attempt, as well as to the suicide attempt itself. Moreover, it is also of critical importance to re-build positive affect within the family, so that the teen views his or her family as a source of support and will reach out to them for help if feeling suicidal in the future. The "family positives" intervention (Miller et al., 1992; for an adaptation see also Berk & Asarnow, 2005) can be used for this purpose. This is a relatively simple intervention, in which the youth and parents are each asked to say three positive things about one another, as well as three positive things about the family.

Before beginning this intervention, youth and parents should be prepped separately, if needed, so that they are able to generate positive comments about each other (e.g., prepare the youth/parent by helping them to remember positive things about each other and underscoring the importance of remembering the good things). The therapist should avoid a situation in which the teen or parents are unable to think about positives in the presence of one another. Positives can include statements about physical appearance, peers, family, personality characteristics, school, and relationships. If youth or parents are feeling so negative that they cannot think of any current positives about one another, the therapist can ask about past situations, such as, "what do you remember most fondly about your son when he was a little boy?" The therapist should then prompt each person to state what he or she finds positive about the family, such as, "we have a lot of fun when we go on vacations together, or "no matter what happens, we are a family that loves each other a lot."

Family Commitment and Engagement

Sometimes parents and teens may be emotionally detached from each other, or the parents display a low commitment to their roles as parents. If family disengagement and lack of commitment were associated with the suicide attempt, then increasing family involvement may be addressed using many of the cognitive and behavioral strategies described in this chapter. One unique strategy for increasing commitment is to ask parents about their role as parents when the teenager was younger. Parents and teens may become alienated from one another during adolescence, and remembering past times when the family was more connected may inspire increased connection in the present. In addition, the teen can be asked to recall a period of time when they were closer as a family and describe the manner in which such family support would be useful in handling future suicidal crises. The therapist can also assign family activities (e.g., attending a movie or dinner together) as homework, to increase positive family interaction and bonding.

Family Communication

It is important to teach families effective communication skills so that they have the skills needed to resolve conflicts that trigger suicidality in the teen and to increase family cohesion and support. The teen and parents should be taught basic communication skills such as active listening (e.g., asking each to repeat back what they heard the other say, prior to giving his or her response, often called the "speaker/listener" technique) and "I" statements. It can also be helpful to identify negative verbal communication strategies, such as interrupting others, lecturing, blaming, name-calling, and putting others down. It is also important to review nonverbal indicators of negative communication, such as not looking directly at the person who is talking. Clinicians can also remind families that "listening does not mean agreeing," but that in order to solve problems, it is important for each person to feel that his or her perspective was heard and understood. It is important that these skills are taught to families both via psycho-education and practice. Role-plays in session are often crucial in helping families to use these techniques effectively, so that they have had sufficient practice with the techniques to be able to use them in emotionally-charged situations. The clinician should start with more neutral or mild disagreements and ensure the family can use the skills effectively with these types of problems before moving onto "hot" topics.

Family Contingency Management

Teens may display oppositional, defiant or uncooperative behaviors, and the parent-teen interactions associated with this problem may be related to teens' suicidal acts. For these behavior problems, a contingency management system may be introduced (Curry et al., 2005). The extent or complexity of the contingency management system will depend upon the specific problems, resources, and capabilities of the family members. Some parents will be able to establish complex token economy systems, whereas other parents may utilize a simple contract system (e.g., "If you do that, then I'll do this"). Family contingency management may also help increase the teen's compliance with homework assignments that are developed during therapy.

Effective contingency management involves several steps. The first step is to specify the target behaviors that are to occur (or not occur) for both the teen and the family. Behaviors should be clearly defined and observable, and the criteria for the behavior occurring or not occurring should be specified (e.g., if the behavior is the teen cleaning his or her bedroom, the parents and teen must first agree upon what tasks will need to be completed for the room to be considered clean). The second step is to establish a monitoring system for tracking the target behaviors. In creating the monitoring system, the therapist and family should decide at what frequency the behavior will be observed and tracked. Formal charts may be useful for this purpose, so the youth has an accurate understanding of his or her progress. The third step is to establish the rewards and/or punishment that will be given if the target behavior occurs or does not occur as well as to discuss the schedule for reinforcement or punishment (e.g., how many times the behavior needs to be performed or not for a reinforcement of punishment to be received). The fourth step is to discuss how the plan will be implemented and troubleshoot any problems. Parents must be consistent with their tracking of behaviors and allotment of rewards and punishments, or risk losing the adolescent's trust. In addition, parents' fears of escalating the likelihood of a future suicide attempt when implementing this plan should be assessed. Family members may be afraid that the teen will attempt suicide if negative consequences or limits are enforced. If parents express this concern, then the therapist assists them in evaluating whether these concerns are legitimate. If these fears are deemed to be reasonable, then increased monitoring and supervision should occur during the period of time that the contingency management protocol is being followed.

High Expectations and Positive Reinforcement

Some family members may have unreasonably high expectations for the teen and offer infrequent positive reinforcement or support (Curry et al., 2005). This may occur because parents lack sufficient information about depression and other types of adolescent psychopathology and thus attribute his or her negative behaviors or poor performance in school to willfulness or defiance. It is important for parents to have realistic expectations of their teen in order to decrease criticism and to increase support and positive reinforcement. Parents should be educated on basic principles of behaviorism and shaping, such as "people tend to engage in behaviors that they get positive outcomes from, so you need to reward the behavior that you want in your son/daughter and not reinforce or ignore those you don't want." For example, providing families with the rationale for reducing high expectations may involve educating the parents that the teen's suicide attempt was related to his or her low self-worth or a sense of helplessness in meeting high standards. In order to identify and negotiate new expectations, teens and parents should discuss the specific area of functioning where teens perceive that the expectations are too high, such as academic, extracurricular, or social activities. The specific ways that parents may reinforce teens should be discussed (e.g., specific praise, general praise or offering a tangible reward), and parents should be encouraged to offer reinforcement for making some or partial progress toward a specific goal.

Later Sessions (Sessions 9–10)

The key intervention utilized in the final phase of treatment is the relapse prevention task (RPT). An outline of the interventions conducted in sessions 9 and 10 is shown in Table 12.7. This task is a guided imagery exercise through both the most recent suicide attempt and a potential future suicidal crisis with a focus on implementing the coping skills learned in treatment. The RPT importantly serves as both a cognitive rehearsal for future coping, as well as an assessment of treatment progress and whether or not termination is appropriate. When the therapist has confidence that the patient will be able to apply his or her new skills to prevent future suicide attempts, termination is indicated. If the patient has difficulty imagining successfully coping with a future suicidal crisis, the therapist uses the RPT to identify areas of difficulty and spends more time with the patient working to solidify relevant interventions prior to terminating treatment. Thus, the treatment may extend beyond ten sessions if it becomes clear that the patient is unable to successfully complete the RPT. The specific procedures used in the RPT are described here (for a detailed description of this procedure, see Wenzel et al., in press).

The task is described to the adolescent as a way of practicing and testing the skills learned in therapy in vivo by applying them to the problems that led to previous suicide attempts in an imagery exercise. Teens and parents are told that the RPT may elicit negative emotions, but that the therapist will talk these through with them before they leave. Some youth may be reluctant to perform the RPT. In this case, it may be helpful to review the rationale for the task. For example, the adolescent can be told, "this task will help us really see if the coping strategies you have learned in therapy will keep you safe in the future and if there are any other skills you need to learn before stopping treatment." Again, a sports metaphor may be helpful, such as "just like an athlete mentally rehearses their performance prior to the game, we also want to make sure you practice your game plan in advance." In cases where the patient refuses to consent to the task, despite a thorough review of his or her concerns with the therapist, we recommend that the therapist and patient simply have a discussion about the coping skills learned and how they might be applied in the future, without engaging in any imagery or emotional provocation.

In the first step of the RPT, the therapist takes the youth through a guided imagery exercise of the index suicide attempt. He or she is asked to imagine the sequence of events that led up to the suicide attempt as well as the associated thoughts and feelings. The patient is instructed to close his or her eyes and to use sensory triggers, such as sights, smells, and sounds, from the time of the attempt to enhance the immediacy of the image. The patient is asked to describe each event to the therapist out loud as he or she imagines it happening and to try to re-experience the emotions that occurred at that time.

In the next step, following this same format, the patient again imagines the sequence of events leading up to the index attempt, but this time also imagines him or herself using the skills learned in therapy to cope with each event. This serves as a test of whether or not the patient can successfully implement adaptive coping strategies.

The final step of the RPT involves imagining a future suicidal crisis. Based on the cognitive conceptualization, the therapist assists the adolescent in imagining a sequence of events that

Table 12.7
Outline of Sessions 9–10

1. Relapse Prevention Task
2. Termination

might occur in the future that would result in him or her becoming suicidal. Once again, the patient is assisted in imagining this scenario in as real and immediate a way as possible and to talk through how he or she would cope with such a situation. At the end of the RPT, the patient is debriefed and his or her reactions to the task are reviewed. If any current suicidal ideation was activated by the task, the therapist assesses suicidal risk, and conducts the appropriate interventions from those described in this chapter. As noted earlier, if the patient cannot imagine successfully coping with a future suicidal crisis, the therapy continues and appropriate coping skills are reviewed. When the therapist feels the patient has made the necessary gains, the RPT is conducted again. Therapy is typically not terminated until the patient performs the RPT successfully.

Termination

The therapist helps the patient and family prepare for termination from the very first session by emphasizing the brief nature of the treatment and encouraging the use of additional mental health services and social supports. The patient should have a plan for ongoing treatment in place to deal with issues that require longer-term treatment once the intervention is completed and suicidal behavior has been addressed. The therapist should take the time to discuss and validate all feelings about termination expressed by the patient and his or her family. The safety plan and interventions that will be used in a future suicidal crisis should be reviewed. It is helpful to prepare patients and families for the possibility of relapse in advance by talking about how they will cope with setbacks, and in particular, how to avoid engaging in hopeless, all-or-none thinking patterns about setbacks if they occur. It is important to remind the patient and family that mood fluctuations and stressful life events are a normal part of life and can be dealt with safely by using the skills learned in treatment. The family should be reminded to go to the nearest emergency room or call 911 if the youth is ever in imminent danger in the future.

Comment

Under optimal circumstances, therapy proceeds as outlined above. However, the therapy must often be modified to suit the needs and capacities of the individual patient. For example, depending on the level of the teen's cognitive development, the emphasis on cognitive versus behavioral interventions may differ. Moreover, teens who are less psychiatrically stable may require a great deal of symptom management and mobilization of outside resources prior to being able to learn coping skills. We recommend that therapists emphasize what works with a given patient and family and not feel pressured to utilize elements of the treatment that they are not responsive to. In addition, although this chapter provides a description of the full range of interventions, clinicians may also want to incorporate individual elements of the treatment (e.g., constructing a hope box), into the approach they are currently using.

CONCLUSIONS

This chapter provides a manual for using a cognitive therapy intervention, originally developed by Beck and colleagues for treatment adult suicide attempters, for treating teens who have recently attempted suicide. The intervention is novel in its approach in that it directly targets suicidal behavior as the primary focus of the therapy, rather than the underlying disorder which has been the standard. The intervention includes a specific set of cognitive-behavioral strategies for suicidal behavior, derived from general principles of cognitive theory and therapy for the emotional disorders (e.g., Beck, 1976; Beck et al., 1979). These strategies include the development of a multi-step safety plan, a cognitive case conceptualization of the suicide attempt focusing on the cognitions that were activated at the time of the attempt, coping cards that list the patient's alternative responses to his or her key suicide-promoting negative cognitions, a hope kit that includes tangible reminders of the patient's reasons to live, behavioral and affect regulation skills, skills to decrease family conflict and build family support, and a guided-imagery relapse prevention task that serves as a cognitive rehearsal of coping skills as well as an assessment of treatment progress. We hope that clinicians will find this article useful as a guide for working with adolescents who have recently attempted suicide, a highly difficult-to-treat population for which at present there are few empirically-validated therapies.

References

American Psychiatric Association (APA). (2003). *Practice guideline for the assessment and treatment of patients with suicidal behaviors.* Washington, DC: American Psychiatric Association.

Asarnow J. R., Carlson, G., & Guthrie, D. (1987). Coping strategies, self perceptions, hopelessness, and perceived family environment in depressed and suicidal children. *Journal of Consulting and Clinical Psychology, 55,* 361–366.

Asarnow, J. R., Tompson, M. C., & Berk, M. S. (2005). Adolescent depression: Family focused treatment strategies. In W. Pinsof & J. Lebow (Eds.), *Family psychology: The art of the science* (pp. 425–450). New York: Oxford University Press.

Beck, A. T. (1976). *Cognitive therapy and the emotional disorders.* New York: Meridian.

Beck, A. T. & Steer, R. A. (1993). *Manual for the Beck Hopelessness Scale.* San Antonio, TX: The Psychological Corporation.

Beck, A. T., Rush, A. J., Shaw, B. F., & Emery, G. (1979). *Cognitive therapy of depression.* Sussex, England: John Wiley & Sons Ltd.

Beck, A. T., Steer, R. A., & Brown, G. K. (1996). *The Beck Depression Inventory* (2nd ed.). San Antonio, TX: The Psychological Corporation.

Beck, J. S. (1995). *Cognitive therapy: Basics and beyond.* New York: Guilford.

Berk, M. S., & Asarnow, J. R. (2005, November). An emergency-room based intervention for adolescent suicide attempters. In G. K. Brown (Chair), *Intervention strategies for suicidal patients: Ideators and attempters.* Paper presented at the 39th annual meeting of the Association for the Advancement of Behavior Therapy, Washington, D.C.

Berk, M. S., Henriques, G. R., Warman, D. M., Brown, G. K., & Beck, A. T. (2004). Cognitive therapy for suicide attempters: Overview of the treatment and case examples. *Cognitive and Behavioral Practice, 11,* 265–277.

Boergers, J., & Spirito, A. (2003). The outcome of suicide attempts among adolescents. In A. Spirito & J. C. Overholser (Eds.), *Evaluating and treating adolescent suicide attempters: From research to practice* (pp. 261–276). New York: Academic Press.

Brent, D. A., Perper, J. A., Moritz, G., Baugher, M., Schweers, J., & Roth, C. (1993). Firearms and adolescent suicide: A community case-control study. *American Journal of Diseases of Children, 147,* 1066–1071.

Brown, G. K., Tenhave, T., Henriques, G. R., Xie, S. X., Hollander, J. E., & Beck, A. T. (2005). Cognitive therapy for the prevention of suicide attempts: A randomized controlled trial. *Journal of the American Medical Association, 294,* 563–570.

Curry, J. F., Wells, K. C., Brent, D. A., Clarke, G. N., Rohde, P., Albano, A. M., et al. (2005). *Cognitive behavior therapy manual: Introduction, rationale, and adolescent sessions.* Unpublished manuscript, Department of Psychiatry, Duke University Medical Center. Retrieved January 31, 2007, from https://trialweb.dcri.duke.edu/tads/tad/manuals/tads_cbt.pdf.

Esposito, C., Johnson, B., Wolfsdorf, B. A., & Spirito, A. (2003). Cognitive factors; Hopelessness, coping, and problem solving. In A. Spirito & J. C. Overholser (Eds.), *Evaluating and treating adolescent suicide attempters: From research to practice* (pp. 89–112). New York: Academic Press.

Friedberg, R. D., & McClure, J. M. (2002). *Clinical practice of cognitive therapy with children and adolescents: The nuts and bolts.* New York: Guilford.

Goldston, D. B., Daniel, S. S., Reboussin, B. A., Reboussin, D. M., Frazier, P. H., & Harris, A. E. (2001). Cognitive risk factors and suicide attempts among formerly hospitalized adolescents: A prospective naturalistic study. *Journal of the American Academy of Child and Adolescent Psychiatry, 40,* 91–99.

Gould M. S., Greenberg, T., Velting D. M., & Shaffer, D. (2003). Youth suicide risk and preventive interventions: A review of the past 10 years. *Journal of the*

American Academy of Child and Adolescent Psychiatry, 42, 386–405.

Hamilton, B. E., Miniño, A. M., Martin, J. A., Kochanek, K. D., Strobino, D. M., & Guyer, B. (2007). Annual summary of vital statistics: 2005. *Pediatrics, 119*, 345–360.

Harrington, R., Kerfoot, M., Dyer, E., McNiven, F., Gill, J., Harrington, V., et al. (1998). Randomized trial of a home-based family intervention for children who have deliberately poisoned themselves. *Journal of the American Academy of Child and Adolescent Psychiatry, 37*, 512–518.

Harris, H. E., & Myers, W. C. (1997). Adolescents' misperceptions of the dangerousness of acetaminophen in overdose. *Suicide and Life-Threatening Behavior, 27*, 274–277.

Huey, S. J., Henggeler, S. W., Rowland, M. D., Halliday-Boykins, C., Cunningham, P. B., Edwards, J., et al. (2004). Multisystemic therapy effects on attempted suicide by youths presenting psychiatric emergencies. *Journal of the American Academy of Child and Adolescent Psychiatry, 43*, 183–190.

Kazdin, A., Rodgers A., & Colbus, D. (1986). The Hopelessness Scale for Children: Psychometric characteristics and concurrent validity. *Journal of Consulting and Clinical Psychology, 54*, 241–245.

Kellermann, A. L., Rivara, F. P., Somes, G., Reay, T., Francisco, J., Banton, J. G., et al., (1992). Suicide in the home in relation to gun ownership. *New England Journal of Medicine, 327*, 467–472.

Kendall, P. C. (2000). Guiding theory for therapy with children and adolescents. In P. C. Kendall (Ed.), *Child and adolescent therapy: Cognitive-behavioral procedures* (2nd ed., pp. 3–27). New York: Guilford.

Kienhorst, C. W. M., DeWilde, E. J., Diekstra, R. F. W., & Wolters, W. H. G. (1995). Adolescents' image of their suicide attempt. *Journal of the American Academy of Child and Adolescent Psychiatry, 34*, 623–628.

King, C. A., Kramer, A., Preuss, L., Kerr, D.C. R., Weisse, L., & Venkataraman, S. (2006). Youth-nominated support team for suicidal adolescents (version 1): A randomized controlled trial. *Journal of Consulting and Clinical Psychology, 74*, 199–206.

Kovacs, M., & Beck, A. T. (1977). An empirical-clinical approach toward a definition of childhood depression. In J. G. Schulterbrandt, & A. Raskin (Eds.), *Depression in childhood: Diagnosis, treatment, and conceptual models* (pp. 1–25). New York: Raven Press.

Lewinsohn, P. R., Rhode, P., & Seeley, J. R. (1993). Psychosocial characteristics of adolescents with a history of suicide attempt. *Journal of the American Academy of Child and Adolescent Psychiatry, 32*, 60–68.

Linehan, M. M. (1993). *Cognitive-behavioral treatment of borderline personality disorder*. New York: Guilford Press.

Linehan, M. M., Armstrong, H. E., Suarez, A., Allmon, D., & Heard, H. L. (1991). Cognitive behavioral treatment of chronically parasuicidal borderline patients. *Archives of General Psychiatry, 48*, 1060–1064.

Linehan, M. M., Comtois; K., Murray, A. M., Brown, M. Z., Gallop, R. J., Heard, H. L., et al. (2006). Two-year randomized controlled trial and follow-up of dialectical behavior therapy vs therapy by experts for suicidal behaviors and borderline personality disorder. *Archives of General Psychiatry, 63*, 757–766.

Marzuk, P. M., Leon, A. C., Tardiff, K., Morgan, E. B., Stajic, M., & Mann, J. J. (1992). The effect of access to lethal methods of injury on suicide rates. *Archives of General Psychiatry, 49*, 451–458.

Miller, A. L., & Glinski, J. (2000). Youth suicidal behavior: Assessment and intervention. In P. Kleespies (Ed.), Empirical approaches to behavioral emergencies (special issue). *Journal of Clinical Psychology, 56*, 1–22.

Miller, A. L., Rathus, J. H., & Linehan, M. M. (2007). *Dialectical behavior therapy with suicidal adolescents*. New York: Guilford.

Miller, S., Rotheram-Borus, M. J., Piacentini, J., Graae, F., & Castro-Blanco, D. (1992). *Successful Negotiation/Acting Positively (SNAP): A brief cognitive-behavioral family therapy manual for adolescent suicide attempters and their families*. New York: Department of Child Psychiatry, Columbia University.

Nock, M. K., & Kazdin, A. E. (2002). Examination of affective, cognitive, and behavioral factors and suicide-related outcomes in children and young adolescents. *Journal of Clinical Child and Adolescent Psychology, 31*, 48–58.

O'Carroll, P. W., Berman, A. L., Maris, R. W., Moscicki, E. K., Tanney, B. L., & Silverman, M. M. (1996). Beyond the Tower of Babel: A nomenclature for suicidology. *Suicide and Life-Threatening Behavior, 26*, 237–252.

Rathus, J. H. & Miller, A. L. (2002). Dialectical behavior therapy adapted for suicidal adolescents. *Suicide and Life-Threatening Behaviors, 32*, 146–157.

Rotheram-Borus, M. J., Piacentini, J., Cantwell, C., Belin, T. R., & Song, J. (2000). The 18-month impact of an emergency room intervention for adolescent suicide attempters. *Journal of Consulting and Clinical Psychology, 68*, 1081–1093.

Rotheram-Borus, M. J., Trautman, P. D., Dopkins, S. C., & Shrout, P. E. (1990). Cognitive style and pleasant activities among female adolescent suicide attempters. *Journal of Consulting and Clinical Psychology, 58*, 554–561.

Rudd, M. D., Joiner, T. E. & Rajab, M. R. (2001). *Treating suicidal behavior*. New York: Guilford Press.

Shaffer, D., Garland, A., Gould, M., Fisher, P., & Trautman, P. (1988). Preventing teenage suicide: A critical review. *Journal of the Academy of Child and Adolescent Psychiatry, 27*, 675–687.

Spirito A., Lewander, W., Levy, S., Kurkjian, J., & Fritz, G. (1994). Emergency department assessment of adolescent suicide attempters; factors related to short-term follow-up. *Pediatric Emergency Care, 10*, 6–12.

Spirito, A., Plummer, B., Gispert, M., Levy, S., Kurkjian, J., Lewander, W., et al. (1992). Adolescent suicide attempts: Outcomes at follow-up. *American Journal of Orthopsychiatry, 62,* 464–468.

TASA. (n.d.) *Treatment of Adolescent Suicide Attempters (TASA).* Sponsored by the National Institute of Mental Health. Retrieved April 9, 2007, from http://clinicaltrials.gov/show/NCT00080158.

Trautman, P. D., Stewart, N., & Morishima, A. (1993). Are adolescent suicide attempters noncompliant with outpatient care? *Journal of the American Academy of Child and Adolescent Psychiatry, 32,* 89–94.

United States Department of Health and Human Services. (2001). *National strategy for suicide prevention: Goals and objectives for action.* Rockville, MD: Author, Public Health Service.

United States Food and Drug Administration. (2004, October). *FDA public health advisory: Suicidality in children and adolescents being treated with antidepressant medications, October 15, 2004.* Retrieved April 8, 2007, from http://www.fda.gov/cder/drug/antidepressants/SSRIPHA200410.htm.

United States Public Health Service. (1999). *The Surgeon General's call to action to prevent suicide.* Washington, DC: United States Department of Health and Human Services.

Wagner, K. D., Rouleau, M., & Joiner, T. (2000). Cognitive factors related to suicidal ideation and resolution in psychiatrically hospitalized children and adolescents. *American Journal of Psychiatry, 157,* 2017–2021.

Weishaar, M., & Beck, A. T. (1990). Cognitive approaches to understanding and treating suicidal behavior. In S. J. Blumenthal & D. J. Kupfer (Eds.), *Suicide over the life cycle.* Washington, DC: American Psychiatric Press.

Wenzel, A., Brown, G. K., & Beck, A. T. (in press). *Cognitive therapy for suicidal individuals: Scientific and clinical applications.* Washington, DC: APA Books.

Wood A., Trainor, G., Rothwell, J., Moore, A., & Harrington, R. (2001). Randomized trial of group therapy for repeated deliberate self-harm in adolescents. *Journal of the American Academy of Child and Adolescent Psychiatry, 40,* 1246–1253.

Chapter 13

The Home Chip System: A Token Economy for Use in the Natural Home

Edward R. Christophersen and Susan Mortweet VanScoyoc

The concept of a *token economy* was first introduced into the literature by Ayllon and Azrin (1968), first in research publications and then in their book, *The Token Economy*. Over the years, token economies have been reported in a variety of adaptations including residential treatment facilities (*The Teaching Family Model*, Wolf, et al., 1995), schools (Ayllon, 1999), and natural homes (Christophersen, Hill, Arnold, & Quilitch, 1972; Barkley, 1990).

What are the indications for recommending a token economy to a family? There are several (Christophersen & Mortweet, 2001).

1. When a child has the skills but is refusing to use them. For example, when child must wear glasses but refuses to or when a child is unwilling to adhere to the various components of a treatment regimen for diabetes.

2. Eliminate undesirable behaviors such as whining or swearing.
3. When a child is just learning a skill or a set of skills to provide the necessary motivation to encourage the child to practice until proficient at the new skills. Sample skills would include academic skills (practicing handwriting), reading skills (encouraging a child to read more), or skills for following a medical regimen like diabetes or asthma management.
4. When a child is learning appropriate social skills and needs the necessary motivation to use the skills consistently. For example, a token economy could be used when a child needs to practice table manners or to practice problem solving skills.

When is a token economy less likely to be successful?

1. When the parents are simply not in control of the child's reinforcers. For example, an older

adolescent who consistently spends huge amounts of time away from the home is not as influenced by parental consequences as a younger child who is home most of the time.

2. When the parents find that they are unable to consistently implement the contingencies requisite for successful behavior modification.

3. When the child lacks the level of skill that the parents are attempting to reinforce. For example, a parent who will only reinforce a spotless room will not be as successful as a parent who is willing to reinforce small steps first such as a made bed or picked up toys.

4. When the behaviors that the parents are attempting to reinforce are not in the child's repertoire. For example, attempting to "reward" a child for appropriate toileting, when the child has not been toilet trained, or when the situation is confounded by constipation.

EVIDENCE FOR USING THE HOME CHIP SYSTEM

The interested reader is referred to Kazdin's two review articles (Kazdin, 1977, 1982) for a very detailed evaluation of the published research on the token economy. The general field of parent management training, which is based largely on the use of the token economy has been evaluated with many randomized controlled experimental trials with children and adolescents. In particular, these techniques have been applied to children with oppositional, aggressive, and antisocial behavior. Kazdin notes that parent management training is "the best established of the evidence-based treatments for children and adolescents" and notes that "there are more reviews of this treatment than there are outcome studies for many other evidence-based treatments" (2005, p. 158).

References

Ayllon, T. (1999). *How to Use Token Economy and Point Systems (How to Manage Behavior Series).* Austin, TX: ProEd.

Ayllon, T., & Azrin, N. H. (1968). *The token economy: A motivational system for therapy and rehabilitation.* New York: Prentice Hall.

Barkley, R. A. (1990). *Attention-deficit hyperactivity disorder: A handbook for diagnosis and treatment.* New York: Guilford.

Barkley, R. A., & Benton, C. M. (1998). *Your defiant child: Eight steps to better behavior.* New York: Guilford Press.

Christophersen, E. R., & Mortweet, S. (2001). *Treatments that work with children: Empirically supported strategies for managing childhood problems.* Washington, DC: APA Books.

Christophersen, E. R., Arnold C. M., Hill D. W., & Quilitch, H. R. (1972). The home point system: Token reinforcement procedures for application by parents of children with behavior problems. *Journal of Applied Behavior Analysis, 5,* 485–497.

Kazdin, A. E. (1977). *The token economy: A review and evaluation.* New York: Plenum.

Kazdin, A. E. (1982). The token economy: A decade later. *Journal of Applied Behavior Analysis, 15,* 431–445.

Kazdin, A. E. (2005). Child, parent, and family-based treatment of aggressive and antisocial behavior. In E. D. Hibbs & P. S. Jensen (Eds.), *Psychosocial treatments for child and adolescent disorders* (2nd ed., pp. 445–476). Washington, DC: American Psychological Association.

Wolf, M. M., Kirigan, K. A., Fixsen, D. G., Blasé, K. A. & Braukmann, C. J. (1995). The teaching-family model: A case study in data-based program development and refinement (and dragon wrestling). *Journal of Organizational Behavioral Management, 15,* 11–68.

The 2006 Home Chip System: A Treatment Manual for Children Ages 3 to 7

The Home Chip System was developed for use by parents who have children with behavior problems. These procedures have been used with preschool-age children, in families with one to six children, with parents whose education ranged from less than high school to postgraduate studies, and with income levels ranging from poverty to upper-income professional. We have experience working with families from a variety of ethnic and racial backgrounds, including Caucasian, African-American, Hispanic, and Asian-American.

The range of problem behaviors has extended from minor, everyday difficulties, such as getting children to bed at night and getting them to keep their rooms neat, to moderate problems such as hitting, temper tantrums and talking back. Our experience is not sufficient to make recommendations regarding the use of this program with such severe problems as substance abuse or autism spectrum disorder.

In the beginning, this program requires dedicated and highly motivated parents who are willing to put forth the effort necessary to teach their children more appropriate ways of behaving. The program also requires that the children be supervised by someone most of the day. We train parents to be teachers. They cannot teach their children if they are not with them. Whether administered by the parents, a nanny, or an alternative caregiver, the program requires that the children be supervised.

The Home Chip System is designed to provide a maximum amount of instruction and feedback to your child through you, the caregiver. Instruction, feedback, and consequences are the tools you will use to train your child in new desirable behaviors, to eliminate already present undesirable behaviors, or both. The system's effectiveness in changing behaviors will depend upon your thoroughness. It will not operate by itself. Its success will depend upon the degree to which you actively observe and reward or punish the behaviors you see your child demonstrate.

It has been more than 30 years since the Home Chip System was first introduced in the literature (Christophersen, Arnold, Hill & Quilitch, 1972), and many professionals are still recommending its use. The most notable is probably Russell Barkley, PhD, who is an expert in the treatment of attention deficit hyperactivity disorder. He included an earlier version of the Chip System as an Appendix in his 1980 book and recommends the use of a Chip System in his 1998 book (Barkley & Benton, 1998) on strategies for dealing with a defiant child.

How the Home Chip System Works

The Home Chip System is based upon two simple, yet thoroughly effective, principles:

1. Behavior that is immediately followed by a good, rewarding consequence continues to occur.
2. Behavior that is followed by an unrewarding or punishing consequence ceases to occur or will occur less often.

Poker Chips

Like money, poker chips themselves have no value. Chips must be given meaning or value in order to become effective. It is only through their power to purchase necessary and enjoyable goods or activities that they gain meaning and become useful. They must always be available for you to give and take. However, poker chips serve as rewards or punishments *only when they immediately follow your child's behavior.* We have had parents use many different items other than poker chips such as tickets, pennies or even pasta wheels! We have found, however, that poker chips work the best as a child will most likely be unable to randomly find the poker chip to add to his or her "stash." Also, they are durable and come in several colors, which can be helpful if a parent is using the token system with more than one child and would like to color code for each child.

Making Chips Powerful

For chips to be used as an effective consequence for behavior, earning chips (like earning money) must be rewarding for your child; your child must feel like she has indeed gained something. Losing chips (like losing money) must be unpleasant or punishing for your child; your child must feel like he has lost something.

Chips will become meaningful for your child as she uses them to buy the "privileges" of having or doing something that she desires. Privileges are items or activities, usually available in your home or community that your child enjoys and can purchase with chips.

Earning Privileges

Privileges can be anything your child likes to do. For example, playing with friends, playing with toys or games, computer time, snacks, and shopping with Mom all might be considered privileges by some children. The privilege to use the computer, for instance, permits your child to use the computer when it is available and he has paid for the time (given you some poker chips). You should decide what constitutes the amount of computer time available per poker chip as well as what computer activities are appropriate for use during that time (games, websites, and chatrooms). For chips to be of value, your child *must be required to spend them for his or her privileges.* Thus, if computer time is on the privilege list, your child should not get to play on the computer unless she spends her chips to purchase the time. Privileges must be available as often as possible when your child has the chips. Again, unless the chips are worth something that cannot be purchased without them, they will not be an effective tool in changing your child's behavior. In other words, if your child can get on the computer to play games or surf the internet at any time, "earning" time with chips will not be very motivating or effective for your child. One solution would be to have the computer available for monitored homework time only, with leisure computer time earned with chips.

Starting a Chip System

If you have more than one child in your home, the procedures can be implemented for each of them. It's better to start the chip system with all of your children at the same time, rather than start with only the child you are the most concerned about. In this way, the children will be able to learn from each other. Just remember to individualize the behaviors that earn and lose chips based on each child's strengths and weaknesses. It is helpful to put a behavior on your list that your child is all ready quite good at so that you will be able to frequently reward your child and increase her investment in this process.

Prior to starting a chip system, you must decide what behaviors you would like to have your child continue to do, such as making the bed or brushing his teeth, and what behaviors you would like to encourage your child to begin doing.

Sit down with your child and make a list of behaviors that you and your child think are positive and suitable for earning chips. It is important to be very specific when choosing behaviors. For example, "clean your room" might not be as clear to your child as providing chips for each of the individual steps involved in cleaning a room. For example, if you instructed your child to pick up the clothes on the floor, give her chips for picking up the clothes. If you instructed your child to pick up the toys, give him chips for picking up the toys. Specifying the steps involved will probably do a much better job than if you just ask you child to clean the room.

The examples below represent behaviors that can earn chips. Fill in behaviors that apply in your home.

Behaviors That Earn Chips

Making bed
Picking up clothes in bedroom
Picking up toys in bedroom
Brushing teeth
Getting dressed on time
Saying please and thank you

Next, you have to agree on how many chips your child will earn each time a household chore has been successfully completed. If you are using this system with more than one child in your family, the point value of similar items on each list should be equal. For example, if "making bed" is on two of your children's lists, it should be worth two chips for both children.

Social Behaviors That Earn Chips

Making bed	+ 2
Picking up clothes in bedroom	+ 2
Picking up toys in bedroom	+ 2
Brushing teeth	+ 2
Getting dressed on time	+ 2
Saying please and thank you	+ 2

One mistake parents usually make is paying their children only for chores. Parents need to find a number of different social skills to pay chips for as well. Please think about a variety of social behaviors that you consider important. Again, it is important to be specific when choosing these behaviors. Some examples are provided below, along with space to add your own.

Social Behaviors That Earn Chips

Sharing with brother	+ 4
Taking verbal feedback without arguing	+ 4
Practicing going to "time-out"	+ 4
Verbalizing a coping strategy	+ 4
Doing homework (per 15 minutes)	+ 8

Each of these behaviors, if completed, results in a chip gain. If not completed, they result in a chip loss. For example, if your child brushed her teeth, two chips would be gained. If she failed to brush her teeth in the allowed time, two chips would be lost. *It is more important to give chips than it is take chips away.* Such behaviors as "helping," or "playing quietly" only earn chips. These are behaviors that are worthwhile to add to your list and to reward consistently, since they are the types of behaviors you would like to see more of every day.

In addition to the behaviors listed above, you might also think of "extra" jobs that earn privileges such as picking up trash in the yard, raking leaves, folding clothes, or dusting. Your child may be capable of doing many such small jobs around the house. It is important that your child share the responsibilities of the house. This is also an excellent time for you to interact with and to teach your child. A list of jobs, made by you in advance, will provide a chance for your child to earn chips when she needs to or when he wants to help. Such a list could be attached to the front of your refrigerator along with the list of behaviors that your child is working on with the token system.

Privileges and Their Value

The privileges listed on your home chip system are privileges your child can "buy" if he has the right number of chips. This list will most likely need to be updated from time to time. You will need to be aware of what your child is doing for fun so you can add those activities to the list as necessary. Most of the activities children naturally do in their spare time are things they enjoy. Thus, these activities can be viewed as privileges, and can be added to the list of privileges. Some examples are:

Privilege	Cost, in Chips (number of chips)
Watching television	5 chips per 1/2 hour
Playing outside	5 chips
Snacks	5 per snack
Going to friend's house	10 chips
Riding bike	5 chips
Playing a video game	5 chips per 1/2 hour
Playing on the computer	5 chips per 1/2 hour

Behaviors that lose chips are behaviors you would like your child to stop doing. For this system to be effective, you *must* take the chips away *immediately* every time one of these behaviors occurs. As mentioned with the behaviors above, it is important to be specific about these behaviors as well. Probably the most frequent behavior that children lose chips for is stalling. So, if you ask your son to pick up his coat and he doesn't respond within five seconds, ask him to give you four chips for stalling. Other examples are provided below:

Behaviors that Lose Chips	Number of Chips Lost
Throwing things	−2
Jumping on furniture	−2
Talking back	−2
Tantrums	−3
Coming downstairs after bedtime	−2
Interrupting	−4
Running in the house	−2

How to Give Chips and Take Them Away

Both giving and taking away chips should be as pleasant as possible. Here are several things you and your child need to do whenever there is a chip exchange.

Rules for Parents

When giving chips remember to:

1. Be near your child and able to touch her (not in the other room).
2. Look at your child and smile.
3. Use a pleasant voice.
4. Make sure your child is facing you and looking at you.

Praise your child by saying something like, "Hey that's great. You're really doing a nice job. That's really helping me."

5. Reward your child with chips and say, "Here are two chips for helping me with the dishes."
6. Describe the appropriate behavior for your child so he knows exactly what behavior he is being praised and rewarded for.

7. Hug your child occasionally—kids love it!
8. Have your child acknowledge you by saying something like, "Thanks, Mom" or "OK."

When demonstrating how to give chips in the office, we always hold the chips between our thumb and first finger, and tell the child he has just earned two chips, for example, for picking up his jacket. As soon as the child places his thumb and fingers on the chips, makes eye contact, and says, "thank you," we release the chips to him.

Children should have some place to keep their chips. This can be any container or bag. In order to discourage children from taking each other's chips, use a different color for each child. Also, make certain that you don't have any extra chips somewhere in your home. Children seem to know exactly where to find extra chips if they are anywhere in the home.

When taking away chips remember to:

1. Be near your child and able to touch her.
2. Look at your child and smile.
3. Use a pleasant voice. Your child should not be able to tell by the tone of your voice or your facial expression whether you're going to give or take away chips.
4. Make sure your child is facing you and looking at you.
5. In a calm manner, *briefly* explain what was inappropriate.
6. Be sympathetic by saying something like, "I know it's hard to lose chips, but that's the rule."
7. Tell the child how much the chip fine costs.
8. Make sure your child gets the chips appropriately (see next section).
9. Prompting the appropriate responses is sometimes necessary by saying, for example, "Come on, give me a smile. That's right."
10. If a chip loss is taken well by your child, give her back one-half of the chip fine, and say, "You gave me your chips so well, I'm going to give you back half of the chip fine!" For example if the fine were two chips, your child would immediately earn one chip back simply by being cooperative when she gave you the two chips.
11. If your child is too mad or upset to give you the chips, don't forget the issue. Place your child in time-out (to cool off) and take the chips out of your child's chip container while she is in time-out.

Rules for Children

When getting chips, children should:

1. Be facing their parents, looking at them, and smiling.
2. Place their thumb and first finger on the chips and acknowledge receiving the chips by saying, "OK," "Thanks," or something else in a pleasant voice.
3. Put the chips in the specified container. (Any chips left lying around are returned to the bank.)

When losing chips, children should:

1. Face their parents, look at them, and smile (not frown).
2. Acknowledge the chip loss with, "OK," or "All right," "I'll get the chips," or something else in a pleasant voice. (Children must keep looking at you and be pleasant.)
3. Give the chips to their parents in a pleasant manner. Most parents find that the exchange works best if they ask their child to "count out the chips." So, for a six-chip fine, children count the chips, one by one, as they place them in their mother's hand.

Practice Giving and Taking Away Chips

Once on the chip system, families frequently encounter instances where a child has done something to earn chips, but hasn't done it very well. This is an excellent time to teach your child how to do it correctly by having him practice doing it correctly. Practicing can be done with both chores and social behaviors.

Practicing with Maintenance Behaviors

When teaching your child how to do a new job correctly or when giving her feedback on a job poorly done, practice is essential. For example, if your child is doing the dishes but, when you check, she is not doing them correctly, the following rules will help you teach your child the correct way.

Practicing with Dish Washing

Table 13.1
Practicing with Chore Maintenance Behavior

Dish Washing Example	Parent Rule
"You're really working steadily and the table looks really clean. Thanks."	Praise related behavior.
"But it looks like you haven't gotten all the food off the plates."	Describe fully the inappropriate or inadequate behavior.
"It's important that all the dishes are clean with no food left on the plates."	Describe the appropriate behavior.
"Because germs can grow on the dishes, and besides, the next time you use the plate you will want it to be clean."	Give a reason for the appropriate behavior.
"Do you understand?"	Request acknowledgment.
"When food is stuck, a good way to get it off is to use the scraper instead or the cloth—like this."	Model: Show child how to do it.
"Now you try it."	Practice.
"Great, you're doing a much better job of getting them clean now."	Praise or feedback.
"When you get done, find me and you will get your chips, plus two for practicing so nicely. You're really doing a good job now."	Praise and reward.

Practicing with Social Behaviors

If your child becomes unpleasant and talks back when he loses points, the following rules will be useful to teach your child the appropriate response.

When to Practice

The best time to practice any behavior is during a pleasant time of the day, preferably when your child hasn't done anything wrong. A great time to practice is when your child needs more chips to purchase an item or activity she wants. This teaches your child—under pleasant circumstances—how to respond to important situations. Prompting and practicing correct responses, however, are still important after a rule violation or a poorly done job has occurred.

When there has not been a rule violation, practice using make-believe violations and a make-believe time-out. For example, if your child says he needs a job to earn some chips, tell him you will give him five chips if he will do a good pretend time-out. If he says, "OK," direct him to go to time-out. When he has completed his pretend time-out, give him the five chips and tell him what a good job he did. This is a good way for your child to earn chips at the same time that he practices important social behaviors.

Table 13.2 Practicing with Social Maintenance Behavior

Talking Back Example	Parent Rule
"You came quickly when I called and I really appreciate that."	Praise a related behavior.
"But the rule is that you don't back-talk after a chip loss. I'll have to take off two more chips for talking back."	Describe fully the inappropriate or inadequate behavior.
"Remember—you're supposed to look at me, be pleasant, and say "OK, Dad" in a nice tone of voice."	Describe the appropriate behavior.
"This way we'll get along better at home and it will help you take criticism better at school."	Give a reason for the appropriate behavior.
"Do you understand what you're supposed to do?"	Request acknowledgment.
"Say it pleasantly and give me a big smile—like this" (parent says "OK" and smiles).	Model: Show child how to do it.
"Now you try it."	Practice.
"That's right, you're looking at me with a pleasant facial expression."	Praise or feedback.
"Great—that's how it's done. You practiced very well. You can have a chip back."	Praise and reward.

You may also practice taking off chips. For example:

MOTHER: *"Jim, let's practice how you're supposed to take a chip loss and you can earn two chips."*

JIMMY: *"OK"*

MOTHER: *"Jim, would you please take two chips off for throwing the ball in the house? Remember the rule is that balls can only be thrown outdoors."*

JIMMY: *"Sure, Mom" (with pleasant facial expression and tone of voice).*

MOTHER: *"That was great! If you can remember to do that the next time you lose chips, I'll give you back half of the chips you lost."*

JIMMY: *"Gee, thanks, Mom."*

MOTHER: *"Let me give you your chips back because we were just practicing and I'll give you four chips for practicing so well."*

Checking Jobs

Checking jobs, whether daily or extra work, is a vital aspect of the chip system. It not only helps you teach your child the right way to do things, it provides a good opportunity for you to interact with your child in an appropriate way. The rules that apply to practice situations also apply to checking jobs. If the job was done correctly the first time, you needn't go through all the steps. Instead, make sure you specifically praise the things done well and give chips.

Giving Chips for Jobs Completed Well

The number of chips given for a job should be decided beforehand; that way, you can reward with extra chips a job done especially well and take away chips for a job performed poorly. All jobs, however, must be done as specified—a poorly done job is not acceptable and must be done again. For this reason, it is good to define how a job is done, then write the description down on the job list so you can look at it whenever a question comes up.

If your child asks you to check the table and all of the steps have been done correctly the first time, praise your child and give her the full chip value. If the job was not done correctly, however, go through the practice components and tell your child that if she corrects the faulty job components, she can get back half the chips that were possible. Be sympathetic, but firm. Encourage your child to do it right this time so she can get the full number of chips. If, when checked again, the job still is not done correctly, it's probably not because the child doesn't know how. Place the child in time-out (without loss of privileges). After the time-out is completed, ask your child, again, to do the steps that weren't done right. Be sure to practice each time before asking the child to repeat the job (see section on the time-out procedure).

If, after the time-out, your child cooperates and corrects the job, give chips for correcting the job. If your child will not cooperate, place him in time-out again. Most children will do what is required of them rather than sit in time-out. The first couple of times they may choose to go to time-out several times in a row—as a test to see if you really intend to follow through. Once in a while, a child will test both you and the rules. Don't give in to such tests, as it may only make it harder to convince your child that your rules are an important part of your family's functioning.

Monitoring Your Child: The 10-Minute Rule

It is important that you be aware of what your child is doing. Periodic checks should be made so you can reward (give chips and praise) such appropriate behavior as playing quietly or working on a job, and punish (take away chips) such inappropriate behavior as fighting, stalling, or getting into things. You don't have to check every 10 minutes on the dot. However, the checks should be done at intervals somewhere between 5 and 20 minutes. This rule should not be used to harass your child. When you go to see what she's doing, you don't need to interrogate her. Instead, look at her behavior and either praise and give chips or take some chips away and give her feedback. If your child is quietly engaged in a privilege, such as playing with a game in her room with the door closed, you don't need to open the door every 10 minutes to see what she is doing.

Punishment: When Chips Don't Work

The use of brief time-outs, when you do not interact with your child in any way until she has calmed down, can be used at two different times: when your child refuses to do a job or a chore and when your child is out of chips.

Time-out means the temporary revoking of all privileges and social interaction. Traditionally, this has been done by having the child stand in the corner or go to his room. We have found, however, that if the time-out "spot" includes places where the child can see what he is missing, it is more effective. The time-out place should not be scary (no closets or dark places)! The best places are a living-room chair, a kitchen chair, or a front step if the child is outside.

The child should be directed to time-out with no more than three words such as "Time-out, stalling," or "Time-out, talking back." No further words should be exchanged until your child has calmed down.

There is no such thing as a time-out within a time-out. Once you have directed your child to a time-out, you should not say another word until she has calmed down—regardless of what he does. Time-outs should be used when your child has lost as many or more chips than she has gained. This may occur at any time during the day. In other words, when your child has no chips, she must go to time-out.

First, practice time outs when your child is not upset so it will be easier for her when a time out actually happens. For example, during a non-emotional time of the day, especially if your child has told you she needs chips to gain access to an activity she wants, she can earn chips for practicing time-out.

Time-Out Procedure

If your child has either refused to do a job or has run out of chips, you need to direct him to time-out. To institute a time-out:

1. Briefly explain to your child that he has lost all of his chips and is in time out.
2. Do not interact with him until he is calm. If he's really upset, he may get very obnoxious, including yelling, calling you names, or telling you that you can't make him do a time out if he doesn't want to.

3. When the initial stay in time-out is completed, your child then has the choice either to earn some chips or to stay in time-out. Many children choose to stay in time-out, hoping you will give in and let them do what they want to. Don't give in. Just let the time-out last as long as the child wants it. It is far better to have a couple of long time-outs (even 30 to 45 minutes!), than to have your child think he doesn't have to follow your rules. Remember, the time out is not a substitute for doing the work.

4. Your child must work until she has earned at least five chips, and may then go about her business. That means she will have to complete some assigned jobs or she will have to ask you for a job that she can do to earn some chips.

Rules for Children in Time-Out

1. While a child is in time-out, no chips are earned or lost.
2. If undesirable behavior occurs while the child is in time-out, ignore it.
3. Social interaction is forbidden during time-out. Instruct other family members to observe this rule and fine the other children each time they interact with anyone in time-out. If the other children are not on the chip system, separate them from the child who is in time-out.
4. Ignore all inappropriate behavior that may follow placement of your child in time-out.
5. As soon as your child is quiet for two to three *seconds,* tell her the time-out is over. Do not remind her why she went to time-out. Do not ask her why she went to time-out. If you're using time-outs to help a child to learn how to calm down, you can't nag her after each time-out.
6. Children of all ages should be started out with these very brief time-outs.
7. As your child learns to calm down when he's in time-out, gradually increase the amount of time between calming down and the end of the time-out.
8. It is critical that your child learns to associate calming down with a time-out.
9. Later, after your child can readily calm down in time-out, you can begin using time-out with her when she is angry or frustrated, and you won't need the chip system anymore.

Example of a Time-Out

The following conversation is an example of when time-out should be used:

FATHER: *"Susie, you were really good about getting home on time, but you forgot to hang up your coat. Remember, the rule is that we all hang up our coats as soon as we get home. Please give me four chips and then hang your coat up."*

SUSIE: *"I don't want to do it right now."*

FATHER: *"I know it's hard sometimes, but we all have to follow the rules. That's back-talk. Remember, you're supposed to say 'OK Dad,' and then go do it. Please give me four more chips for back-talk and we'll try it again."*

SUSIE: *"I'm not going to give you any chips."*

FATHER: *"Right now, you're a little upset so you'll have to go to time-out and cool off."* As soon as Susie is quiet, father says, *"You're really being quiet, that's great. You're out of time-out now."*

Susie would then be asked to return the four chips to the bank. As soon as she relinquishes the four chips appropriately, she'll be given two of the four back because of her cooperation. Then, father would say again, "Susie, please hang up your coat for me."

Helpful Hints for Parents

1. *Nothing good is free.* For chips to be powerful and useful as consequences for behavior, it is absolutely necessary that all privileges be purchased with chips.
2. *If it bugs you, it's worth improving.* If your child does something that annoys you, it probably annoys other adults too. Explain this to your child, set a chip consequence, fine this behavior, and reward a more appropriate one. Thus, any behavior that bothers you should probably be modified. You should define it, instruct your child about the appropriate behavior and provide feedback.
3. *Baby sitters.* Have a baby sitter you can call on short notice. There will undoubtedly be a time before a family outing when one of your children has no chips to pay for the outing. Since it's not fair to make the rest of the family stay home, you'll need someone to stay with your child, somewhere to take him and drop him off, or you may have to take him with you but deny him any and all privileges. If you allow your child to participate in a privilege he can't purchase, you are weakening the whole system.
4. *Be realistic about behavior change.* Don't be discouraged when a behavior doesn't change overnight. Change will happen more quickly if you are consistent with both taking away chips and giving chips. Frequent practice can also be helpful for changing behavior.
5. *Be patient.* Keep in mind that your child has, on the average, 70 more years to live. A couple of months teaching her some critical skills don't seem like such a big deal when you put it in this perspective.
6. *Be prepared.* Prepare your child for the right response before you tell the child what he did wrong. Example: "Tommy, I'm going to tell you something that might make you a little angry, but if you keep looking at me, stay pleasant, and take it well, you'll earn an extra five chips." Try it—it works.
7. *Be sympathetic.* When chip fines are given, remember you can express your sympathy with your child's unfortunate situation at the same time that you stay firm in applying the chip fine. Reassure the child who is receiving a lot of chip fines that when you take away chips it doesn't mean you are mad; it only means she is behaving in a manner unacceptable to you.
8. *Refrain from all nagging.* Don't use unenforceable threats, warnings, emotional pleading, or anger as methods of changing behavior; data indicate these do not work. Also, nagging, tantrums, and anger by a parent make life very unpleasant for the whole family. Firm but unemotional, even sympathetic, feedback works best.
9. *Chips and praise should go together.* Chips are not powerful just because they are chips. They must be *made* to be powerful. *That's the secret to making your chip system work.* To make chips powerful, they must be the *only* way the child can get his privileges. When you give chips, also give praise. And, if it is worth a few words of praise, it couldn't hurt to give a few chips.

Phasing Out the Chip System

The prime criterion used for deciding when to phase out the chip system should be your child's overall behavior. Your child doesn't need to be "perfect" before the chips are taken out. Rather, when your child's behavior has been satisfactory to you over a period of a month, and she has clearly learned how to take feedback, it is a good time to begin phasing out the chips.

If it is obvious that you phased out the chips too soon, you can always reinstitute them as soon as necessary. In order to reinstitute the chips, just pick a job that your child completes when asked and give your child the correct number of chips for doing the job when asked.

Trial Days

While you are still using the chips on a daily basis, initiate trial days off the chip system. The following steps should be followed for any trial day.

1. Explain to your child that you would like to try a day off the chip system.
2. Stress that if things go well, you'll have another trial day the next day, too.
3. Explain that the child must follow the rules just as if he were on the chip system.
4. Explain what will happen if the rules are not followed: You will be using time-out for any misbehavior. If time-out is used more than two times for the same behavior, the next day cannot be a trial day. The chips may be started again at any time during any day.
5. Prompting the right response from your child can be very effective in obtaining or regaining cooperation, as the following example shows:
6. Mother: "Michael, I'm going to give you four chips for helping me bring in the groceries. You remember, don't you, that you would have earned twice as many chips if you had carried in the groceries without being asked first."
   Michael: "Yes, I understand. Thanks, Mom."

It is important for parents to remember that not all trial days are successful; it may take some time before the chips can be completely phased out. Chips can always be used again, whether it's been one day off the system or four weeks. After your child once knows how you want her to behave, it is up to you to follow through when a rule is broken.

And, after you have phased out the use of the chips, you will still need to make sure that you are reinforcing your child(ren) for appropriate behaviors and implementing consequences for inappropriate behaviors.

Concluding Remarks

When your child is on the chip system, breaking a rule should result in a chip loss. When he is off the system, breaking a rule should result in time-out. If these procedures are not followed by you, your child will not follow the rules. Praise for desirable behavior is also a must, whether you are on or off the system. If being good doesn't have a reward (attention, praise or extra privileges), the desired behavior will not occur as often. When phasing out the chip system, all the procedures for practicing, checking jobs and time-out should still be followed consistently with praise, rather than chips.

The implementation of a chip system provides the necessary structure so parents and children interact in predictable ways with predictable consequences. Over time, parents learn to provide appropriate consequences in a matter-of-fact, consistent, and unemotional manner. Children learn how to earn the privileges they desire and to avoid the behaviors that prevent them from earning those privileges. In this way, the chip system can make your family's time together more satisfying and enjoyable.

Chapter 14

A Manual for the Family Treatment of Anorexia Nervosa

James Lock, MD, PhD, and Daniel le Grange, PhD

Few evidence-based treatments are available for anorexia nervosa (AN). Among those that are most promising, at least for younger adolescent patients, is a particular form of family therapy, family-based treatment (FBT), devised by clinician researchers at the Maudsley Hospital in London in the 1980s and manualized and studied subsequently in various other locations (LeGrange & Lock, 2005).

Anorexia Nervosa (AN) is seen by many as the paradigmatic illness for the application of family therapy. Historically, structural and strategic family approaches have been used to help adolescents with AN (Minuchin, Rosman, & Baker, 1978; Palazzoli, 1974). Employing techniques derived from these types of family therapy as well as feminist therapy, clinical researchers at the Maudsley Hospital devised a family treatment specifically tailored to the needs of adolescents with AN (Dare & Eisler, 1997). The approach is highly practical and initially focuses exclusively on problems related to improving eating and promoting weight gain in the adolescent with AN. The adolescent

and family are not seen as responsible for the illness as AN is "separated" or externalized from patient and family. The therapist takes a consultative rather than leadership role with the family, leaving specific decisions about treatment up to the parents. The aim here is to empower parents, not the adolescent with AN, to take needed action to abate the behaviors associated with AN. The approach aims to change directly only problems in the family that interfere with their success in weight restoration and normalization of eating. The approach includes a family meal that allows the therapist to help the parents in vivo their approach to helping their child eat. It also provides an opportunity to identify other related problem areas (e.g., avoidance of making demands, anger, and inadequate food choices) that interfere with weight gain. The family meets weekly and reviews the patient's progress on a weight chart and discusses what worked and did not work related to changing eating and weight loss behaviors. A keen focus is kept on these weight restoration processes and examination of other family or adolescent issues is deferred until weight and behaviors are nearly completely normalized.

When the patient's weight is near normal and eating is better, treatment focuses on beginning to return control of eating back to the adolescent. Under parental guidance, the adolescent typically, although gradually, establishes an age appropriate level of independence around food and other weight related issues (e.g., exercise and food choices). Only when eating and weight are no longer central therapeutic concerns does the treatment focus on general adolescent issues, and then only insofar as they have been thrown off course by the advent of AN. Therefore, this part of treatment is generally brief.

EVIDENCE FOR FAMILY-BASED TREATMENT FOR ANOREXIA NERVOSA

The substantive evidence in support of FBT for adolescent AN comes from several randomized clinical trials examining variations of FBT. Although these trials are generally small in scale, their findings are consistent that this particular form of family treatment is effective for adolescents with AN. The initial study by Russell and colleagues (1987) found that an adolescent subset of 18 patients who had been ill with AN for less than 3 years had significantly better outcomes when treated with family treatment compared to individual supportive therapy; however, adult patients and adolescents with longer duration AN did not differ in outcome in respect to therapy type (Russell, Szmukler, Dare, & Eisler, 1987). Two other studies from the Maudsley group, used FBT for adolescents for outpatient treatment only that suggested that FBT was viable without first hospitalizing patients. More tentatively, these studies also suggested that patients with highly critical (i.e., those with high levels of expressed emotion) families did better when the parents and the adolescent were seen separately (Le Grange, Eisler, Dare, & Russell, 1992; Eisler, Dare, Hodes, Russell, Dodge, et al., 2000). In the first U.S. trial to use a form of family therapy based on the Maudsley approach, Robin and colleagues (1999) compared Behavioral

Family Systems Therapy or BFST to a developmentally oriented psychodynamic therapy (Ego-Oriented Individual Therapy) aimed at enhancing adolescent self-esteem, self-efficacy, and assertiveness (Robin, Siegal, Moye, Gilroy, Dennis, et al., 1999; Robin, 2003). These authors found that at the end of one year of treatment, BFST was superior in terms of improved weight gain and menstrual return. However, at follow-up one year later, no differences between the groups remained. Recently, a study comparing a six-month/10 session dose of FBT to a 12 month/20 session dose, found that there was no difference in the efficacy of the two doses on weight gain or changes in psychological concerns related to eating and weight (Lock, Agras, Bryson, & Kraemer, 2005).

Taken together, the data suggest that about 80% of typically referred adolescent patients with short duration AN will remit using FBT (Couturier & Lock, 2006). Further, two studies suggest that these effects are enduring at the long term. Eisler et al published a five year follow-up on their original cohort of subjects and found that patients treated with FBT continued to be substantially improved over those who received individual therapy (Eisler, Dare, Russell, Szmukler, Le Grange, et al., 1997). Lock et al, in a four year follow-up, found that the gains made by the subjects in their large Randomized Control Trial were maintained in terms of weight gain and improvements in eating related psychopathology (Lock, Couturier, & Agras, 2006). Further, the vast majority of subjects were in school or working. However, significant problems with anxiety and depression affected about 30% even though eating related symptoms had abated.

One of the significant developments that took place in 2001 related to FBT was the publication of a manualized version of the Maudsley approach to adolescent anorexia nervosa (Lock, & Le Grange, 2001; Lock, Le Grange, Agras, & Dare, 2001). This version was piloted and then used in the largest randomized clinical trial of adolescent AN published to date. The description of treatment strategies that follows is a summary of that manual. Details and further illustrations of the approach can be found in the full-length manual that follows.

Manual for Family-Based Treatment for Adolescent Anorexia Nervosa—Short Version

Purpose of This Manual

This manual contains background information essential to the understanding of adolescent anorexia nervosa (AN) and its treatment with family therapy. It presents a treatment program, including the details of specific sessions and phases of therapy that is based on research that has demonstrated effectiveness. The manual derives from several controlled trials of family treatment for AN initially at the Maudsley Hospital, London and subsequently studied at Stanford University, Department of Psychiatry, Child Division and Lucile Salter Packard Children's Hospital. This manual is intended for use by qualified therapists who have experience in the assessment and treatment of eating disorders in adolescents. The therapist in training under the guidance of experienced clinicians may also use it. It is not intended as a self-help manual. The treatment described should be conducted with appropriate consultation and involvement of professionals in pediatric medicine, nutrition, and child psychiatry.

The overall perspective of this therapeutic approach is to see the parents as a resource in the treatment of adolescent patients with AN. Mobilizing parents and family members as a resource is the most important theoretical position that sets this approach apart from other family and individual therapies for AN. Parents play an important role throughout the three phases of this treatment. Thus, the *first* phase of treatment attempts to reinvigorate parental roles in the family system, particularly as it is related to the patient's eating behaviors. This is considered the key therapeutic maneuver in this phase of family treatment. Therapy is almost entirely focused on the eating disorder and its symptoms and begins with a family meal. The therapist's goal in this phase is to develop a strong parental alliance on the one hand and to align the patient with a peer or sibling sub-system. The families are encouraged to work out for themselves the best way to re-feed their anorexic child. The *second* phase begins when the patient accepts parental demands to increase food intake and begins to experience steady weight gain. At this point, family therapy focuses on the relationship of other family problems in relationship to the effect these issues have on the parents' task of supporting steady weight gain in the patient.

The theoretical understanding or overall philosophy of the Maudsley approach is that the adolescent is imbedded in the family, and that the parents' involvement in therapy is vitally important for ultimate success in treatment. In anorexia nervosa the adolescent is seen as regressed. Therefore, parents should be involved in their offspring's treatment, while showing respect and regard for the adolescent's point of view and experience. This treatment pays close attention to adolescent development and aims to guide the parents eventually to assist their adolescent with developmental tasks. In doing so, fundamentally working on other family conflicts or disagreements have to be deferred until the eating disorder behaviors are out of the way. Normal adolescent development is seen as having been arrested by the presence of the eating disorder. The parents are temporarily put in charge to help reduce the hold this disorder has over the adolescent's life. Once successful in this task, the parents will return control to the adolescent and assist the adolescent in usual negotiation of predictable adolescent development tasks, as appropriate.

The Maudsley approach differs from other treatments of adolescents in several key ways. First, as pointed out above, the adolescent is not viewed as being in control of her behavior, instead the eating disorder controls the adolescent. Thus in this way only, the adolescent is seen as not functioning on an adolescent level, but instead as a much younger child who is in need of a great deal of help from her parents. Second, the treatment aims to correct this position by improving parental control over the adolescent's eating (also read *eating disorder*). This control has often been lost because parents might feel that they are to blame for the eating disorder or the symptoms have frightened them to the extent that they are too afraid to act decisively. Third, the Maudsley approach strongly advocates that the therapist should primarily focus her/his attention on the task of weight restoration, particularly in the early parts of treatment. The Maudsley approach, as opposed to Minuchin's approach, tends to "stay with the eating disorder" for longer, that is, the therapist remains alert not to become distracted from the central therapeutic task which is to keep the parents focused on refeeding their adolescent so as to free her from the control of the eating disorder.

Setting up Treatment

It may seem unusual to make special mention of the initial telephone contact. However, as this is time-limited treatment and success depends to a large extent on the therapist's ability to make a powerful connection with the family, and given the formidable task at hand, these initial telephone contacts are crucial for the successful outcome of this process. By setting up the initial family meeting, the therapist should achieve two aims with the phone contacts: (1) Establish that there is a crisis in the family, and begin the process of defining and enhancing parental authority around management of the crisis; and, (2) Explain the context of treatment, that is, treatment team and medical monitoring. The therapist's first goal is to have every family member attend. The theoretical rational for having all family members present is to aid in the therapist's assessment of the family, as well as to maximize the opportunity to help the family—the family plays a role in both the maintenance and the resolution of the eating disorder. If everyone is not present, the therapist risks losing both power and information.

To demonstrate the seriousness the therapist attaches to the patient's illness, he/she should convey the central therapeutic message to the parents in an elaborate letter to the family prior to the first face-to-face meeting. This letter should once more emphasize the seriousness with which the therapist views the patient's illness and how important it is for the entire family to attend this initial meeting. A follow-up call the evening prior to the appointment by the therapist to remind the family of the upcoming meeting will greatly enhance attendance. This call will also emphasize the seriousness that the therapist feels for the problem at hand.

Session 1: The First Face-to-Face Meeting

The first face-to-face meeting with the family is critical because it sets the tone for the entire first phase of therapy. The therapist has prepared the family through the initial telephone and written contacts that are designed to communicate the importance of everyone's presence and the seriousness of the therapy that the family is about to engage in.

There are three main goals for the first session:

- To engage the family in the therapy
- To obtain a history about how the AN is effecting the family
- To obtain preliminary information about how the family functions, that is, coalitions, authority structure, conflicts

In order to accomplish these main goals, the therapist undertakes the following therapeutic interventions:

1. Weigh the patient
2. Greet the family in a sincere but grave manner
3. Take a history that engages each family member in the process
4. Separate the illness from the patient
5. Orchestrate an intense scene around the seriousness of the illness and in recovery
6. Charge the parents with the task of re-feeding
7. Prepare for next sessions family meal and end the session

Weigh the Patient

Why: Weighing the patient does not just serve an instrumental goal; it also strengthens the relationship between therapist and patient by helping the patient through a potentially stressful process. As the therapist communicates his/her understanding of this difficult process to the patient, and so strengthen his/her relationship with the patient. The therapist is therefore able to use both the weight and relationship aspects that emerge from this process in the family therapy sessions.

How: Prior to beginning the family session, the therapist must weigh the patient. Weighing the patient prior to the onset of each meeting should be the therapist's responsibility. The therapist should be at hand to monitor the patient's response to any weight change, and address her response to these changes. The patient should be greeted, separated, and asked to join the therapist. As they walk to the weighing in area, the therapist should ask if the patient has any particular concerns or problems that should be discussed during the upcoming session. In future sessions, this process will be repeated and should become the expected routine opportunity for the patient and the therapist to have a few minutes apart from the family as a whole to allow for communication and support for issues the adolescent may have difficulty bringing up without the support of the therapist.

Second, the therapist should record the weight on a weight chart, and this information should be conveyed to the family. We recommend that these weights be plotted on a weight chart in the presence of the family. In this way, the patient's weekly weight will help determine the direction each treatment session will take, that is, if her weight has gone up, the therapist will use this information to congratulate the parents on their efforts and reinforce a continuation of this success. Should the patient's weight stay at a low level or drop, the therapist should use this information to reinvigorate the parent's efforts to re-feed their youngster. In addition, the family should be provided with a copy of the weight chart at every session. This should serve as another visual reminder of their daughter's progress (or lack thereof) in regaining her lost weight over time. Because many patients with AN become overly fixated on specific weights or numbers it is not helpful to focus on targets in this type in this therapy. Instead, the emphasis should not be on specific weights, but rather on the direction of weight gain or loss.

Greet the Patient and Her Family

Why: Engaging eating disorder patients and their families in treatment is often a profound challenge and the outcome of treatment is affected by the degree to which the therapist will succeed in this task. To emphasize the seriousness of the illness, the style in which the therapist conducts the first greeting is most important, that is, intensely, gravely, empathetically, warmly, sincerely, and with foreboding. The therapist must make sure that he/she meets each family member, gets to know what he or she does whether it is work or school related, and check that each family member knows why the family is attending. The therapist should treat every member of the family with the same degree of respect, and should make special efforts to let everyone feel that their presence at the meeting is valued.

How: The therapist invites the family into the room and greets each family member by a handshake or clear eye contact. The therapist is serious and conveys this attitude through facial expression, tone of voice, and calm demeanor. Each family is asked to take a seat of their choosing. Sometimes it is difficult for the therapist to focus adequately on each family member. There may be a tendency to spend more time on the parents at the expense of the patient and siblings. This problem may arise in part because the therapist is aware that the need to stir the parents to action toward the end of the session is paramount and is therefore preparing for this. However, not focusing adequately on each family member would be an error because at the beginning of the session the entire family needs to be engaged, as they are all needed in the process of helping with recovery.

Take a History That Engages Each Family Member of How AN Is Effecting Each Family Member

Why: The therapist now turns to the way in which the family members view the eating problem. The therapist should get a detailed description from each family member including the patient of how each perceives the anorexic member's state of ill health. The therapist has to succeed in this task, so that he/she can highlight the harmful effects of the illness and set the stage for orchestrating an intense scene regarding the patient's illness. The therapist uses a circular style of questioning in order to engage the whole family and to help guard against a single-family member or only a few members taking over the session. The purpose of this history taking is not just to gather more information, but also to enlighten family members among themselves about how the illness is effecting them. In this sense, it is not about history so much as about what is happening to the family currently which are the result of things that have happened in the past as a result of AN. This information is critical to the therapist as they prepare for the other interventions of this session that depend on some knowledge of the impact of AN on the family.

How: Circular questioning is often very helpful in getting an idea from each family member how they experience the illness, that is, instead of asking father or mother how much they worry about their daughter not eating, the therapist can ask the patient or one of the siblings this question. For example, turning to a sibling the therapist may say: "How do you know that mom is worried?" and "How can you tell dad is worried?" Similarly, asking mother "What does your husband do when your daughter struggles to eat," or asking dad "What does your wife typically do to encourage your daughter to eat more." The way in which each family member describes the problem influences the therapist's response to the family, that is, the therapist reflects the family's comments back to the family in such a way so as to amplify the seriousness of the problem and the family's sense of having done all it could do to help, but to no avail. It is also important to spend some time on a direct discussion of "who's to blame for the AN," with the aim of this intervention to dispel and contradict existing beliefs about this. It is also important that the therapist spend time addressing the patient, specifically in terms of acknowledging her current skills, power, and her achievements. Again, the successful conclusion of this maneuver depends on the therapist's ability to sufficiently get a detailed history from the family.

Separate the Illness from the Patient

Why: In stressing that the patient has little control over her illness, the therapist tries to enable the parents to take drastic action against the illness, and not their daughter, when ordinarily they might be reticent to force food onto such an obviously frail looking adolescent. Therefore, it is important that the therapist models his/her support of the patient who has been overtaken by this illness. All of the information about how devastating the illness is and how the parents have to work hard at combating its effects may perturb the patient and she may fear that the therapist is exaggerating the problem. She may also fear that she is not being understood and that the therapist is about to unleash the family on her, which is true. This is an important challenge for the therapist who has to show the patient that while her dilemma is understood, at the same time she needs to gain weight, which is the exact opposite of her wishes. By stressing that AN is not identical to the patient herself, the therapist can distinguish the support for the developing adolescent, while at the same time insist on seeing AN as a problem for the patient. This strategy is key in maintaining engagement with the adolescent while attacking AN. Failure to achieve this separation can increase resistance to the treatment on the patient's part.

How: The therapist should ask the patient to list all the things the illness has given her as well as taken away from her. As s/he listens to this list, the therapist must show as much warmth for the patient and as much distress and fear about the symptoms as possible and may say: "I am saddened that this terrible illness has interrupted your life to this degree, that it has taken your freedom away, and it has left you without much control of what you do." In doing this, it is vitally important for the therapist not only to show sympathy for the family, but also an understanding of the patient. The therapist must model an uncritical attitude toward the patient's symptoms, and must simultaneously show warmth toward the patient and as much distress and fear about the symptoms and their consequences and may say "I know that you are more frightened of eating, sometimes, then of dying. Dying seems a long way off, food is right in front of you." It is essential that the therapist attends to and modifies any parental and sibling criticism of the patient. The therapist may point out that: "The symptoms don't belong to your daughter, rather, it is this terrible illness that has overtaken her and is determining almost all of her activities. For instance, it is AN that makes her hide food, or dispose of food, or makes her behave in deceitful ways. In other words, it is the illness that gets your daughter to do all these things that you find so upsetting. The daughter you knew before this illness took over is not in charge of her behavior, and it is your job to strengthen your daughter once more."

Orchestrate an Intense Scene Regarding the Patient's Illness

Why: Next the therapist wishes to raise parental anxiety/concern by orchestrating an intense scene about the seriousness of AN in order to increase their sense of responsibility to take on a dreadful task where others have had limited success. In this sense, anxiety is a useful motivator, while guilt and blame are not. Successful restoration of their daughter's health through weight gain depends on the parents' unified action in the re-feeding process in much the same way as competent and caring nursing staff would have if the patient had been admitted to a specialist inpatient unit. The therapist is summarizing his/her findings and is now going to deliver his/her salvo. That is, the therapist should model grieving over the past treatment failures in the context of the present treatment. The therapist is therefore stirring up the family in order to call on their energy sources.

How: The therapist should now orchestrate an intense scene that neither scapegoats the patient, blames the parents, nor exempts the siblings. The focus of this trepidation should be the patient's weight, the failed previous attempts at weight restoration, the medical and emotional problems likely to occur if AN persists, and an emphasis that the family is the last resort for the patient. For example, if the patient has been in hospital, the therapist should alarm the family about the potential for rapid weight loss. If weight gain in the hospital has been unsatisfactory, this should be grieved over. The inability of past health care professionals' efforts should be treated respectfully, but held out as further evidence of the dire position the family finds themselves in. Regardless of the specifics of each patient and her family, the therapist should impress upon the parents that: "Most couples have a variety of ways in which they approach everyday issues and dilemmas in their families. You as a couple may also have some issues that you differ on, and that is okay. However, when it comes to working out a plan about how to nourish X back to health, you cannot afford to disagree at all, you have to work together all the time. The slightest disagreement between the two of you will make it easy for the eating disorder to stay in charge of your daughter's life and defeat her. You have to act as if you are one person in order to succeed." Upon gathering information from the family about how they experience the illness, the therapist then tells the family what it is he/she hears the family is telling them (reflection), but in such a way so as to amplify (increase) the seriousness of the illness. The therapist should be genuine and purposeful in his/her expression of the "horror, despair, panic and hopelessness of the family." The therapist may find it helpful to show his/her empathy by holding close to the actual medical seriousness of the illness, the patient's corpse-like appearance, and the horror of the illness. It may be helpful for the therapist to think of other non-eating disorder cases of dying children. To illustrate this concern, the therapist may say something akin to the following: "Your child is dying of this disorder." Also, the therapist must work hard not to accept the anorexia nervosa façade that everything is all right. Paradoxically, this could very well be a pitfall for experienced therapists who could be seduced by their shared familiarity with the illness. On the other hand, less experienced therapists may let the horror of the illness overwhelm them and consequently become immobilized. The therapist must try to raise the family's activation energy as habit. Family structure, and patient resistance are all aspects that may inhibit parental ability to take charge of re-feeding their daughter.

Charge the Parents with the Task of Re-Feeding

Why: After the therapist has described the difficulties and failures of past efforts to help the patient and the consequences of inaction, s/he must next help the family to see that no matter what other treatments may be available in the short term finally the patient will return to the family. This prepares the family for the charge that the therapist is about to make which is that they need to re-feed their daughter. The family will likely be horrified, angry or resentful with the therapist's suggestion that they ought to help restore the patient's health. The reason that the family is the best resource for re-feeding their daughter include that they know her best, they are the most invested in her well being and future health, that they have shown evidence of being good parents in the past, and that as an adolescent, their daughter still needs her family.

How: The therapist should now make a case for the family being the major resource for their daughter's recovery. The therapist should first point out what the other treatment alternatives are (e.g., hospitalization, individual therapy, residential treatment) and how that may soon put the family in the same predicament as before, that is, a severely underweight offspring. Although the therapist should leave the decisions to how to accomplish the re-feeding to the parents, it may help to offer them some ideas to consider, for example, organizing meals so that they can monitor them more effectively by having two breakfasts (before school), an early dinner, and a late supper. S/he also alerts the parents not to become engaged in discussions about diet foods, and to emphasize that they should nourish the patient according to her profound state of malnutrition, and not according to the wishes of AN. The therapist should press upon the parents that for the first few weeks of treatment it may be necessary for the patient to be absent from school and be under parental supervision 24 hours per day. Similarly, the therapist may advise the parents that one or both of them might need to take a leave of absence in order to accomplish the task of re-feeding.

Prepare for the Family Picnic and End the Session

The therapist should end the session with great sympathy and sorrow, but also a sense of optimism that the parents will be able to work out a way to save their daughter's life. Thus, the therapist leaves the family with a sense of responsibility to take on this awesome task of re-feeding their daughter. He/she will invite the family to return within a few days and ask them to bring a picnic lunch with enough food for the patient and everyone else—not based on the patient's wishes but rather on her level of starvation. In other words, the parents should make a decision as to an appropriate meal to serve their starving offspring.

End of Session Review

As should be the case at the end of each treatment session, the lead therapist should communicate/review the previous aspects with therapy and consultation team members.

Session 2: The Family Meal

The second session involves a family meal. At the end of the first session, the parents were instructed to bring in a meal for their daughter with AN that they felt met the nutritional requirement to help with her starved state. In Session 2, the therapist hopes to build on her/his understanding of the patient and family as well as provide hope that the family can succeed in re-feeding their daughter. The assessment of the family is not a single occurrence; rather, further understanding comes throughout treatment. With the family meal though, the therapist wants to start his/her assessment of the family's transactional patterns around eating, help persuade the parents to have their daughter eat one bite more than she is prepared to, while making sure the patient feels supported by her siblings through this ordeal.

The major goals for this session are:

- Continue the assessment of the family structure and its likely impact on the ability of the parents to successfully re-feed their daughter.
- To provide an opportunity for the parents to experience that they can succeed in re-feeding their daughter.
- To assess the family process specifically around eating.

In order to accomplish these goals, the therapist will undertake the following interventions during this session:

1. Weigh the patient.
2. Take a history and observe the family patterns around food preparation, food serving, and family discussions about eating especially as it relates to the patient.
3. To help the parents convince their daughter to eat at least one mouthful more than she is prepared to, or to help set the parents on their way to work out among themselves how best they can go about in re-feeding their daughter.
4. To align the patient with her siblings for support.
5. End of session review and close session.

Weigh the Patient

The session begins, as all sessions in the first two phases will, with the patient being weighed by the therapist. A report of this weight to the family will help set the tone of the session. If the patient is doing well, then the tone will be more optimistic; whereas, if there is a decline in weight or lack of progress, the tone may well be more foreboding.

Take a History and Observe the Family Patterns around Food Preparation, Food Serving, and Family Discussions about Eating Especially as It Relates to the Patient

Why: The assessment of the family is obviously not a single occurrence; instead it is an ongoing process that brings an enriched understanding as treatment progresses. Generalizations of interaction patterns (e.g., cross-generation problems, poor parental alliances, importance of separation of identity) in families are often confusing. The therapeutic meal offers the therapist an opportunity to observe in vivo these family processes specifically as they are brought to the fore during a meal.

Knowledge of the family structure, that is, the often-repeated patterns of communicating, controlling, nurturing, socializing, forming boundaries, making alliances and coalitions, and solving problems, is gained throughout the family meetings, but may become more obvious during the family meal. The family meal provides strong exposure to the family's characteristic organization. Similarly, an understanding of the significance of the family patterns and the patient's symptoms should lead to the therapist's effectiveness in producing family changes. Symptoms are not believed to be the result of a specific family structure. However, this does not exclude the fact that there may be patterns of family interaction that render a family powerless in the presence of symptoms. Therefore, a patient with an eating disorder cannot improve unless and until there is a change in dietary patterns. In other words, anorexic patients must gain weight to get better. Family therapy is effective not because it undoes a hypothetical family etiology, but rather because it changes the way a family responds and manages their daughter's eating disorder.

With adolescent patients, the aim is to set up a meal regimen similar to that in a well-functioning inpatient treatment setting for eating disorders. The parents must be coached to set up a culture such that eating and completing a meal occurs within a set period of time, while the expectation for that occurrence is relentless and powerful. In other words, there is no alternative for the patient other than to comply with her parents' wishes.

How: First, the family is instructed to proceed in laying out/dishing up the picnic lunch. The therapist does not participate in the meal, instead, he/she takes part in learning more about the family style around eating by observing the family ritual, and by asking questions about eating. For example, the therapist may ask the parent who is dishing up whether that is typical of the pattern at home, or whether the food they brought represents the kind of meal they would have had as a family lunch in their dining room, who prepares the food at home, who does the food shopping, and so on. The reason for this inquiry is to help the therapist and family understand what potential changes in these activities would be advisable.

Assist Parents to Convince Their Daughter to Eat at Least One Mouthful More Than She Is Prepared to (Or Set the Parents on Their Way to Work out among Themselves How Best They Can Go about Re-feeding Their Daughter)

Why: One aim of the family picnic is for the therapist to help the parents make their daughter eat at least one mouthful more than she is prepared to. This symbolic act is important and the family meal may have to last as long as it takes to achieve this goal. The therapist seldom has to achieve more with the family meal as the effect is striking and the patient now knows that her parents have a new resource in re-feeding her. Thereafter the parents feel more empowered with the knowledge that they may find it easier to get their daughter to eat more, and although the struggle may continue for several more months, parental power to enforce more food intake alters the relationship among the patient, parents and food. The therapist hopes to enforce change by disrupting old and familiar patterns, taking advantage of the family's disorientation in the strange setting of the family therapy and under the impact of the therapeutic bind.

The therapist has to help the parents delve into their resources about appropriate feeding of a growing child and can say: "It is full cream milk and pasta with a cream sauce that will make the difference, not a salad."

How: The therapist suggests that the parents sit on either side of the patient and advises them not to discuss the type or amount of food to be eaten, but to take action by filling the daughter's plate, and so on. The therapist consistently coaches the parents by making repetitive and insistent suggestions how to act uniformly so as to compel the parents to increase gradually the monotonous force applied to their daughter, that is, to get her to eat. While "coaching" the parents it is sometimes necessary and useful for the therapist to physically stand behind the parents and provide them with specific suggestions, much like a prompter. It is often helpful to remind the parents of a time when their daughter was even younger and ill in bed with a bad head cold and the parents tried to get her to eat or to take her medicine. The therapist may say "You would have found a way to get her to eat," or "You know how to feed a starving child and you don't need expert nutritional advice" in an attempt to bolster their confidence in this task. This procedure is sometimes inelegant, humiliating and inappropriate given their daughter's age, but getting her to eat that one mouthful more than she was prepared to often marks a turning point.

Align the Patient with Her Siblings for Support

Why: Cross-generation instead of interparental alliances are often observed in families with an anorexic youngster. The role of the therapist is to allow the parents to work out a way to operate together as a team (interparental alliance) in order to re-feed their adolescent offspring. The therapist should oppose unhealthy family structures, especially those that confuse communication, disrupt powerful parental control, obscure clear cross-generation boundaries, and/or interfere with the maintenance of clear separateness of identity.

How: While the therapist is supportive of the joint parental efforts to re-feed their daughter, the therapist must demonstrate to the patient that he understands her dreadful predicament, that is, being consumed by her eating disorder. Having the therapist unleash her parents to take away her only sense of identity/power, and feeling entirely unsupported while this is going on around her, may initially overwhelm the patient. The therapist will say to the patient (and indirectly addressing her siblings), "While mom and dad make every effort to fight your illness and nourish you back to health, you will think that they are being awful to you. You will need to be able to tell someone just how bad things are for you, that is, you will need someone like your brother/sister/school friend who could listen to your complaints." Likewise, the therapist will turn to the patient's siblings and encourage them to be supportive of their sister, not in her efforts to be anorexic, but in comforting her when she feels overwhelmed by the turn of events.

End of Session Review and Close Session

The session should be ended on an optimistic note, congratulating the parents and the family on their efforts, almost regardless of their actual material success. The parents must experience the session as giving them more hope and encouragement about what they can do to help their child. Most sessions should end with a positive note, though where there has been slippage or failure to gain needed weight, more cautionary reminders may also be made in order to keep the family vigilant about the seriousness of not following through on their re-feeding initiatives.

The Remainder of the First Phase
(Sessions 3–8)

Most of the remainder of this phase is characterized by the therapist's attempts to bring the patient's food intake under parental control by expanding, reinforcing and repeating some of the tasks initiated at the beginning of therapy. What the therapist has to achieve here, in addition to continuing the work begun in Sessions 1 and 2, is to review with the parents, on a regular basis, their attempts at re-feeding the patient and systematically advise the parents how to proceed in curtailing the influence of the eating disorder. Sessions are characterized by a considerable degree of repetition as the therapist may go over the same steps week after week to get the parents to become consistent in their management of the patient's eating behavior and the eating disorder's attempt to defeat these efforts.

Unlike the more structured nature of the first two meetings, the following sessions may seem less systematically organized, and may not follow a pre-specified order. However, a combination of the following four goals will apply to almost every session until the conclusion of the first phase of treatment.

There are three goals for this part of treatment:

- Keep the family focused on the eating disorder
- Help the parents take charge of their daughter's eating
- Mobilize siblings to support the patient

In order to accomplish these goals, the following interventions will be appropriate to consider during the remainder of treatment for Phase 1:

1. Weigh patient at the beginning of each session
2. Direct, re-direct, and focus therapeutic discussion on food and eating behaviors and their management until food, eating, and weight behaviors and concerns are relieved
3. Discuss, support, and help parental dyad's efforts at re-feeding
4. Discuss, support and help family to evaluate efforts of siblings to help their affected sibling
5. Continue to modify parental and sibling criticisms of the patient
6. Continue to distinguish adolescent patient and her interests from those of AN
7. Close all sessions with recounting of progress

These goals will be applied in sessions three through ten in any order, with their momentary applicability or appropriateness determined by the family's response to the initial interventions (sessions one and two). For the purpose of clarification, however, we will outline a description of each goal separately, even though in practice, they may overlap to a considerable degree.

Weigh the Patient

Why: As in the first two sessions, weighing the patient is an important opportunity to assess the patient and her progress. The pattern of weight gain can be quite variable. In one family, who readily take up the task of re-feeding and who figure out quickly how to accomplish this, weight gain may occur swiftly. On the other hand, many families struggle with a variety of issues which prevent them from achieving the re-feeding of their starving daughter. For example, parents may have trouble working together. They may disagree on the strategy to employ. One of them may not make it a priority to assist with re-feeding. Parents may try to avoid taking their daughter out of school even though she is not eating because they so value her accomplishments there. Siblings make undermine their ill brother or sister by becoming unruly in some manner themselves. Most often, the parents are extremely reluctant to take on the strong will of their child with AN because they know what they are up against and do not want to face this challenge. In some cases, one parent may be over-involved with the accomplishments of their affected son or daughter and be unwilling to challenge their behaviors. For all of these reasons, and many more like them, the weight gain course may be quite variable.

How: The therapist's own resilience to stay with the eating disorder symptoms will send a powerful message to the parents that, for now, this is the focus of treatment. The therapist starts every session by first recording the patient's weight. This is carefully plotted on a weight chart. Weight progress, or lack thereof, is shared with the entire family.

Direct, Re-Direct, and Focus Therapeutic Discussion on Food and Eating Behaviors and Their Management until Food, Eating, and Weight Behaviors and Concerns Are Relieved

Why: As stated before, the primary challenge for the parents during the first phase of treatment is to engage successfully in the task of re-feeding their anorexic daughter. Whereas initially the therapist may have to work hard to convince the parents that drastic action is required, for the remainder of Phase 1 and in most instances, the therapist has to keep the family focused on the eating disorder. Parents may become fatigued or the patient may gain weight initially creating the illusion that the immediate crisis has been removed. Because AN can become intractable and can be wearying to continue to confront, therapists and families alike may be tempted to relax their efforts too soon. However, this would be an error as a mind that is preoccupied with AN thoughts usually takes every opportunity to reassert itself.

How: The usual reaction to the third session is for the parents to gain more control, although weight gain may not yet be evident. One exception may be for dehydrated patients who could quickly gain several pounds after the first visit. Regardless of weight gain, the therapist may provide basic dietary instructions and coach the parents in terms of their re-feeding skills from Session 3 onward. This is done by eliciting from the family their large, but often unused, store of knowledge about what constitutes healthy eating and sufficient amounts of high-caloric foods suitable for a starving person, as well as their particular understanding of their child. Parents soon become inventive and begin to create high-density meals. Although discussions around dieting should be discouraged, when they do occur, the aim is to encourage the parents to debate the value of a meal of 1,000 calories or more, instead of getting locked into unproductive and futile arguments with their daughter about the negligible caloric content of a salad of lettuce leafs or a fat-free yogurt. The emphasis of weight gain should be in the overall context of achieving a weight that the patient's healthy body "knows is right," that is, through a return of healthy skin and hair, return of menses, and an increase in bone density. In other words, the therapist should see weight gain less in term of "norms" or numbers on a scale and more in terms of a particularly patient's health. The therapist should refrain from setting a specific target weight. Instead, the goal of a healthy body should be used to guide the patient toward a healthy weight. This weight is essentially a range that the patient can sustain without undue dieting and, if female, one at which menses is comfortably maintained.

After the family meal, feeding will remain a preoccupation for the next several sessions, even when the patient is gaining weight under the new regimen. The therapist has to insist that the parents should remain relentless until they are convinced that the patient no longer has any doubts that she will not be able to return to anorexic behavior while a part of the parents' household. Consequently, the therapist will stress the need for regular, dietetically balanced food intake; for example, vegetarianism may be temporarily suspended. Other symptoms (such as binge eating and purging) should also be subject to strict parental control. As is the case with dietary control, this control should be emphasized as a temporary measure. The intention is for the parents to demonstrate that they can achieve control, and if necessary, remove the possibility for their daughter being able to make herself sick again. This may include keeping their daughter occupied after a meal (e.g., watching a favorite movie on television), supervised bathroom visits, locking the kitchen if possible, and so on. This may also include visiting local pharmacies to inform them of the possibility that their daughter is abusing laxatives and to ask that they be contacted if she attempts to purchase them.

Once the weight chart has been explained and discussed, the therapist should carefully review events surrounding eating during the past week. The family's strategies to bring about weight gain should dominate discussions, especially in the absence of significant symptomatic improvements. The therapist will ask each parent, the patient and her siblings to tell him/her how the past week has been and how they have gone about the task of re-feeding. The therapist should discourage broad statements such as: "it's been an okay week," or "it was difficult." Instead, he/she will turn to each parent separately and ask them to relay in great detail what happened at mealtimes, and in the same style of circular questioning outlined before, check with every family member in turn whether that is also the way they would describe events. Discrepancies should be lingered over and the therapist should search for clarification. The therapist should be able to construct a clear picture of what happens at meal times, as well as between mealtimes, so that he/she can carefully select those steps parents have taken that should be reinforced, and those that should be discouraged.

Discuss, Support, and Help Parental Dyad's Efforts at Re-Feeding

Why: One of the most important aspects of this treatment at this particular juncture is for the therapist to make sure that the parents are working together as a team. The parents' success in re-feeding their daughter can often directly be contributed to their ability to work as a team in this process. Because the aim of the therapy is develop, enrich, and support the parents in their efforts to care for their ill adolescent, the ability of the therapist to provide assistance in this is crucial. At the same time, the therapist may be tempted to "take over" the parental role by directing or over-controlling the re-feeding process. This hazard should be avoided because the ultimate message of the therapy is that the family, not the therapist, is the major resource for recovery.

How: The therapist might have to emphasize to the parents that although she/he understands and respects that they (the parents) may have differences of opinion, as many couples may have, parents' cannot afford to differ at all in how they should re-feed their daughter. The therapist should exercise extreme vigilance in checking with the parents on a weekly basis how they are doing in this regard. By carefully reviewing their attempts at re-feeding as, described above, she will also check with everyone how mom and dad are doing as a team. The therapist will make a point in addressing the parents as the authoritative team to reinforce for them that they are indeed in charge. Consistently addressing the parents as the key decision makers in relation to their daughter's health matters also reinforces for their daughter and her siblings that mom and dad are in charge in this arena. Making decisions jointly as a couple may in fact be uncharted territory for some parents. Reminding the parents that they should work together and that they should be "on the same page, on the same line, and on the same word, at all times when it comes to their daughter's eating" should be done at several time points at this early part of treatment.

Discuss, Support and Help Family to Evaluate Efforts of Siblings to Help Their Affected Sibling

Why: To reinforce healthy cross-generation boundaries, and to prevent the siblings from interfering with the parents' task of re-feeding, consistent support of the patient by her siblings should be encouraged. Healthy boundaries between the siblings and their parents make the parents' immediate task less difficult, while this also prepares the groundwork for successful resolution of the eating disorder and the launching of a healthy adolescent into young-adulthood.

How: Similar to the stated aim for this part of Phase 1, the therapist should be consistent in his/her encouragement of the siblings not to interfere with their parents' task, but rather support their sister through this ordeal. The therapist will say to the siblings that: "While mom and dad make every effort to fight your sister's illness and nourish her back to health, she will think that they are being awful to her and she will need to be able to tell someone just how bad things are for her, that is, she will need someone like yourselves who could listen to her complaints. She will also need you to comfort her when she feels that things are too rough for her and she gets too scared about eating and weight gain."

The therapist will want to discourage siblings from rushing to their parents' aid in feeding the patient or attempt to deter them from pursuing their task of re-feeding the patient. In addition to having explained to the family that the job of re-feeding belongs to the parents, and supporting and comforting the patient during this time are the tasks of the siblings, the therapist should reinforce the siblings in this role throughout treatment. For instance, efforts by siblings to either jump to the parents' rescue while they (the parents) try to insist that the patient eats more, or when they try to discourage parents from pushing too hard, should be prevented.

Continue to Modify Parental and Sibling Criticisms of the Patient

Why: It has been shown that parental criticism of the anorexic offspring can have a negative impact on the family's ability to remain in treatment as well as the eventual outcome in treatment. Consequently, it is of great importance to address parental criticism we believe are either due to parental guilt about the eating disorder, a reaction to the eating disorder symptoms per se, or indications of a poor premorbid relationship between the adolescent and her parents. Sessions in this part of treatment are therefore characterized by attempts to absolve the parents from the responsibility of causing the illness, and by complimenting them as much as possible on the positive aspects of their parenting of their children.

How: We have already made mention of the fact that modeling by the therapist of an uncritical acceptance of the patient is an essential therapeutic task. This is achieved in part by externalizing the illness, that is, the therapist must convince the parents that most of the patient's behavior around eating are in fact outside of her control and that it is the illness that has overtaken her behavior in this respect. In other words, the therapist must consistently point to the fact that the patient cannot be identified with the illness. This will help foster an understanding of the patient's behavior and reduce any parental criticism of the patient. Changing parents' behavior in this regard can be difficult, but persistence on the therapist's behalf may pay dividends in the end. For instance, some parents may say, in response to anorexic behaviors from their daughter, "she is making it so difficult for us, we make an effort to get the foods she likes, and then we catch her trying to throw it in the trash," or "we are desperate now, because if we just turn our backs for a second, she'll give her food to the dog, or stick it in her pockets," or "I've had it with X, I have to be with her 24 hours a day, because if I dare let her out of my sight, she's up and down the stairs exercising." What these examples demonstrate is that in all three cases, the anorexic behaviors have been identified with the patient. Another way of reading or understanding these passages is that "I am trying my best (the parent), and just look how deceitful or ungrateful our daughter is." As pointed out before, parental anger, frustration or criticism can have deleterious consequences for the successful resolution of the eating disorder. In guiding the parents through this difficult period, the therapist should remember that families have very different ways of parenting and different circumstances that will influence how this process is worked through. It is important to remember that each family should be encouraged to work out for themselves how best to re-feed their anorexic child.

Continue to Distinguish Adolescent Patient and Her Interests from Those of AN

Why: As discussed in session one intervention, it is important that the therapist and the family keep in mind that they are struggling to combat the effects of AN and not the independent thinking and will of a developing adolescent person. If the therapist fails to keep this a focused aspect of the treatment during this phase, the hope for developing an alliance with the patient is greatly diminished and her resistance to the treatment enhanced.

How: Again, this intervention is described in session one. However, as Phase I continues, the therapist may stress the need to recognize that more of the effort of eating is safely being taken up by the healthy part of the patient. This can be done by saying things like: "It seems to me that your parents reported that they needed to encourage you less to eat and that you are more interested in fighting back AN yourself;" or, alternatively asking something like: "As you have been progressing you are taking more of your life back. Have you noticed that your thoughts are less preoccupied by food and weight?" The therapist may ask the patient to gauge her progress figuratively. For example, by drawing a Venn diagram that shows how much of themselves remains preoccupied by AN. At least part of every session should be devoted to these periods of observations, questions and assessments.

Close Session and End of Session Review

As was the case for Sessions 1 and 2, the lead therapist should continue to review each treatment session with the rest of the team for the remainder of the phase. At the end of each session, the following information should be conveyed to the treatment and consultation team: patients weight progress, development of any new symptom (e.g., purging, over exercise, etc.), new diagnostic concerns (e.g., anxiety disorder, depression, suicidality, etc.), overall sense of family progress with illness, and discuss any problems between team members (i.e., medical team not informing parents of progress or concerns).

Beginning Phase 2: Helping the Adolescent Eat on Her Own (Sessions 9–14)

The mood displayed by the therapist in Phase 2 is different from the somber and sad tone characteristic of most of Phase 1. By the time the family moves into Phase 2, the patient and her family would have demonstrated progress in terms of weight regain. This advance should be reflected in the therapist's mood when he/she embarks on this next step in treatment. In addition, unlike the more structured nature of treatment interventions concerning re-feeding the adolescent up to this point, guidelines for the therapist's style/technique from here onward is less circumscribed. From a developmental perspective, the eating disorder can be seen as having interfered with the patient's normal adolescent development. Therefore, the therapist's task now is to help get the patient "back into" adolescence. It should be noted that the parents also need to get "back into" adolescence—that is they need to examine their own lives with the view toward their daughter growing up. The specifics of this process are highly individualistic and there is seldom a prescribed way to proceed. Instead, we will provide broad guidelines about therapeutic procedures the therapist should begin to introduce toward the latter part of this treatment phase.

How Does the Therapist Assess the Family's Readiness for the Second Phase?

Given the above summary of the second phase of treatment, the following is offered as an approximation of the criteria that should be met in order to signal readiness for the second phase of treatment:

- Weight is at a minimum of 90% IBW.
- Patient is able to eat without undo cajoling by parents, and parents report no significant struggles getting the patient to eat regular meals.
- Parents report that they feel empowered in the re-feeding process, that is, the parents demonstrate a sense of relief that they can manage this illness.

How Does the Treatment Team Change in Phase 2?

For Phase 2 the treatment team remains intact, that is, the Family Therapy team plus the Consulting Team. As the eating disorder dissipates treatment begins to resemble regular family therapy for adolescence, and the involvement of the Consulting Team, for example, the pediatrician or the nutritionist, may become more secondary. However, the reappearance of eating disorder symptoms might still necessitate maintaining the active involvement of the Consulting Team. Therefore, all team members should be kept abreast of the patient's progress. The relationship among the Family Therapy team itself though, remains essentially unchanged from Phase 1 to Phase 2.

The major goals of the second phase of treatment are:

- Maintain parental management of eating disorder symptoms until patient shows evidence that she is able to eat well and gain weight independently
- The return of food and weight control to adolescent
- Termination with patient and family

In order to achieve these goals, the therapist will need to undertake a the following kinds of interventions:

1. Weigh patient
2. Continue to support and assist parents in management of eating disorder symptoms until adolescent is able to eat well on her own
3. Assist parents and adolescent in negotiating the return of control of eating disorder symptoms to the adolescent
4. Encourage family to examine relationships between adolescent issues and the development of AN in their adolescent
5. Continue to modify parental and sibling criticism of patient, especially in relation to the task of returning control of eating to patient
6. Continue to assist siblings in supporting their ill sibling
7. Continue to highlight difference between adolescent's own ideas and needs and those of AN
8. Close sessions with positive support

Although the treatment goals are the same for all needed sessions of this phase, the emphasis of each session changes as one moves toward the end of this phase. For example, sessions may start out very similar to that of Phase 1 with weight gain being the primary goal, but the emphasis will shift toward weight maintenance as control over eating is handed back to the patient. Finally, the therapist will begin to focus more on adolescent issues as she/he makes a transfer from Phase 2 to Phase 3.

Weigh Patient

Why: As in previous sessions, continued close monitoring of weight using the weight chart is an important mechanism for providing feedback to the patient and family on their progress.

How: At this point, the patient and therapist should have developed some increased rapport such that the weighing process becomes increasingly acceptable. The intimacy of sharing the vulnerable information of weight change should lead to greater trust overall.

Continue to Support and Assist Parents in Management of Eating Disorder Symptoms until Adolescent Is Able to Eat Well on Her Own

Why: Weight gain remains fragile at the early stage of the second phase of treatment, and optimal weight has not yet been achieved. Therefore, the therapist has to make sure that the parents do not relax their vigilance in so far as the re-feeding process is concerned. Although this task is very similar to that described in Phase 1, the therapist should note the shift in emphasis here. Whereas until now the therapist's task was that of helping and coaching the parents to get their daughter to eat more, the therapist's role here shifts more toward that of greater delegation. That is, the therapist wants to consolidate the parents' trust in their own abilities to make appropriate decisions in the process of re-feeding their daughter.

How: Similar to the therapist's regular review of the parents' efforts at re-feeding their daughter that earmarked much of the first phase, the therapist should start this phase of treatment with the same goal in mind. The therapist will insist that the parents remain relentless in their efforts to restore normal weight until they are convinced that the patient no longer doubts their ability to prevent her from starving herself. The therapist has to show determination to stay with the eating disorder symptoms in order to send a powerful message to the parents that, for now, re-feeding is the focus of treatment. At every session, the therapist has to carefully review events surrounding eating and discuss weight gain (or lack thereof) with the family members. The family's strategies to bring about weight gain should dominate discussions for as long as it is needed.

Assist Parents and Adolescent in Negotiating the Return of Control of Eating Disorder Symptoms to the Adolescent

Why: Once the patient is relatively free from the eating disorder, it is timely for the parents to allow the patient to assert her independence in this respect which is part of the development of healthy adolescent independence. Also, the gradual phasing out of parental supervision should serve as a trial period to see whether the adolescent can cope with eating adequately on her own, without the reappearance of eating disorder symptomatology thwarting her progress. The therapist's responsibility here is to assist the parents and the adolescent in bringing about a careful and mutually agreed upon handing over of responsibility in this domain from the parents to the adolescent. This process is orchestrated against the backdrop of each family's unique rituals or habits around regular eating activities before the eating disorder changed the family's meal times. Although the parents may seek guidance from the therapist about how to proceed with handing control regarding eating back to the patient, it is ultimately the parents *in collaboration* with the patient, who should decide how to proceed with this process. This is a delicate maneuver as the therapist should balance the involvement of the patient, who might jump at the opportunity to regain responsibility in food choices, the parents, and her/himself in terms of the decision-making process.

How: As stated before, the task of re-feeding (as described in Phase 1) is continued during the second phase, although with a gradual change in emphasis. Soon in the second phase, the therapist will guide the family toward *relinquishing* their control over the patient's eating. This can only be done if the patient's weight has mostly been recovered and the therapist is reassured that improvement will continue even when the parents begin to exert less vigilance. Parents may chose to gradually lesson their control over this process in several ways, for example, by letting the patient dish up for her at mealtimes while the parents continue to supervise this activity. Alternatively, parents may allow the adolescent more of her *own* food choices, as long as these selections represent healthy and adequate quantities of food. Another way to move forward is for the parents to leave the patient to her own devices when it comes to one or two meals per day, while still supervising the main meal of the day. Ultimately, the parents and the patient would want to arrive at an age appropriate decision which is in keeping with each family's unique set of rules about food shopping, food preparation, joint family meals versus individual responsibility and tastes, and so on.

Continue to Modify Parental and Sibling Criticism of Patient, Especially in Relation to the Task of Returning Control of Eating to Patient

Why: The reason that family criticism is suspected to contribute to poorer outcome has been enumerated above. In the context of Phase 2, the issue of family criticism is more directly focused on the return of eating to the adolescent. There is a renewed opportunity for parents and siblings to reproach the adolescent with AN and thereby compromise her best efforts. This may undermine the patient's attempts to return to healthy eating and can trigger greater resistance to help from her family.

How: The basic mechanisms for modifying parental and sibling criticism have been described above.

Continue to Assist Siblings in Supporting Their Ill Sibling

Why: Again, the basic reason for this type of intervention have been previously articulated. However, it may seem that at this point, sibling support is less vital. The case has been made that siblings should support their ill sibling, but she is clearly getting better, so they may feel their work is done. It is true that the need for their specific support in relation to helping the adolescent with AN to put up with the re-feeding efforts of her parents does diminish in this phase. Nonetheless, the adolescent has not yet recovered and still needs support, especially when she advocates for more autonomy. Siblings are still important in helping her to sustain herself during this process.

How: The strategies for involving peers have been illustrated earlier.

Continue to Highlight Difference between Adolescent's Own Ideas and Needs and Those of AN

Why: It is important that the difference between AN thoughts and goals and those of the adolescent continue to be explored.

How: The basic strategies are presented above. However, in this phase, the therapist can emphasize the differences between AN thinking and goals and those of the adolescent through the negotiating process of regaining control of eating from the parents. Thus, the therapist encourages the adolescent to set her own goals for recovery—for example returning to a dance class that AN deprived her of because of her severe malnutrition. In addition, the therapist should explore failure to achieve such goals as a way to invigorate the adolescent's own wish to differentiate herself from AN.

Close Sessions with Positive Support

Why: As in previous sessions, the attitude of the therapists at the conclusion of sessions is warm and generally congratulatory so that guilt, powerlessness, and feelings of inadequacy are minimized

How: As in previous sessions, the therapist summarizes the main achievements of the family while footnoting the shortcomings. This is done efficiently, but with warmth as the family leaves. The therapist may take care to say good-bye to each family member as they leave the room in order that they continue to feel recognized and valued.

Termination

Why: As important as greeting the family at the onset of treatment is the process of respectful bidding adieu. This process should clearly end the therapeutic relationship by conferring on the family the sincere confidence that they can proceed with likely success if future problems arise. The treatment for AN using the family model described in this model lasts approximately one year. Although the early interventions are the most intense and most closely spaced, the involvement with the family is significant over this period. The early use of the authority of the therapist to engage the family in the seriousness of the illness, as well as the use of paradoxical interventions throughout the therapy, make the relationship with the therapist that much more intense. Over Phase 2 great effort is made to decrease the dependence on the therapist while also increasing both the patient's and the family's autonomous functioning in line with the ultimate goal of a successful termination. The method of termination employed here is one of many that could be used. The key concern is that the family has an opportunity to review the therapy and say goodbye to the therapist; while the therapist has an opportunity to lend the family optimism and support in the process of separation.

How: The therapist should reserve about ten minutes to conclude the therapy by saying goodbye to each family member. This should mirror the first session's momentous and careful greeting of each family member. Attention should be paid to each family member's involvement and praise should be given for the work committed on behalf of the family. The demeanor of the therapist should include a genuine warmth, a comforting quality, as well as a subdued optimism. Family members should each be given an opportunity to bid the therapist farewell. The therapist's aim is to encourage the family's abilities to proceed smoothly and successfully undertake any problems that are ahead.

References

Couturier, J., & Lock, J. (2006). What constitutes remission in adolescent anorexia nervosa: A review of various conceptualizations and a quantitative analysis. *International Journal of Eating Disorders*, 39, 175–183.

Dare, C., & Eisler, I. (1997). Family therapy for anorexia nervosa. In: D. M. Garner & P. Garfinkel (Eds.), *Handbook of treatment for eating disorders* (pp. 307–324). New York: Guilford Press.

Eisler, I., Dare, C., Hodes, M., Russell, G., Dodge, E., & Le Grange, D. (2000). Family therapy for adolescent anorexia nervosa: the results of a controlled comparison of two family interventions. *Journal of Child Psychology and Psychiatry*, 41(6), 727–736.

Eisler, I., Dare, C., Russell, G.F.M., Szmukler, G. I., Le Grange, D., & Dodge, E. (1997). Family and individual therapy in anorexia nervosa: A five-year follow-up. *Archives of General Psychiatry*, 54, 1025–1030.

Le Grange, D., & Lock, J. (2005). The dearth of psychological treatment studies for anorexia nervosa. *International Journal of Eating Disorders*, 37, 79–81.

Le Grange, D., Eisler, I., Dare, C., & Russell, G. (1992). Evaluation of family treatments in adolescent anorexia nervosa: A pilot study. *International Journal of Eating Disorders*, 12(4), 347–357.

Lock, J., Agras, W. S., Bryson, S., & Kraemer, H. (2005). A comparison of short- and long-term family therapy for adolescent anorexia nervosa. *Journal of the American Academy of Child and Adolescent Psychiatry*, 44, 632–639.

Lock, J., & Le Grange, D. (2001). Can family-based treatment of anorexia nervosa be manualized? *Journal of Psychotherapy Practice and Research, 10*, 253–261.

Lock, J., Couturier, J., & Agras, W. S. (2006). Comparison of long term outcomes in adolescents with anorexia nervosa treated with family therapy. *American Journal of Child and Adolescent Psychiatry, 45*, 666–672.

Lock, J., Le Grange, D., Agras, W. S., & Dare, C. (2001). *Treatment manual for anorexia nervosa: A family-based approach.* New York: Guildford Publications, Inc.

Minuchin, S., Rosman, B., & Baker, I. (1978). *Psychosomatic families: Anorexia nervosa in context.* Cambridge, MA: Harvard University Press.

Palazzoli, M. (1974). *Self-starvation: From the intrapsychic to the transpersonal approach to anorexia nervosa.* London: Chaucer Publishing.

Robin, A. (2003). Behavioral family systems therapy for adolescents with anorexia nervosa. In A. Kazdin & J. Weisz (Eds.), *Evidence-based psychotherapies for children and adolescents* (pp. 358–373). New York: Guilford Press.

Robin, A., Siegal, P., Moye, A., Gilroy, M., Dennis, A., & Sikand, A. (1999). A controlled comparison of family versus individual therapy for adolescents with anorexia nervosa. *Journal of the American Academy of Child and Adolescent Psychiatry, 38*(12), 1482–1489.

Russell, G. F., Szmukler, G. I., Dare, C., & Eisler, I. (1987). An evaluation of family therapy in anorexia nervosa and bulimia nervosa. *Archives of General Psychiatry, 44*(12), 1047–1056.

Chapter 15

Strengths-Oriented Family Therapy (SOFT): A Manual Guided Treatment for Substance-Involved Teens and Families

James A. Hall, PhD, Douglas C. Smith, PhD, and Julie K. Williams, PhD

This chapter was developed to assist in the evaluation plan of the Strengthening Communities for Youth (SCY) initiative funded by the Center for Substance Abuse Treatment (CSAT IU79 TI 13354), a division of the Substance Abuse and Mental Health Services Administration (SAMHSA). The opinions presented here are those of the authors and do not represent official positions of the government. We gratefully acknowledge SAMHSA's role in both expanding the range of available services to adolescent substance abusers and their families in eastern Iowa, as well as supporting the development of this treatment approach.

STRENGTHS-ORIENTED FAMILY THERAPY

This chapter describes Strengths-Oriented Family Therapy (SOFT), an efficacious treatment for adolescent substance abuse. Strengths-Oriented Family Therapy blends solution-focused therapy (Berg & Miller, 1992a; deShazer, 1988), skills training ap-

proaches (Hall, Schlesinger, & Dineen, 1997; Spoth, Redmond, & Shin, 1998) and case management approaches (Hall et al., 1999; Hall, Carswell, Walsh, Huber, & Jampoler, 2002) into a comprehensive outpatient program for adolescents who abuse substances. In this chapter we will discuss the rationale, development, and core session content of the SOFT model. SOFT was designed to comprehensively address the diverse needs of adolescents presenting for substance abuse treatment. Each component of SOFT is supported by empirical research. We begin by describing the components of SOFT and the research base for each of these components. Next, we explain the development of the SOFT manual. Finally, we review the core session content for implementing SOFT.

SOLUTION-FOCUSED THERAPY

Solution-Focused Therapy (SFT) (Berg & Miller, 1992a; deShazer, 1988; Walter & Peller, 1992) posits that clients are continually changing and working on their own goals the best way they know how. SFT is a task-oriented therapy, and the primary role of the therapist is to be the client's *solution coach*. That is, the role of the therapist is to ask the right questions that will direct the client toward goal clarification and the means by which to achieve each goal. Treatment planning is termed *solution planning* in our approach, and this important distinction reflects the subtle nuances of correctly using solution-focused interviewing techniques. That is, the focus of *solution planning* is always on specific, concrete actions that the client is willing to take to address problems. *Solution planning* is directed by the client's perceptions of their goals for treatment.

At this time, very few studies have evaluated the efficacy of solution-focused therapy approaches with adolescents, but some descriptive work outlines case histories when such models have been adapted for children and adolescents (Selekman, 1997). Nevertheless, the approach appears promising with teens for several reasons including: (1) the continual praise for past successes and emphasis on mutuality may engage teens to work on personally meaningful goals, (2) the task-oriented nature of the approach may assist in goal planning and development of a *future orientation* that is important for teens, and (3) the general avoidance of *problem talk* may make teens feel less singled out as the identified patient within their family system. Thus, embedding solution-focused therapy within SOFT is likely to be effective and acceptable with adolescent substance abusers.

FAMILY-BASED MODELS FOR ADOLESCENT SUBSTANCE ABUSE

Other family-based models already exist for the treatment of substance abuse (Hamilton, Brantley, Tims, Angelovich, & McDougall, 2001; Henggeler, 1999; Henggeler, Schoenwald, Borduin, Rowland, & Cunningham, 1998; Liddle et al., 2001) and various studies have described these family treatment models as efficacious with adolescent substance abusers (Dennis et al., 2004; Liddle & Dakof, 1995; Waldron, 1997; Williams & Chang, 2000). SOFT, however, is distinguished from existing family therapy models in several ways. First, SOFT contains a pre-treatment motivational enhancement session that includes parents (Smith & Hall, 2007). Thus, parental motivation for treatment is also targeted, and treatment starts

with presenting both a clear rationale for treatment, empathizing with parental frustrations, and orienting families to treatment processes. We emphasize parental involvement due to studies suggesting parents want more information about their adolescents treatments, and due to feedback from parents and community professionals that they are pleased with this approach (White, Godley, & Passetti, 2004). Second, the heavy emphasis on solution-focused techniques and language in SOFT is not replicated in existing family therapy models. Finally, skills training exercises provided in a multifamily group augment conjoint sessions and provide an additional platform for family work. Including multifamily group therapy in SOFT allows the model to be replicable in publicly-funded programs. That is, limited staff resources often dictate the use of efficient modalities for providing as much service to as many families as possible. These unique components of SOFT form the rationale for evaluating it as a distinct treatment model.

SKILLS TRAINING

Cognitive-Behavioral skills training approaches are rooted in social learning theory and usually involve the teaching, modeling, and in vivo practicing of new skills. Based on previous research, skills training approaches appear to be efficacious for treating adolescent substance abusers (Dennis et al., 2004; Kaminer & Waldron, 2004; Sampl & Kadden, 2001). An inherent assumption of skills training is that specific skills can be taught and, once acquired, a client can use one or more skills to modify substance using behaviors and consequences. In the SOFT model, skills training activities were delivered in both conjoint family sessions as well as in multifamily group settings. In SOFT, skills training content is delivered both during family sessions (i.e., role play assignments with counselor observing, follow-up homework) and during multifamily group sessions.

CASE MANAGEMENT

In recent years, clinicians and researchers have increasingly focused on ecologies of adolescent substance abusers. That is, greater attention has been given to environmental barriers to treatment and how multiple systems in the clients' life impacts their substance using behavior. Many of the aforementioned family therapy models for adolescent substance abuse focus on multiple systems. Case management models are useful in linking clients to needed services, advocating for client needs, and navigating the often times fragmented social service delivery system. The use of case management services with adolescents leaving residential substance abuse treatment have been shown to significantly increase service utilization and impact relapse rates when compared to those receiving continuing case as usual (Godley, Godley, Dennis, Funk, & Passetti, 2002). In SOFT, the therapist also assumes case management responsibilities when they would benefit the treatment of the teen.

SUMMARY

Strengths-Oriented Family Therapy (SOFT) is an integrative model responsive to the needs of heterogeneous adolescent substance abusers presenting for treatment. Integrative models are increasingly becoming important (Kaminer, 2001) as the treatment and research community have begun to recognize that no one-size-fits-all program is likely to be flexible enough for the diverse needs of adolescents and families presenting with substance-related concerns. Despite some shared features with other family-based interventions, the unique features of SOFT include a heavy emphasis on solution focused language, a formal strengths assessment, a pre-treatment motivational session, and family integration into both conjoint and multifamily group sessions.

SOFT DEVELOPMENT AND EFFICACY

Overview

The SOFT therapy manual was written to facilitate the evaluation of this intervention in a randomized longitudinal study. This section outlines the developmental efforts in this project, including: the process by which the manual was written, the supervision strategies used to ensure integrity, and the evaluation design of the randomized study, and findings to date on the efficacy of SOFT. The foundation for the SOFT model was the family therapy model used by the senior author in his counseling practice with adolescents and their parents. This clinical model combines skills training, with heavy doses of positive reinforcement and a focus on family dynamics.

Treatment Manual Development

Strengths-Oriented Family Therapy was developed as part of collaboration between staff members at a community not-for-profit substance agency and university-based clinical researchers. Initial didactic trainings with therapists focused on family therapy and solution focused techniques. The therapy manual was developed in close collaboration with project therapists. That is, therapists frequently met with clinical researchers to discuss the feasibility of implementing the family content in their community based setting until agreements were made on exact delivery format. These collaborative efforts are typically recommended for those entering the process of behavioral therapy development (Rounsaville, Carroll, & Onken, 2001).

Initial and On-going Supervision

Once therapy manuals were developed, therapists tested the SOFT model with two voluntary families prior to the onset of our study. These cases were closely supervised to ensure that the model was being used as specified and to identify problems or issues in the procedures outlined in the manual. The two main SOFT therapists in our longitudinal study completed co-therapy with these initial families. Therapists were supervised by reviewing audio taped sessions with particular emphasis on engaging (and re-engaging) clients into the treatment process, the clients' clinical issues, appropriate case management activities for the clients, use of solution focused language, and the use of appropriate family therapy techniques. After these initial cases, supervision continued on a weekly basis to prevent therapist drift. Therapists also were trained to enter time spent on therapeutic activities into a web-based management information system, which was routinely audited to ensure that clients were receiving both the appropriate session content as well as the expected dosage. Later in the study, an instrument using client self-report was developed and administered to document treatment fidelity. The second author (DCS) was the primary clinical supervisor of these therapists.

Evidence-Based Findings for the SOFT model

Research Design. In this project families ($n = 103$) were randomly assigned to receive either SOFT or The Seven Challenges ® (7C) (Schwebel, 1995,

2004). Adolescents completed baseline measures prior to treatment intake and then were reassessed at 3, 6, 9, and 12 months following intake using a battery of reliable and valid instruments. Parents or legal guardians were interviewed at baseline, 6, and 12 months. Participants were paid $20 for each assessment with bonuses for timely completion and for completion of all follow up assessments. Data were collected between June 2003 and August 2005. (For a full description of study procedures see Smith et al., 2006.)

Substance Use Outcomes. Strengths-Oriented Family Therapy (SOFT) was found to increase abstinence rates and substance use disorder symptom remission rates at the three and six month follow up waves (Smith, Hall, Williams, An, & Gotman, 2006). Even among those adolescents that did not attain full abstinence or symptom remission we saw significant reductions in the amount of use and substance related problems. These findings held even after controlling for post-treatment time spent in controlled environments (i.e., detention). In short, SOFT was efficacious at reducing drug use and substance-related problems through the six month follow up wave.

Despite this encouraging evidence on the efficacy of SOFT, we saw no differences *between* SOFT and 7C in terms of efficacy at reducing substance use frequency or substance related problems (i.e., dependence and abuse symptoms). Based on previous research that also found few differences between treatments, we were not surprised that SOFT was not more efficacious than 7C. Furthermore, we attribute this finding to three factors. First, unlike studies comparing well-implemented study treatments to poorly specified treatment as usual (TAU) condition, our community collaborators implemented this promising manualized program as their standard treatment. That is, for the 7C condition didactic training in the model was provided to staff by the model's author, Dr. Robert Schwebel, and clinical supervision was provided by the Project Director (second author of this paper). Thus, we believe that 7C as delivered here was both a potent and well-implemented intervention and this neutralized our ability to demonstrate that SOFT was superior to a TAU condition. Second, during one period in our study therapist turnover in the 7C condition forced us to cross over our two therapists completing SOFT into providing 7C. This therapist cross-over may have introduced some *model bleeding* into the 7C condition and it is also possible that the more established therapists may have been more

skilled than previous 7C therapists. (We should note, however, that therapists in the SOFT group were not significantly different from 7C therapist in terms of effectiveness.) Finally, statistical power was low for this study. Thus, despite some seemingly clinically significant group mean differences on some variables, we cannot be certain that we would reliably replicate these due to low statistical power.

Retention in Treatment. Another key finding in our preliminary study was that families randomly assigned to the SOFT condition were more likely to have longer treatment episodes, which is important as treatment length is often associated with better outcomes. Treatment length was longer for SOFT even after accounting for differences in program length between SOFT and 7C. As seen elsewhere, family inclusion and case management activities may have been effective in retaining youth in treatment (Henggeler, Pickrel, Brondino, & Crouch, 1996).

Impact on Family Cohesion. Adolescents receiving SOFT also reported significant increases in family cohesion at the three month follow up wave. However, these increases in family cohesion disappeared at subsequent follow up waves. This initial increase and later decrease could reflect the focus on positive family activities and communication during the treatment episode when much time is spent together as a family, but it is unknown why these families did not maintain gains in family cohesion after treatment.

Treatment Satisfaction and Breadth. At the three month follow-up sessions, we investigated both treatment satisfaction and the number of distinct treatment activities completed by adolescents in our study. Adolescents in SOFT reported significantly higher satisfaction with treatment, and also received more distinct types of services than adolescents in 7C. For SOFT participants, the average scores on the 14-item *Treatment Satisfaction Index* (TXSI) and 20-item *Treatment Received Scale* (TRS) were 11.96 (*sd* = 4.09) and 9.63 (*sd* = 4.60). Although we cannot account for why satisfaction scores were higher among SOFT participants than for 7C, we are encouraged by both these findings as the SOFT model appears to be both well-received by adolescents and encourages the use of multiple treatment modalities (i.e., family activities, case management activities) not occurring in some traditional office-based therapies.

Summary and Future Research. In our preliminary studies, we found encouraging results suggesting SOFT is a feasible and efficacious treatment model for use with adolescent substance abusers. In our current research we are addressing the limitations of these findings by investigating the long-term results of SOFT through the 12 month follow up wave, investigating the impacts of the intervention on other psychosocial outcomes (i.e., criminal behavior, family functioning, school functioning), and investigating the cost effectiveness of the model.

INTRODUCTION TO THE TREATMENT PROTOCOL

Integrated models of adolescent substance abuse treatment (using multiple intervention strategies) are quickly becoming the norm in the field—in part, due to the recognition of the great heterogeneity among adolescent substance abusers. The Strengths-Oriented Family Therapy (SOFT) model integrates the Social Work *Strengths* philosophy, solution-focused therapy, skills training, and ecologically-minded family therapy (Berg & Miller, 1992b; Henggeler & Borduin, 1990; Saleebey, 1992).

All treatment models contain implicit theories of how to elicit change in clients (Liddle, Rowe, Dakof, & Lyke, 1998) and SOFT is no exception. The blending of skills training, family inclusion, the social work Strengths Perspective, solution-focused therapy, and case management form the backbone of this intervention. *The pervasiveness of solution-focused influence, formal strengths assessment, the family skills training multifamily groups, and the pre-session motivational sessions with teens and parents are among the features that give our model a unique flavor when compared to other family-based treatment models.* In this section, the theories and practice models influencing SOFT intervention are reviewed and SOFT's assumptions are identified.

The Social Work Strengths Perspective

The Social Work Strengths Perspective is based on the belief that people are most successful in solving problems and creating change in their lives when they focus on their strengths and become meaningfully involved in directing their own treatment. When people encounter difficult situations they naturally turn to their strengths and resources to find solutions (Saleebey, 1992). Only when people become overwhelmed or stuck do they seek help from others (i.e., professionals) outside their normal range of resources. The extension of this philosophy to teens and families should be apparent. Sometimes the multiple developmental challenges of adolescence *overload* the coping abilities of both the teen and family (Schulenberg, Maggs, Steinman, & Zucker, 2001). Assisting the teen and family to discover or rediscover their personal strengths is a vital step in helping them get back on track to creating solutions to problematic situations. When the professional focuses on what a family or teen is already doing well, the clients usually feel empowered by messages of self-reliance and creative solutions to their problems.

Brief Solution-Focused Therapy (BSFT)

Brief Solution-Focused Therapy is a model originally developed by the late Steven de Shazer and Insoo Kim Berg, the co-directors of the Brief Family Therapy Clinic in Milwaukee, Wisconsin (Berg & Miller, 1992a; deShazer, 1988). Additional applications of Solution-Focused Therapy to special populations exist (Berg, 1994; Selekman, 1997; Walter & Peller, 1992). However, very little has been written applying Solution-Focused Therapy with adolescents (Corcoran, 1997; Selekman, 1993) and even less empirical research has evaluated the effectiveness of solution-focused techniques with adolescents. Nevertheless, for reasons that are described below we expect this component of the SOFT model to be especially pertinent to adolescents in substance abuse treatment.

BSFT Overview. Brief Solution-Focused Therapy is based on the philosophy that change is inevitable and ongoing. Beyond being continuous, change has what de Shazer describes as a "ripple effect"—change leading to more change. In this philosophy, clients are viewed as the experts on what is required for them to change and presumes that the process of change is unique to each individual client. *In this model there is no such thing as resistance on the part of clients. Clients are always seen as being willing to work on some goals even if they are not the goals that are most important to the therapist.* This approach has interesting implications for the substance abuse field, which has traditionally conceptualized substance abusers as being *in denial about problems* and more recently varying on *readiness to change* (DiClemente & Prochaska, 1998; Prochaska, DiClemente, & Norcross, 1992).

BSFT considers cooperation as inevitable and leaves it to the therapist to negotiate and assess until a *right* method for change is agreed upon. In viewing clients as *experts* on change, BSFT therapists adopt a respect for clients through believing they possess their own unique solutions to creating positive changes in their lives. In a dialogue between therapists and clients, emphasis is placed not on the problem but on the client's strengths, resources and abilities. Unless a teen sees the past as the way to change, therapists and teens do not dwell on the problematic past. *Instead*, they move on to deal with the here and now and development of goals for future change. De Shazer (1988) and his colleagues have suggested some general principles that guide the brief solution-focused model:

1. If it ain't broke, don't fix it (look at what is working and do more of it),
2. Once you know what works, do more of it, and
3. If it doesn't work, don't do it again. Do something else.

Thus, emphasis shifts from delineating problems through detailed, problem-focused interviews to de-emphasizing problem history in favor of having fruitful discussion to generate ideas for solving problems. In short, in solution-focused therapy the *why* of the problem is less important to treatment than specific steps needed to overcome the problem.

Useful Solution-Focused Questions. Questions are the tools used to both assess for strengths and develop solutions within BSFT models. In some ways these questions become the key element in creating the expectation of a positive future. The Brief Family Therapy Clinic developed the *Five Useful Questions*, which have become a hallmark of the model:

1. *Pre-session change question:* This question is grounded in the belief that changes occur constantly and the reality that clients often experience some change between the time the appointment was made and the actual first session. *I often notice that, with many people, between the time the appointment is made and the actual meeting, things are often better. Have you experienced this?* Answers to this question can provide therapists with insights into a client's strengths and coping style.
2. *Exception finding questions:* These questions are used to generate ideas for future solutions and can be asked in many ways. *When was the last time you did not have this problem?* This question is often followed with a question that highlights personal coping, such as, *What were you doing differently back then when this was not a problem?*
3. *Miracle question:* This question is an effective tool for moving beyond problem-talk to solutions. The question will vary from client to client, but its basic components are included here. *Suppose you go home tonight and go to sleep, and while you're asleep a miracle happens. And the miracle is that all the problems that brought you here today are solved, but you're sound asleep and don't know this miracle has taken place. When you awaken in the morning, how will you know this miracle has happened? What will you be doing differently?* Answers to this and subsequent follow-up questions should prove helpful in creating small, behavior-oriented goals.
4. *Scaling questions:* These questions are useful in measuring client progress before, during, and after interventions and to determine levels of client motivation, confidence, and hopefulness. These questions ask clients to assess their perceptions subjectively on a scale of one to ten. *On a scale of one to ten, with one being the worst things have ever been and ten meaning your problems are solved, where would you put yourself today?* Follow-up questions to scaling question responses can focus on helping clients determine the next steps in working towards their goals. *You say you are a four. What would you be doing differently if you were at a five?*
5. *Coping questions:* These questions are often used when a client's life situation has not improved, but the therapist needs to credit whatever skills the client has utilized to cope with this lack of change. *How have you managed to get through this? How have you kept things from getting even worse?* These questions are designed to challenge the client's belief system and confront feelings of uselessness and hopelessness.

Use of BSFT in SOFT. Typically, in initial sessions of BSFT specific questions are used as tools to help clients identify their own strengths and positive coping skills. In our SOFT model, therapists assess client and family competencies using the Strengths and Resources Assessment (SRA). This process highlights both personal strengths and environmental resources that can be used later to address needs and accomplish goals. After the initial SRA assessment, we engage the client in a process of setting realistic, measurable goals by developing a solution plan.

Goal Development

Establishing goals is important in moving away from the problem and toward active solutions (Walter & Peller, 1992). Goals must be concrete and behaviorally described so that goal attainment can be measured. In fact, one of the strengths of this model occurs when therapists and clients establish criteria that can be evaluated for progress within treatment and as treatment outcomes. Goal development is one of the most important components of a cooperative therapist-client relationship. Therapists should remember that goals may change as life circumstances and client perceptions change. The qualities of well-formed goals include:

- *Saliency to the client:* The client is invested and believes goals are attainable.
- *Small, and achievable:* Small goals enable a client to be successful, which increases confidence and may have a special relevance to treatment of alcohol and substance abuse.
- *Concrete, specific, and behavioral:* These qualities enable both client and therapist to monitor progress.
- *The presence rather than the absence of something:* As it is much easier to *do* than *not do*, the issue becomes what will the client be doing *instead* of engaging in the problem?
- *A beginning of something, rather than the end:* Goals must be stated as a start, rather than some vague ending such as *sobriety* or *happiness.*
- *Realistic and achievable within the context of the client's life:* On-going treatment may reveal a need to establish more realistic goals.
- *Perceived as hard work:* This principle enhances the dignity of the task and enables the client to accept setbacks given the amount of work involved.
- *In the client's own words:* Using the client's own language in goal development increases the saliency of the goal to the client.

SOFT Key Assumptions. So, based on these theoretical foundations, we developed assumptions, goals and treatment techniques for the SOFT model.

SOFT Assumption #1. The therapist should use specific language in sessions to focus on strengths, abilities, influences and treatment outcomes.

Central to the Strengths Perspective is the belief that clients are most successful when they identify and use their strengths, abilities, and assets. The process of enumerating and using personal strengths allows clients to appreciate their own past efficacy, encourages motivation, and sets the stage for identifying and achieving goals. In SOFT, we find this approach to be useful with teen clients in substance abuse treatment who are mandated to attend treatment. Such clients may receive an extra benefit from articulating their strengths because it detracts from them being the identified client, promotes a view of self efficacy by concretely promoting the means to change, and possibly promotes a therapeutic alliance with a therapist. A recent analysis of client's statements in therapy sessions found that increased articulation of abilities, the need to quit, and reasons to quit predicted less drug use at follow-up (Amrhein, Miller, Yahne, Palmer, & Fulcher, 2003).

SOFT Assumption #2. Clients will participate most fully in treatment if they are in charge of goals, as opposed to having goals dictated by others.

All goal setting is guided by the clients' perceptions of their own needs. The role of the SOFT therapist is to assist the teen and family in clarifying goals such that they are action-oriented, behaviorally specific, positively worded, realistic, and attainable. Such a task orientation is especially appropriate for male adolescents who may be more oriented to working on goals than talking about feelings (Corcoran, 1997).

SOFT Assumption #3. Task-oriented, solution-focused therapy promotes a future orientation in adolescents and enhances problem solving skills.

In adolescence, people are inching toward adult roles in occupational functioning, romantic relationships, and other social relationships. *One assumption of our model is that assisting clients with goal development in small manageable tasks increases the client's feelings of self-efficacy and also helps foster the belief that future goals may be obtained.*

SOFT Assumption #4. Mutual development of goals appeals to adolescent autonomy and thus, enhances engagement.

Adolescence is a developmental transition during which increased autonomy is achieved (Steinberg & Silverberg, 1986). Teens are likely to bicker with parents over things that are seemingly small to themselves, but represent parental values (Steinberg, 2001). Similarly, teen clients may see things entirely different than adult therapists. Thus, the focus on mutual development of goals is very developmentally appropriate and could increase teen engagement in therapy. *Thus, an assumption of our model is that when the teen's solutions and goals are given some weight, it conveys respect, fosters independent thinking, and increases engagement.*

SOFT Assumption #5. When clients are reinforced for what they are already doing, they perceive treatment as a positive experience and self-efficacy is enhanced.

Families are often relieved when in treatment they are told to do what they have done in the past to resolve their difficulties. This approach elevates the family to expert status in the treatment, and engages them into the treatment process by recognizing past successful coping efforts. Past coping that was successful can be praised and exploration of how it applies to current problems is facilitated. This positive approach toward problem solving assists in engaging families, leads to greater satisfaction with the treatment process, and increases confidence in problem solving skills.

SOFT Assumption #6. Changes in family communication and family cohesion will impact subsequent substance use.

Past studies of treatment of disruptive behavior disorders have shown that parent training interventions are effective in increasing parenting skills, which in turn, had an impact on teacher reports of disruptive behaviors (Dishion, French, & Patterson, 1995). Other research in the adolescent substance abuse field has shown that changes in parenting and family cohesion during family therapy were associated with reductions in substance use (Godley, Kahn, Dennis, Godley, & Funk, 2005; Schmidt, Liddle, & Dakof, 1996). In a similar vein, our skills training module multifamily group should increase positive communication, family communication, and family problem solving which should have an impact on the youth's substance use.

SOFT Assumption #7. Family involvement in sessions will *reunite* adolescents who have become distant from parents due to drug use, and begin *uniting* clients with poor bonds to their parents in the first place.

Parents and youth are often disengaged from each other at the onset of treatment due to both the effects of adolescent substance use on parental trust, and past relationship difficulties that may have even contributed to the development of substance abusing behaviors (Diamond & Liddle, 1999). Family-based treatment is presented as a positive family activity that can increase trust, communication, and cohesion.

SOFT Assumption #8. While the SOFT therapist is the primary relationship in treatment, treatment is coordinated with others in a fluid way.

The SOFT therapist serves as the consistent figure in the client's treatment experience and is thereby able to organize fragmented and poorly coordinated resources. This consistency is especially salient for clients involved with multiple systems, or those with high psychiatric co-morbidity. A strong relationship allows the SOFT therapist to advocate for the client as necessary. Far from being an exclusive relationship, however, the client and therapist will involve many other persons in the search for resources. Informal and formal resources are explored with an emphasis on creative problem solving strategies that work.

SOFT Assumption #9. View the community as a resource, not a barrier.

The Strengths Perspective assumes that a creative approach to community use will lead to discovery of needed resources. In working with formal resources, such as housing agencies and job training programs, therapists assist clients by modeling and practicing behaviors that increase the likelihood of a successful contact. Whenever possible, therapists will encourage clients to explore informal resources, including friends, neighbors, electronic media, and other clients as sources of assistance.

SOFT Assumption #10: Conduct case management as an active, community-based activity.

Office-based contacts are supplemented with meeting with clients in community settings, such as their home or work site. For the therapist, this activity will inevitably lead to an increased appreciation of the challenges clients face in making changes resulting from a better understanding of their ecological surroundings. For the clients, these meetings provide an opportunity to develop and master skills where they actually live. In turn, this focus helps clients to break an all too prevalent reliance on institutional settings for assistance.

STRENGTHS-ORIENTED FAMILY THERAPY SESSIONS

Overview

This section reviews the major activities of Strengths-Oriented Family Therapy (SOFT) family and Multifamily Group sessions. Families engage in SOFT by completing a two-session comprehensive assessment program. Then, families complete five bi-weekly family therapy sessions and ten multifamily group sessions. Family sessions are 90–120 minutes in duration and groups last two hours. One month after the completion of these 15 sessions, the family completes a booster session.

The major activities included in SOFT are completing a placement assessment and engaging into treatment, completing a *Strengths and Resources Assessment,* developing a solution plan, participating in multifamily groups that emphasize skills training and family communication, and case management and monitoring associated with the later stages of treatment. Although SOFT has required activities and these session outlines exist, it is a flexible approach in that therapists will set aside their agendas if it appears that the family has urgent business to address. When dealing with crises, however, the SOFT model focuses on past successes in coping and action steps that can address the problem instead of extensive excessive history taking.

GETTING STARTED: STRENGTHS-BASED ASSESSMENT AND REFERRAL

Strengths-Oriented Family Therapy treatment starts by completing a two session assessment protocol. The first session involves completing a comprehensive assessment where in-depth information is collected on current functioning. This session is the only time during SOFT treatment when history taking about current problems is permitted, as this assessment is used for placement purposes. During this session teens are interviewed separately from parents, and parents complete collateral assessment forms. We recommend using a standardized assessment for which interpretive guidelines exist that may be used to provide a solid rationale for a treatment recommendation—such as the Global Appraisal of Individual Needs—Intake (GAIN-I; (Dennis, Titus, White, Unsicker, & Hodgkins, 2002).

Strengths-Based Assessment Feedback

After completion of the comprehensive assessment, the therapist provides feedback in the second session including drug treatment recommendations using our strengths-based approach, called Strengths-Oriented Referral for Teens (SORT) (Smith & Hall, 2007). This assessment feedback is given in a one-hour session that is attended by both the teenager and the parent. We typically split this session into three segments each approximately 20 minutes in duration. Each segment contains approximately the same format including: a scripted orientation statement, a review of client strengths, discussion of concerns, and recommendations. In the family segment, the therapist summarizes the session and works to build consensus among the family on what should be done next. In the sections that follow we give detailed descriptions of what we do in the teen, parent and family segments of this session.

Scripted Introductions. When introducing either the parent or the teen segment we comment on their expert status, praise their attendance, and briefly orient them to what will be done in the session.

Teen Segment

Below is a brief scripted introduction we use with teens, which can be paraphrased as long as key points are retained (i.e., expert, praise for attendance, review format):

> Today we're going to review the assessment you completed the other day. We want to focus on both the good things you told us about yourself as well as some areas where you have trouble so that we get the whole picture. Remember that we told you before doing the assessment that the purpose was

to figure out how we can best help you. Then we'll tell you what ideas our group came up with here that may be beneficial to you. Remember, you're the expert on your own life and these are only suggestions. We'll also ask you what you think will help you. You and I will meet for 20 minutes alone. Then I'll meet with your parent alone for 20 minutes. Finally, all of us will meet together to make a decision about where to go from here. Any questions?

Strengths Review. During the placement assessment, we ask the adolescent several *yes/no* questions about their personal strengths—including an open-ended question about what they consider to be their most important strengths. The therapist reviews these responses with the client using active listening skills (i.e., open-ended questions, empathy) and gets the client to elaborate on their strengths.

Reviewing strengths is an important exercise. First, it communicates with the client that the assessment is not completed to find out what is wrong with them. In fact, we often tell clients that the rationale for reviewing strengths is that we want to find out the good things about them. Second, when client strengths are reviewed the counselor can learn about valuable reasons that the client wants to quit using substances. For example, when asked to elaborate about reporting that he was good at sports, one client talked about his love for baseball and being a starter on his high school team. He also reported being on the verge of ineligibility because of his falling grades and drug use. This information was used later in the session when discussing treatment recommendations. Finally, reviewing client strengths in SORT facilitates rapport building in a productive and focused manner. That is, rather than extended periods of small talk, SORT therapists build rapport by highlighting their clients' positive attributes and expanding on their strengths and interests. In short, strengths reviews are important precursors to discussing concerns and ultimately exploring the need for behavior change.

Discussion of Concerns. Great caution is taken with how we frame problematic areas we have identified with the GAIN-I. Specifically concerns are framed out of personal concern for them, using concrete examples from the assessment, and giving a rationale for why those responses are concerning. For example, we may say something like:

We are concerned about your responses to the questions about depression, because you met the criteria for being depressed. For example, you said that you were having significant problems with trouble sleeping, feeling hopeless, losing weight, feeling easily irritated and annoyed, and losing interest or pleasure in things you once enjoyed. We're concerned about this because all these statements are signs of depression, and people living with depression often turn to drugs or other things to make themselves feel better instead of doing healthier and safer things to cope with their feelings. What do you think about what I just said?

The reader should note several things about this format for presenting concerns. First, concrete examples of client responses from the assessment were used to assist the counselor in defining what is meant by *depression*. This specification is especially important with teens that are developing cognitively and may have a poor understanding of abstract terms like *depression* or *emotional problems*. Second, a rationale was presented for why these responses were concerning (i.e., people with depression sometimes self-medicate and need coping skills). Finally, the concern was followed by an open-ended question to engage the teen about the information that was presented—thus allowing the teen to give feedback and multiple opportunities for the clinician to gauge treatment readiness. Furthermore, even though the counselor will be assertive in giving recommendations and relying on their professional knowledge, efforts are always made to elicit dialogue with clients on their perception of the referrals, express empathy when they are frustrated with the referrals, and remind clients that they are the decision makers.

We recommended that the counselor prioritize concerns before the SORT session and limit the discussion of concerns to 3–4 major points. This brevity is especially important with clients who raise a lot of red flags during the assessment. For example, if a client meets several mental health diagnoses it would be more efficient to discuss them together and build up to the recommendations for mental health treatment to be made later. As this session begins the treatment process, we try not to overwhelm the client with a litany of problems. Prioritizing into major themes for treatment planning purposes becomes a necessity with multiproblem teens.

Giving Recommendations. Recommendations should flow from the concerns that were discussed with the client, so the client knows why recommendations are being made. Counselors should refer back to this information and also to any information gained from this session that is indicative of the client's motivation for treatment. For example, if a client elaborates on problems they have been having with alcohol and the legal trouble it has caused them, the counselor can state that coming to substance abuse treatment will assist them with preventing any future legal problems.

Once the counselor has briefly laid out the reason for making the referral they should give details about the SOFT model and include information on: what the client will do in the program, past experiences referring to the program, program duration and cost, and contact information (i.e., names, phone numbers, web links, etc.) on how to engage in the program.

The last component of giving recommendations is assessing for the client's readiness to use these services. One strategy frequently used in giving assessment feedback is to ask a scaling question about how ready the client is to use a particular service. Below is an example script on giving a referral, explaining some details and, assessing the client's motivation with a scaling question which is illustrated in the following dialogue:

COUNSELOR: *Because of the things we've mentioned before like you getting into repeated trouble with the law because of substance use and having lots of friends that use (tying referral back to concerns), I'm going to recommend that you attend our 8–10 week outpatient treatment program. In this program you'll come in once a week and meet with an individual counselor who will work with you on identifying and meeting your personal goals (details about program duration). You and your family will also be attending a group once a week with other families and talking about your progress and how your family can support you. I think this will be especially helpful to you as you mentioned that your family has been fighting and arguing almost every week. I'll also help you get set up, but first let me ask you a question: On a scale of 1 to 10 where 1 is not willing at all and 10 is completely willing, how willing are you to do this? (scaling question)*

TEEN: *A two. I'm not going. I don't think I need it at all.*

COUNSELOR: *It sounds like you are frustrated with this referral because you don't think*

you need treatment? (empathy) What would have to happen to you for you to think you need treatment? (open-ended question) For example, would you have to get another legal charge such as an OWI?

TEEN: *I'll go because my P.O. will make me, but I'm not going to like it.*

COUNSELOR: *It sounds like you're feeling some pressure to go to treatment. (empathy) Tell me more about that? (open-ended question)*

TEEN: *My P.O. told me I'd have to do whatever you recommended, and that pisses me off. He's always trying to find out things that are wrong with me and trying to "fix" me.*

COUNSELOR: *I'm really impressed with your honesty (positive feedback), because it is difficult to speak openly with people like me who can make decisions that affect you, and you're smart enough to realize I am in that position. I also want to let you know that even though you're feeling this pressure, you still have to make the decision to come to treatment. The cool thing is that when you're done with treatment you can take credit for your improvements. (supporting self-efficacy) I'm also impressed with your responsible attitude toward keeping your probation officer happy. (positive feedback) You seem willing to make sacrifices when you know they'll help you meet your overall goals. That's a great strength.*

TEEN: *Whatever. Just tell me what I have to do.*

Reviewing Confidentiality/Consents. We recommend explaining the parameters of confidentiality for the adolescent and obtaining appropriate signatures of consent before meeting with the adolescent's parent or guardian. Not only do we obtain the teen's consent to speak with their parents, we also collect appropriate written consents to referral destinations from the client. Clinicians who are not used to routinely including parents in adolescent drug treatment have voiced some discomfort and confusion about how much to talk to parents. We alleviate some of these concerns by orienting the teen and parent to the format of the sessions and confidentiality guidelines prior to completing the initial assessment. Thus, before attending the SORT session, the teen is aware that they have confidentiality rights and that they decide the extent to which parents have access to the assessment results. We reiterate our confidentiality rules during the SORT feedback session:

> OK. Next, I'm going to talk to your mom and pretty much talk about the same things I just shared with you. Before I do that, I want to let you know that as a teenager you have a legal right to confidentiality. Is there anything we discussed that you do not want me to share with your mom? I'll also need you to sign this form to give me permission to share the results of your assessment.

In our experience, clinicians with little experience including family members in the assessment process have been pleasantly surprised by the amount of information that teens are usually willing to share with their parents. From time to time, we point out to adolescents who want to limit information that such limitations may be confusing to their parents when we give treatment recommendations. For example, if a client is being referred to residential treatment and does not want us to share his daily use of cocaine for the past three months, his mother could possibly question our clinical judgment and the rationale for the referral. When situations like this arise we give as much detail to parents as permitted by the teen. We also communicate with the teen that we respect their desire for confidentiality, but we also inform the teen that their parent may be confused about the referrals we make. Due to state and federal laws and regulations, we have encountered situations in which we have been explicitly forbidden by the teen to discuss personal use and recommendations. In these situations, we discuss in detail with the teen what feedback we may provide to the parent and sometimes we are forced to use general language. We also discuss the benefits and possible consequences of disclosing assessment information to parents. One question we frequently use is: *How do you think your parents would react if they found out about this?* Balancing the teen's right to confidentiality with family inclusion is a pervasive issue in family-based treatment with adolescents.

Parent Segment

When discussing the adolescent's assessment results with parents or guardians, we follow the same basic progression as when talking with teens. We discuss some of the key differences in the brief sections that follow.

Scripted Introductions. We orient the parent to the session in a similar manner as we do the teen with one major difference. In addition to praising the parent for being in treatment, we remind them that they continue to have influence with their teens. We acknowledge this continuing influence as many parents believe that they do not have influence and we believe that teens thrive when they remain connected with their parents even during adolescence. Below is the scripted introduction we use with parents:

> We appreciate your coming in today to talk about your child. We feel that it is important to let you know that in many studies of teens that come to treatment for a variety of problems, having an involved parent or guardian is usually associated with greater success. In fact, most research shows that parents have a tremendous amount of influence on their teenage children, even though the teen may give you no indication that you are reaching them. Today we're going to review the assessment your child completed the other day. We want to focus on both the good things you and your child told us as well as some areas where your child may be having some trouble. This way we get the whole picture. Then we'll tell you what ideas our group came up with here that may be beneficial to your child. Remember, our attitude here is that you and your child are the expert on your child's life and these are only suggestions. We'll also ask you what you think will help you. Our meeting will take about 20 minutes and then all of us will meet together to make a decision about where to go from here. Do you have any questions?

Strengths Review. Strengths are reviewed in the same manner with the parents as with the teen. We recommend a couple strategies when discussing the client's strengths. First, we remind parents that the strengths being reviewed are based on the teenager's self-report, and that we need parental feedback so we can better understand the client. For example, we might say something like: *Johnny said one of his strengths was doing well at school. What do you think about that?* Second, during the strengths review with the parent, we find several opportunities to praise the parents for helping develop some of these strengths in their children. The counselor capitalizes on these opportunities for praising the parents, which helps them build rapport with parents. Reviewing strengths with parents also gets them to consider the teen's strengths which they may not have thought about in a while, especially if the teen has been struggling.

Discussion of Concerns. When discussing concerns with the parent, we present concerns in the same manner. What we may do differently with parents is talk about what services and remedies they have already tried. If they have given consequences for misbehaviors or indicate that they have addressed substance using behavior at home, we praise them for their efforts.

Giving Recommendations. When giving recommendations to parents we may add some discussion of our impression of the teen's receptivity to the recommendation—which is amazingly encouraging for many parents. We also assess their perception of the need for services just as we do with teens. Without the teen, we talk with parents about family resources for treatment including health insurance coverage and the fees for drug treatment.

Conjoint Segment

During the last portion of this session, the counselor meets with the teen and parent together. This segment is flexible and the major purpose is to paraphrase agreements and summarize key themes in the session (i.e., strengths, concerns, recommendations). In this segment, we try to reconcile discrepant information gathered from parents and teens. We end on a positive note by summarizing strengths and supporting decisions made during the session which then maximizes the impact of the session.

Techniques

In this section brief descriptions of techniques used to give assessment feedback are provided. Although these skills can be used in on-going therapy programs the examples here are tailored to the task of reviewing assessments and giving treatment recommendations.

Motivational Enhancement Techniques. The major techniques used from motivational enhancement when reviewing assessment results are: expressing empathy, using open-ended questions, challenging discrepant information, reflecting, and summarizing. Table 15.1 outlines the major techniques that are used

by giving a brief description of the skill, examples of proper and improper usage of each skill, and the purpose of using each skill. Research evaluations have confirmed that these types of skills are important components of motivational interviewing (Moyers, Martin, Manuel, Hendrickson, & Miller, 2005). An astute reader may notice that while the strengths-based feedback session uses these techniques, the session is goal-oriented with the explicit goal of giving recommendations. SORT therapists have the difficult task of conveying their professional opinions (i.e., treatment recommendations) using the *spirit* of motivational interviewing in a one hour session.

Solution-Focused Techniques. Solution-focused techniques used while giving strengths-based feedback on assessment findings include: coping questions, scaling questions, exception-finding questions, and giving praise. Table 15.2 summarizes these skills by giving a brief description of the skill, examples of correct and incorrect use, and the purpose of using the skill. More detailed examples of these skills and a flowchart of when they are appropriate exists elsewhere (Walter & Peller, 1992).

Other Techniques. Giving positive feedback is a skill that cuts across many different models of therapy. In giving assessment feedback, we do not limit ourselves to only commenting on client strengths by reviewing and elaborating on their self-endorsed strengths. Counselors are also to look for spontaneous ways to praise clients *throughout* the SORT session. These opportunities will arise naturally as the counselor uses active listening skills. Positive feedback takes many forms, ranging from brief *way to go* statements to rather elaborate behaviorally specific feedback. We define positive feedback broadly as any statement that compliments a client for a strength, effort, or trait, or reinforces positive behaviors.

STARTING THERAPY

Upon completion of the initial two-session placement assessment, called Strengths-Oriented Referral for Teens (SORT), families that engage in SOFT move into the treatment planning phase of therapy. The first three sessions of the actual SOFT program are outlined in the sections that follow.

TABLE 15.1 Motivational Interviewing Skills Used in Giving Feedback from Assessments

Skill Definitions	Purpose	Correct Example	Incorrect Use
Empathy: statements that convey understanding of the client's experience. Empathy statements involve tentatively labeling their experience.	Build rapport. Diffuse frustration.	"It seems like you're a little frustrated and wondering why everybody is making a big deal out of you being caught at a party."	"I understand you feel upset right now because getting caught at a party is no fun. I know because it happened to me once." (Assuming)
Open-Ended Questions: cannot be answered with a short answer (i.e., yes/no, factual answer).	Exploration. Goal definition.	"What would be the first sign you'd notice if marijuana use was becoming more of a problem for you?"	"Do you think you'll have problems in the future?" (Closed Question)
Reflecting: responses to client statements that demonstrate to the client that the therapist is listening to them.	Conveying understanding.	Client: "Pot is not a problem for me, but alcohol is messing me up." Therapist: "So, alcohol is the main reason you're here."	Therapist: "So, you currently think pot is not a problem for you even though your P.O. sent you?" (Confrontational)
Challenging Discrepancies: exploring discrepancies between two or more different client statements, objective behaviors, or desires. Therapist presents purpose to better understand client.	Eliciting change talk. Clarifying goals.	"I'm confused. On one hand you said you really want to do better in school, but on the other hand you go to school high. Tell me more about this?"	"Don't you think you'd do better in school if you quit using?" (Leading Closed-Ended, Conveying expert opinion)
Summarizing: Summarizing is reflection, but involves tying more than one concept together.	Wrapping up sessions. Transitioning to new themes.	"Today we talked about your strengths, concerns we have like your legal trouble and family situation, and we discussed some possible strategies to deal with these concerns."	"It seems to me that we've made some progress today." (Too general; does not review separate themes. Client perspective on progress also not elicited.)

TABLE 15.2 Solution-Focused Techniques Used in SORT

Skill Definitions	Correct Example	Incorrect Use	Use(s) in SORT
Coping Questions: ask clients how they have been managing even though they are experiencing tough times.	"You've had a lot going on lately with the death in your family, being on intensive probation, and dealing with depression. What *have you been doing* to keep yourself going through this difficult time?"	"You've had a lot going on lately with the death in your family, being on intensive probation, and dealing with depression. What keeps you going?" (Doesn't ask for specific actions.)	Elicit successful coping. Elicit strengths.
Scaling Questions: ask a client to rate something on a scale with defined endpoints.	"On a scale of 1–10, where 1 is not ready at all, and 10 is ready to roll, how ready are you to go follow up with this recommendation?"	"How ready are you to use this recommendation?" (Not specific; will likely elicit a vague reply)	Measuring progress. Exploring client perception.
Exception Finding Questions: ask clients when something was not so much of a problem.	"Can you tell me the last time when depression wasn't such a problem for you? (Alternative wording: was even a little bit less of a problem?)"	"How long have you been depressed?" (Not specific; focused on the problem.)	Elicit successful coping. Elicit examples of strengths to praise.

Session 1: Orientation and Start of Strengths and Resources Assessment

The purpose of this session is to orient the client to the SOFT model, build initial rapport, complete the SOFT contract, complete and process the *Immediate Concerns Checklist*, and (time permitting) begin the *Strengths and Resources Assessment*. Client orientation to SOFT is accomplished in one session through a number of short tasks. By the end of this session, each family will be have an even better understanding of the treatment they are receiving, address immediate concerns they have with the therapist, and begin the process of identifying their unique strengths.

Task 1: Introductions and welcoming the family. In the beginning of the first session the therapists introduce themselves, greet the family and give a brief overview of what the first session will be like. The therapist should summarize that the purpose of the session is to become familiar with one another, explain the SOFT program to the family, find out about any immediate concerns, and if time permits, begin a Strengths and Resources Assessment.

Task 2: Orientation and contracting. This task involves orientation to the SOFT model and ends once the family has heard an overview of the philosophy of SOFT, the program sessions and tasks, as well as the expectations of both the family and therapist. We provide an example script for the orientation to SOFT below:

> Now let me start telling you a little bit about Strengths-Oriented Family Therapy (SOFT) and what you can expect of me in our interactions over the coming weeks. The philosophy of SOFT is that your family has much strength and skills that will help you be able to develop and accomplish goals that will make your life better. That is, we want to make sure that you are the one making the plans for your future, with us here to provide guidance along the way. I'm not going to tell·you what to do, but I will help you set your goals and make detailed plans for achieving them. My job is to ask questions that are helpful to you in figuring that out.
>
> These are the actual things we are going to do over the next few weeks . . . [Describe the tasks (i.e., complete Strengths and Resources Assessment, Develop Solution Plan, Multifamily Groups, etc . . .]
>
> Now let's discuss the expectations you can have of me . . . and these are the expectations I have of you . . ."

Task 3: Address immediate concerns. The Immediate Concerns Checklist is a brief questionnaire intended to determine the immediate needs of the family that is just beginning treatment. An *immediate concern* is defined as any concern that is so pressing that the family wants immediate assistance with its resolution.

Although the main premise of this model is to focus on strengths right from the beginning, families are sometimes dealing with crises and beginning with a strengths assessment may be perceived as ignoring their serious and immediate concerns. The principle behind the use of *Immediate Concerns Checklist* is to briefly acknowledge the family's immediate concerns, document them for later solution planning, and gauge the family's perceptions of the concerns using scaling questions. That is, for each immediate concern, therapists ask a scaling question where the endpoints are *we can table this concern temporarily* and *this is life or death.* This process permits the therapist to prioritize concerns and empathize. Although some therapists may be uncomfortable with this delay in addressing problems, we contend that the use of the *Strengths and Resources Assessment* will be rapport building just as much as dealing with client *crises*. Once a therapist becomes comfortable with the process, they often find that it works well. If the family indicates that several of the problems do not require immediate attention, the therapist begins conducting the *Strengths and Resources Assessment*.

If the family has indicated that they are *immediately concerned* with something, the therapist gathers more detail by using coping and exception finding questions, and empathic listening. The therapist makes notes on the *Immediate Concerns Checklist* and assists the family in developing a triage plan with concrete activities that mirror what we describe below as *solution planning*. In future sessions the therapist revisits these concerns using the *Individual Solution Plan*. Once immediate concerns are addressed satisfactorily and an initial plan is developed, and if time permits, the therapist will begin with the family. Remember, even at this point it is critical to share the rationale underlying the treatment process with the client. That is, the client will benefit from receiving a brief rationale for why these activities are important in their treatment. They will appreciate the help and their inclusion in the planning process. We provide an example script for identifying immediate concerns:

> Next we'll go over the Immediate Concerns Checklist. It is intended to be a quick look at where you want *immediate help*. If you would like to speak about any of these concerns now, then we will spend some time talking about these in more detail. Otherwise, we'll proceed with the Strengths and Resources Assessment, which is designed to give us a better understanding of your strengths, so we can use these strengths to help us with solution planning.

Task 4: Begin Strengths and Resources Assessment (SRA). This structured assessment may take 1–2 hours to complete but the SRA represents one of the first major therapeutic interventions used in the SOFT model. Additionally, the SRA gives structure to rapport building that is essential for a solid working relationship and the SRA provides a positive focus for communication.

Definitions. For the purposes of this assessment, *strengths* will be defined as any positive behaviors or coping mechanisms, motivations, positively focused goals or desires, or internal resources the person describes. *Resources* are external sources of strength, including friends, relatives, social service agencies or community organizations. Therapists should review these definitions with the client prior to starting this activity.

Client-driven. We recommend that the client has final say in what is included as a strength or resource. We also recommend that the therapist not question whether or not something is, in reality, a strength or resource. The therapist may make a professional decision to recommend the inclusion of some strength or resource, but must confirm with the client about whether or not it is recorded. Ultimately the client makes the choices and decisions.

The Strengths and Resources Assessment Form. The specific strengths, skills and assets are categorized in nine separate life domains including: life skills, finance, leisure, relationships, living arrangement, occupational/educational, health, internal resources, and recovery. (See Table 15.3 for sample page of Strengths and Resources Assessment Form.) Each domain has several suggested strengths listed on the left-hand side of the page, with room for comments on the right. These suggested strengths and life domains were developed by adolescent counselors working with teens to ensure that they were developmentally appropriate. A comment section is used extensively to describe details of the client's strengths and successes in each life domain, which the therapists elicit by using open-ended questions.

During the assessment, most listed skills, assets, and strengths under each life domain should be covered. Specific skills which are not already listed under each life domain may be added on one of the *Other* lines. Specific details of client's strengths and successes relative to each topic should be recorded. Documentation may include examples, dates, special interests, and abilities. Using non-descriptive terms such as *yes* or *no* should be avoided.

Table 15.3
Sample Page of Strengths and Resources Assessment

LIFE DOMAINS	STRENGTHS-ORIENTED FAMILY THERAPY Strengths and Resources Assessment				
JOB—SCHOOL:	1 ----------- 2 --------- 3 --------- 4 --------- 5 ---------- 6 ----------7 ---------- 8 ----------9				
Occupation: (Full-time/ Part-time, Experience/Skills, Work Ethic/ Assets, Satisfaction)	doesn't hold job or go to school; expresses no or little interest in job or school;	seldom holds job or attends classes; vague plans for work or school;	sometimes holds a job or attends classes; plans for work or school goals with action;	holds regular job or attends classes; works toward goals;	holds regular job or attends classes; completed some job or school goals;
	(Teen)				
Education: (Years of School, Training, Progress Towards Goals, Sat- isfaction, Volunteer Activities)	(Parent)				
	(Family)				

Introducing the Strengths and Resources Assessment. Conducting the *Strengths and Resources Assessment* is an opportunity for the therapist to set the tone for the relationship. Up until this point, clients have typically spent most assessment sessions discussing their problems in-depth, and have likely held a dim view of the assessment process. In fact, they may have both animosity for the assessment process and a difficult time *not* talking about problems.

The therapist can introduce the *Strengths and Resources Assessment* to the client as *something different* and suggest that it may be a challenge. The therapist should then move on to say that instead of focusing on problems, this assessment will focus on what the client does well, both now and in the past. *The therapist tells the client that they are doing this so that the therapist can gain a deeper understanding about the client's strengths, which will assist them in helping the client plan their treatment goals so they can get what they want to get out of treatment.* Imparting this introduction to the assessment will help set the stage for the discussion of positive aspects of the client's life, and help put them at ease. The following Script highlights how to introduce someone to a Strengths and Resources Assessment:

> At this point, I'd like to introduce you to the SOFT Strengths and Resources Assessment. This assessment is probably a bit different from those that you might have encountered in the past. Instead of talking about problem areas that you may be facing, this assessment is focused on looking at the areas of your life in which you do well.

Describe the definitions for strengths and resources, and provide basic examples (i.e., refer to definitions above and feel free to put in simpler language).

> The first area that we are going to discuss is Life Skills. These include household activities such as cooking, cleaning, and taking care of yourself, interaction with society in general such as the TV or the internet or reading, and getting yourself places using public transportation, getting a driver's license and recruiting rides. Tell me about any of these things that you enjoy or do well.

If needed, you could use questions as *Follow-ups Probes:*

> Tell me about how you get places around town including school, your friends' homes and entertainment like movies? What do you do for yourself when you are going to go out and meet people?

If you have to use a closed-ended question, follow it up with an open-ended one: What do you like about *using public transportation? What are your favorite things to do on the internet?*

Techniques used during the Strengths Assessment. When moving into the assessment, each section should be presented in a general and open-ended format, allowing the client to initiate the flow of information. Presenting the life domain and asking the client open-ended questions allows the client to share with the therapist most easily. For example, the therapist may introduce each domain by saying something like: *Tell me about things that you do well in this area of your life.*

Remember, the client may not be accustomed to talking extensively about successes. Many strengths, skills, and assets have been underutilized or not been identified for most people. Also, many teens are not introspective and may have difficulty eliciting strengths. Younger teens may need many examples of what we consider to be strengths, because the word *strength* may be too abstract for their level of cognitive development. These occurrences should not be viewed as failures of the model, but rather as special situations where slight adaptations may be necessary to assist the client in completing the *Strengths and Resources Assessment.* That is, the counselor may need to be more directive in identifying strengths and ask the client for confirmation that they too do indeed perceive these as strengths.

As the client may also talk a lot about problems and difficulties, the therapist should refocus on when things did go well by using *exception finding questions.* For example, if the teen claims to have no strengths academically, the therapist might say: *Tell me about the last time when you were doing well at school? What were you doing differently then?* The goal is to identify past strategies that worked in the hopes of including them on the solution plan, which is the next treatment activity. If the client holds their ground and claims to have never done well in a particular domain, therapists slightly alter the question and ask: *Tell me about the last time things were even a little better in school than they are now?* If the client continues to maintain that things have always been awful in a particular domain, we recommend that the therapist not dwell on this. Instead, the therapist offers help in that area and briefly mentions that they would like to address this domain again when planning out goals. In thinking ahead to the solution plan, the therapist jots down client responses to exception finding questions, as client responses will naturally flow into possible activities to include on the solution plan. Solution-focused theorists claim that this is powerful because the family is both reinforced for past successes as well as actively suggesting treatment plan activities.

Again, we recommend that the therapist spend very little time, if any, on identifying or addressing past deficits or current problem areas. The therapist can write brief notes on the *Immediate Concerns Checklist* for later use during goal setting, but maintain a positive focus on the Strengths and Resources Assessment form itself. They may respond empathically when these situations arise, so that the client does not perceive the counselor as missing the boat. Nevertheless, counselors should only touch on these briefly and indicate to the client that while these areas will likely be addressed when goals are discussed, this assessment is about finding out their strengths.

The life domains do not necessarily need to be presented to the family in the order they are written. Rather, as the family talks about their various strengths, the therapist's role is to write out these strengths on paper. Skipping around between domains is permissible as long as the counselor maintains a conversational feel to the exercise. In other words, it would be a mistake to rush through this systematically for the sake of getting it done, but rather it should flow easily and be conversational. If the assessment is robotic or too structured, the client will not garner the full benefit of the activity, because they will pick up the tone of the therapist that it is just something to get done.

Therapists should generally focus on the recent past in the client's life when gathering information for the Strengths and Resources Assessment, though going back further may be necessary for some topics. For example, if the client has not had any positive experiences recently with a topic, ask them to think back to a time when they did well in that area. Also, information from these earlier periods can be included to *round out* the picture of the client's functioning. Dates should be provided when this earlier information is included.

Incorporating Parents. Parents and guardians can be flexibly integrated into the *Strengths and Resources Assessment.* The SOFT model places no mandate on whether or not the assessment must be initially completed in a conjoint session (i.e., with parents present) or in an individual session (i.e. having the parents integrated later). Sometimes starting with the adolescent alone is beneficial when family conflict is high or when parents are extremely frustrated with their teen's behaviors leading up to treatment. Frustrated parents may have a blaming style and only see the negative aspects of the teen's behavior and the presenting problem. Thus, one result of SOFT's *Strengths and Resources Assessment* is to reframe the teen's behaviors for the parent that lead to more productive interactions that are supportive of reduced drug use.

Completion. The Strengths and Resources Assessment should generally be completed within a couple of sessions to facilitate the timely development of a treatment plan. As the relationship between client and therapist progresses, the assessment may be reviewed as a tool in goal planning or to add new information. It is possible that the *Strengths and Resources Assessment* is not completed in the first session and you have to revisit it in the beginning of the second session.

Session 2: Completion of Strengths and Resources Assessment and Start of Solution Planning

Purpose. The purpose of this session is to continue reviewing the family's strengths in several life domains, continue praising them for things they are doing well, and begin solution planning based on questioning regarding what they would like to accomplish in treatment.

Goals. By the end of this session, the family will have completed the *Strengths and Resources Assessment,* and will have begun to develop the *Solution Plan.* They should have identified several family/personalized goals, including the identification of steps or activities that they believe will help them achieve these goals.

Session Task 1: Check-in, review last session, and orient family to the second session. In the beginning of this session, the therapist welcomes the family and begins by asking a variation of the pre-session change question such as: *What is working better for you since last week?* The purpose of this question is to communicate our belief that things are changing for the better all the time and to direct the client toward thinking positively. If the family says nothing has changed or actively describes how things are worse, the therapist will make note of these difficulties and use *exception-finding questions* and *coping questions* to direct the conversation back to strengths and resiliencies. The therapist will also then explain that they will be discussing strategies for dealing with these concerns after finishing the assessment. If they do tell the therapist about how things are better, it is important that the therapist follows up with a question about what the client has been doing differently to achieve these positive results. *This focuses attention on the client's role in bringing about this change.* The therapist highlights this, and may propose to the family that *hard-working* be added as a strength to the *Strengths and Resources Assessment.*

Task 2: Finishing the Strengths and Resources Assessment. If the *Strengths and Resources Assessment* was not completed during the first session, the first part of this session should be used to summarize what was already discussed on the *Strengths and Resources Assessment* and finish the life domains that were not completed in the first session. Upon completing the *Strengths and Resources Assessment* the therapist summarizes what the family has reported. That is, they briefly discuss the strengths that were mentioned and ask the family if they missed anything. The therapist then makes brief mention of the goals that the client has already mentioned for therapy either inadvertently through problem talk or something that was directly mentioned as a goal by the client.

Task 4. Begin Solution Planning. The *Family Goal Worksheet* (see Appendix), along with the handout on identifying goals, is given to the family prior to the solution planning process. Typically this task is given at the end of the first session as between session homework. To begin solution planning, the therapist should engage the family in a discussion of what goals the family would like to achieve over the next several weeks that they are in treatment as well as the long-term goals for the adolescent and family. Keep in mind that these are *the family's* goals, not the goals of the therapist. In keeping with the SOFT model, goals must be established from the family's perspective in order to have meaning for the family. Some useful questions for starting solution planning are: *When therapy has been successful for you and we've had our last session, what will you be doing differently?* and *If someone you know were to see you in a month and notice how well you were doing, what would that person see you doing?*

During solution planning, therapists alter the wording questions. For example the question above on how someone else would know the client is doing well can be modified to alternative vantage points including: of a fly on the wall, a CIA operative tapping the client's phone, or someone the client hasn't seen in a while. The same alterations can be done with the end-points of scales on scaling questions. For example, end points we've used have included *no way I'm doing this* to *jumping up and down and doing cartwheels*. Alternating the wording of these simple questions often injects humor into the process.

As the family begins to highlight goals, the therapist documents the basics of each goal in writing, assuming that they are *works in progress* to be more precisely defined over the course of the session, and then come back to each one in turn. Initially, the therapist may ask for some clarification as the client offers the goals, but is best off getting a list of things the client is interested in achieving before getting too involved in the details of any single goal. To draw out the client's ideas, use questions such as: *What else are you considering? What other things would you like to do for yourself? What things will you have accomplished in your sessions with me to know that this was a success? What other changes do you want to achieve in the next several weeks?*

Goals can be anything the client wants to work on, either short- or long-term. A goal might include something the client wishes to attain in the future, but does not wish to or cannot work on right now. Because these are the client's own goals, they do not necessarily have to be *realistic* to the therapist, though they do have to be legal and ethical. For example, a teenager may have long-term aspirations to be either a rock star or a professional athlete. Although the therapist may know that this goal will be difficult to accomplish in outpatient treatment, the therapist's role is to validate the goal and explore the steps necessary for accomplishment.

Adolescents vary in how much of a future orientation they have. Although our approach is largely centered on the *here and now*, the solution plan may contain little tasks that will inch the client closer to long-term goals. Goals can be revised or changed as family members or individuals work on attaining them. The adolescent client might realize that the goal he first established, to be a rock star, is a very long way off. He or she might revise the goal to something more attainable in the short-term, such as; to practice playing music four times a week for an hour or by November 31st to speak with a performer he or she admires in order to find out what it takes to achieve their level of success. This level of concreteness is always desired when setting goals.

Walter and Peller (1992) stated that well-defined goals are (1) in the client's language (2) worded in the positive, (3) outlines of the process to achieve them, (4) in the here and now, (5) as specific as positive, and (6) in the client's control. Table 15.4 summarizes these criteria with sample goals that either meet or do not meet these criteria. SOFT counselors review goals using these criteria in supervision.

SOFT therapists should work with clients to brainstorm solution ideas a creative and imaginative process. During initial solution planning, therapists do not need to evaluate the value or reality base of ideas. Questioning which generates lists of previously successful solutions,

Table 15.4
Examples of Well-Defined Goals

Criteria	Doesn't Meet Criteria	Meets Criteria
1. In client's language	"Meet all the requirements of probation by June 10."	"Get done with my P.O. by June 10th."
2. Worded positively	"Not use drugs or alcohol."	"Will continue doing activities that support a drug and alcohol free lifestyle."
3. In process form	"Will achieve lifelong abstinence."	"Will remain drug free until June 10th."
4. In the here and now	"I will avoid or learn to cope with high risk situations."	"I will drive my own car to any gathering where I feel that alcohol or drugs will be present, so I may leave if I feel I may use."
5. Specificity	"My probation officer will leave me alone."	"I will have done everything I can to get my P.O. to leave me alone."
6. In the client's control	"I'll just quit."	"I will be spending more time playing guitar and finding a job."

possible successful solutions, or even totally outrageous or unsuccessful solutions can increase engagement between therapist and client by initiating a creative process that is mingled with humor.

The Solution Plan. After the *Family Goals Worksheet* is completed, the therapist can then help the family develop more precisely defined goals, and determine whether any of these goals may need to be broken down into sub-goals before moving on with the *Solution Plan.* The goals should be worded positively, entailing the achievement of something, rather than the stopping of some behavior, or *getting rid* of something. For example, if the family lists *using drugs less* as a goal, the therapist should help the family reword this goal to entail the actions that are involved in meeting that goal. This rewording can be accomplished by saying something like: *What will you be doing* instead *when you are using drugs less?* We have found it counterproductive to work toward a goal of not doing something. Goals should describe something the family wishes to attain, something to be achieved in the future. Additionally, goals should be time limited, rather than ongoing. A useful solution focused question that can be used to put a time limit on goals is: *As you leave here today, what little part of this goal can you work on today?* Ongoing goals may be converted to time limited ones for this process.

Documentation of goals on the *Solution Plan* is the next step in the treatment process (see Table 15.5). This worksheet will help the family organize the activities they must perform to accomplish each of his goals. By creating this activity plan, the family should be able to see the whole picture, keep track of what activities have been accomplished, what the schedule is for each activity, and what is left to do before the goal is achieved. Remember, this *Solution Planning*

Table 15.5:   SOFT Solution Plan

Date _____

Name _____

Client Number _____

SOFT Therapist

Goal _____

LD _____

#	Activity	Person Respon- sible	Identi- fied Date	Review Date	Target Date	Review Date	Out- come Code	Comments
___	_____	_____	_____	_____	_____	_____	_____	_____
___	_____	_____	_____	_____	_____	_____	_____	_____
___	_____	_____	_____	_____	_____	_____	_____	_____
___	_____	_____	_____	_____	_____	_____	_____	_____
___	_____	_____	_____	_____	_____	_____	_____	_____

Outcomes Codes: C - Completed   R - Revised   NC - Not Completed

_____   _____   _____   _____
Client   Date   SOFT Therapist   Date

512

process is to assist the family, and this completion of this form should not be an impediment to the family in attaining goals. Assist the family as needed. If the form presents complications, the therapist can complete it and enter information on it. The therapist would want to talk about and explain the elements, or sections, of the form to the family. These sections are integral to the process of *Solution Planning*. Who physically completes the form is not as important.

Goals. Goals which the family wishes to work on should be transferred from the Family Goal worksheet to an Individual Solution Plan worksheet. The life domain that the goal is derived from should be indicated at the top of the Individual Solution Plan worksheet.

Activities. Next, the therapist will help the family to operationalize goals. Operationalizing a goal means breaking it down into small, achievable pieces, that we will call activities. When operationalizing each goal, the therapist should keep in mind the following questions: *What are all of the smaller* activities *that need to be completed in order to achieve this goal? How will the client go about completing each of these activities? What is the first step? Who will the client need to contact? When will the client work on each activity? How long will each activity take?* Think of all the details that may need to be covered.

Example Activities

- Decide on type of employment to be done.
- Read employment section of newspaper each day.
- Interview for three jobs per week until hired.

The aim is to have the family take ownership of goals and activities, and become invested in completing them. To that end, if the family is put in charge of figuring out how to accomplish these things through a series of questions, they should become much more invested than if the therapist were to make the plans for them. The SOFT model incorporates solution-focused questioning techniques to encourage the client to work through the problem solving process on their own, with the therapist orchestrating the discussion. *What do you think is the first thing you'll need to do to work on this goal? What else? What is the next thing? How will you do that? Who will you need to contact in order to complete that activity? When do you want to start this? How long do you think that will take? When do you want to have this done?* Thus, the therapist becomes the catalyst of the goal planning process, rather than being the problem solver.

When evaluating the proposed solutions each solution is rated on a scale of 0 to 5, with 0 representing no chance of success, 1 representing a slight chance of success, 3 representing a moderate chance of success, and 5 representing a high chance of success. This approach enables the therapist-client team to eliminate all but realistic solutions. Involving parents or referral sources in the solution rating process may be important in determining likelihood of success, because the teen has a sounding board for the feasibility of their ideas. Questions such as "*What do you think your mom's rating would be?*" may prove helpful.

Evaluating movement toward goals is essential to therapists and clients staying on track. Using the 0-to-5 rating scale to evaluate confidence, satisfaction, and progress may prove helpful. Therapists should acknowledge the hard work clients do and the positive direction of movement. Treating any failure as simply a *setback* to be overcome is also important. The therapist plays an essential role in this problem-solving process by expecting success and highlighting successes, however small, throughout the process.

The amount of detail required will vary by client, and the therapist should make a clinical judgment about how much detail to discuss and to write down on the Solution Plan. The client family's abilities to articulate specific activities will be evident to the therapist, and some modifications may need to be made for particular adolescents. Younger adolescents may not be able to clearly articulate steps to solve their problems and may need a more directive approach from their counselor. That is, instead of asking the client what they need to do differently to solve the problem, they may have to be more suggestive and say something like: *Many clients that have had similar problems have found that doing _____ is helpful. What do you think about trying that?* In this way, the therapist still has agreement and collaboration from the teen, but is more directive in goal planning.

In our experience, one pitfall of using this model with teens is that some teens will have difficulty setting concrete goals, or may oversimplify what they have to do to achieve their goals. We find this especially true of clients that are pressured into treatment by probation or another source and have few personal reasons for wanting to be in treatment. Consider the following dialogue between a therapist and a client when they attempt to set goals:

THERAPIST: *Today, I'd like to get a sense of what kinds of things you'd like to work on here and make some specific plans for how you will achieve your goals. When you leave here successfully and treatment has been successful, what will you be doing differently?*

CLIENT: *My probation officer wants me to quit using drugs.*

THERAPIST: *What can you differently to stop using drugs?*

CLIENT: *I don't know. I'll just stop.*

THERAPIST: *But how, specifically will you do this?*

CLIENT: *I just won't use drugs.*

THERAPIST: *What will you be doing instead of using drugs?*

CLIENT: *Nothing. I'll just stop. I can quit anytime.*

In the dialogue above the client is holding their ground that they do not have to do anything differently in order to stop using. For clients like this one, we have found that stopping drug use is actually not their goal. A more accurate goal for this client is likely to be that they want to get off of probation, but do not necessarily want to stop using drugs. In the following dialogue, more attention is paid to the client's cues leading to a more accurate goal definition.

CLIENT: *My probation officer wants me to quit using drugs.*

THERAPIST: *It sounds like the main reason that you want to quit using drugs is to please your probation officer, but you're not so sure that you want to quit. (Empathy)*

CLIENT: *Yeah. I don't really think I need treatment to quit using drugs and alcohol. I'm just here because I have to be here.*

THERAPIST: *Nobody likes to be forced into counseling, but I'm impressed that you're here even though you don't want to be. A less responsible kid would just blow this off. Since you don't want to quit using drugs, would you like to work on getting off of probation?*

Another approach that is useful with younger or resistant teens is explaining the rationale of setting clear goals and activities. The key purpose of this is reminding the teen that in this model they have a lot of say over what they will work on in treatment and that the process is important because it will give them a framework for thinking about all problems, not just the ones they are bringing to treatment with them now.

So, what are the key principles to remember when completing the Solution Plan with your clients?

Person Responsible. We emphasize the importance of naming those persons who should be accountable for the accomplishment of the activity. The Person Responsible for each Activity is generally the family or client. If it is not a family goal, the individual person responsible should be named. However, the therapist or another person or organization that is assisting the client achieve an Activity may be listed here.

Dates. The setting of dates in relation to activities is an *important* part of the Individual Solution Plan process. Dates serve both to remind clients of the Activities they need to complete and as a review mechanism for the therapist. Each of the five dates listed below are critical, and the reasoning behind them is explained in the following paragraphs.

1. *Identified Date:* date the Activity is identified by the family and therapist.
2. *First Review Date:* date on which the therapist will contact the family to review progress towards completion of the Activity.
3. *Target Date:* date by which it is planned that the Activity will be completed.
4. *Second Review Date:* date on which the therapist will contact the client to review completion of the Activity.
5. *Terminated Date:* date on which the Activity is no longer being worked on between the family and therapist. At this point the Activity has either been completed, revised, or not completed. This provides more clarity and matches the table.

Identified Date. Indicate the date that the activity is written on the Individual Solution Plan in the Identified Date column. This date indicates how much planning is involved from the beginning of the process, and what activities were added later due to some further planning or discovery from completed activities. As activities are added to the Solution Plan, the dates are indicated in this column.

Target Date. Enter the Target Date for the activity to be completed in this column. The target date sets a realistic completion date for the activity that is negotiated between the client and therapist. In some cases, for the therapist and client, it may not be possible to identify an absolute target (completion) date for some Activity. For instance, the completion of the Activity may be based on information which is going to be obtained in the course of completing other Activities. In these cases, the therapist may leave the date open pending completion of the other Activity.

Target dates should not be based on an artificial construct, such as seeing clients once a week. Target dates should be set based on how long it should realistically take to complete an activity.

Review Dates. Enter the Review Dates *AFTER* the review has been completed. Review dates are particularly important for both the family and therapist. The Review Date prompts the therapist to contact the family to *remind* them about goals and activities, help them monitor progress towards them, and identify barriers that have arisen relative to completion of an activity. This date often may serve as the added impetus to actually complete the activity.

Termination Date. Enter the date that the activity was completed, revised, or eliminated in the Terminated Date column. At the same time, indicate the Outcome Code for the activity. Activities that are revised should be terminated, and then re-written on the Individual Solution Plan with a new set of dates. If this activity was a prerequisite for other activities on the Individual Solution Plan, at this time the target date for those activities should be set, and this process continued.

The use of specific dates at every point (identification, target, review and termination) is intended to structure and prompt a client's organization of those Activities which lead him toward the completion of Goals. Terms such as *on-going, weekly,* etc. defeat this structure and organization and should never be used. These terms imply the need to not review Activities. This approach can lead to stagnation and lack of initiative because the client cannot see any progress and completion of goals. Instead, such goals and activities should be converted into time limited goals for the purpose of the Solution Planning process.

If a client has (1) gone through several cycles of successful accomplishment of a Goal, and (2) seems to have thoroughly integrated the Activities associated with this Goal, then it might not be necessary to continually repeat the Goal, at least in a formal case management setting. This is what we want! The client/family is now completing goals on their own through use of the Individual Solution Planning process.

Example Timeline

The following timeline should put the discussion of dates in some visual perspective. Target dates should be determined at the same time an Activity is Identified (||). The First Review

Date (*) should be completed a day or two before the Target Date. The Second Review (**) should be completed on the same day as the Target Date or within one day following that date.

Changes to Goals and Activities

Goals and activities can be changed at any time. People change and so do their goals. When the client's goals change, or when things do not go quite as planned, the therapist should work with him to modify the plan to work around the change. We do not see failure, only feedback. If something is not working, try something different. Remember to indicate the appropriate dates when activities are revised or eliminated.

Outcome Codes. Outcome codes are useful in monitoring the progress of activities. If an activity is completed, we write in the code *C* and we can move on to other business with the client. If the activity has been revised, we write in the code *R*. An activity could be revised when new information comes to the client's or your attention, or if the situation changes. If an Activity is not completed by the target date—we write in the code, *NC*.

Changes to goals and activities. Goals and activities can be changed at any time. People change and so do their goals. When the client's goals change, or when things do not go quite as planned, the therapist should help the client modify the plan to work around the change. We continually tell the client that the SOFT model does not include failure, only feedback. If a particular solution is not working, try something different. Remember to indicate the appropriate dates when activities are revised or eliminated.

Managing family dynamics. The therapist must rely on family therapy techniques in determining whose goal is being articulated during solution planning. Because the *Solution Plan* is being made in the context of family therapy, it is important to assess the willingness of the teen and other family members to work on the goals that are being discussed. If disagreements arise about the goals that should be the focus of treatment, the therapist needs to actively intervene between the parents and the teen by identifying other points of view and negotiating a solution. Reframing the disagreements with a positive spin often eases the tension between parents and their adolescents.

For example, a father suggests that he would like to see the teenage client "be a leader more than a follower." In this situation, the therapist will first have to clarify the meaning of this statement by using solution focused questioning: "What will he be doing differently when he is a leader and not a follower?" Then, the therapist will have to elicit the teen's view of this goal by saying something like: "What do you think of the goal your father has for you?" These subtle opportunities point out to the teen the positive motivation of the parent for the teen's success. While many teens see their parents' actions as hindering their freedom and autonomy, we often remind the teen that the motivation of their parents for such actions is usually driven out of care. For example, the therapist might say, "Did you know your dad cared about you so much that he did not want to see you following other kids?" Restating the treatment goals of a parent with a twist can enhance the positive feelings in sessions that are also cultivated by focusing on positive goals and strengths. Solution planning is a structured activity during which many directive family therapy techniques are used.

Sessions 3–4: Monitoring Solutions and Providing Case Management

Purpose. The purpose of sessions three and four is to provide ongoing support, structure, and feedback to assist families in completing their goals, and to provide families with ongoing skills training through the SOFT Multifamily Group meetings. Clinicians should also be looking at environmental interventions and case management strategies whenever they are appropriate. These techniques are appropriate when altering the client's environment will promote success in treatment, or when reducing or eliminating barriers to treatment attendance and future success.

Task 1: Reviewing goals. Therapists continue to use solution-focused language to address goals on client's solution plans. Much like the second session of the intervention, the third and fourth sessions will open with a question about what positive changes have occurred since the last meeting. Sessions proceed as task-oriented and focus on progress on current goals and identifying new goals.

Task 2: Case management activities. Adolescents frequently benefit from ecological interventions that enhance their possibilities for success. Case management activities are often appropriate, especially when adolescent clients are involved with multiple systems (i.e., criminal justice, child welfare, school disciplinary proceedings) or face significant treatment barriers. Below are some examples of common case management tasks used with adolescents in the SOFT approach. This list is by no means exhaustive, as therapists frequently do many creative environmental interventions. The list of common activities is followed by a case vignette illustrating the creative use of a home visit.

Example Case Management Activities

1. Initiating a meeting with school administrators regarding placing a client in an alternative school.
2. Making a court appearance to focus on achievements of a client in treatment.
3. Making a home visit with clients that do not have telephones and have missed appointments.
4. Traveling to detention to meet with a client that has been placed to discuss residential placement and transitioning back into aftercare services.
5. Driving around town to assist clients in completing job applications.
6. Assisting a parent in obtaining an involuntary commitment for a child that is possibly a danger to him or her self or others due to substance abuse.
7. Writing a "personal" letter of reference for a client that has limited references available.
8. Following up with other referral sources on the client's progress and attendance in their services.
9. Facilitating a referral to another provider to address medication or specialized assessment needs.

Case Management Vignette

Alex was a 16 year old client that began missing office visits. His father worked odd hours at a local factory and was frequently difficult to reach, as the family had no phone. The SOFT therapist drove to the client's mobile home and initiated an informal session with the client and his dad, who were at home playing cards. The therapist was invited by the family to join the card game, and during this informal "session" was able to build much rapport with the client and also engage the father and son into a meaningful discussion of how things were going recently. The client and his father set an appointment and discussed treatment expectations in their home environment and subsequently began a pattern of more regular treatment attendance. The therapist in addition to this visit had frequent contact with the client's probation officer to inform him of the client's progress, which also aided in retaining the client in treatment.

Session 5: Family Relapse Prevention Planning

Purpose. The overall purpose of this session is to begin the process of terminating the family's treatment by formally acknowledging their completion of primary treatment. At this point in treatment, the family will have completed ten multifamily group sessions and four two-hour family sessions. In this session, the progress since last session is reviewed, the Solution Plan is reviewed, a family relapse prevention plan is made, continuing care plans are discussed, and a booster session is scheduled.

Task 1: Check-in. The therapist opens the session in typical fashion by reviewing what progress has been made since the last session. Questions that presume positive changes have occurred are used.

Task 2: Review Solution Plan. The last session of primary treatment is used to review the Solution Plan for a final time. The therapist documents the completion status of various goals. The emphasis of the final review is on praising client accomplishments in a genuine manner that promotes the family's sense of achievement.

Task 3: Create family relapse prevention plan. The last major treatment activity in primary treatment is the creation of a family relapse prevention plan (see Table 15.6), which we modified from the Family Support Network treatment (Hamilton et al., 2001). Much like the Solution Plan, the family relapse prevention plan outlines specific actions that will be taken by each family member to prevent a relapse.

Our modifications to Hamilton and colleagues' (2001) plan highlight our dedication to solution-focused language in two key ways. First, most activities on the relapse prevention plan are natural extensions of the solution plan. Thus, we emphasize to them that they are continuing

Table 15.6
SOFT Family Relapse Prevention Plan

> **Instructions:** The entire family can take an active role in helping prevent future substance use. We ask that each of you commit to continuing to work on the tasks you identified in treatment. Use the worksheet below for documenting these commitments.

Commitments	
Communication: "I will *continue to* improve my communication by doing…"	Teen: Parent(s):
Improving Trust: "I agree *to continue* to improve trust and be more trustworthy by doing…"	Teen: Parent(s):
Positive Activities: "I will *continue doing*… , which are positive activities for me."	Teen: Parent(s):
Concerns on Warning Signs: "I will listen to concerns from all family members by…"	Teen: Parent(s):
If the family has a concern "I agree to …"	Teen: Parent(s):
Continuing Support: "I agree to ….as a means of continued support ."	Teen: Parent(s):

_____   _____   _____   _____
Client Signature   Date   Therapist Signature   Date

_____   _____
Parent Signature   Date

what they already started as well as reiterate that these are activities they identified as their own medicine. Second, unlike more traditional substance abuse programs that directly refer to 12-Step based support groups as standard practice, we allow the family to determine their own appropriate aftercare activities as part of mutual goal development. Thus, our modifications to the relapse prevention plan included making this more apparent by eliminating specific reference to support groups.

Several themes addressed during family treatment are reassessed and commitments are secured from each family member to continue to use the communication skills used during treatment. Specifically, the family relapse prevention plan addresses specific actions that will be taken in several areas, including: maintaining trust in each other, communicating, using fair fighting strategies, identifying warning signs that the client may again use substances, identifying a plan the teen will implement if family members raise concerns, and identifying other supports that may be beneficial to maintaining progress. The therapist and family complete the relapse prevention plan together and a copy is given to the family to take with them. In this relapse prevention approach, adolescents are often encouraged by the fact that their parents are asked to make commitments to change in ways that are supportive of the adolescent's goals.

Task 4: Discuss need for continuing care. After the family relapse prevention plan has been completed, the therapist transitions to a discussion of continuing care options. For youth that have struggled with goals or had difficulty maintaining abstinence during the program, we frequently recommend on-going contact in a structured continuing care program which can include several options. For substance dependent adolescents, we may encourage attendance at self help meetings either in the community or sponsored by the drug treatment agency. We recommend formal continuing care treatment services (i.e., continuing care groups) for adolescents who are diagnosed with a more chronic substance abuse problem. Since the SOFT model does not assume all adolescents have a chronic substance use disorder (i.e., dependence or addiction), we consider many options for follow up care (e.g., sports programs, church, etc.) and for some clients may not need continuing care at all.

Task 5: Schedule booster session. A booster session is scheduled with the family, which occurs approximately one month after their primary treatment services have ended. Although additional contact will be made with the family, a certificate is given to the family to recognize their accomplishments and acknowledging that their primary treatment services have been successfully completed.

Session 6: One Month Post-Treatment Booster

Purpose. The purpose of the booster session is to monitor the family's progress since termination of primary treatment services. The main tasks include checking in with the teen and family and completing a brief review of the Family Relapse Prevention Plan.

Task 1: Checking in. The session opens by asking the family what is better since the last time they met with the therapist. Therapists follow this opening question with additional questions on what actions the family has taken to create these reported improvements. If the family has committed to the monthly continuing care group, the therapist inquires about their attendance and elicits feedback on how the group is going. If the family has not committed to this group and the therapist has recommended continuing care, the therapist reintroduces this option. However, therapists are sensitive to the families' preferred format of continuing care. That is, for some youth, formal continuing care groups may not be the best method for maintaining on-going support if clients are actively engaged with informal supports (i.e., sports participation, church groups).

Task 2: Review Family Relapse Prevention Plan. The Family Relapse Prevention Plan is reviewed by the therapist. Particular emphasis is on ways in which the plan has been successfully implemented. When the plan is working well, general praise is given to the family and each family member is praised for their role in continued work toward their initial goals. An example of general praise would be when the therapist might say: "I'm really proud of you for keeping up with this plan. Unfortunately, many adolescents begin using substances again after treatment, but you are doing all the right things to keep that from happening." For example, the therapist may give specific praise:

> Remember how difficult it was for you to introduce your parents to your friends at the beginning of treatment? Currently, your parents know all your friends and have said this is why they trust you so much more. You have gone up from a three on the trust scale to a nine on the trust scale. I commend you for your part in making things better for your whole family.

When plans are going well and adolescents remain on course for meeting their goals or maintaining achieved goals the primary purpose of this session is to provide encouragement and brainstorm any potential bumps in the road that may occur.

Sometimes families report increased problems during the booster session, and raise serious concerns. The most common problems typically reported are additional legal charges or continued substance use. If adolescents have continued to use drugs, the therapist will assess if continued abstinence is still a goal of the adolescent and family. Therapists may express concern for the adolescent and may give examples of what may happen if the adolescent continues using, but ultimately they remind the client that it is their responsibility to determine their own goal. If remaining substance free is a client goal, then the therapist revisits the successful coping strategies used during treatment when the client was completely or mostly substance free. Praise for previous successes is paramount to encouraging them to continue their work on this goal. Some review of the antecedents of substance use may be necessary to determine what additional goals should be addressed through continued contact with the therapist. More family sessions are encouraged if the adolescent and family feel they need additional support.

Task 3: Termination or engagement. For families that are stable and reporting continued success, the end of the booster session is a final opportunity for the therapist to summarize accomplishments. In keeping with SOFT's solution-focused roots, emphasis is on reiterating that their actions during treatment lead to the change. Families are also told that they may experience previous problems such as continued substance use or increased family fighting. Families are instructed to monitor whether they are still using the coping skills that were learned or revisited during treatment. They are also given instructions on how to reengage in treatment if they feel that problems are too much for them to handle as a family. The therapist ends the session on an inspirational note by saying, for example: "I'm so pleased that you met all your goals during treatment. It is so nice to see families that have been so successful in treatment. I have really enjoyed working with all of you."

For families that are continuing to struggle, the end of this booster session involves obtaining consensus about what plan should be implemented. After the family's current goals have been clarified, options for continuing care are discussed. In spite of the family's reported difficulties, the therapist remains upbeat and recognizes the achievements that have been made in treatment. The therapist points out these accomplishments to underscore the point that treatment has been successful in some ways, but other goals are still in progress or are no longer important family goals.

SOFT Multifamily Group Sessions

In addition to the six conjoint family sessions, families attend ten weekly multifamily group sessions. Clients usually begin group after their initial session as described in the previous section. Groups are two hours in duration, and are scheduled during the evening to accommodate work and school schedules. The SOFT multifamily group curriculum focuses primarily on family communication skills training, but also includes common skills training techniques (i.e., refusal skills, anger management, problem solving) also found in other interventions for adolescent substance abusers (Sampl & Kadden, 2001). What distinguishes SOFT from other skills training approaches, however, is that family members are involved in these interactive skills trainings groups. We now include detailed descriptions of the multifamily group sessions.

Multifamily Group Topics

The main topics for the group are: (1) Giving and Receiving Positive Feedback; (2) Assertive Listening; (3) Giving and Receiving Constructive Criticism: (4) Coping with Using Peers; (5) Problem Solving; (6) Family Problem Solving; (7) Health Relationships and Fair Fighting; (8) Stress Management; (9) Anger Management; and (10) Preventing Future Use.

Guidelines for Group Management

Several group therapy skills are needed to run successful SOFT multifamily groups. Although an in-depth discussion of group therapy skills is outside the scope of this chapter, we briefly discuss methods for monitoring group and family dynamics, and balancing when to stay on task versus flexibly addressing issues that may arise.

Group and family dynamics. Therapists need to monitor both group and family dynamics during multifamily groups. Specifically, directive approaches are needed to intervene when (a) parents are skeptical about progress or (b) adolescents or parents are badmouthing each other in group sessions. That is, group should never be used as a platform for family dyads to criticize each other. Group leaders address this early when reviewing group rules such as "refraining from put downs." Despite our best efforts, however, occasionally family members will make disparaging comments to each other or to other group members. When this occurs counselors should remind group members of the group rules and the role of group in family treatment (i.e., to improve family communication by focusing on solutions). At times, therapists may need to address such incidents during family sessions and underscore the need for everyone in group to feel safe.

The SOFT multifamily groups often include role-playing activities where family members are learning (or revisiting) skills. During role-plays, the therapist should monitor the tone of the role-play and praise efforts to bend toward the other's point of view. Such flexibility is difficult among conflicted family dyads when entering treatment and this is clearly a sign of progress. Another useful technique in role-plays is to have the teens role-play with other adults in the group besides their parents. Mixed family role-plays are useful for (a) preventing highly conflicted families from reenacting ineffective communication patterns, and (b) fostering rapport among group members.

Responsiveness to family concerns. SOFT multifamily groups are highly structured and include check-ins by each group member, a brief skills lecture outlining the rationale for the skill in substance abuse treatment, in vivo practice of the skills presented, and weekly homework assignments. Therapists should master the skills lecture materials and activities for each session so they may seamlessly stay on task and address group dynamics within the structure of the sessions. This approach ensures that core concepts are covered with all families receiving SOFT.

Nevertheless, one reality of conducting group treatment is that clinicians often have difficulty proceeding when families talk about issues that they want to discuss instead of proceeding with the group curriculum. SOFT is responsive to client requests to talk about problems in group, which usually occurs during the check-in period at the beginning of group. For example, one family may want to discuss an adolescent's recent use with the group to obtain peer feedback on what to do. Group therapy skills such normalizing the experience for families, obtaining peer feedback and support, and focusing on how the group can help with such problems are all proposed curative factors of group therapy and should be used during check-in periods (Yalom & Leszcz, 2005). Spending some time addressing such relevant issues adds to the credibility of the SOFT multifamily group. When addressing these concerns in group, however, the therapist must maintain their solution-focused orientation and return to things that can be done to address such problems. Therapists will also relate issues brought up by families to past or future group content to reinforce the value of the group activities in solution finding.

Check-ins. At the beginning of group, all group members are asked to give a brief progress report to the group on how they are doing that week. Both parents and adolescents respond to a set of standard questions about: their efforts to stay drug free, positive changes made during the week, goals, successful handling of high risk situations, and efforts to use the skills training activities outside of the group. During the check-in the therapist remains attuned to anything that may be followed up on with solution-focused language for the purposes of identifying current successful coping, give clients credit for changes made, and refining or identifying the client's goals.

Skills lectures. Each week an interactive lecture on each skill is given prior to starting role play practice exercises. During these mini-lectures the therapist presents the rationale for the activity and frames its importance within the context of family-based treatment for adolescent substance abuse. The therapist also demonstrates (i.e., modeling) the skill or skills for this lesson and, following the demonstration, the therapist asks the families for positive feedback: *So, what did you like about the approach I just used?* Reinforcing the modeled behavior is one strong intervention which helps many families learn the skills efficiently.

Practice exercises and homework assignments. Upon completion of the interactive lectures, each family is given an opportunity to practice the skills within the group and with the therapist present for guidance and troubleshooting. As mentioned previously, the therapist's role during these role plays is to ensure that a positive tone and appropriate *real life* examples are used during the role play activities. Homework, usually involving practice of the skills at home in between groups, is assigned and discussed during the next week's check-in.

Group evaluation. Participants complete a group evaluation form that assists the therapist with identifying any concepts that were unclear, the participants' ratings of how useful sessions were, and suggestions for improvement of the group.

What follows are step-by-step instructions for conducting the ten multifamily group sessions:

SOFT Multifamily Group Session 1: Giving and Receiving Positive Feedback

Welcome families/check-ins. New group members should be introduced to the group by the facilitator, who will provide a brief overview of the topics to be covered and group rules. As the group progresses, we recommend enlisting family members that have been in group a while to help with orientation by describing group activities and how they have personally benefited from the group. For example, the therapist may ask for a volunteer by saying, "Can I get a volunteer to explain what types of activities we do in group and how they have been helpful to you so far?" Upon welcoming families, the therapist passes out the check-in sheet and has clients review the check-in questions. Each member is asked to report on each question. If a group member raises an immediate concern, the therapist may address it at this time.

Provide rationale for session topic. Family communication is often interrupted when adolescents are using drugs. Rekindling relationships is hard work, but giving each other well-deserved positive feedback can often help. Below are some key points that therapists address as a rationale for the session topic:

- Parents often feel like the adolescent does not appreciate them.
- Adolescents may feel like parents only focus on negative behaviors.
- Praise is something we have control over and can increase. Thus, we can increase positive feelings among family members during treatment, which is a stressful time.

In addition to making these points, ask the group to list all the reasons they think it is important to discuss giving family members positive feedback as a session topic in substance abuse treatment.

Skills lecture talking points. In these sessions, we will focus on three types of positive feedback including: behavioral, personal or relationship. Behavioral feedback is praise that is based on a person's action (e.g., You did a good job paying attention in class today.). Personal feedback is praise based on something specific about the person (e.g., I really like the shirt you are wearing today.). Relationship feedback is praise based on a relationship with you or others (e.g., I really like working with you or I liked the way you and your brother completed that task together).

Giving and receiving positive feedback is not always as easy as it sounds. If we tell somebody something positive about himself or herself, we might feel embarrassed. When someone tells us something positive about ourselves, it might be even more embarrassing, or we might feel like we don't deserve it.

Tips for giving positive feedback. Here are some key tips for families to consider when giving positive feedback.

1. *Be sincere.* Being honest will make it easier for the person to accept what you are saying.
2. *Watch your body language.* If you are saying that someone made a good dinner, your behavior and face should say the same thing. If you make a face or look away while you are giving feedback, it will appear less sincere.
3. *Use feeling words.* Don't try to give an explanation for the wonderful things someone did. Tell them, "I liked your help, I'm glad you're here!"
4. *Choose the right time and place.* Make sure the person you are talking to is able to listen to you. Don't give feedback when a person is too busy to listen to what you are saying.

Tips for receiving positive feedback. Here are some key tips for families to consider when receiving positive feedback.

1. *Acknowledge that you heard it.* If you say nothing, the other person won't know if you are ignoring him/her or if you just did not hear. A good way to acknowledge positive feedback is to say, "Thank you."
2. *Don't disagree.* Even if you feel that you don't deserve the compliment, don't argue. When you disagree, you invalidate what he/she just said. A compliment is another person's opinion and it deserves to be respected.
3. *Don't put yourself down.* If someone says, "You look good in that dress," don't say, "Yeah but I wish I was thinner." The other person is trying to be positive, so don't change the mood.

Therapists demonstrate some of these behaviors by asking for a volunteer to either give them positive feedback or receive positive feedback from them. In addition to these points, family members are asked to brainstorm other techniques they have used in the past to give or receive compliments.

Practice exercises. In group, each parent-child pair will practice both giving and receiving positive feedback from each other stemming from real family situations. They practice giving each type of feedback (i.e., behavioral, personal, relationship). The recipient is asked to track whether or not the feedback appeared genuine based on three ways to define behavior (i.e., what we see or hear) known as the *three V's:*

- Visual-what you are observing while it's being said
- Vocal-how it is being said
- Verbal-what is being said

Therapists circulate during this activity and listen to each dyad. Upon completion of the activity the therapist leads a large group discussion about how the activity went. Group members are asked to give examples of feedback they gave to other family members, and therapists praise correct uses of positive feedback. Therapists also ask group members how receiving the feedback felt.

Explain homework assignment. The homework assignment is to give positive feedback to your parent or teen at least once per day over the next week. Therapists indicate that they will monitor progress on this assignment at the next group session during check-ins.

Session evaluation and adjournment. The last activity of the group is evaluating the group. Participants are asked a series of questions: (1) What did you like about today's session; (2) What did you find least helpful about today's session; and (3) What suggestions do you have for future sessions to make them better meet your needs?

SOFT Multifamily Group Session 2: Assertive Listening

Welcome families/review homework/check-ins. Families check in using the standard SOFT multifamily group questions. When asking what is better since last week, therapists frequently discover that some families will immediately report successful experiences with giving positive feedback. If the check-in questions do not elicit discussion of the homework, therapists ask families how well they adhered to the homework assignment. To keep the conversation positive they initially ask for examples of positive experiences. Some key points to remember when following up with families are:

- Ask for the specific wording of the praise.
- Reiterate what type of positive feedback was given (i.e., personal, behavioral, relationship).
- Ask the recipient how they received the feedback.

- Praise their efforts to use the skills, even if they still need practice using the skill.
- Give specific examples of how wording could be better.

Provide rationale for session topic. When we introduce the topic for this session, we give several reasons why it is important to address assertive listening in family treatment for adolescent substance abuse. Some reasons to discuss when introducing this topic are:

- Listening is a skill that can be taught and practiced.
- Listening is hard work and bad listening habits can develop, especially during tough and stressful times.
- Breakdowns in communication are common when teens are using drugs. Teens often become more secretive when using, which can lead to negative family interactions.
- On the flipside, teens often report that their parents are preoccupied with work or other things and do not take the time to listen to them.

Skills lecture talking points. Below are the key points to address when discussing what skills are needed to listen well.

- *Show that you are listening non-verbally.* Your body language should reflect that you are listening to the speaker. Make eye contact, nod, or turn your body towards the speaker. Even if you are distracted, don't show it. Don't look around at other people while you are listening. Don't laugh inappropriately or talk to someone else.
- *Show that you are listening verbally.* Use the assertive skills of *paraphrasing* and *checking for understanding.*
  - Paraphrasing means repeating back to the speaker in your own words what you thought he/she said: "What I heard you say was … (repeat what you heard them say)" or "So you are telling me …" or "So if I'm getting you right."
  - *Checking for understanding* means asking the other person if you are correct in what you heard: "So, is that what you said? Do I understand you correctly?" Unless the speaker states that the listener did indeed understand the message, the speaker repeats (in a kind voice) what the listener seemed not to understand and then the listener paraphrases a second time and then checks for understanding again.
- *Do not interrupt the speaker.* Constant or inappropriate interruptions do not allow the speaker to finish his or her message, which prevents you from hearing everything he or she wants to say. Occasional interruption is alright, because otherwise the speaker may feel that you are not listening.
- *Do not evaluate nor interrupt what the speaker is saying.* If the speaker asks for your evaluation or interpretation, then give it. Otherwise, concentrate on what the person is saying, not on what you want to say. Thinking about what you'll say prevents you from concentrating on what is being said. Also, temporarily postpone judgment of the speaker's comments until you fully understand what they are saying. That is why we include checking for understanding to the listener focuses on the message of the speaker rather than on a debate.
- *Agree with speaker often.* This assertive skill is often used to diffuse anger especially when someone is criticizing you aggressively. If you can agree with some point the speaker is making, the speaker will feel you are listening and will probably listen better to your response. For example, you may say "You've got a make a good point that I have been having a hard time getting to school on time and the grade in my first hour class is low."
- *Praise the speaker often.* Even though you might not agree with what the speaker says, try to praise something about the speaker's idea or how the speaker talked. You might even praise the speaker for taking the time to tell you what s/he feels. Do not compromise yourself, however, be honest.

- *If distracted, set a time to talk later.* If you feel you are unable to listen at that moment, suggest another time when you can give your undivided attention. It is ok for someone to say, "This is a really bad time because.... (provide reason). Can we talk about this (set time) so I can pay attention?" Note that this skill should not be inappropriately used to continually delay important discussions.

When discussing these skills, therapists ask for volunteers in the group to demonstrate proper use of the skills. Prior to the role-play, therapists ask the audience to write down verbatim what the therapist said when using the skill.

Practice Exercises. Parents and teens first role-play together in pairs using the vignettes provided. One person uses the assertive listening skills, while the other records the listeners' visual, vocal and verbal behaviors (i.e., Three V's). Once role-plays with parents are done, each parent-teen dyad takes a turn role-playing with the whole group observing. When they role-play for the group, we recommend that they use a real life conversation they have had in the past week, but not one that was such a heated argument that they may not be able to complete the exercise. Therapists guide the group process by reminding them to give positive feedback for positive behaviors observed, which reinforces the content from the first session. Group members are temporarily asked not to comment on what is being done wrong, and the therapist takes on the task of making suggestions for improvement. In order to give balanced feedback, a suggestion for improvement is always preceded by positive feedback on something done well. For example the therapist may say "I like how you maintained eye contact with her when she was talking and nodded. That really showed you were attentive. Great job! One suggestion I have for you is to remember to ask them if your understanding was correct after you have paraphrased. That way you make sure you avoid misunderstandings."

Often teachable moments come up when processing these vignettes with families. In addition to teaching basic listening skills, therapists usually find that this exercise often leads to discussions of the various pressures faced by both teens and parents. The focus should be on instilling empathy in both teens and parents for each other. For example, for teens it is good to highlight the real pressures of the adult world in order to instill empathy for their parents.

Group members may also find the vignettes are funny or similar to experiences they have had in their own lives. We recommend that therapists encourage families to use real life exercises that are more applicable, and can help them explore by asking them openly about things they typically discuss at home. When group members make fun of the vignettes or find them humorous laugh with them, or challenge them to write better ones to use in future sessions.

Explain homework assignment. The second homework assignment is for families to have at least one 20–30 minute conversation where they have each other's undivided attention and consciously practice their listening skills. The speaker rates the listener's assertive listening skills on a 1–5 Likert scale where 1 is *not attentive at all* to 5 is *very attentive,* and writes down one positive listening behavior. The listener can also identify something that s/he did that was positive and they can even identify one thing that s/he would do differently next time (i.e., self improvement feedback). They are instructed to be very specific about what was said or observed during the conversation and to bring these notes to the next group session for use in the practice exercise on giving constructive criticism. Speakers are asked to postpone giving immediate criticism (negative feedback) to listeners as this will be the topic of the next session. However, they are encouraged to give positive feedback immediately on the positive things that they noticed the listener doing. (Practice tip: If a family has a family session scheduled in between groups, the therapist should check in with the family to monitor progress of this assignment.)

Session evaluation and adjournment. Written session evaluations are completed and returned to the therapists. The therapist ends session on a positive note by giving positive feedback. Several options can be considered, and as long as the feedback is specific, positive and genuine, the therapist has many choices.

SOFT Multifamily Group Session 3: Giving and Receiving Constructive Criticism

Welcome families/check-ins/homework review. If new families start treatment they are welcomed and the group leader orients them to group by having each family member briefly introduce themselves by giving them their name and telling the new member one thing that has improved since they have started group. Then each member discusses the check-in questions. The check-in questions may prompt some discussion of the homework assignment (i.e., using assertive listening). The therapist should remind the group to focus on the positive, postpone giving criticism and highlight the success in the stories shared. Be prepared to redefine these skills if, during the check-in discussion, family members appear to be confused or uncertain about the listening skills introduced in the second group session.

Provide rationale for session topic. The topic of this session is how to give constructive criticism to others. *We provide several reasons why this important topic is included in substance abuse treatment.*

- Parents and teens often forget that *how* you communicate is just as important as *what* you communicate.
- Sometimes the ways we say important things make others less receptive to our well-intentioned feedback and contribute to hurt feelings.
- Parent-teen conflict can be very high when teens are using substances. Sometimes, bad communication habits develop that carry over to when the teen is not using.
- Parents and teens should not shy away from telling each other when they want to give each other feedback about things that the other is doing that concerns them.
- This session will focus on how to keep these discussions positive and productive so families may solve problems more efficiently.

Skills Lecture Talking Points

Giving negative feedback. Below are general guidelines for giving constructive criticism to another person:

1. Remember, that the purpose of criticism is usually *to express your disappointment* with some action by another, or *to request a change* in their behavior. The purpose is *not* to make the other person feel bad. This approach requires you to *stay calm* and *think about how to word your concern so that the recipient of the constructive criticism accepts it.*
2. State the criticism as *your understanding,* not an evaluation of the other person in general.
3. *State the reason you are giving constructive criticism* positively (i.e., out of concern) and try to give *praise statements* before and after you state your criticism.
4. Suggest a *change in the other's behavior, not their person* (that is, specific: visual, vocal, verbal, etc.). Focus on the behaviors and avoid vague "you" language. For example "I'm disappointed that you (specify what the person did)."
5. *Use "I feel" or "I think" statements.* Do *not* be aggressive by saying, "You are wrong and (continue to attack the person)..." Instead, we suggest that you say "When you say that, I feel hurt inside."
6. *Choose the right time and place.* Make sure the person you are talking to is able to listen to you. Do *not* give constructive criticism when a person is too busy, and try *not* to criticize someone at the end of a hard day of work or school.
7. *Consider the risks of criticizing someone?* There is a lot of wisdom in the old cliché that one must pick their battles. Giving too much constructive criticism, even if

well-intentioned, may be viewed by another as someone being politely overcritical. As a general rule, use more praise and positive feedback than constructive or aggressive criticism.

Receiving constructive criticism. Receiving constructive criticism can be challenging. Below is a list of points to remember when someone approaches you with constructive criticism.

1. *Stay calm.* Use techniques like counting to 10, take deep breathes, or ask for a few minutes to think about the feedback. Severe reactions such as yelling, leaving without saying anything or slamming doors will likely only escalate conflicts and will not be effective for solving your family's problems.
2. *Dwell on the positive.* Remind yourself that the constructive criticism is being delivered out of concern for your safety or well-being.
3. *Be polite and monitor your voice tone.* For example, if someone says, "You really look tired, are you okay?" try not to say, "Yeah, I'm fine. Now mind your own business!" The other person may be concerned about you, so try to listen and not lash out.
4. If confused, *ask for specifics* and purpose of feedback.
5. *Reflect your feelings* about criticism, if appropriate. If you disagree with the feedback try not to attack the sender, but rather comment on specifically why the criticism is not fair.
6. Use *active listening* to convey understanding of criticism.
7. *Try not to thank* the other person for the criticism. Thanking the other person may sound insincere and they may actually think you are just trying to avoid the conversation.
8. *Attempt to agree* with some aspects of the criticism, especially before making a counterpoint. Even if you feel that you don't deserve the criticism, try *not* to argue. For example, you may say "I agree that I still need to work on turning in all my assignments on time, but I have made some improvements and I'm upset by what you said because I do not feel like you are giving me enough credit for how far I have come." This type of reply is generally less threatening than others.

Practice exercises. The therapist first instructs parents and teens to give each other constructive criticism on the use of listening skills during the homework assignment. By this time the group may be cohesive enough that a volunteer may be comfortable role-playing this with the entire group prior to pairing off into parent-teen dyads. The therapist and group can then give feedback on the constructive criticism. (A great joke can be made here about giving feedback on the feedback.)

After giving constructive criticism on the past week's homework, the teen and parent then take 10 minutes to practice giving and receiving constructive criticism to each other by using a relevant real life situation. Therapists remind families to select minor conflicts rather than issues that have been explosive for them in the past. Families record their observations of the other member, and are asked to prepare to share the demonstration with the rest of the group. Therapists circulate to each dyad to answer questions, praise the appropriate use of skills, and (if applicable) interrupt inappropriate use of skills. When interrupting inappropriate use of skills they follow the same general guidelines presented above, which further reinforces the use of the skills through appropriate modeling.

Explain homework assignments. Prior to the next session, family members are asked to give constructive criticism to each other one time during the week. The speaker and recipient are both asked to use the skills discussed during group. The situation can be minor (i.e., not a "big" talk about a serious issue). Teens and parents rate each other on two factors: how well the other gave constructive criticism and how well the other received the constructive criticism. They are asked to rate these communications immediately following the task, but asked to postpone giving immediate negative feedback to each other. They are free to give each other positive feedback on how they worded or received constructive criticism.

Session evaluation and adjournment. Written evaluations of the session are completed and collected by the therapist.

SOFT Multifamily Group Session 4: Coping with Using Peers

Welcome new families/check-ins/review homework. Check-ins proceed as described previously. Therapists praise all efforts to complete homework during check-ins and involve other group members by asking them to also make comments and offer praise to other family members. When reviewing homework, both parents and teens present the constructive criticism they gave to the other by reviewing specifically what they said and their ratings on the receptiveness of the other. Prior to commenting on the use of the skill, the therapist also elicits the recipient's reaction to how the constructive criticism was worded by reviewing their reaction. Then, the therapist praises efforts to see each other's points and elicits group feedback on the family's topic and performance.

As the group matures and becomes more cohesive, the check-in period is an appropriate time for the therapist to request other families to offer peer support and advice on issues that families raise. Opportunities arise to praise families both for seeking help when they are stuck, as well as praising families that have shared some of their coping techniques that have been successful in the past. SOFT therapists should remind group participants that they should view each other as resources as they have likely had similar experiences.

Provide rationale for session topic. We believe that the safest way to avoid substance use is to avoid situations where you know that substances will be present. However, sometimes teens simply cannot avoid situations where alcohol or other drugs are present. *Peer refusal skills* are strategies for avoiding use when one encounters a situation where they are offered alcohol or other drugs. Additionally, some teens will resist the idea that they must avoid all friends who use alcohol or other drugs, as is commonly suggested in treatment. Teens keep different kinds of company; they usually can describe the major differences between *using* buddies and friends. *Using buddies* are peers with whom the relationship centers mainly or solely around using alcohol and other drugs. *Friends* are peers with whom the teen has had a fairly long-term relationship with common interests beyond simply using alcohol or other drugs. Friends may use heavily or occasionally when teens enter SOFT. Therapists should empathize with any objections they may raise to eliminating using buddies from their peer groups. For example, if a teen says something like, "This is stupid. I can hang out with using buddies and it won't affect whether I use or not" and "I like hanging out with them." An appropriate (initial) therapeutic response would be empathizing by saying something like "It sounds like you really enjoy being with these folks. What do you like about them?"

When facilitating the discussion above, note that these ideas are key points that should be addressed, but presentation format may vary according to personal style. We recommend rather than simply reading "lecture notes" that the therapist put all italicized definitions appearing above on a flipchart and having families define these terms. It is also beneficial for therapists to ask open questions such as "Can anyone tell me the difference between a *using buddy* and a *friend*?" Additionally, provocative questions such as "On a scale of 1–10, where 1 is *not confident at all* and 10 is *completely confident*, how confident are you right now that you would not use pot if I was holding a blunt?" This introduction is great for presenting the rationale for content focusing on increasing both their confidence and skill set in turning down offers to use drugs.

Skills Lecture Talking Points

We provide several suggestions for maintaining relationships with friends who may still be using alcohol or other drugs:

- If you are serious about ceasing to use drugs or alcohol, you may benefit from talking to your friend(s) about your commitment to not using drugs or alcohol.
- If your friend truly cares about you, they will recognize the difficulty that you have had (i.e., consequences, risks you took) and will respect your decision not to use.
- Your friends will benefit from hearing that you value their friendship even though you are no longer using drugs or alcohol.
- Tell your friends that you do not want them to offer you drugs, take you places where they know the primary activity is drug use, talk about how much fun they had when they got loaded, or use around you when simply hanging out.

Therapists should role play a conversation with a friend where these key points are discussed. Therapists can work with one teen in group to describe the friend that they want to retain by asking questions about how long they have known this friend, what types of drug-free activities they envision doing with that friend. Then, they ask the teen to role-play their friend. Below is a narrative example of what a teen might say to their friend:

John, we've been friends for a long time, and I like hanging out with you. I really don't want to use drugs right now because of my probation, my goal of going to college, and how my family feels about it. I'll need your help if I'm going to pull this off. I'd appreciate it if you not use around me, not take me to parties, and not talk about times you are using. What do you think?

Please note that therapists will have to emphasize to teens that they should use wording that sounds genuine. Depending on the responses of the friend to these initial comments, the group and therapist brainstorm appropriate responses to the potential reactions from friends. Teens in the group are also asked how they think their friends would react if they were to approach them.

In addition to dealing with friends, there are several techniques that a teen can use to avoid substance use in situations where there is potential to be offered substances.

1. *Seek more information.* Preventing offers to use drugs is often the best way of avoiding use. Thus, if you're friends or peers are asking you to go somewhere to "hang out" and you don't know if drugs or alcohol will be present, ask some simple "who" "what" and "where" questions. For example, by asking who will be there you may know that someone that uses drugs frequently will be present. Asking what you will be doing, if there is any doubt, can also clarify what your friends want to do.
2. *Decline assertively.* The best way to say no is to be direct and not hesitate when someone asks you directly if you want to use drugs or alcohol. If you sound tentative, or do not sound genuine your friends may question your commitment to not using.
3. *Provide a reason.* It may make your friends and acquaintances uncomfortable that you not use alcohol or other drugs around them and it may be best to give them a reason for your decision. However, use your discretion. If you think that the other party will make fun of you no matter what reason you provide, you don't have to explain yourself.
4. *Suggest an alternative activity.* Think of something else that you'd rather be doing and suggest that your friends or acquaintances come with you instead of going off to use substances.

5. *Have a plan for leaving.* It is best to think ahead if you are unsure that the evening will take you to a place where drugs will be present. It may be best to drive yourself to ensure that you can leave if you want to and prevent yourself from either using drugs or being transported in a car by an impaired driver.

Practice exercises. Using the vignettes that are provided, teens and parents role-play the refusal skills. In addition to the teen role-playing the skill, parents are asked to role-play the skills, and told that the purpose of their role-play is to have a better appreciation of what we are asking their teens to do. Time permitting, the parents and teens can also simulate a discussion where the teen discusses their decision not to use drugs or alcohol with a close confidant.

When processing reactions to this activity, teens are asked how well the vignettes reflect real world situations where they may encounter substances. If they indicate they do not, which frequently happens, they are asked to provide specific examples of how things are different, where they typically receive offers to use drugs, and the relevance of these skills.

Explain homework assignments. Teens are asked to identify one friend that they feel will be supportive of them not using alcohol and drugs, and have a discussion with them where they request that friend's support. If any situations come up where they are offered alcohol or other drugs, they are to practice the refusal skills learned during this group.

Session evaluation and adjournment. Session evaluations are completed and collected by the therapist.

SOFT Multifamily Group Session 5: Problem Solving (Adolescents Only)

Welcome new teen members/check-ins/review homework. In this session, adolescents come to group without their parents. During check-ins, in addition to the standard questions, they are also asked what positive changes their parents have made in the past five weeks. This question reinforces our message that we are anticipating parents to participate and support them, and challenges the perception many teens have that treatment is only targeting their behavior. If this discussion takes off, counselors may use their discretion to extend the check-in time and use this session as more of an open processing group where they spend time getting more acquainted with adolescents without their parents present. (Therapists will see substantial overlap between decision making skills presented in this group session and family problem solving skills covered in session 6, which permits continuity without loss of coverage if teens are talkative and a good discussion ensues.)

During check-ins teens are also asked if they approached a friend to ask for support in quitting, and also asked if there were any situations where they were offered drugs. Any efforts to complete these assignments are praised and teens that have yet to complete the assignment are asked if they feel the assignments are relevant. Additionally, scaling questions such as "On a scale of 1 to 10 where 10 is completely ready to 1 being not ready at all, how ready are you to talk to a friend." It is also often useful to discuss what discussions, if any, teens had with their parents about this assignment. It is often useful to ask teens here whether or not their parents currently know about their friend's current substance use (if any), as well as if the discussion last week made them nervous. Essentially, this reinforces that this group period is their time and they are free to speak about how family treatment is going for them. Thus, one of the benefits of reviewing this assignment without parents present is that teens may speak more freely about whether or not friends are actually using when parents are absent.

Provide rationale for session topic. In this session, teens will be discussing decision making skills. Therapists use a flip chart to ask teens why they think it is important in substance abuse treatment to address problem solving skills. Therapists guide this brainstorming activity and highlight the following key points:

- Many teens in substance abuse treatment have been using drugs as their main coping strategy and just ignored making important decisions.
- Everyone gets stuck sometimes and has trouble deciding what to do.
- Some decisions are bigger than others, and more difficult to make.
- Critical thinking skills can be applied to many situations (e.g., business, school), and not just personal decisions.
- When important decisions are made, teens gain self-confidence and things get better. Problems don't seem as big after repeated successes.
- We should give ourselves credit for making important decisions. Sometimes people get paralyzed, which is often a sign that they are overwhelmed with the importance of the decision.

Skills lecture talking points. We try to make a logical progression in the decision making process, and these steps can be used with many different types of decisions. Key points that are discussed include:

- *Clearly defining the decision that needs to be made.* For example, what are the choices that you are currently—Identify the issue or decision clearly?
- *Take time to think about your decision.* Do not be rushed or impulsive. On the other hand, for many people it is useful to set a date by which they want to finalize a decision.
- *Brainstorm options and alternatives.* When making an important decision, look at all your choices. Ask yourself if there are there any other ways you can solve this issue that you haven't thought about yet. Write down all the options you think of no matter how silly or extreme they seem. As a goal, try to generate between five and ten new alternatives.
- *Get the facts or information about your options and alternatives.* Gather any information that will assist you in making an informed decision. This often includes getting the input of someone you respect such as a counselor, parent, teacher, coach, or other individual you trust.
- *Weigh the pros/cons.* In weighing the pros and cons, think about your strengths and resources we identified earlier in treatment. Also, think about the potential consequences, both good and bad, of each option you are evaluating.
- *Prepare to make your decision.* Make detailed plans for (a) how you will carry out your decision, and (b) think ahead about what you will do if one the option you selected is not positive or productive. Decide ahead how you will know if it is working!
- *Evaluate your decision.* Consider how it worked out. Have you achieved what you wanted to achieve? Were there any consequences, good or bad, that you didn't consider previously?
- *Reward yourself!* If you're decision is working well, do something nice for yourself that you enjoy. Consciously say that you are doing this because of your success with this decision. If your decision did not turn out the way you thought it would and feel as if you have failed, give yourself credit for getting in the ring, do something nice for yourself, and try a different option.

Practice exercises. Therapists ask teens for examples of important decisions that teen often have to make, the group selects one by voting, and the entire group goes through all the decision-making steps. Specific attention should be paid to how the teens are evaluating the outcomes of the decision, which is easily accomplished by using the solution focused questions such as, "If you achieve your desired outcome from this decision, how will you know that it worked? What will you be doing differently?" Additionally, therapists should spend time both brainstorming appropriate individuals that can provide advice and examples of appropriate self-rewards. If time permits, the therapist asks for a volunteer that may need assistance with a current decision, and the group assists that member in going through the steps.

Explain homework assignments. Teens that are making an important decision are asked to obtain input on the decision from their parents. They are asked to temporarily suspend judgment on the advice they get, and observe their parents reactions. For example, did their parents become preachy, or did they appear surprised? Additionally, teens are instructed to consider how well their parents listened to them about the decision they faced. Finally, they are instructed that if this activity does not go well, they may call their therapist in between now and the next group to discuss the outcome. They are reminded that some issues may be better to speak with privately with their therapists rather than in the group, as we do not intend for them to embarrass or attack their parents in group.

Session evaluation and adjournment. Session evaluations are completed and collected by the therapist.

SOFT Multifamily Group Session 6: Family Problem Solving

Welcome new families/check-ins/review homework. Families are welcomed and check-ins proceed as previously described. Teens and parents are asked if they have completed the previous week's homework assignments where teens requested advice from parents on a current decision they are making. If time permits, therapists should review feedback obtained from session evaluations by providing a summary of suggestions and processing these suggestions with the group.

Provide rationale for session topic. When families solve problems together it enhances their sense of cohesion. Usually when problems concern the safety and overall well-being of children the parents will have non-negotiable rules and standards for children to follow. These rules are usually in place to protect teens and teens should try to identify the good intentions behind parents' rules. However, as teens get older, it is very important that they have an increasing say in family problem solving. Thus, it is important to discuss how to negotiate and decide on solutions when solving family problems. The negotiation skills that are presented in this group may be applied to many situations including: the use of substances (including alcohol), communication, trust, honesty, and many other situations.

Skills lecture talking points. One of the keys to successful family communication is the family's ability to solve conflicts. Everyone has conflicts, but there are numerous suggestions that may help assist you and your family in better dealing with these situations as they arise. Listed below are some guidelines for productive problem solving.

1. *Identify the issue/concern:* Be specific on what the problem is. Knowing the *real* issue or concern is half the battle. In this process of solving family issues, *no one is to blame.*
2. *Get everyone's point of view:* All persons involved in the situation have a point of view and needs to be considered when effectively issue solving and decision-making.
3. *Brainstorm possible solutions:* By brainstorming the family generates options or alternatives surrounding the identified issue or concern. Make a list, be creative; *no idea is invalid even if they seem silly.*
4. *Evaluate the solutions:* Ask what each family member thinks of each option. Discuss what may happen if you choose an option, as well as how difficult you think it would be to try a particular solution. Eliminate the options the family is unwilling to try, but try to compromise.
5. *Pick a solution and evaluate progress:* Once your family has decided on a solution, try it out. Have a clear definition in mind of how you will know whether or not it is working so you can evaluate it. Select an appropriate interval of time to check back

on how your solution is working. If the solution selected is not working, go back to your original list of solutions and select another option.

Practice exercises. Families are instructed to select a current problem and use the steps described in the skills lecture to address this problem. The therapist circulates to monitor discussions and answer questions.

Explain homework assignments. Families are asked to use the family problem solving skills as opportunities permit during the following week.

Session evaluation and adjournment. Session evaluations are completed and collected by the therapist.

SOFT Multifamily Group Session 7:
Healthy Relationships and Fair Fighting

Welcome new families/check-ins/review homework. Check-ins proceed as described previously. Therapists praise all efforts to complete homework during check-ins and involve other group members by asking them to also make comments and offer praise to other family members. When reviewing homework, both parents and teens are asked to share about their efforts at using the family problem solving techniques. Prior to commenting on the use of the skill, the therapist also elicits the recipient's reaction to how the constructive criticism was worded by reviewing their reaction. Therapists also weave the comments made in the previous week's evaluations about the usefulness of the topic. For example, if group members rated the topic as not being very useful, therapists may capitalize on this by investigating what types of things they would like to examine with remaining weeks in group. This flexibility both shows that we are sensitive to their needs and not merely trying to fit them into our program. Therapists should also continue to elicit peer support for clients that disclose difficulties during check-ins.

During this particular session, it is appropriate to extend check-ins and informal processing discussions when group cohesion is high. That is, this group is primarily a review of many of the communications skills exercises previously completed. The therapist should be prepared to follow the agenda of structured activities in case the group has little productive discussion during the check-in period. However, the therapist is allowed the latitude to condense the skills lecture and practice exercises if a cohesive working group has developed.

Provide rationale for group topic. The purpose of this session is to review broad principals of healthy relationships that can be applied to both family life, as well as other types of relationships. The purpose of this session is to review previous concepts we have introduced, as well as discuss some principles of fair fighting.

Skills lecture talking points. Healthy relationships bring happiness and health to our lives. Unfortunately, sometimes our bad habits cause our relationships to deteriorate. Some habits we have already discussed have included giving positive feedback, giving constructive criticism, and assertively listening to each other. Beyond these simple skills there are also several key tips for maintaining healthy relationships:

1. *Keep expectations realistic.* No one can be everything we might want him or her to be. Sometimes people disappoint us, and having healthy relationships means making an effort at accepting people as they are.
2. *Talk with each other.* We can not say enough that communication is essential in healthy relationships! It means _____
3. *Take the time.* Really be there.
4. *Genuinely listen.* Don't plan what to say next while you're trying to listen. Don't interrupt.
5. *Ask questions.* Ask if you think you may have missed the point. Ask friendly (and appropriate!) questions. Ask for opinions. Show your interest. Open the communication door.

6. *Use "I" statements.* Say, "I feel frustrated that I am grounded for a week" rather than, "You are always grounding me for a week." Say, "I am happy that you care for me" rather than "It's nice to know some parents still treat their teens as children."

7. *Share information.* Be generous in sharing yourself, but don't overwhelm others with too much too soon.

8. *Be flexible.* Most of us try to keep people and situations just the way we like them to be. It's natural to feel apprehensive, even sad or angry, when people or things change and we're not ready for it. Healthy relationships mean change and growth are allowed!

9. *Take care of you.* You probably hope those around you like you so you may try to please them. Don't forget to take time for yourself. Healthy relationships are mutual!

10. *Be dependable.* If you make plans with someone, follow through. If you have an assignment deadline, meet it. If you take on a responsibility, complete it. Healthy relationships are trustworthy!

11. *Fight fair.* All relationships have some conflict. It only means you disagree about something, it doesn't have to mean you don't like each other! When you have an issue or concern:

    - *Negotiate a time to talk about it.* Don't have difficult conversations when you are very angry or tired. Ask, "When is a good time to talk about something that is bothering me?"
    - *Don't criticize.* Attack the problem, not the other person. Open sensitive conversations with "I" statements; talk about how you struggle with the problem. Don't open with "you" statements and avoid blaming the other person for your thoughts and feelings.
    - *Don't assign feelings or motives.* Let others speak for themselves.
    - *Stay with the topic.* Don't use a current concern as a reason to jump into everything that bothers you. Don't use ammunition from the past to fuel the present.
    - *Apologize when you make a mistake.* Say, "I'm sorry" when you're wrong. It goes a long way in making things right again. Admit mistakes.
    - *Don't assume things.* When we feel close to someone it's easy to think we know how he or she thinks and feels. We can be very wrong! Check things out.
    - *Ask for help if you need it.* Talk with someone who can help you find resolution—like your RA, a counselor, a teacher, a minister or even parents.
    - *Accept a non-solution.* Each problem discussed may not lead to a resolved ending. Be prepared to compromise or to disagree about some things.
    - *Don't hold grudges.* You don't have to accept anything and everything, but don't hold grudges—they just drain your energy. Studies show that the more we see the best in others, the better healthy relationships get.
    - *Everyone can win.* The goal is for everyone to be a winner. Relationships with winners and losers don't last. Healthy relationships are between winners who seek answers to problems together.
    - *You can leave a relationship.* You can choose to move out of a relationship. Studies tell us that loyalty is very important in good relationships, but healthy relationships are NOW, not some hoped-for future development.

12. *Show your warmth.* Parents should know that lack of warmth predicts substance use by adolescents. Teens should know that parents become warmer if they reduce their substance use during treatment.

13. *Keep your life balanced.* Other people help make our lives satisfying but they can't create that satisfaction for us. Only you can fill your life. It is ok to participate in activities that don't involve your parents, friends or significant others such as clubs, hobbies, sports, or other activities. When you step out of your primary relation-

ships with such activities you paradoxically have more to share with them. Stay close with the ones you love, but maintain balance!

14 *Be yourself!* It's much easier and much more fun to be you than to pretend to be something or someone else. Sooner or later, it catches up anyway. Healthy relationships are made of real people, not images!

15. *Relationship skills exist.* Our belief is that you can practice these principles and learn to have healthy relationships if your relationships are not currently satisfying. Seek a neutral person to discuss your relationships and explore why they are not satisfying and, more importantly, what you can do to improve them.

Role-play demonstration. The therapist uses the scripts below for examples of healthy relationships and teen-parent communication. The therapist solicits a volunteer to role-play either the teen or the parent for the healthy communication. For the unhealthy communication, the therapist reads the exchange between the teen and parent by raising his/her voice, standing in a threatening stance, and including other threatening non-verbal expressions. The idea is to allow them to recognize communication that they have seen in their own family or in other families. For the script exemplifying health communication, the therapist should recruit an unrelated parent and teen to role-play the healthy communication exchange. During this demonstration, the parent and teen are asked to use calm voice tones.

Unhealthy communication

Andy: You are on my nerves! You are always bugging me about stuff. You just can't stop judging me. I told you that I do not want to discuss my friends, the clothes I wear, or the person I am dating. You're just all up in my business that doesn't concern you. I *don't care* what you say. It is my choice who I hang with and what I wear.

Mom: Shut-up! As long as you live here, you will follow my rules. Believe it or not, I know some important stuff, but you *don't ever* listen. Sometimes, talking to you is like talking to a wall.

Healthy communication

Andy: I was really angry when you talked about my friends and the clothes I wear, because I feel like you're not giving me enough credit for the times when I do have good judgment. I was also hurt because it *seems like* you do not trust me. Mom I take your advice about many things in my life, but I feel like I do not want to discuss this right now, because we talked about this the whole day.

Mom: Andy, I am sorry. I feel really bad that you think that I do not trust you, because I really am learning to trust you and know you have good judgment in choosing your friends most of the time. I am only trying to help. I do not want to keep talking about these issues, and will drop them. When you are ready to speak with me about anything I will be here for you.

Practice exercises. For the in-session practice exercise, the therapist asks each parent-teen dyad to work in pairs and identify a recent mild or moderate conflict between them and to describe this situation in writing. After each pair has developed a problem situation description, the therapist reviews each situation and asks each participant (parent and teen) to identify their goal in that situation. Goals are written for each participant with the situation description and the pairs are again asked to work together—this time to create a healthy communication exchange, based on their goals. The therapist moves about between the dyads and comments on their progress. After each pair has developed a healthy communication exchange (and it's written down for each participant), the therapist asks each pair to demonstrate their healthy communication for the group. Before each demonstration, the therapist asks the group members to observe the role-play for behaviors that were effective and to describe why these behaviors were effective. The therapist then guides the demonstrations so that negative behaviors are not included. After each demonstration, the therapist asks the group what they liked about the demonstration and why. After the positive feedback, the therapist asks the parent and teen separately, "If you had to demonstrate this situation again, what is one thing that you would change?" This approach to corrective feedback helps clients learn a non-aggressive approach for giving feedback. Finally, the therapist summarizes the demonstration and provides additional positive feedback.

Explain homework assignments. The homework assignment for this week is to practice this healthy communication exchange two or three times. Each pair is also asked to identify one other conflict situation and to follow the same procedures that they did in class to develop the healthy options of communication.

Group evaluation and adjournment. Session evaluations are completed and collected by the therapist.

SOFT Multifamily Group Session 8: Stress Management

Welcome families/check-ins/review homework. Follow the same procedures as in previous sessions.

Provide rationale for group topic. The therapist introduces the topic of stress management by coving the following major points:

- Stress management skills are important for both parents and teens.
- Teens often use drugs to cope with anxiety and depression. Additionally, teens experience many pressures as they grow up (i.e., grades, peers, romantic relationships, preparing for adult roles).
- Parents need to attend to their self-care as they often face multiple roles (e.g., elder care, job stress, child in substance abuse treatment). (Note—it is important for the teen to hear this as they frequently are unable to empathize with their parent's experience.)
- Having some stress is normal and healthy. It shows that we haven't just checked out and that we care about the things that are going on in our lives. Stress is maladaptive when we become so overwhelmed that we get paralyzed.

Skills lecture talking points. Dealing with daily stressors can be overwhelming. Although we can't control what life throws at us, we can control our response. We can gain control over the following things:

- Frequency of positive thoughts. We can actively practice positive thinking. For example, you can wake up and consciously say to yourself something like "Today is going to be a great day."
- Frequency of negative thoughts. We can interrupt ourselves when we catch ourselves dwelling on negatives.
- Looking for the good in all situations. Even when bad things happen that are out of our control, we must look for what good can come out of them.

When you face what at first seems like an overwhelming problem or set of problems, ask yourself the following questions:

1. Is this an issue or concern that someone close to me has experience? Am I willing to turn to them for advice?
2. What can you do today or this week to make these stressors a little better?
3. If you are facing a lot of concerns or issues, can you prioritize them?

4. On a scale of 1–10 where 1 means *no big deal at all* and 10 means *this is life or death* how would you rate the problem or problems?
5. In the past, what did you do to get through the same or similar situations?
6. What will you be doing differently when you are dealing with your stress more appropriately?

Demonstration. Therapists first ask both parents and adolescents to generate a list of situations that cause stress for teens and parents. Although the initial instructions are to talk about common stressors in general, therapists can ask if group members have had these experiences and (more importantly) how they coped. Then, therapists generate a second list about things that are relaxing to them that may help assist them with dealing with stress.

During this activity, therapists can pose provocative questions that instill empathy in parents and teens for each others situations. For example, side comments like, "These teens (or parents) really have a lot of stressors," or "Does it surprise you that parents have all these stressful situations to deal with?" An additional question to ask is, "What can you do as a (parent or teen) to help your (parent or teen's) reduce their stress?"

Practice exercises. First, parents and teens interview each other with vignettes of stressful situations where they analyze the stressful situation using the series of six questions to ask about the stressful situation. After analyzing an impersonal situation, they are asked to identify one positive self-statement they personally may use when things are getting overwhelming.

Explain homework assignments. Parents and teens are asked to use their positive self statements 1–2 times per day over the next week. They are asked to pay attention to the situations they experience that prompt their use of the self statements.

Session evaluation and adjournment. Session evaluations are completed and collected by the therapist.

SOFT Multifamily Group Session 9: Anger Management

Welcome new teen members/check-ins/review homework. Check-ins proceed as previously described. Therapists continue to praise all efforts to complete homework during check-ins and involve other group members by asking them to also make comments and offer praise to other family members. Both parents and teens are asked to share about their efforts at using positive self-statements. Therapists continue to elicit peer support for clients that disclose difficulties during check-ins.

Provide rationale for session topic. Many teens have difficulty expressing their anger in healthy ways. Anger is a natural emotion that can be dealt with in a constructive and productive manner. When anger isn't properly dealt with it can contribute to problems such as drug use or problems at school, work, or home. Therapists then engage adolescents by asking, "What has been your experience with anger and drugs and alcohol?" and also brainstorming situations that make them mad. Therapists write down these anger provoking situations on a flip chart for later use in the group.

Skills lecture talking points. Therapists make several key points about anger in a brief skills lecture. Therapists engage family members into the discussion by asking questions that prompt discussion of these points. For example, when discussing the physical and emotional cues of anger, therapists may ask questions such as, "How does your body feel physically when you are angry?" In short, although we present talking points below, these points are covered in an interactive discussion with the families during SOFT multifamily groups. Therapists ensure that the following points are discussed:

- Anger is a useful emotion in that it can propel you to take action about something. Dealing with anger inappropriately, however, can have negative effects.

- Some people take their anger out on other people, and others hold their anger inside. Both approaches can have negative side effects.
- Sometimes we get mad when we assume that others are deliberately trying to make us mad or do not care about our feelings. Making these assumptions will only make us mad in response.
- Assertive management of anger requires that we recognize anger and calmly and directly indicate why we are angry and what we would like to change. Assertive management requires that we do the following things:
  - Face our anger and don't avoid it.
  - Identify the feelings at the root of the anger.
  - Use "I statements" to express the feelings of anger.
  - Confront the events that stimulated the anger.

In addition to assertive management when dealing with interpersonal situations that provoke anger, there are several techniques that can be used to quell anger. For example, deep breathing and progressive relaxation techniques work for many people. Second, people can talk themselves down using a trigger word such as "relax," which they can say repeatedly in conjunction with slow breathing to calm themselves. Third, it is best to avoid using harsh words or taking rash actions in the heat of the moment that will compound the problem and lead to other consequences. Fourth, it often helps to look at the situation from a different angle. Try to inject some humor into the situation or think about what good may come from this situation.

Therapists here ask teens for an example situation that is something that commonly makes teens mad. Then, they brainstorm possible reactions the teen may have, both positive and negative. After identifying all the reactions, they brainstorm the possible consequences associated with each action. Therapists note the connections between this approach to addressing anger and earlier sessions on problem solving strategies.

Practice exercises. Teens and parents complete an exercise analyzing a situation that occurred to the teens that made them angry in the past. Therapists instruct families not to use family situations for this activity that are highly charged. The therapist should circulate to monitor conversations, provide support, and answer questions.

Explain homework assignments. Teens are asked to use the anger management skills during the week as situations present.

Session evaluation and adjournment. Session evaluations are completed and collected by the therapist.

SOFT Multifamily Group Session 10: Preventing Future Substance Use

Welcome new teen members/check-ins/review homework. Therapists welcome families, facilitate check-ins, and review homework as described in previous sessions.

Provide rationale for session topic. Continued substance use is common among adolescents leaving substance abuse treatment, even after making internally motivated decisions to quit using. In this program teens have explored relevant goals, and most have identified that substance use will interfere with meeting their other life goals. Families need to recognize the risk factors for continued use so that they may make efforts to prevent this from occurring.

Skills lecture talking points. Therapists engage the families in a discussion that covers the following main points about continued substance use. We view a return to substance use not as an isolated event, but rather as a process marked by several common warning signs, including:

- inadequate skills to deal with social pressure to use substances;
- frequent exposure to "high-risk situations" that have led to drug or alcohol use in the past

- desires to test personal control over drug or alcohol use
- recurrent thoughts or physical desires to use drugs or alcohol
- overwhelmingly stressful situations or emotional problems

The therapist then generates a list of triggers that may prompt kids to use substances after treatment. If anyone in group has had personal experience with previous substance abuse treatment. For example, they may say something like, "Let's generate a list of reasons why teens may go back to using substances." After generating a list of triggers, the therapist completes a second brainstorming activity where parents and teens are asked how they will cope with such triggers. Some families will have already completed their family relapse prevention plans with their individual counselors prior to attending this group. Therapists should ask these families if they are comfortable sharing some of their ideas from that session with the other families.

Practice exercises. Therapists facilitate a group discussion where they analyze the continued use potential of two fictitious clients. Therapists make personal connections between the experiences of the fictitious clients' and those of the group members. Parents are asked in this session what they would do if their child were in this situation, or how they could see themselves helping.

Explain homework assignments. Since this is the last multifamily group session, the therapists do not assign homework for this session.

Session evaluation and adjournment. Session evaluations are completed and collected by the therapist.

Implementation and Supervision of SOFT

Overview

In this section we review recommendations for implementing and supervising the Strengths-Oriented Family Therapy (SOFT) model. We begin by discussing supervision strategies, therapist training, and on-going clinical supervision and adherence monitoring. Then, we discuss common program issues (i.e., client's arriving high on drugs, level of care transfers, confidentiality, etc.).

Therapist selection. Selecting the therapist is an important implementation task for any treatment model. We recommend several desirable characteristics for potential SOFT therapists:

- minimum completion of a bachelor's degree in human services (with Master's degree preferred),
- some experience working with adolescent substance abusers,
- experience providing family therapy,
- willingness to provide out-of-office case management, and
- the willingness to adhere to a manualized treatment protocol including receipt of direct feedback from audiotape reviews.

Interview questions should reflect these priorities. In our experience, candidates who have superior clinical skills may be screened out because they may endorse practice models at odds with SOFT techniques. For example, some experienced candidates were screened out for having a philosophy not conducive to providing case management activities and for concern over following a manualized treatment.

Therapist training. Initial didactic trainings on the use of solution-focused questioning in family therapy are provided by clinical supervisors. Training addresses the philosophy of the solution-focused model, procedures for the core session content (i.e., strengths assessment and orientation, solution planning, relapse prevention planning, and case management). These supervisors include several training techniques, including: demonstration, lecture, and role-play practice for fundamental skills. Following this initial training, we recommended that supervisors closely monitor the first few cases either by actually observing treatment sessions or by reviewing sessions through video or audio recordings. Once clinicians have attained mastery level of the concepts, they are considered certified in SOFT and future supervision should focus on continual use of the skills.

Documentation of treatment activities. As an adjunct to live supervision, we recommend that supervisors conduct periodic documentation audits. We audio record every session so that the supervisor can select a session at random or by plan for review (i.e., audit). In a documentation audit, supervisors can efficiently assess whether or not therapists are providing case management, developing detailed goals on Solution Plans, and including family members in most conjoint sessions.

Supervision and adherence monitoring. Clinical supervision focusing on model integrity was provided weekly in our initial study on the efficacy of SOFT. Our supervisor conducted both individual (once weekly for an hour) and group supervision (once weekly for two hours). During supervision, clinicians answered a standard set of questions about their use of the model, which were meant to assess clinician adherence to the model and brainstorm solutions to client problems when clinicians felt stuck. These supervision questions included:

- What strengths did the client identify during the Strengths and Resources Assessment?
- Give 2–3 examples of concrete activities a client identified on their Solution Plan.
- What does the client have to be doing differently to consider treatment successful?
- What past coping strategies have worked for this client?
- Are there any goals on the treatment plan that the client has low commitment to fulfilling and possibly need revision?
- What family interventions have you done with this family this week?
- What homework did you give the client for this week?
- What difficulties did you encounter maintaining a strengths and solution focus this week?
- What examples do you have of the SOFT model working well this week? What is it about the SOFT model that is working?
- What case management have you done, or are you planning to do with this family?

In addition to using these questions, we also reviewed audio recordings of sessions in group supervision. In these recordings, therapists presented a short segment (i.e., 5–10 minutes) of an actual session that reflected family interventions and use of solution-focused techniques. We found that use of these techniques made supervision more time efficient and allowed for adherence monitoring to occur during clinical supervision during which other programmatic issues also arose (i.e., level of care transfers, programmatic issues).

Client-rated treatment integrity. A client-rated adherence measure can be used as an additional source of data on treatment integrity (see Table 15.7). Items on our questionnaire ask for ratings on a five-point, Likert-type scale ranging from *rarely* to *often*. Scores range from 12–60, with higher scores indicating higher treatment adherence to the SOFT model. When administering this instrument, clients are instructed that their therapists do not have access to their replies.

Program Issues

Abstinence. Although we allow clients to determine their own goals, we often have to be realistic about the pressures adolescent clients face to immediately abstain from drugs and alcohol. Whether or not it is a goal that adolescents are committed to, we challenge adolescents to remain abstinent during the duration of the program. This is especially important if a third party referral source such as a probation officer or child welfare worker is involved. Despite this recommendation to remain abstinent during the program we openly acknowledge that abstinence may not be one of the client's goals, as goals in solution-focused treatment are sup-

Table 15.7
SOFT Client-Report Treatment Integrity Measure

(Item stem) How often did your counselor...	Intervention Measured
ask you to answer questions using a scale (i.e., "On a scale of 1–10 how well did your week go," etc...)?	Solution-Focused Language
praise you for the positive things you were already doing well, or recommend that you do more of the things that worked well for you in the past?	Solution-Focused Language
ask you to tell him or her about your strengths as a person?	Focus on Strengths
help you define specific steps to solve your problems (i.e., ask you what you needed to do differently to solve your problems)?	Solution-Focused Language
meet with you outside of the office (i.e., job hunting, at a court date, at your home, etc...)?	Case Management
include family members in family sessions or group sessions with you?	Family Involvement
talk with you and your family about family communication or other family issues?	Family Communication
include your ideas on your treatment plan or solution plan?	Mutual Goal Development
point out strengths of yours that you hadn't thought of before?	Focus on Strengths
meet with another professional (i.e., probation officer, school official, etc...) to tell them about how you were doing?	Case Management
tell you about and help you follow through with other referrals such as going to see a mental health counselor, attend self help groups, or going to another service?	Case Management
spend more time discussing how your problems began rather than how you could do things differently to solve your problems? **(Reverse Scored)**	Maintaining Here and Now Focus

posed to emanate from the client. Thus, many times, the adolescent's primary goal is getting out of legal or family trouble. Reducing or eliminating one's substance use is often a task lower in the client's hierarchy of goals.

Arriving to sessions intoxicated. According to our program guidelines, adolescents can participate in sessions only if they are free from substances (i.e., not intoxicated or under the influence). If substance use is detected, our clinicians do not allow the adolescent to attend group or family sessions. We explain to adolescents at the beginning of the treatment program that we expect them to come with a clear mind so they can benefit the most from each treatment session. We also explain that we are concerned that the presence of an intoxicated teen in group could lead to cravings by other group members. Adolescents are instructed to return when clean and a follow-up phone call from the clinician is used to process any embarrassment or reluctance to come back to group.

Discharges and level of care transfers. When clients appear unresponsive to outpatient treatment, we recommend that the clinician consult with his or her supervisors about the appropriate course of action. Reasons for transferring up a level of care include continued or escalating use of substances or deteriorating mental health conditions which prevents them from benefiting from treatment.

Nonattendance. Adolescents who miss family sessions, but continue to attend group sessions, are required to attend a family session prior to returning to the group. This approach prevents adolescents from attending group sessions without participating in *working sessions* with their therapists. Client files are kept open for up to one month past last contact, and after two no-shows a phone call from the clinician is made to attempt to engage the family with the understanding that if a client does not make (and keep) an appointment within a certain time period (usually 2–3 weeks), they will be discharged. Therapists must offer a home visit before discharging a client for not attending office sessions.

References

Amrhein, P. C., Miller, W. R., Yahne, C. E., Palmer, M., & Fulcher, L. (2003). Client commitment language during motivational interviewing predicts drug use outcomes. *Journal of Consulting and Clinical Psychology, 71*(5), 862–878.

Berg, I. K. (1994). *Family based services: A solution-focused approach.* New York: W. W. Norton & Co., Inc.

Berg, I. K., & Miller, S. D. (1992a). *Working with a problem drinker: A solution-focused approach.* New York: W. W. Norton & Company.

Berg, I. K., & Miller, S. D. (1992b). *Working with the problem drinker: A solution-focused approach.* New York: W. W. Norton.

Corcoran, J. (1997). A solution-oriented approach to working with juvenile offenders. *Child and Adolescent Social Work Journal, 14*(4), 277–288.

Dennis, M. L., Godley, S. H., Diamond, G., Tims, F. M., Babor, T., Donaldson, J., et al. (2004). The Cannabis Youth Treatment (CYT) Study: Main findings from two randomized trials. *Journal of Substance Abuse Treatment, 27*(3), 197–213.

Dennis, M. L., Titus, J. C., White, M. K., Unsicker, J. I., & Hodgkins, D. (2002). *Global Appraisal of Individual Needs (GAIN): Administration guide for the GAIN and related measures.* Bloomington, IL: Chestnut Health Systems.

deShazer, S. (1988). *Clues: Investigating solutions in brief therapy.* New York: W. W. Norton & Company.

Diamond, G. S., & Liddle, H. A. (1999). Transforming negative parent-adolescent interactions: From impasse to dialogue. *Family Process, 38*(1), 5–26.

DiClemente, C. C., & Prochaska, J. O. (1998). Toward a comprehensive, transtheoretical model of change: Stages of change and addictive behaviors. In W. R. Miller & N. Heather (Eds.), *Treating addictive behaviors* (2nd ed., pp. 3–24). New York: Plenum Press.

Dishion, T. J., French, D.C., & Patterson, G. R. (1995). The development and ecology of antisocial behavior. In D. Cicchetti & D. J. Cohen (Eds.), *Developmental psychopathology: Risk, disorder, and adaptation* (Vol. 2, pp. 421–471). New York: Wiley.

Godley, M. D., Godley, S. H., Dennis, M. L., Funk, R., & Passetti, L. L. (2002). Preliminary outcomes from the assertive continuing care experiment for adolescents discharged from residential treatment. *Journal of Substance Abuse Treatment, 23*(1), 21–32.

Godley, M. D., Kahn, J. H., Dennis, M. L., Godley, S. H., & Funk, R. R. (2005). The stability and impact of environmental factors on substance use and problems after adolescent outpatient treatment for cannabis abuse or dependence. *Psychology of Addictive Behaviors, 19*(1), 62–70.

Hall, J., Schlesinger, D., & Dineen, J. (1997). Social skills training in groups with developmentally disabled adults. *Research on Social Work Practice, 7*(2), 187–201.

Hall, J., Vaughan, M., Vaughn, T., Block, R., Huber, D., & Schut, A. (1999). Iowa case management for rural drug abuse: Preliminary results. *Journal of Case Management, 1*(4), 232–243.

Hall, J. A., Carswell, C., Walsh, E., Huber, D., & Jampoler, J. (2002). Iowa case management: Innovative social casework. *Social Work, 47*(2), 132–141.

Hamilton, N. L., Brantley, L. B., Tims, F. M., Angelovich, N., & McDougall, B. (2001). *Family support network for adolescent cannabis users, Cannabis Youth Treatment (CYT) series, volume 3.* Silver Spring, MD: Substance Abuse and Mental Health Services Administration.

Henggeler, S. W. (1999). Multisystemic therapy: An overview of clinical procedures, outcomes, and policy implications. *Child Psychology and Psychiatry Review, 4*(1), 2–10.

Henggeler, S. W., & Borduin, C. M. (1990). *Family therapy and beyond: A multisystemic approach to treating the behavior problems of children and adolescents.* Pacific Grove, CA: Brooks/Cole Publishing Company.

Henggeler, S. W., Pickrel, S. G., Brondino, M. J., & Crouch, J. L. (1996). Eliminating (almost) treatment dropout of substance abusing or dependent delinquents through home-based multisystemic therapy. *American Journal of Psychiatry, 153*(3), 427–428.

Henggeler, S. W., Schoenwald, S. K., Borduin, C. M., Rowland, M. D., & Cunningham, P. B. (1998). *Multisystemic treatment of antisocial behavior in children and adolescents.* New York: Guilford Press.

Kaminer, Y. (2001). Adolescent substance abuse treatment: Where do we go from here? *Psychiatric Services, 52*, 147–149.

Kaminer, Y., & Waldron, H. B. (2004). On the learning curve: the emerging evidence for supporting cognitive-behavioral therapies for adolescent substance abuse. *Addiction, 99*(Supplement 2), 93–105.

Liddle, H. A., & Dakof, G. A. (1995). Efficacy of family therapy for drug abuse: Promising but not definitive. *Journal of Marital and Family Therapy, 21*(4), 511–543.

Liddle, H. A., Dakof, G. A., Parker, K., Diamond, G. S., Barrett, K., & Tejeda, M. (2001). Multidimensional family therapy for adolescent drug abuse: Results of a randomized clinical trial. *American Journal of Drug and Alcohol Abuse, 27*(4), 651–688.

Liddle, H. A., Rowe, C., Dakof, G., & Lyke, J. (1998). Translating parenting research into clinical interventions for families of adolescents. *Clinical Child Psychology and Psychiatry, 3*(3), 419–443.

Moyers, T. B., Martin, T., Manuel, J. K., Hendrickson, S. M. L., & Miller, W. R. (2005). Assessing competence in the use of motivational interviewing. *Journal of Substance Abuse Treatment, 28*(1), 19–26.

Prochaska, J. O., DiClemente, C. C., & Norcross, J. C. (1992). In search of how people change: Applications to addictive behaviors. *American Psychologist, 47*(9), 1102–1114.

Rounsaville, B. J., Carroll, K. M., & Onken, L. S. (2001). A stage model of behavioral therapies research: Getting started and moving on from stage I. *Clinical Psychology: Science and Practice, 8*(2), 133–142.

Saleebey, D. (1992). *The strengths perspective in social work practice*. White Plains, NY: Longman.

Sampl, S., & Kadden, R. (2001). *Motivational enhancement therapy and cognitive behavioral therapy for adolescent cannabis users: 5 sessions, Cannabis Youth Treatment series (CYT), volume 1*. Silver Spring, MD: Substance Abuse and Mental Health Services Administration.

Schmidt, S. E., Liddle, H. A., & Dakof, G. A. (1996). Changes in parenting practices and adolescent drug abuse during multidimensional family therapy. *Journal of Family Psychology, 10*(1), 12–27.

Schulenberg, J., Maggs, J. L., Steinman, K. J., & Zucker, R. A. (2001). Development matters: Taking the long view on substance abuse etiology and intervention during adolescence. In P. M. Monti, S. M. Colby, & T. A. O'Leary (Eds.), *Adolescents, alcohol and substance abuse: Reaching teens through brief interventions* (pp. 19–57). New York: The Guilford Press.

Schwebel, R. (1995). *The seven challenges: Challenging ourselves to make wise decisions about alcohol and other drugs*. Tucson, AZ: Viva Press.

Schwebel, R. (2004). *The Seven Challenges Manual*. Tucson, AZ: Viva Press.

Selekman, M. D. (1993). *Pathways to change: Brief therapy solutions with difficult adolescents*. New York: Guilford Press.

Selekman, M. D. (1997). *Solution-focused therapy with children: Harnessing family strengths for systemic change*. New York: The Guilford Press.

Smith, D. C., & Hall, J. A. (2007). Strengths-Oriented Referral for Teens (SORT): Giving balanced feedback to teens and families. *Health and Social Work, 32*(1), 69–72.

Smith, D. C., Hall, J. A., Williams, J., An, H., & Gotman, N. (2006). Comparative efficacy of family and group treatment for adolescent substance abuse. *The American Journal on Addictions, 15*(6), 131–136.

Spoth, R., Redmond, C., & Shin, C. (1998). Direct and indirect latent-variable parenting outcomes of two universal family-focused preventive interventions: Extending a public health-oriented research base. *Journal of Consulting and Clinical Psychology, 66*(2), 385–399.

Steinberg, L. (2001). We know some things: Parent-adolescent relationships in retrospect and prospect. *Journal of Research on Adolescence, 11*(1), 1–19.

Steinberg, L., & Silverberg, S. B. (1986). The vicissitudes of autonomy in early adolescence. *Child Development, 57*, 841–851.

Waldron, H. (1997). Adolescent substance abuse and family therapy outcome: A review of randomized trials. *Advances in Clinical Child Psychology, 19*, 199–234.

Walter, J. L., & Peller, J. E. (1992). *Becoming solution focused in brief therapy*. New York: Brunner/Mazel.

White, M. K., Godley, S. H., & Passetti, L. L. (2004). Adolescent and parent perceptions of outpatient substance abuse treatment: A qualitative study. *Journal of Psychoactive Drugs, 36*(1), 65–74.

Williams, R. J., & Chang, S. Y. (2000). A comprehensive and comparative review of adolescent substance abuse treatment outcome. *Clinical Psychology—Science and Practice, 7*(2), 138–166.

Yalom, I. D., & Leszcz, M. (2005). *The Theory and practice of group psychotherapy*. New York: Basic Books.

Chapter 16

Multiple Family Groups to Reduce Youth Behavioral Difficulties

Lydia Maria Franco, LMSW,
Kara Marie Dean-Assael, MSW,
Mary McKernan McKay, PhD, LCSW

Oppositional Defiant Disorder (ODD) and Conduct Disorder (CD) continue to be the most common reason for referral to child mental health care in community clinics (Frick, 1998; Kazdin, 1995). Estimates of childhood conduct problems suggest that 5% to 10% of children, ages 8 to 16 years, have persistent oppositional or aggressive behavioral problems (Rowel, Maughan, Pickles, Costello, & Angold, 2002). In urban, low-income communities, prevalence rates for youth externalizing behavioral difficulties range from 24% to 40% which is more than four times the national estimates and makes this a significant mental health problem facing these communities (Gorman-Smith, Tolan, Henry, & Florsheim, 2000). ODD and CD are of great concern because of their high degree of impairment and poor developmental trajectory in children (Applegate, Lahey, Hart, Biederman, Hynd, Barkley, Joseph, et al., 1997; Lahey, Pelham, Stein, Loney, Trapani, & Nugent, in press).

Family factors have been consistently implicated in the onset and maintenance of childhood behavioral difficulties and appear to be among the most powerful predictors of the development of ODD and CD (Dishion & Andrews, 1995; Loeber, Farrington, Southamer-Loeber, Moffit, & Caspi, 1998). Parental child management skills, discipline practices, family communication and interactional patterns have been repeatedly linked to the development and maintenance of childhood disruptive behavioral difficulties (Keiley, 2002; Loeber & Stouthamer-Loeber, 1987; Tolan & McKay, 1996; Tolan & Henry, 1996). In addition, children may develop behavioral difficulties in the presence of family conflict, lack of parent-child bonding, stressors, and inadequate behavioral limits (Keiley, 2002; Kumpfer & Alvarado, 2003; Patterson, Reid, & Dishion, 1992). Kazdin and Whitley (2003) also emphasize specific family factors tied to urban living, socioeconomic disadvantage, social isolation, high stress and lack of social support, may undermine parenting and contribute to the development of childhood conduct problems (Kazdin, 1995; Wahler & Dumas, 1989). However, parenting in context, especially involvement with peers in school and community, has been linked to positive child mental health (Keiley, 2002). Therefore, supporting families and bolstering key areas within the family that support positive mental health is critical.

A SOLUTION: MULTIPLE FAMILY GROUPS

Based on this empirical literature, a Multiple Family Group (MFG) service delivery model was developed to address the numerous needs of children and families, particularly in low-income, urban environments. This model is based upon previous research involving hundreds of urban parents and their children (Tolan & McKay, 1996; McKay, McCadam, & Gonzales, 1996; McKay, Harrison, Gonzales, Kim, & Quintana, 2002; McKay, Chasse, Paikoff, McKinney, Baptiste, Coleman, et al., 2004). The multiple family group approach incorporates empirical findings for intervening at a family level to reduce childhood behavioral difficulties (Dishion & Andrews, 1995; Loeber & Farrington, 1998; Loeber & Stouthamer-Loeber, 1987). In addition, the MFG approach also incorporates an understanding of the urban environment and the obstacles that it presents to parenting (Halpern, 1990; McKay et al., 1996). MFGs provide an opportunity for parents and children to share information, address common concerns and develop supportive networks (O'Shea & Phelps, 1985; McKay, et al., 1996). An MFG is defined as: (1) a mental health service that involves 6 to 8 families; (2) an intervention that is facilitated by trained clinicians; (3) a treatment where at least two generations of a family are present in each session; and (4) psychoeducation and practice activities that foster both within family and between family learning and interaction (O'Shea & Phelps, 1985).

Four broad conceptual categories related to parenting skills and family processes form the basis for the MFG model. The categories—Rules, Responsibility, Relationships, and Respectful communication (4 Rs)—were named via collaboration with urban parents of youth evidencing behavioral difficulties to summarize the evidence base in a manner that: (1) increases the understanding of urban parents about the importance of specific aspects of family life in the remediation of childhood behavioral difficulties; and (2) enhances the relevance of addressing parenting and family processes while simultaneously reduces

parental or family blame for youth conduct difficulties. In addition, two other categories, stress and social support, were added to this MFG model as these factors impact child urban use and outcome.

This MFG model targets both child behavioral symptoms and functioning, but is also meant to impact parental skills and family processes that appear to be critical to enhancing youth mental health over time. In addition, MFG is meant to address issues that are potentially related to early drop out and interfere with achieving outcomes for youth within urban communities (e.g., high levels of stress, damaging influences within the community or peer group, and negative attitudes toward mental health care) (Cunningham & Henggeler, 1999; Kazdin & Whitley, 2003). Additionally, this MFG model takes into account research findings about the factors that influence engagement and retention of minority children and families in social services and research interventions. Firstly, families of color often associate seeking mental health services with stigma (Alvidrez, 1999; McKay et al., 2001). Secondly, parents of children with mental health difficulties have reported fears of being blamed for their child's problems and these fears may in turn influence decisions to continue in services over time (McKay & Bannon, 2004). Finally, mutual support, help from peers, and normalization of family struggles with child mental health needs may create greater receptivity to treatment and may potentially engender family-level change necessary to reduce child disruptive behavioral difficulties (Brannan, Heflinger, & Foster, 2003; Koren, Paulson, Kinney, Yatchmonoff, Gordon, & DeChillo, 1997). This MFG model is specifically tailored to address the issues that impact inner-city service delivery and thereby improve engagement, retention, and effectiveness of services to urban youth and families of color.

PRELIMINARY EVIDENCE

McKay and colleagues have conducted a series of studies testing the effectiveness of MFGs within child mental health clinics serving low-income youth exhibiting disruptive behavioral difficulties (McKay, et al., 1996; Stone, McKay, & Stoops, 1996; Mckay, Gonzales, Quintana, Kim, & Abdul-Adil, 1999; McKay, et al., 2002). Dr. McKay and her colleagues have also employed MFGs as part of a core service delivery strategy in research investigating delinquency (Tolan

& McKay, 1996; Tolan, Hanish, McKay, & Dickey, 2002) and youth HIV risk behavior (Madison, McKay, Paikoff, Bell, 2000; McKay, McKay, Chasse, Paikoff, McKinney, Baptiste, Coleman, et al., 2004; Baptiste, Paikoff, McKay, Madison-Boyd, 2005). In these studies, McKay and her colleagues, including members of the community, refined guidelines for intense collaboration with parents and providers that had been used successfully in prior prevention studies (McKay, et al., 2000; Madison, et al., 2000). Parent consumers assisted in the development of the focus of each session and helped to define session activities and language used in explaining core content areas. Further, during each of the pilot studies, providers within an urban child mental health center made recommendations for changes to the intervention protocol after each session.

In one study, a sample of 88 consecutively accepted disruptive youth at an urban mental health center were involved in a test of MFGs. At baseline, a Conners Parent Rating Scale (CPRS) was completed. Families were referred to 3 MFGs until they were filled ($n = 34$). The next 54 families whose children presented with conduct difficulties were followed and serve as a comparison in this quasi-experimental study. Of 34 children in MFG, 20 children (59%) were still in services by the 16th group meeting. In comparison, of the 54 children assigned to individual/family therapy, only 21 (39%) were still in service after the 16th week of the study (McKay, Quintana et al., 1998). Child mental health outcomes as measured by the CPRS were compared for children participating in a MFG with those in comparison services. Below

are the results of the entire sample of youth as completion of the CPRS was built into standard clinic procedures and those that had dropped out prematurely were contacted via telephone to complete the rating scale (100% completed assessments). Table 16.1 summarizes the results. Participation in the MFG was associated with a significant decrease in total disruptive behavior scores and in conduct problems, impulsivity, learning problems, and hyperactivity.

An earlier study set the stage for the study detailed above. In this study with disruptive youth in an urban mental health center, significant decreases in child mental health symptoms, as measured by the CPRS, were noted from pre- to post-test in the following areas: Conduct Problems ($t = 2.36$; $p < .05$); Hyperactivity ($t = 2.3$; $p < .05$); Impulsivity ($t = 1.9$; $p < .05$) and; Learning Problems ($t = 1.9$; $p < .05$) (Stone & McKay, 1996). Only four target youth of the 21 were missing posttest assessments.

With this sample, we also examined service use. There were 138 children with disruptive behavioral difficulties who were referred to an urban child mental health clinic were consecutively assigned to three multiple family groups until the groups were full. The remaining youth and their families were assigned to standard services (consisting of individual or family therapy). The families who participated in the MFGs attended a mean number of 7 sessions ($s.d. = 3.3$) during the 16-week study, compared with an average of 4 sessions ($s.d. = 3.2$) for families who participated in family therapy and an average of 3 sessions ($s.d. = 2.7$) for those youth who participated in individual

Table 16.1 Summary of child mental health outcomes (MFGs relative to comparison services)

	MFG ($n = 34$)		Comparison ($n = 54$)		
	Pre-test	Post-test	Pre-test	Post-test	F
	Mean (S.D.)	Mean (S.D.)	Mean (S.D.)	Mean (S.D.)	
Total Disruptive Behavior	27.0 (15.7)	19.2 (11.9)	31.0	29.7	12.2**
Conduct Problems	10.0 (6.9)	7.1 (5.2)	11.7 (5.6)	11.1 (5.6)	8.7**
Impulsivity	5.8 (3.2)	4.0 (2.6)	6.0 (2.1)	5.8 (2.4)	7.8**
Learning Problems	6.4 (4.9)	4.7 (3.4)	7.5 (2.9)	7.5 (2.8)	16.0**
Hyperactivity	14.6 (8.6)	10.9 (6.9)	17.9 (6.1)	16.9 (6.4)	8.8**
**$p < .01$					

- "Rules" sessions emphasize family organization, consistent discipline practices, and parental monitoring/supervision. (Sessions 3 & 4)

- "Respectful Communication" sessions emphasize family communication, resolving family conflict, and positive parent/child interaction. (Sessions 5 & 11)

- "Responsibility" sessions emphasize family interconnectedness and parents' positive expectations for their children. (Sessions 6 & 10)

- "Relationships" sessions emphasize family warmth and attachment, within family support, and time spent together. (Sessions 7 & 9)

- "Stress" sessions identify stressors, how they affect the family, how they hinder families from doing the 4 Rs, and how to help alleviate it. (Sessions 8 & 12)

- "Social Support" sessions emphasize how parents and children can better support each other; identify when they need support, and how to access it. (Sessions 13 & 14)

Figure 16.1 Main Content Areas of MFG Model

psychotherapy ($F = 15.6$, $df = 2,136$, $p < .001$) (McKay, et al., 2002).

With the support of a recently awarded NIMH research grant, this MFG model will be studied across 10 child mental health clinics in New York City through 2011. Additional findings and research will be published as it becomes available.

DESCRIPTION OF THE MFG MODEL

The MFG model is a series of 16 weekly sessions for an hour and a half each time. There are two sessions devoted to each of the core content areas plus an additional four sessions focused on factors that potentially impact the ability of families to incorporate new behaviors that may enhance youth mental health (i.e., stress and social support) (see Figure 16.1). Additionally, the first two sessions focus on orienting families to the group, outlining group rules, and identifying family strengths. The last two ses-

sions allow time to complete a post-test and have a group ending party. If needed, a pre-test should be completed prior to the first session of group. These content areas are not intended to be discrete; rather, this model is intended to have the topics build upon each other. The proposed intervention is relatively intense in terms of dose but lengthy interventions are necessary, particularly for urban families who experience significant stressors and have access to fewer resources (Wahler & Dumas, 1989; Webster-Stratton, 1985). The intensity is necessitated by the high risk nature of the context in which families reside, as well as by the long-term nature of the child mental health care effort undertaken.

- "Rules" sessions emphasize family organization, consistent discipline practices, and parental monitoring/supervision. (Sessions 3 & 4)
- "Respectful Communication" sessions emphasize family communication, resolving family conflict, and positive parent/child interaction. (Sessions 5 & 11)

- "Responsibility" sessions emphasize family interconnectedness and parents' positive expectations for their children. (Sessions 6 & 10)
- "Relationships" sessions emphasize family warmth and attachment, within family support, and time spent together. (Sessions 7 & 9)
- "Stress" sessions identify stressors, how they affect the family, how they hinder families from doing the 4 Rs, and how to help alleviate it. (Sessions 8 & 12)
- "Social Support" sessions emphasize how parents and children can better support each other; identify when they need support, and how to access it. (Sessions 13 & 14)

This model is ideally targeted for children between 7 and 11 years of age. We expect that the core content and family practice exercises related to each of the MFG core elements (e.g., 4 Rs) will be the same for children spanning this age range. For example, there is an emphasis on the importance of creating opportunities for children to express themselves and assisting parents to ask their children questions while encouraging expression via listening (as opposed to responding too quickly or criticizing the youth) across the targeted age range for youth. However, as seen in the MFG manual, this is not a scripted model that does not allow room to apply to the individual needs of the child and family. There are opportunities to adjust messages, content, and process to the age of the child. However, the MFG model has been designed to provide multiple opportunities during each session to directly apply content to the realities of family life. In addition, discussions are meant to help family members try to determine what changes at the family-level need to be made to support their children, address the behavioral difficulties that they are evidencing, and problem solve around family-specific obstacles.

Each session is divided into segments that generally follow this outline:

Family Social—A time at the beginning of each session where food is provided and families are encouraged to socialize with each other. Although this is an informal time, some sessions introduce icebreakers or other activities, such as a "stress thermometer" to assess and discuss stress affecting families that day.

Homework Review—Homework from the previous session is reviewed and discussed at this time. Families can be encouraged to complete homework through incentives, such as sticker awards or periodic raffling of a prize.

Topic Discussion/Group Discussion—This is the segment of the session where a new topic is introduced by the facilitators. This is the only time where the facilitator is leading discussion and providing information. As sessions continue, the facilitator should encourage families to participate more in the discussion. Both children and parents should be included in discussions and activities.

Family Activity/Family Practice—This time gives families an opportunity to practice what they have learned for that session in their individual family units. Facilitators will travel around to each family unit providing suggestions and support. Generally, there is also time after this exercise to discuss what each family has worked on in the larger group (Group Discussion/Family Discussion). Some sessions also ask families to role-play different situations based on the topic for that day.

Homework Assignment—The last few minutes of each session is allotted for homework assignment which is usually a continuation of what was learned in that session. It is emphasized that homework helps families to practice and integrate the core concepts (4 Rs) into their daily lives.

FACILITATOR RECOMMENDATIONS

As noted earlier, these are large groups consisting of 6–8 families with any number of family configurations (e.g., a family can be the grandmother, mother, and child or a family can be the father, child, and siblings, etc.). Therefore, it is recommended that these groups have a minimum of two facilitators to provide families with enough support. We also encourage clinics to use trained parent consumers (e.g., parent advocates) to be the co-facilitator with a clinician as we have seen that families relate well to these parent facilitators and can help in retaining participants.

In order to ensure the success of these groups, active engagement skills must be used with the participant families. From the first contact with families, facilitators should determine potential barriers that will prevent families from attending the group. Some common barriers include transportation problems, lack of childcare, scheduling conflicts, stigma around receiving mental health care, negative past experience with providers, crises, and so forth. Facilitators must actively use problem-solving skills to encourage the ongoing participation of families. Additionally, we recommend that facilitators contact families mid-week between sessions to check in, address any problems that may arise, encourage homework completion, and remind families to attend the next session. As the sessions continue, a buddy system may help where families are paired up to assist each other by providing support and updating each other if a session was missed. This system also encourages families in building new social support networks which is a goal of the later sessions. By the end of the group, we encourage families to meet outside of the group or to have a planned event, such as a potluck, to encourage families to continue providing support for each other. Lastly, a system of incentives can help retain families in the group. Food is often a strong incentive, along with transportation money, providing childcare, periodic prizes, and homework sticker awards.

References

Alvidrez, J. (1999). Ethnic variations in mental health attitudes and service use among low-income African American, Latina, and European American young women. *Community Mental Health Journal, 35*, 515–530.

Applegate, B., Lahey B. B., Hart, E. L., Biederman, J., Hynd, G. W., Barkley, R.A., et al. (1997). Validity of the age-of-onset criterion for attention-deficit/hyperactivity disorder: a report from the DSM-IV field trials. *Journal of American Academy of Child and Adolescent Psychiatry, 36*, 1211–1221.

Baptiste, D., Paikoff, R., McKay, M., & Madison-Boyd, S. (2005). Collaborating with an urban community to develop an HIV and AIDS prevention program for black youth and families. *Behavior Modification, 29*, 370–416.

Brannan, A. M., Heflinger, C. A., & Foster, E. M. (2003). The role of caregiver strain and other family variables in determining children's use of mental health services. *Journal of Emotional and Behavioral Disorders, 11*, 78–92.

Coleman D, Bell, C., McKay, M., McCadam, K., & Gonzales, J. (1996). Addressing the barriers to mental health services for inner-city children and their caretakers. *Community Mental Health Journal, 32*(4) 353–361.

Cunningham, P. B., & Henggeler, S. W. (1999). Engaging multiproblem families in treatment: Lessons learned throughout the development of multisystemic therapy. *Family Process, 38*, 265–286.

Dishion, T. J., & Andrews, D. W. (1995). Preventing escalation in problem behaviors with high-risk young adolescents: Immediate and 1-year outcomes. *Journal of Consulting Clinical Psychology, 63*, 538–548.

Frick, P. J. (1998). *Conduct disorders and severe antisocial behavior*. New York: Plenum Press.

Gorman-Smith, D., Tolan, P. M., Henry, D. B., & Florsheim, P. (2000). Patterns of family functioning and adolescent outcomes among urban African American and Mexican American families. *Journal of Family Psychology, 14*, 436–457.

Halpern, R. (1990). Poverty and early childhood parenting: Toward a framework for intervention. *American Journal of Orthopsychiatry, 60*, 6–18.

Kazdin, A. E. (1995). *Conduct disorders in childhood and adolescence* (2nd ed.). Thousand Oaks, CA: Sage.

Kazdin A., & Whitley, M. (2003). Treatment of parental stress to enhance therapeutic change among children referred for aggressive and antisocial behavior. *Journal of Consulting Clinical Psychology, 71*, 504–515.

Keiley, M. K. (2002). Attachment and affect regulation: A framework for family treatment of conduct disorder. *Family Process, 41*, 477–493.

Koren, P. E., Paulson, R., Kinney, R., Yatchmonoff, D., Gordon, L., & DeChillo, N. (1997). Service coordination in children's mental health: an empirical study from the caregiver's perspective. *Journal of Emotional and Behavioral Disorders, 5*, 162–172.

Kumpfer, K. L., & Alvarado, R. (2003). Family strengthening approaches for the prevention of youth problem behaviors. *American Psychologist, 58*, 457–465.

Lahey, B. B., Pelham, W. E., Stein, M. A., Loney, J., Trapani, C., & Nugent, K. (in press). Validity of DSM-IV attention-deficit/hyperactivity disorder for younger children. *Journal of American Academy of Child & Adolescent Psychiatry.*

Loeber, R., & Stouthamer-Loeber, M. (1987). The prediction of delinquency. In H. C. Quay (Ed.), *Handbook of juvenile delinquency* (pp. 325–416). New York: Wiley.

Loeber, R., Farrington, D., Southamer-Loeber, M., Moffit, T., & Caspi, A. (1998). The development of male offending: Key findings from the first decade of the Pittsburgh Youth Study. *Studies on Crime and Crime Prevention, 7*, 141–171.

Madison, S., McKay, M., Paikoff, R. L., & Bell, C. (2000). Community collaboration and basic research: Necessary ingredients for the development of a family-based HIV prevention program. *AIDS Education and Prevention, 12*, 75–84.

McKay, M., Gonzales, J., Quintana, E., Kim, L., & Abdul-Adil, J. (1999). Multiple family groups: An alternative for reducing disruptive behavioral difficulties of urban children. *Research on Social Work Practice, 9*, 593–607.

McKay, M., Pennington, J., Lynn, C. J., & McCadam, K. (2001). Understanding urban child mental health service use: Two studies of child, family, and environmental correlates. *Journal of Behavioral Health Services & Research, 28,* 1–10.

McKay, M., Myla, E., Harrison, J., Gonzales, L. K., & Quintana, E. (2002). Multiple-family groups for urban children with conduct difficulties and their families. *Psychiatric Services, 53,* 1467–1468.

McKay, M., Chasse, K., Paikoff, R., McKinney, L., Baptiste, D., Coleman, D., et al. (2004). Family-level impact of the CHAMP Family Program: A community collaborative effort to support urban families and reduce youth HIV risk exposure. *Family Process, 43,* 79–93.

McKay, M. M., & Bannon, W. M., Jr. (2004). Engaging families in child mental health services. *Child and Adolescent Psychiatric Clinics of North America, 13,* 905–921.

O'Shea, M., & Phelps, R. (1985). Multiple family therapy: Current status and critical appraisal. *Family Process, 24,* 555–582.

Patterson, G. R., Reid, J. B., & Dishion, T. J. (1992). *Antisocial boys.* Eugene, OR: Castalia.

Rowel, R., Maughan, B., Pickles, A., Costello, E. J., & Angold, A. (2002). The relationship between DSM-IV oppositional defiant disorder and conduct disorder: Findings from the Great Smoky Mountains Study. *Journal of Child Psychology and Psychiatry 43,* 365–373.

Stone, S., McKay, M., & Stoops, C. (1996). Evaluating multiple family groups to address the behavioral difficulties of urban children. *Small Group Research, 27,* 398–415.

Tolan, P. H., & Henry, D. (1996). Patterns of psychopathology among urban poor children: Comorbidity and aggression effects. *Journal of Consulting and Clinical Psychology, 64,* 1094–1099.

Tolan, P. H., & McKay, M. (1996). Preventing serious antisocial behavior in inner-city children: An empirically-based family intervention program. *Family Relations, 45,* 184–155.

Tolan, P. H., Hanish, L. D., McKay, M., & Dickey, M. H. (2002). Evaluating process in child and family interventions: Aggression prevention as an example. *Journal of Family Psychology, 16,* 220–236.

Wahler, R. G., & Dumas, J. E. (1989). Attentional problems in dysfunctional mother-child interactions: An interbehavioral model. *Psychological Bulletin, 105,* 116–130.

Webster-Stratton, C. (1985). Case studies and clinical replication series: Predictors of treatment outcome in parent training for conduct disordered children. *Behavior Therapy, 16,* 233–243.

Multiple Family Group
Treatment Manual

Session Outline

Session 1: What Are Multiple Family Groups?

Overall Goal

- To familiarize families with the group process.

Session Objectives

- Help families understand the purpose of the group.
- Help families feel comfortable in the group.
- Help families to identify their concerns.
- Have each group member speak at least once during the session.
- Assist families in identifying goals for future work in the group.

Materials for session

- Scavenger hunt list
- Newsprint with statements for discussion
- Blank newsprint to write down group rules
- Markers—so group members can sign group rules
- Newsprint with 4 Rs listed on it

Introduction for Facilitators

The primary goal of this session is to create a comfortable atmosphere. As much as possible, highlight families' concerns. Try to have each member of the group speak at least once. In addition to facilitating the group process, facilitators should make efforts to connect with each family during the beginning and end of each group meeting. A good analogy to use with the group would be one that says the group will come to resemble a family. The practice of making changes in the group can then be translated to making changes in the home. Make sure to distribute a workbook per family. Explain that families will be using this workbook throughout the duration of the group and that it should be brought to session every time.

Part I: Family Social (20 min.)

Families will partake in refreshments and utilize this time to get to know each other by playing the Scavenger Hunt game:

Scavenger Hunt Instructions

1. Each family member is given a list of things to find (e.g., find another person not in your family born the same month as your first born).
2. Family members must then approach members of other families and attempt to find people with the similarities listed. *No yelling across the room!!*
3. Families are then asked to return to their seats and share the information they have found.

Note: If you notice some family member not participating in activity it is your job as the facilitator to engage them.

Part II: Discussion (15 min.)

Facilitators ask families (children first), *"Why do you think you are here?"* Facilitator then explains that the group is meant to give both parents and kids support and encouragement while they are making changes so that kids will do well. Emphasize that parents are the experts on their children but that we all need to partner together to help find different ways of helping children do better. It's a forum to help address some of the difficulties that kids are having.

Each family is then asked, *"What is an example of a difficulty you are currently having within your family?"* Discuss answers.

(Note: Facilitators should write on newsprint ahead of time the bolded statements for each of the three points below and place at the head of the room for discussion.)

During the discussion facilitator will point out:

- *Families are the place that kids are likely to get the most help* because they care about you and because you spend most of the time with them.
- This group focuses on strengths while working on some of the things that are going on. The assumption is that *everyone has strengths,* both parents and kids. *We have to build on those strengths to create change.*
- The exercises and activities in the group are meant to help kids and parents practice new ways of behaving and thinking so that when you try these at home, you can be more successful. *Activities help us practice our new ways of behaving and thinking.*

Part III: Confidentiality and Rules (10 min.)

Talk about *confidentiality.* After kids and parents define the term, ask kids whether it is acceptable to talk about what happens in group with their friends at school. Consensus should be "What's said in the group stays in the group."

Discuss and create a list of group *rules. These rules are to be written on newsprint and should be posted during each group session. Have all families sign the rules once completed.*

Rules to be included:

1. What's said in the group stays in the group
2. No cross talk (only 1 person speaks at a time)
3. Respect each other (comments and opinions)
4. No swearing and/or derogatory statements
5. Turn off all electronic devices (cell phones, Gameboys, etc.)
6. No physical or verbal aggression

Facilitators should ask families if they have any questions about the group process.

Part IV: Family Discussion (10 min.)

Ask families to identify the key ingredients of a strong family. *What makes a strong family?* (e.g., family members get along)

- Write group member ideas on board as you go along
- Identify as many points of agreement among members as possible

Part V: 4 Rs (20 min.)

Write the 4 Rs on the board.

The 4 Rs are meant to be the building blocks of a strong family:

- Rules
- Responsibility
- Relationships
- Respectful Communication

Identify these areas as being the most influential in helping kids to address some of their difficulties. As the group discusses these ideas, relate the groups' responses to the concepts behind the Rs. (Refer families to "The 4 Rs" handout in their workbook.)

Define each of the 4 Rs and then *ask the group* why these would be important.

Ask why they think rules is listed on the board as one of the 4 Rs?

- *Ask group members, why are rules important?* Rules organize the family. They also organize a child's life in other areas like school, in the neighborhood, etc. Parents play a huge part in deciding which rules are right for which age child. Also, parents have to set up systems for knowing when rules are being followed and when they are not. They also have to decide how they are going to tell their kids when they are doing a good job following the rules, and what to do if kids are not. Some rules work fine in a family, while others don't work well at all.

Ask why they think responsibility is listed on the board as one of the 4 Rs?

- Kids have *responsibilities* within families as do parents. What are some of the things that kids are responsible for? What are parents responsible for within your families? Everyone has some say in how a family runs. Parents and kids have different responsibilities within the family, but each contributes to the things that are going well, and each member has the responsibility to help fix those things that are not going as well.

Ask why they think relationship is listed on the board as one of the 4 Rs?

- *Relationships are the cement of the family.* Relationships represent how much each member cares about the other. By building more positive relationship with each other, children will be more likely to behave well.

Ask why they think communication is listed on the board as one of the 4 Rs?

- *What is good communication? Good communication is the foundation for spending positive time together.* By communicating, parents are able to know what their kids are doing and feeling. Kids can feel better supported by their parents. Here we emphasize respectful communication to show that there are certain physical expressions and ways of speaking a person can show they are listening (e.g., not interrupting, eye contact, not rolling eyes, etc.).

Ask: "How do you think these 4 Rs can help your family?"

If anyone feels that this group can't help them, then ask: "How can we, as a group, support this family with coming to group?" "Is this family committed to trying it?" Summarize discussion and ask families to think about why they are coming to the group and how some of the discussion fits in with what they want to work on.

Part VI: Explanation of Sessions (10 min.)

Briefly explain to participants how sessions will be structured, what will be covered, the reason and use for the workbook (that it must be brought to group every session, etc.).

Part VII: Homework (5 min.)

Ask families to work together to create one goal or identify one thing to work on as a family. The objective is to have them think about this together as a family (emphasize that all members participate) and come to a decision as a family. Have families write down their goals in the "Family Goal" Handout in their workbooks.

Session 2: Building on Family Strengths

Overall Goal

- To help families identify strengths.

Session Objectives

- Reframe role of child and parent as being competence based.
- Create a context for more positive interaction between children and parents.
- Help families adjust to Multiple Family Group format and feel comfortable in the group.
- Help families to identify their own strengths of the family.

Materials for session

- Group rules
- Sock or Ball for icebreaker
- Newsprint with 4 Rs written on it

Introduction for Facilitators

This session could prove to be somewhat difficult for families where conflict level is high. The goal of this session is to validate families' reason for help seeking and recognize that significant difficulties exist. However, the primary emphasis here is that change occurs as a result of families' efforts, not by magic. Therefore, the family will need to draw on their own resources and the ideas of facilitators and other group members to make changes that will benefit their children. This is a process that takes time and will not happen overnight.

The technique of reframing will be initiated and continued throughout group. Reframing is a means by which facilitators elicit greater participation by children in the group process as well as give importance to their input.

Immediately after this session, facilitators should note the strengths that each family identified and add strengths they observed. Facilitator should keep these notes and continually remind families of the expertise that they bring to discussions and family life. Further, these lists can be used at the end of group to help families to recall where they started and what they have built upon together.

Part I: Family Social (15 min.)

Parents and children have time to get to know each other and have refreshments before session begins. Parents and children can sit with each other or separate from each other during this time. Facilitators can help facilitate casual conversation within the group or allow families to just hang out with each other if everyone seems comfortable.

Part IIA: Ice Breaker/Group Exercise "Name Juggling" (15 min.)

Note: Before playing this game it is important to sets firm rules with what is acceptable play (i.e., no throwing the ball hard/at someone's face, only ask appropriate questions, etc.). It may be helpful to make sure that children are sitting in between adults and not together.

When introducing this group exercise, facilitators should emphasize that this is a game that will help us to get to know each other but also highlight things we are good at or like about each other. Emphasize that the things we are good at are what we call strengths.

This activity will be a good way to get the families reacquainted. Instead of having everyone reintroduce themselves, try this activity.

- Have everyone stand in a circle. Give one person a sock/ball. They will throw it to another person in the circle.
- That person then picks another person to throw it to.
- When you throw the ball you say: "Here *name of person receiving ball.*"
- The person who receives the ball then says "Thank you *name of person throwing.*" This person must then say *one thing they like about their family.* They then throw the ball to someone else and repeat.

This is a fun activity and really helps people loosen up, remember each other's names and learn something about each other that they may not have ever paid attention to. Remember to emphasize to the young kids that we throw softly so that we can catch it.

Part IIB: Discussion of Family Strengths (10 min.)

Introduce the idea that any changes that are going to take place with kids require that they use all the strengths that they and their families have accumulated. That is why we start with helping families identify what is working in their family and what strengths each family member has.

Ask children/family members if they were surprised to hear the strengths their family members reported. Then acknowledge that strengths can be hidden from others in the family when people make mistakes or are angry at each other.

Part III: Homework Review (10 min.)

Review previous session's homework. Ask family members if they found the assignment easy or difficult to complete and why. Have each family explain what their family goal is from the homework assignment. Have each family explain how each member came to agreement on this goal. Make sure to have children respond to this question as well. At this early point in the group, families may not be communicating with each other. This may be a good time to incorporate the 4 Rs into the family goals. Briefly explain the 4 Rs from the last session.

Part IV: Discussion of the 4 Rs (10 min.)

Facilitator says: "As you can remember from the last session there are 4 concepts that we know can help families work well together." Ask members: Do you remember the 4 Rs? (Newsprint/poster with the 4 Rs should be posted in the room). Have people in the group volunteer to explain what they are. Facilitators may prompt by asking: What are some things that may get in the way of talking to each other and getting along with each other? Emphasize respectful communication and relationships as these two Rs will help as we begin discussing the difficulties families have. You can then have a brief discussion about the answers received. Facilitators should make note that all issues brought up will be discussed throughout the duration of the group.

Part V: Discussion of Topic (10 min.)

Facilitators can say: "Something that can get in way of families doing well is STRESS." Stress is something that happens to everyone adults and children. We also know that stress can get in the way of seeing strengths in each other and ourselves. Ask children and parents to volunteer to briefly answer the question; "What is stress?" Facilitator should emphasize that children experience stress as well.

Part VI: Group Activity (15 min.)

Facilitator introduces stress thermometer that will assist each member of the family to rate their level of stress. Facilitator then hands out "Stress Thermometer" to each member and has them complete it at this time. Have children and parents volunteer what they rated and what is causing them significant stress at this time.

Note: If there are any significant issues, facilitators should address these issues afterwards if it can't be done in the group.

Have group members volunteer solutions for stress relief to those who have volunteered. Facilitator should then introduce some of the tips on the "Stress Tip Sheet" and explain the different techniques. Facilitator should highlight stress tips from the handout that are pertinent to those stressors being discussed by the families. Facilitators do not have to explain each technique. Families may volunteer additional tips which can be written in on their handout.

Facilitators should inform members that the thermometer will be distributed to check stress levels at the beginning of each session.

Part VII: Homework Assignment (5 min.)

Have each parent identify strengths for each of their children and then ask children to do the same for their parent. Have them write this in the "Family Strengths" Handout in the workbook. Encourage family to use stress tips with family members.

Session 3: Rules for Home and School

Overall Goals

- To help families understand what are rules and how they are important.
- To help families establish clear rules and know what to do when they are followed or not followed.

Session Objectives

- Families clarify the set of rules that are operating in the family.
- Rules are used to create structure and should not be punitive.
- Families clarify the consequences for not following the rules.
- Families use rewards or praise for following the rules.
- Parents come to understand that children learn how to follow rules at home first. This is a necessary step to actually following the rules at school.

Materials for session

- Group rules
- 4 Rs
- Stress thermometer
- Family Board Game

Introduction for Facilitators

This is often a critical unit for families as the primary reason that they often seek service is to address behavior problems that children experience. Parents may feel defeated in that they have attempted to make changes previously without successful results. Therefore, there can be a tendency to disregard new ideas as not having the potential to work because of their negative experiences. An additional difficulty often revolves around the lack of clarity of rules. Parents assume that "my kids know what I mean." While global expectations might be communicated over and over again, specific rules, consequences, and rewards are rarely laid out. Parents and kids can work together to better specifically define global expectations to form a set of specific routines. Additionally, parents sometimes expect that their children know how to act or respond to situations, often saying, "he knows better," yet these expectations have not been clearly communicated to the children.

Part I: Family Social (20 min.)

Parents and children have time to get to know each other and have refreshments before session begins. Parents and children can sit with each other or separate from each other during this time.

Stress thermometer is reintroduced and handed out to be completed. Families should then be asked if anyone had any high ratings on their thermometer and if so would they like to *briefly* share what's been going on. For the last ten minutes of this time, have families participate in an icebreaker.

Icebreaker

- Pose this question to all participants and have everyone respond: "If you were on a desert island what is one thing you wish you had with you?"

Part II: Homework Review (5–10 min.)

Ask members if they had any difficulty completing the homework assignment. If so, why? Help problem-solve ways families can build time in to do homework. Have members share the strengths they identified for their family members. Ask if they previously noticed these strengths.

Part III: Discussion of Topic (10 min.)

- Facilitator should post group rules up in the room. Reiterate the group rules and use this as a lead into the discussion of why families need rules.
- Ask, "*Why are rules important in a family?*" Relate the need for rules in a family to rules in society. A useful analogy would be the implementation of traffic lights to keep us all from crashing. Some reasons why rules are important are: rules help keep everyone safe; rules help you understand what is and is not acceptable, etc.

Part IV: Family Activity (15 min.)

- Participants should break into separate family groups for this activity. Refer families to the "Family Board Game" in their workbooks. Facilitators should distribute the Family Board Game player pieces to each family. *The goal of this game is to have families come up with a list of rules the family is using currently.* The board game allows each member to participate and as they land on different categories (e.g., bedroom, kitchen, school, etc.) the family is supposed to write down each rule that pertains to that category. The families should use the "Family Rules" handout for Session 3 to write down their list of rules.

Part V: Group Discussion (10 min.)

- Each participant should stay within their respective family groups. Now that each family has a long list of rules at home, have them offer to share some rules from their lists. Then raise the following points for the families to consider.
  a. Who is responsible for making the rules in the family?
  b. Are children involved in that process?
  c. Are there different rules for kids of different ages?
  d. How do families know when the rules need to be changed?

Part VI: Family Practice Exercise (20 min.)

- Have each family review the long list of rules they developed from playing the "Family Board Game." Using the "Family Rules" handout, each family should then mark which rules are easiest and most difficult to follow. Then have each family pick the three most important rules they feel they can try to work on. These rules should also target behaviors that they want to change. Keep in mind that these rules should be manageable for the families to problem solve during the length of this 16 week program. Suggest to families that at least one of the three rules should come from their difficult list.
- Once each family has developed their list of three rules, explain to the whole group that children learn rules at home first and this is how they can then follow rules at school. Emphasize that rules always need to be accompanied by rewards and consequences. These rewards and consequences are often the things that need to be changed when rules are not working.

Note: Facilitators can walk around to individual family groups and help families write their rules as well as discuss rewards/consequences. Facilitators can help families by prompting them with the following questions: *Kids can be asked: "What is the rule?" "Why does your family have* this rule?" *Parents can be asked: "How do you know when the rule has been broken?" "What specifically happens when the rules are followed? Broken?"*

Emphasize that *rewards are not just about spending money and buying children things* but that rewards can come in the form of praise and privileges (e.g., more TV and phone time, etc.).

Other information that is important to keep in mind when thinking about rules:

- Rule should be stated in a positive way. For example, instead of "No Screaming," write "Talk Calmly."
- Rules are clear, concise, and age specific.
- There shouldn't be too many rules.
- Rules need to be followed by everyone in the home.
- Consequences for following and not following the rules should be delivered consistently.

Send families home with this concept: "A rule is only as good as what happens afterwards."

Part VII: Homework Assignment (5 min.)

Have families go home and try to implement the three rules as discussed in this session. Encourage families to write on their "Family Rules" handout their experience of the three rules during their week. Write consequence and reward for each rule and how it worked or didn't work for them.

Session 4: Problem-Solving Broken Rules

Overall Goals

- Examine family rules more in depth.
- Provide families with tools to change and/or fix rules that are not working.

Session Objectives

- Families clarify set of rules that are operating in the family.
- Rules are more clearly identified for children.
- Parents examine their own behavior in relation to rules. (Are parents clear and consistent?)
- Consequences (positive and negative) for not following the rules are clarified.
- Rewards for following the rules are clarified.

Materials for session

- Group rules
- 4 Rs
- Stress thermometer
- Tools for fixing rules

Part I: Family Social (20 min.)

Parents and children can spend time with each other and have refreshments before session begins. Parents and children can sit with each other or separate from each other during this time.

Stress Thermometer is distributed and families should rate their stress level for today. Families should then be asked if anyone had any high ratings on their thermometer. If so, would they like to *briefly* share what's been going on? Process concerns that come up within the group. If any issues are too complicated to discuss in the group, make sure to discuss it with that participant after the group.

Part II: Homework Review (10 min.)

Facilitators should ask families how they did with the homework from last week. Ask families to take out their "Family Rules" handout. Review with families if this homework was easy or difficult to complete. Give stickers (or another form of reward, such as certificate, raffle, etc.) to those who completed the homework.

Part III: Group Discussion (20 min.)

- Facilitators should use the homework exercise to begin a discussion about what happened over the week with their family rules: "How did the rules work in your family this week?" "How difficult was it to be consistent with this rule?" "How difficult was it to implement consequences or rewards?" "What are some things that helped you or stopped you from implementing it consistently?"
- Facilitators should emphasize that those rules that are working are the strengths of the family and won't be changed because they seem to be working fine. However, the rules that are not working are the focus of the group today.

- Facilitators should highlight some of the common reasons that "rules become broken."
  - They are not clear or specific and sometimes too wordy.
  - There are too many rules and the child has a hard time remembering all of them.
  - They are not appropriate for the child's age.
  - Nothing happens if the child follows the rule—no rewards.
  - Nothing happens if the child does not follow the rule—no consequences.
  - Rewards and consequences are only given on certain occasions and not on others (e.g., a parent has a difficult day so they are more willing to punish behavior or a parent has a really stress-free day so they are willing to overlook breaking the rule).

Part IV: Family Activity (15 min.)

After group discussion, facilitators should separate each family into individual groups. Facilitators then introduce the "tools for fixing rules." Families will create a toolbox to help change and/or fix any rules that need to be changed to work better in their families.

- *Family Toolbox:* Refer families to the "Toolbox" pages in their workbooks. Have families read through these pages and to help them to understand that on each tool is a statement that will help them fix their rules. Parents and kids should work together to cut and color the tools. Each family should paste the actual toolbox picture on a Ziploc bag where they then can put their tools. This becomes their Family Toolbox.

Part V: Family Practice Exercise (20 min.)

Families remain in their individual family groups from the last activity. Each family identifies a rule from their list of three that is not working. Ask one family to volunteer to role play a situation when this rule is not working. Invite the other group members to help this family problem-solve or fix the rule with the "tools" from their toolbox. Have additional families role-play out situations if time permits. Make sure to process each role-play after it is completed and address any concerns from parents. Focus on recurring issues that arise across families.

Part VI: Homework Assignment (5 min.)

During the week, each family should sit down and fix one of the rules that are broken in their family and report on their progress next week. Each family should use the "Rules Rule!" handout in their workbook.

Session 5: Respectful Communication

Overall Goal

- To enhance communication between parents and children.

Session Objectives

- To enhance parents' ability to communicate with children in a manner that they will attend to and understand.
- To enhance parents' ability to listen to their children and be more available to them.
- To enhance children's ability to discuss concerns with their parents more freely.
- To enhance children's ability to actually hear what their parents are trying to communicate to them.

Materials for session

- Group rules
- 4 Rs
- Stress thermometer

Introduction for Facilitators:

The goal of the unit is to increase communication between parents and kids. Communication is the foundation for spending positive time together: solving problems and finding out what is going on in each other's lives. Good communication becomes especially important as kids get older and as they tend to spend more time away from parents. If parents are going to be able to keep track of where their children are spending their time, what is going on in school, and who their friends are, communication is essential.

This session involves a lot of group participation and discussion. Facilitators should be mindful of leaving enough time for the discussion questions, group exercise, and a thorough explanation of the homework.

During the discussion questions when children and parents are separated into groups, be sure to clearly state that each group will meet for a stated amount of time and will come back and share with the whole group. One facilitator will be with each sub-group. This separation will give kids and parents an opportunity to be with other kids and parents and to get support from their peers.

Part I: Family Social (20 min.)

Parents and children have time to catch up with each other on the weeks events and have refreshments before session begins. Parents and children can sit with each other or separate from each other during this time.

Stress Thermometer is distributed and families should rate their stress level for today. Families should then be asked if anyone had any high ratings on their thermometer. If so, would they like to *briefly* share what's been going on? Process concerns that come up with the group. If any issues are too complicated to discuss in the group, make sure to discuss it with that participant after the group.

For the last ten minutes of this time, have families participate in the following activity while they are still able to socialize and have refreshments.

Activity:

1. To warm the group up to tonight's exercise, start the session off with a round of the telephone game. Facilitators should write down a statement to use prior to the group session so they remember it. It should be complex but not too difficult for latency age children to remember. (Example: "Strong families communicate with each other.")
2. Discuss the outcome of the activity with the families. What was the ending statement? How close to the original statement was it? What reasons can the families provide to why the ending statement was not the same as the starting statement? What does this game teach you about communication?

Part II: Homework Review (15 min.)

Review previous session's homework. Ask family members if they found the assignment easy or difficult to complete and why. Problem-solve ways to help families do homework. Have each family discuss what rule in their family was broken in their family, and how did they go about trying to fix it? Ask members if they were successful in fixing their broken rule, why or why not? If not, what steps can they take to fix the rule? Have group members assist each other in finding alternate ways to fix broken rules.

Part III: Discussion of Topic (20 min.)

Indicate that the group will begin working on the next R, "Respectful Communication." Explain that although this may be new for some participants, it can also be a reintroduction for others. Ask group, *What does respect mean to kids and parents? Why would the word respect be in front of communication?*" Discuss active listening and clear communication (i.e., parents may say to kids, "don't you think you should have known to do that . . ." instead of saying, "I would like for you to . . ."). Discuss the importance of effective communication, tone of voice and voice level, body language and eye contact. Have facilitator act out what active listening is and then call on some parents and children to do so as well. Facilitator should use the "Express Yourself Skills Script" and refer families to the "Express Yourself Skills" handout in their workbooks.

Part IV: Group Exercise (30 min.)

For the following exercise, children and parents are divided into separate groups. A facilitator should go with each group and ask the following questions. A list of answers should be generated for these questions. Each participant should use the "Communication Questions" handouts in their workbook. Facilitators should distribute extra handouts to make sure all participants have their own. Facilitators should also write some answers on the board.

Questions for Children

1. How do you know when your parents are listening to you?
2. What can you do so that your parents feel that you are listening to what they are saying to you?
3. What kinds of words should you use when you are asking your parent for something? (e.g. "please," "thank you," "may I," etc...)
4. When is the best time to ask them for something that you really want?
5. Can you think of times when you really want to talk with your parents? If so, when? If not, why not?

In your everyday life, outside of your parents:

6. Who is the best listener in your life?
7. Who gives you the best advice?
8. Who do you wish would quit lecturing you?
9. What is the difference between lecturing and communication?

Questions for Parents

1. How do you know when your children are listening to you?
2. What can you do so that your children feel that you are listening to what they are saying to you?
3. When is the best time for your children to ask you for something they want?
4. When is the worst time for your children to ask for something?
5. Can you think of times when you really want to talk with your children? If so, when? If not, why not?

In your everyday life, outside of your children:

6. Who is the best listener in your life?
7. Who gives you the best advice?
8. Who do you wish would quit lecturing you?
9. What is the difference between lecturing and communication?

(Leave last 10 minutes of this section for group discussion.) Parents and children are then rejoined and the answers are discussed. Question to consider for discussion: *Are we communicating with each other the best way we possibly can?* Aspects of effective communication should be highlighted if not identified by the group. Include: Eye contact, asking appropriate questions, responding in a way that encourages more talk: active listening, not giving advice, etc.

Part V: Homework Assignment (5 min.)

Have parents and children get information from each other about one or more *positive* event(s) that occurred during the day for everyday during the week. Parents and children must list these events on their "How was your day?" handout.

Activity: Express Yourself Skills for Kids

"We are going to learn our Express Yourself Skills today and then practice them because it is very important that we learn helpful ways to express ourselves. You will also use these when you talk with your family. Expressing yourself means talking so that you get your ideas across and listening to people so that they can get their ideas across to you. Sometimes it is not easy, which is why we are going to practice today."

"There are four parts of your body to remember when you express yourself. Your back, eyes, mouth, and ears."

"We use our *backs* to stand or sit up straight. Let's all practice standing up straight. (Everyone should be standing up in a circle and facilitator will demonstrate.) That's right. Now, what happens when you talk with your back bent like this? (Everyone demonstrate.) That's right. No one pays attention to what you are saying because they cannot see your face. And you can't fill up your lungs with air."

"Now once we get our backs straight, we can use our *eyes* to look at people. Let's all practice looking at each other in their eyes. Look around the circle. What would happen if I tried to talk to you (choose someone) and I was looking down at the floor? (Demonstrate). That's right. You might think I was scared or embarrassed or shy. You wouldn't think that what I have to say is important. So, when we use our eyes to look at the person we're talking to, they know that we are serious and want them to pay attention." (Facilitator be aware of cultural values regarding eye contact.)

"Now we use our mouths to what? That's right, talk. But when we talk, we need to speak in a strong and clear voice. What would you think if I talked to you like this (mumble something)? Yeah!! You wouldn't know what I was talking about, right? You wouldn't be able to understand me. Now what if I talked to you like this (yell something). Right. I would get on your nerves. You wouldn't want to listen to me. But if I use a nice strong, clear, voice, you would be able to understand me and you would listen."

"So, when we are expressing ourselves, it helps if we put all of this together and stand up straight (demonstrate), look at others in the eye (demonstrate), and talk in a strong and clear voice (demonstrate)."

"Now, what was the last body part that we use? Can you remember? That's right, your ears. What do you think they're for? Yep; to listen to other people. It is just as important for you to listen to what other people say as it is for you to say what you have on your mind. If we do a good job of listening, then when it's our turn to talk, that person will probably listen to us too."

"Sometimes you might want to talk to your parents and they are busy. So, try to stop and ask them if it's a good time to talk. If it's not a good time for them, ask, 'When's a good time for us to talk?'"

"Okay, now we are going to practice expressing ourselves. Each of us is going to say our name, our favorite food, favorite hobby, and what you want to be when you grow up. Remember to stand up straight, look others in the eye, and speak clearly."

Session 6: Responsibility at Home and School

Overall Goals

- Families develop a better understanding of how maintaining responsibilities contributes to enhanced family functioning.

Session Objectives

- Roles of parents and children are clarified within each family.
- Each family member is given credit for the contribution that they already make to the family.
- Expectations for children are clarified.
- Parents identify areas where they need additional support and problem solve about ways to obtain necessary resources.

Materials for session

- Group rules
- 4 Rs
- Stress thermometer
- Newsprint or board and markers
- Responsibility Handout

Introduction for Facilitator

The responsibilities of children in the family are often focused on at this point. It is important to integrate the prior messages regarding enforcement and distribution of rules, parent and child responsibilities, and that families cannot function unless everyone maintains their responsibilities in the family, the community, and at school. Facilitators should have puzzle pieces cut and ready to distribute for Family Practice Exercise, along with any other materials families will need. Facilitators should be aware of time constraints in this session as there is a lot to cover.

Part I: Family Social (15 min.)

Parents and children have time to spend time together and have refreshments before the session begins. Parents and children can sit with each other or separate from each other during this time.

Stress thermometer is also handed out and discussed during this time.

Part II: Homework Review (10 min.)

Review homework from last week. Have each family volunteer examples of positive events from their lists. What was it like for kids to ask their parents about their day? What was it like for parents to ask their kids about their day? Was it easy or difficult to focus on positive things?

Part III: Discussion of Topic (10 min.)

- Introduce the next unit of the program, *responsibility*. Each family has members that perform different roles (role is your function—a parent, a child, an aunt, a caregiver, a sibling) and with each role comes responsibilities. Each member of a family is responsible for making the family "work." *(Note: Begin discussion with children to make sure they understand the concept and remain engaged with the group.)* Ask children what it means to have responsibility. Then ask if they can give any other words that mean the same as responsibility (e.g., "to do," "jobs," "chores," "assignments").

- Continue the above discussion with parents. Ask what does responsibility mean to them? Definitions of responsibility includes: sense of obligation to perform your role (as a child, parent, etc.); duty; accountability; dependability; reliability; excellence.
- With each role comes lots of different things we expect parents and kids to do. There are expectations that the society or the outside world places on us (e.g., kids have to go to school until 16; parents have to provide basic needs for kids) and then there are the expectations that we place upon our own families. In the family, parents have many expectations for their children. *How does this translate to responsibility?* The expectations parents have for children often become their responsibilities.

Part IV: Group Activity (20 min.)

- As a larger group, identify appropriate family roles and the responsibilities for each of those roles (e.g., parents are responsible for providing food for their children; children are responsible for completing their homework). Facilitator should write responses on the board. Make sure to have children and parents respond to these questions. Prompt families by asking: *What are a child's responsibilities? What are parents' responsibilities? What are parents' expectations of kids and themselves? What are kids' expectations of parents and themselves?* It is helpful to see what children think is expected of them and compare this with what the parent says.
- Attempt to facilitate a discussion around the listed roles by highlighting the following points:

  a. There are some responsibilities within the family that only parents can fulfill.
  b. Level of responsibilities change as children get older.
  c. How do we help kids to be responsible? (How do they learn that responsibility pays off at home?)
  d. What are some of the obstacles to getting our jobs done, as both parents and kids?

Part V: Family Practice Exercise (15 min.)

Have families do the following practice exercise (at this point, families should be responding more directly to each other and relying on the facilitators less for decision making in the group).

Directions

- Hand out the puzzle pieces.
- The pieces are then divided evenly amongst each family member.
- Participants then need to write one task on each puzzle piece that they think they are responsible for at home.
- Once everyone has written something down, they share their answers.
- Now participants can start to put the puzzle together. Paste the puzzle pieces together on the "Responsibility Puzzle" page in the workbook.

It is important for the groups to realize that just like a family cannot function unless everyone maintains their responsibilities; the puzzle cannot be completed unless everyone communicates and comes to an agreement, so that all the pieces can be put together to complete the puzzle!

Group Discussion (15 min.)

First emphasize that each member deserves credit for the contribution they already make in the family. Then have family members role-play situations where responsibilities need to be readjusted for the larger group for assistance from other families. (In this role-play the parents will role-play as the children and the children will role-play as the parents.) After families receive these suggestions, have them role-play the situation again more positively while in their respective roles (parent as parent; child as child). Try to have as many families as possible get the opportunity to role-play. *Refer families to the "Readjusting responsibilities" handout.*

Part VI: Homework Assignment (5 min.)

Have each family review the list of responsibilities on the "Responsibility Puzzle" used in session. Each member (parent and child) should pick a responsibility that needs to be readjusted and try to implement it at home. They will report how it went at the next session. Remind families that there is an extra "Responsibility" information sheet in their workbook for them to review.

Session 7: Relationships

Overall Goal

- To build more positive "Relationships" between family members.

Session Objectives

- To help families understand the importance of their relationships.
- To help families develop a consistent time that parents and children spend together.
- To help families schedule fun activities that will promote a positive family atmosphere.
- To help families spend more quality time together.

Materials for session

- Group rules
- 4 Rs
- Stress thermometers
- Monthly calendar for families to plan activities together (in members' workbook)
- Handouts of local resources for family activities

Introduction to facilitators

This session is very important for all of the families. A lot of families may have strained relationships with their children and we want to help families to begin repairing those relationships by helping them understand how important they are to each other and to also have fun with each other.

Part I: Family Social (15 min.)

Parents and children have time to spend time with each other and have refreshments before session begins. Facilitators can help facilitate casual conversation within the group or allow families to just hang out with each other if everyone seems comfortable.

Stress thermometers are also distributed during this time.

Part II: Homework Review (5–10 min.)

Were families able to complete the last homework? Have families volunteer which responsibilities they worked on. How were they able to readjust them? What worked and what didn't work? Have other families volunteer suggestions.

Part III: Discussion of Topic (10 min.)

Facilitators should acknowledge that much of the group meetings thus far have concentrated on solving problems and fixing rules that had become "broken." What we know to be equally important for kids to do well is having positive relationships with their parents and siblings. Research has shown that kids really want to be close to their parents. If they learn important things from their parents, they are more likely to make better choices in their lives.

Part IV: Group Discussion (15 min.)

Facilitators should facilitate the following discussion with families and be open to any responses they may have while keeping the goals in mind.

- What does it mean to have a good relationship with someone?
- Why would having good relationships in the family be just as important as things like rules or getting our chores done?
- What would it mean to have a good relationship between a parent and a child?
- What are some things that parents and kids like to do with each other?
- Ask kids what types of activities they would like to do with their family—could be something they used to do and don't anymore or something completely new.
- Discussion: One way of improving relationships is to spend more quality time together with each other.

Part V: Family Activity (30 min.)

Facilitators should have families separate into their respective family groups.

Note: Facilitators can walk around to individual family groups and help families generate ideas for family activities by asking the following questions: *"Tell me the last time you had fun with each other? What did you do?"* or *"What kinds of activities are the most fun for you as a family?"*

- Families will split up into individual groups and come up with a series of fun activities that they can do together over the next month that do not cost much money. For example: Eating dinner together, using time to talk about things (time on train or bus together), praying together, family karate, going to Riverbank Park, playing board games, etc. During this time, have families develop some rules around "Family Time" (e.g., no arguing during family time, do not take away family time as punishment, etc.). *Families should include in the calendar new activities as well as ones they already do together.*
- Facilitators refer families to the calendar in their workbooks. Individual families complete calendars in order to identify family time on a weekly basis.
- Facilitators provide a handout/list of local resources for families to use for suggested activities in the community. Two lists can be provided: One for kids only activities and one for family activities.
- As a larger group, families should discuss:
  - What are some rules around Family Time?
  - What are the obstacles to spending time together?
  - What issues get in the way of having fun together?
  - How easy or difficult is it to have fun together if you have been angry with each other?

Part VI: Homework Assignment (5 min.)

Have families go home and implement their plan(s) to spend time together this week and have them write at the bottom of their "Family Calendar" any obstacles that come up for them. Families should also take some time to examine how well their rules are working this week.

Session 8: Dealing with Stress at Home

Overall Goal

- Families understand how using the 4 Rs can relieve stress in their lives.

Session Objectives

- Families can identify the stressors that hinder the 4 Rs.
- Families will feel support from the group and have opportunity to share experiences that have been stressful in their lives.
- Parents and kids will become more aware of the stressors each one faces.
- Families will have the opportunity to practice supporting and communicating with each other in hopes of alleviating stress.

Materials for session

- Group rules
- 4 Rs
- Stress thermometer
- Popsicle sticks
- Stress handout

Introduction for Facilitator

In this session, families identify significant stressors in their lives. It may be difficult for parents not to identify their children as being stressors in a way that makes children feel as though they are being blamed. During this session, help families to reframe those concerns. Make sure to allow children the opportunity to voice their own concerns and stressors. Throughout this session refer back to the 4 Rs as much as possible to help families integrate these concepts within their lives.

Part I: Family Social (15 min.)

Parents and children have time to have refreshments and socialize with each other.

Facilitators should explain to families that the thermometer will not be distributed today as the focus of today's session is on stress. Any significant stressors can be addressed individually after the group.

Part II: Homework Review (5 min.)

Ask families to volunteer to explain how they spent their family time this past week. Any successes? Any difficulties? Help families problem-solve solutions for each other. Encourage families to continue spending family time together.

Part III: Group Discussion (15 min.)

Have kids answer the following question: "*What is stress?*" Write answers on the board so that you can refer back to them. Follow up questions might be: "*Where does stress come from? How do you know when you are stressed?*" Have parents answer the questions as well. At this point, the facilitators can begin to talk about how stress can hide family strengths and make it difficult to get along as a family. *Remember that a child's behavior can look exaggerated when seen by a parent who is under a lot of stress. Also, a parent's stress can negatively impact the child.*

Stress should be seen as an indicator that a change needs to occur in a situation. Problems can be solved more easily when people work together. The key to this is good communication and family support. For this to occur, each family member must be willing to listen when someone else calls for help and be willing to ask for help if they need it. Refer parents back to the session on "Respectful Communication" when explaining this.

Help families to understand this discussion with the following metaphor:

Each family member is like a twig, by itself it can be easily broken. When placed with a bundle of twigs, it cannot be broken. The same is true of families working together.

Have families illustrate this point by distributing a bundle of Popsicle sticks to each participant (including children). Have each participant try to break one Popsicle stick first, then have them attempt to break the whole bundle. It should be more difficult to break the bundle which illustrates the point that families who work together are stronger.

Part IV: Group Exercise (15 min.)

The goal behind this exercise is creating awareness and sensitivity to the pressures faced by individual family members. Separate the parents and children into their respective groups. Have each member write on their individual "Stress Checklist" stressors that they face on a daily basis. Then have each group member offer examples that the facilitator will write on the board or on newsprint (children discuss amongst the children and parents discuss amongst the parents).

While still in groups, the facilitator should recite the lists to the entire group membership. The facilitators should elicit questions and discussion around these stressors: *Parents, were there any stressors on the children's list that surprised you? Children, were there any stressors on the parent's list that surprised you? Children, do you think that your parents knew about these stressors?*

Part V: Family Practice Exercise (35 min.)

Families should then break up into their individual family groups. Each member should have their "Stress Checklist" from the previous exercise. Give families five minutes to discuss the stressors on their lists. Encourage open communication and active listening between members. Based on their individual lists, families should come up with family stressors and write these on the "Family Stress List" in their workbooks.

Have families pick one particular stressor from their lists and tell them that they will role-play these stressors in front of the whole group. Try to have as many families role-play as time permits. The family should role-play the situation for at the most five minutes as they would normally address it. Once completed, have the rest of the group assist this family in problem-solving the situation. *The families should keep in mind the 4 Rs when offering suggestions. (At this time, the facilitator may need to review the 4 Rs briefly.)* Encourage participation by all members, children and parents alike, in problem-solving. Then have the family do the role-play again for at the most five minutes by using the recommendations given by the group.

The task for facilitators is to try to keep this exercise from becoming a blaming session in which the kids are belittled.

Refer families to the "Stress Tip Sheet" that was used in Session 2 and also the "Tips for Taking Care of Yourself" sheet in the workbooks.

Part VI: Homework Assignment (5 min.)

Encourage families to continue to practice the solutions role-played in the group at home and to use the stress tips as a way to address any other stressful situations that may occur. Families should work on the "Family Self-Care Plan" as homework. Refer families to the worksheet in their workbooks.

Session 9: Building Families Up

Overall Goal

- To strengthen "Relationships" between family members.

Session Objectives

- To help increase more positive family interactions.
- To help parents understand that building positive interactions helps to encourage more positive behaviors in the child.
- To encourage acknowledgement of family strengths which also builds unity and pride.
- To give parents examples of how to reward by using praise and acknowledgement (which can help in enforcing rules).

Materials for session

- Group rules
- 4 Rs
- Stress thermometer
- "Build Me Up" Handout
- Certificates

Introduction to facilitators

It's important to remind families that this session is a follow up to the first session on Relationships. This may be a good time to check in with families to see if their relationships have improved at all with each other. A short discussion could be beneficial to everyone about this.

Part I: Family Social (15 min.)

Parents and children have time to have refreshments and socialize with each other. Stress thermometer is also distributed at this time.

Part II: Homework Review (5–10 min.)

Review homework assignment from last session. Have families volunteer their Family Self-Care Plan. Have families talk about their experience in completing the handout. Are they able to do these things on a regular basis? What kind of support do they need to be able to do so?

Part III: Discussion of Topic (10 min.)

Families should be praised for all of the hard work they are doing in the group. Let them know that today is mostly going to include family activities so that they can bond and have fun together. Remind kids and parents that relationships are easier if there is a focus on the positives within each other rather than the negatives.

Part IV: Family Activity (40 min.)

Start activities as a large group with the "Build Each Other Up" exercise and then separate into separate parent and child groups for the Certificate exercise.

- "Build each other up"

Parents and kids write their name on the Build Me Up Handout. They then pass the paper to their right, and write one POSITIVE quality about the person whose name is on the paper in front of them. The papers get passed around the room until each person has the original paper with their name on it. (At the end of this activity, all members should have a paper with a list of good qualities about themselves.) Discuss the activity and ask if anything on their list was surprising? Have some members volunteer qualities that surprised them.

(*Note*: Facilitator can suggest the members to post their list of strengths somewhere at home where they can refer to it especially in moments of stress and low self-esteem.)

- "Certificates"

The group splits up into separate parent and child groups. The children have to make a certificate acknowledging a positive quality about their parent and the parents do the same for the children. (Each family should have at least two certificates—one for the child and one for the parent—but can make more for the remaining members of the family if time permits.) Have each family present their certificates to each other in front of the group.

Example: "Best Kid is awarded to (*name of child*)" and parent signs/dates.

Part V: Family Discussion (10 min.)

Review with parents and kids the positive qualities that facilitators have observed in the families. Ask parents and kids what they got out of today's activities.

Group members are asked to summarize their experiences over the last few weeks as sessions focused on positive aspects of kids, parents, and family life.

- Was it difficult to focus on positive things instead of negative things?
- How did it feel to focus on positive things?
- Does it seem as important as working on the difficulties that families must confront?

Facilitators make sure to end the discussion with an explanation of how building positive interactions within the family helps to encourage more positive behaviors in the child and decrease negative behaviors. Ask families if they have noticed any changes in the family (or specific child) that emphasizes this point (for example, a parent may have been spending more quality time with their child and noticed that the child does not need requests repeated as much). Facilitators can prompt families to explain any progress they have seen in their Session 1 "Family Goals" or in Session 3 "Important Rules."

Part VI: Homework (5 min.)

Have families hang up their certificates. Families should pick a time during the week in which they will create a Family Flag that they will show to everyone at the next session. Refer them to the Family Flag Handout in their Workbook.

Session 10: Everyone Does Their Share to Solve Family Problems

Overall Goal

- Each family member shares "responsibility" for family functioning and resolving conflicts that arise.

Session Objectives

- To help families share responsibility for solving commonly occurring family conflicts.
- To help each family member identify new ways that they might relate to each other.
- To interrupt commonly occurring conflicts.
- To help parents encourage more positive behaviors in their children by including them in problem-solving.

Materials for session

- Group rules
- 4 Rs
- Stress thermometer
- R balls for "family practice" exercise

Part I: Family Social (20 min.)

Parents and children have time to socialize with each other and have refreshments before the session begins. Stress thermometers are distributed and discussed at this time.

Part II: Homework Review (10 min.)

General check in: Ask members are there any concerns, comments, or questions on the information covered so far. Review some of the skills and tips learned in previous sessions and how they can be applied to every day living. Have families share their Family Flag from last week's homework.

Part III: Discussion of Topic/Group Discussion (20 min.)

- Every member of the family has responsibility for the operation of the family. In addition, when conflicts occur, every family member has the responsibility to help resolve it. *Ask: What is a recent family-related problem you have had? What was the child's responsibility here (ask the child)? What was the parent's responsibility here?*
- If parents are not able to offer a recent problem, facilitator can prompt the group by providing their own example: "A child was angry at their parent for not telling them that they were moving. The parent didn't feel the child needed to be included in this decision. The child was angry that he would lose contact with friends, have to change schools, and start over." Have children explain how this would have affected the child. Encourage a discussion between families about this issue.
- Parents always have more responsibility than kids, but if you involve kids in the process, you are teaching them valuable skills that they will use all through their lives. Ask child: *How do they feel when they are/aren't included in the decision making process in their home?* Ask the group: *What does this teach a child when you include them in problem-solving for the family? Emphasize that children don't need to be involved in everything (e.g., issues with finances, etc.) but it helps to include them in things that affect them (e.g., decisions over changing schools).*

Part IV: Family Practice Exercise (20 min.)

- Do the "Juggling for Solutions" exercise. This exercise highlights the family's ability to work together to problem solve and how each member is responsible for keeping the family afloat. (Note: This is a fun exercise that can literally show families what happens when one person doesn't participate or support the rest of the family. Take your time in explaining this exercise and translating this to families' practical life experiences.)
- You will need a set of Rs balls for each family member. Each ball represents family stressors.
  Note: If a family is small (2–3 members), combine them with another family.
  - Identify each ball as a family stressor or a responsibility (e.g., completing homework, doing chores, coming in at curfew, paying bills, etc.). Label them.
  - Hand balls one at a time to the leader who immediately throws each ball to the next designated person until all balls are in use. (It should appear as if family members are juggling with each other.)
  - When a family member drops a ball, the family must stop throwing the ball and begin to work together to problem solve the stressor indicated by the dropped ball.
  - Have families practice once to make sure they understand what to do.
  - Allow families ample time to complete activity so they can practice working together to problem solve.

Part V: Group Discussion of Activity (15 min.)

- Bring all families together to discuss the exercise. Have families comment on what they saw and how that translates to their lives and stressors. Generalize to everyday life how families can work together and be supportive of one another. Emphasize how families can use the 4 Rs to work better together and problem solve any issues that arise. Facilitator may need to review what the 4 Rs are. How did this exercise help them work together as a family?
- The message is: "If you communicate as a family, you can handle whatever stress comes along."

Part VI: Homework Assignment (5 min.)

Have families set a goal to continue to use the 4 Rs to work together to solve any family problems that may arise within the week. Have families use the "4 Rs Review" handout in their workbooks. At next session, families will report a problem that occurred and how they used all the concepts learned to solve it.

Session 11: Everybody Gets a Chance to Be Heard

Overall Goal

- To further enhance family communication.

Session Objectives

- To enhance parents' ability to communicate with children in a manner that they will understand and respond to.
- To strengthen parents' ability to listen to their children and be more available to them.
- To enhance children's ability to discuss concerns with their parents more freely.
- To strengthen children's ability to actually hear what their parents are trying to communicate to them.

Materials for session

- Group rules
- 4 Rs
- Stress thermometer
- Crayons (various colors) and Paper

Introduction for Facilitators

This session consists of a lot of activities. When completing the first activity it is important to make note if the adults tended to take over and become more directive.

The drawing exercise should illustrate how important communication is to completing a task as a family. The difference between the two end products should be significant in highlighting how working together is better than working as a group that doesn't communicate. The family drawing exercise may be used as an illustration of how parents are most often listened to while we have to learn how to actively listen to our children, as was done during the practice exercise.

Part I: Family Social (15 min.)

Parents and children have time to catch up with each other on the week's events and have refreshments before session begins. Parents and children will complete and discuss stress thermometer at this time.

Part II: Homework Review (5–10 min.)

Review homework from last week. Ask families, children first: Did any problems arise during the week and if so where they able to utilize the concepts learned to solve them? Why or why not?

Part III: Review (5 min.)

Review with the group the components of respectful communication (i.e., eye contact, asking appropriate questions, responding in a way that encourages more talk: active listening, not giving advice, etc.). Have either a child or a parent act this out.

Part IV: Group Discussion (10 min.)

Ask the following questions of the children first, and then later the parents:

- How does it feel not to be listened to? Remember to ask them how it feels not being listened to by their teacher, parents, friends, siblings, etc. Is there a difference? If so, what? What makes a good listener? (For parents, use examples of boss, their partner, etc.)

Part V: Family Activity (15 min.)

Do a family drawing exercise to illustrate how lack of communication impacts the family's functioning:

- Distribute crayons to the family members, giving each family member a particular color—no swapping colors or crayons.
- Place one large sheet of paper in front of family—*no talking*.
- Instruct families they are to draw one picture as a family, not several individual pictures, of either a house, a small family, or a park, for approximately five minutes.

Note: Remind families that there is *NO talking* during this exercise. They are to attempt to communicate with each other without words! During the process part, make note if the adults tended to take over and become more directive.

Facilitators call time and each family unit discusses how the process went for them. After first discussion:

- Crayons are rotated and a new sheet of paper is given. This time the families may talk as they draw the picture. At the end of five minutes, time is called and families process how this drawing session went. The two pictures are compared and the differences highlighted.
- Come back to larger group and share how the experience went.

Part VI: Family Practice Exercise (10 min.)

Note: Remind families to remember their "Express Yourself Skills" when completing this exercise. Refer families to the "Express Yourself Skills" sheet in their workbooks.

1. Practice Exercise:
   - Each family will work on this exercise individually.
   - Each child is told to talk to his/her parent for approximately five minutes. Prompt them on topics which may include their day at school, an outing with a friend, the last movie they saw, what they would like to do on vacation or for their birthday.
   - Parents are instructed to listen and empathetically respond in a primarily non-verbal manner using eye contact, head nods, short appropriate questions. In short, anything that will encourage the child to elaborate more on his/her topic. Avoid judgmental statements, giving advice, and criticism.
   - Come back to the larger group and process how this exercise went. How did it feel different from the parents' perspective? From the children's perspective?

Part VII: "Family Communication Game" Activity (20 min.)

This is a very fun activity and engages both the parent and the children in talking about how they communicate with each other. The facilitator should have children and parents separate into different groups. Facilitator distributes the sheets with child questions on them to the children and the same for the parents. Each participant should have his/her own set of sheets with questions. Give each participant about 5–10 minutes to write in the answers on their sheets. After everyone completes their packets, then have each family discuss the answer to each question. (For example, kid's packet asks "who is your best friend?" and the parent packet asks "who is your child's best friend?" Compare responses.) This game can also highlight areas where parents and kids are not communicating. Emphasize that parents can better monitor their kids if they are communicating with each other.

Part VIII: Homework Assignment (5 min.)

Practice the listening exercise at home at least once during the week. Take a few minutes one day during the week where parents and kids sit down together. Kids should talk with their parents about a topic of their choice.

Session 12: Who Can We Turn To (Building Supports)?

Overall Goal

- To assist families in recognizing, building, and relying upon support networks.

Session Objectives

- Parents see themselves as support for one another.
- Kids see their parents as supports for them.
- Families can identify the need for building supports in their lives.
- To be able to identify times when support is needed.

Materials for session

- Group rules
- 4 Rs
- Stress thermometer
- M&Ms

Part I: Family Social (20 min.)

Parents and children have time to have refreshments and socialize with each other. Stress thermometer is distributed and discussed.

Part II: Homework Review (5–10 min.)

Review homework from last week. Ask families, children first: Was it easy or difficult to practice the listening exercise at home? What are some of the things that made it difficult? Did it become easier to communicate with each other as the week went by? Why or why not?

Part III: Group Discussion (40 min.)

Facilitators should use the homework as a discussion starter for the session. Ask families to keep in mind the stressful events of the week. *Do families feel that they need additional supports to address these issues? If so, where will they get the support?* If families have already given examples of using supports, highlight those examples. Facilitators should identify when group members provide support for each other.

M&M Support Game

Each member (parents and children) is to identify up to five people (can include agencies) in their lives that they turn to for support. They should give specific names. The facilitator gives an M&M to the member for each person they mention (up to five). For those participants that have very few supports, members with five M&Ms should help that member identify other possible supports (e.g., church, school, community members, group members, etc.). (This activity is a visual exercise in how much or little support families have in their day to day lives.)

Move on to group discussion by asking the group about the supports in their lives:

- How have they utilized these people?
- Where do you find new sources of support?

- When we find these new supports, do we know how to go about obtaining and utilizing them?
- *Do we need support when we are not in crisis?*
- How do kids support their parents and vice versa?

(Families are allowed to eat their M&Ms after this exercise is completed.)

Discuss with families how to pick appropriate sources of support. Not everyone is helpful. We want to make sure parents and children alike have positive, responsible sources of support. Ask families about the qualities they want in people (and agencies) who will be their supports. Facilitator can start off by giving examples: trustworthy, responsible, resourceful, experienced, etc.

Facilitators should make sure children participate in this activity. Have children volunteer examples of possible people they can turn to when in need. Encourage children to look towards their parents for support (along with other adults and not just peers). Encourage parents to be open to providing this support for their children (being open to listening, providing positive feedback, etc.). Facilitators should refer families to the "Positive Sources of Support" sheet in their workbooks.

Part IV: Family Practice Exercise (15 min.)

Families separate into their individual families. Facilitators should briefly review the 4 Rs with the entire group. Ask families to identify one area where they currently need extra support. (Some examples could be child's problems in school, personal mental health, financial stressors, etc.). Ask families, "How would you use the supports you just identified in helping you with this problem?" Emphasize importance of all family members working together to solve problems. Have families write up their list of supports on the "Resources for Support" Handout. This should include both the personal supports mentioned in the M&M game and any additional sources in the community. Have at least one family volunteer what they worked on. Have all families give suggestions to those who may be struggling with this exercise.

Part V: Homework Assignment (5 min.)

Have families continue to identify possible supports in their lives. Encourage them to use at least one support during the week when stressful things happen.

Session 13: Dealing with Environmental Stressors/Finding Resources: Part One

Overall Goal

- To help families understand how environment stressors affect the family.

Session Objectives

- Families are better able to identify stressful situations that come from the outside but impact the inner workings of the family.
- Families will feel support from the group and have opportunity to share experiences that have been stressful in their lives.
- Families are given the opportunity to identify the strengths that help them deal with stress.
- Help families locate resources/solutions to some of their identified stressors.

Materials for session

- Group rules
- 4 Rs
- Stress thermometer
- List of updated resources in the community

Introduction for Facilitators

Try to keep family members, particularly parents, from focusing on the stress from inside. Help them see how environmental stressors impact their children which in turn bring the stress within the home. The idea is that we don't lay all the blame on the children but also recognize how living in a stressful environment affects our families. Facilitators should consider the needs of the families when selecting resources to give to research. Facilitators should put in a mid-week call to families to encourage them to complete the assignment. *Facilitators should develop a list of agencies in the community that the families will contact as part of the homework assignment.*

Part I: Family Social (15 min.)

Parents and children have time to have refreshments and socialize with each other. Stress thermometer is distributed and filled out during this time.

Part II: Homework Review (5–10 min.)

Review homework from last week. Ask families, if they were able to identify any additional support systems after leaving the session. Were they able to utilize any of their supports during a "stressful" event that may have happened during the week? Why or Why not?

Part III: Family Check-In (15 min.)

There should be time during this session to ask families how they are progressing in the 4 Rs areas. Touch base with families on how rules, family time, and communication building are working. Try to problem-solve with families and give them the opportunity to discuss with you after the session or on the phone during the week. *At this point, explain to families that there are only three more sessions left before the group ends. Briefly highlight how each family has improved throughout the course of the group. Briefly discuss feelings towards termination. Explain that families have been relying on each other for support and can continue to do so after the group is over.*

Part IV: Discussion of Topic (10 min.)

Re-introduce the topic of stress. Ask group members to define stress. Remember that we have talked about this in Session 8. We have talked about stress in the home, and today we will be talking about stress from outside the home. Did anyone experience anything stressful last week outside of the home (e.g., on the subway, at work, in the store, etc.)? Have families explore how things that happen outside of the home (i.e., neighborhood, city, state, nation, etc.) impact their family.

Part V: Group Exercise (15 min.)

Separate the parents and the children into two separate groups. Ask children/parents to tell their group about a stressful day that occurred recently in which there were environmental stressors. Prompt the group by giving them examples of recent stories/events that have impacted the family by causing them more stress. This can be both local as well as national/international events (e.g., a fight in their neighborhood, child abduction, gang wars, New Orleans, 9/11). After each group has discussed this separately, have them offer examples to the other group. It's important to emphasize to parents that children experience stress as well. Encourage discussion around these issues.

Part VI: Group Discussion (20 min.)

After this discussion of stress, have families identify where we find our external sources of support as a group. This may include the church, extended family, school, mental health professionals, and community centers. Facilitators should ask the group, "How do we access these resources?"; "How are these resources helpful?" Be sure to include in the discussion something about what keeps families isolated from accessing these support systems. "What stops families from accessing these sources of support?" (Facilitators should note specific barriers to services such as stigma, difficulty managing systems, not having access, etc.) Make sure to include children in this discussion and that above all, their parents are their primary sources of support.

When there is difficulty finding services or there are no services, it's important for families to know how to advocate for themselves. Families can turn to their elected officials for help in developing services. Ask families if they know who their elected officials are and how to contact them if needed. {Facilitators may want to find this information ahead of time and distribute it to families.}

Note: Facilitator can also remind participants that they too can be a resource for other people or each other (e.g., volunteer work, community involvement, etc.).

Part VII: Homework Assignment (5 min.)

Facilitators will give out a list of resources in the areas in which families reside. Divide the list so that each family has at least 2 agencies/organizations to research and to report back next week. Distribute the "Community Resource Log" Handout to each family. Review the handout and brainstorm around how to ask agencies for this information. If there is time, have some parents practice asking the questions they would ask the agencies. Have families write in what they learned on the handout.

Session 14: Dealing with Environmental Stressors/Finding Resources: Part Two

Overall Goal

- To establish supports and community resources to cope with stressors.

Session Objectives

- Families are better able to identify stressful situations that come from the outside but impact the inner workings of the family.
- Families will feel support from the group and have an opportunity to share experiences that have been stressful in their lives.
- Families are given the opportunity to identify the strengths that help them deal with stress.
- Help families locate resources/solutions to some of their identified stressors.

Materials for session

- Group rules
- 4 Rs
- Stress thermometer
- Binders
- Picture (from magazine, etc.)
- Markers/crayons
- Construction paper
- Glue
- Scissors
- Hole puncher
- Yarn/string (colorful)

Introduction for Facilitator

Be prepared for the possibility that group members will want to continue looking for more resources in their community. Have a resource directory ready. It is important to acknowledge that some of our families are under so much stress that they may not have been able to complete the assignment. They should not be made to feel as though they failed.

Part I: Family Social (20 min.)

Parents and children have time to have refreshments and socialize with each other. During this time, the facilitators will also ask the families how they feel about the group's termination. Remind families that there are only two sessions left for the group. Facilitators should address any concerns from both the parents and the children. The facilitator should ask the families how they plan to stay in touch with each other. Ask families to start thinking about ways to stay connected with each other.

Part II: Homework Review (10 min.)

This session is a continuation of the previous week. Have each family talk about their experience in contacting agencies.

- Did anyone find out anything new?
- Can the group utilize these resources?
- Have the group share what they found and explain that today the group will be making their own resource directory.

Part III: Group Discussion (20 min.)

Promote a discussion around the process of researching these community resources.

- Was it an empowering experience?
- If there were negative experiences, what did you do?
- *Was it disheartening to find out about lack of resources?*
- *How do we mobilize as a family, group, and as a community to get services? How do these resources address the stressors identified by families?*
- Can their needs be met by any of these agencies?

Ask members: What do you do when you face too many barriers in finding resources? Do you give up? What are some things you can do to overcome these barriers? Facilitators should emphasize importance of continuing on in their search and not giving up. Oftentimes, families have had many negative experiences which prevents them from finding help when they need it. Emphasize here the importance of advocacy (e.g., get name of person spoke to and ask to speak to supervisor—"If you can't help me, then transfer me to someone who can."). Emphasize here communication skills learned in past sessions. Make sure to ask children the same questions as their experiences may be very different from their parents. How can children manage the systems in school to find help?

For those families that weren't able to do this assignment, facilitators should attempt to elicit the families own personal knowledge of resources to add to the directory.

Part IV: Family Practice Exercise (30 min.)

Create a Family Resource Manual

Distribute a small binder or folder to each family. The families should be given materials they can use to decorate the binders. As the families are decorating the binders, a facilitator should collect all the completed "Community Resource Logs" that each family worked on for homework. Facilitators will photocopy the logs and distribute a complete set of copies to each family to place in the binders. Facilitators should also give families some blank logs so that families can add additional resources as necessary. Facilitators should also provide their own resource directories for the families to include in the binders.

Supplies needed: Binders; pictures from magazines (note: pull pictures from magazines ahead of time rather than bringing in whole magazines as this can be too distracting. Be sure to include both symbolic pictures, phrases, and culturally diverse photos); crayons, markers, glue, scissors, hole puncher, additional paper (construction and regular paper).

Part V: Homework Assignment (10 min.)

Encourage families to use the "Family Resource Manual" when problems arise.

Use any remaining time in the group to continue a discussion around the termination of the group. Remind families that there are only two more sessions. Have families complete the "My Group" sheet in their workbooks for homework.

During this time the facilitator should also suggest that the families meet together outside of the group, such as having a pot-luck for the families. Encourage families to continue communicating with each other after the group is over. Highlight that families have been relying on each other for support in the group this whole time. Emphasize that the families have learned many skills they can continue to use.

Session 15: How Did the Group Go?

Overall Goal

- To complete the post-test measures and facilitate families' termination of the group.

Session Objectives

- Administer the post-test measures.
- Group members summarize the things that have changed and the areas that continue to need work within their family.
- Help families have a healthy termination with each other and the group.

Materials for session

- Post-test Measures
- Group Contact List
- "Children Learn What They Live" Handout.

Part I: Family Social/Discussion (15 min.)

Have families enjoy their refreshments at the same time as they discuss their feelings about the group and its end.

Part II: Assessments (75 min.)

Distribute assessment battery. Read aloud questions for those who need assistance in understanding them. Give periodic short breaks. Allow parents and kids to take as much time as necessary.

Session 16: Ending Party

Overall Goal

- To end the group and acknowledge the families for their hard work with a party.
- Encourage families to continue to rely on each other for support.

Session Objectives

- Compile a listing of family names and numbers to distribute to each family so that they can stay in contact with one another.
- Families plan for a group event away from the clinic which they plan themselves.
- Have fun!
- Eat food!

Materials for session

- Certificates of Completion
- Materials for the party (radio, games, etc.)
- My Group Handout
- Family contact sheet

Have Fun! Eat!

Have families discuss the "My Group" homework sheet. Facilitators should also ask families the following questions about their experience:

- Did they enjoy the activities? Homework Ideas for greater participation?
- How do you feel about the length of the group?
- What other help do you need to continue doing well?
- Is there anything else you would like to share about the group?

You can use this opportunity to highlight the strengths of each family. Please review all the tools/skills the families now have to handle problems as they arise.

Use the following questions to highlight what they can do in the future:

- How can families handle problems in the future?
- What resources do families feel are available?
- What potential hurdles do families foresee?

Encourage families to continue communicating with each other after the group is over. Highlight that families have been relying on each other for support in the group this whole time.

Encourage families to set up a group event (such as a potluck meeting) on their own. Have families share contact information with each other. Have the group pick one point person to help in organizing this event.

Facilitators should take time during this session to talk with individual families about their future treatment goals and what modality, if any, may best meet their current needs.

Read: "Children Learn What they Live" aloud in the group.

Index